PRACTICAL
OBSTETRIC PROBLEMS

Practical
Obstetric Problems

IAN DONALD

M.B.E., M.D., B.S.(Lond.); B.A.(Cape Town);
F.R.C.S.(Glasg.); F.R.C.O.G.; F.C.O.&G.(S.A.)

*Regius Professor of Midwifery, University of Glasgow.
Formerly Reader, University of London, Institute of
Obstetrics and Gynæcology, Hammersmith Hospital.
One time Reader in Obstetrics and Gynæcology, St.
Thomas's Hospital Medical School, London*

Fourth edition
(Reprint)

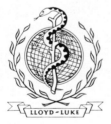

LLOYD-LUKE (MEDICAL BOOKS) LTD
49 NEWMAN STREET
LONDON
1972

First Edition	.	.	1955
Reprinted	.	.	1956
Second Edition	.	.	1959
Reprinted	.	.	1960
Reprinted	.	.	1961
Third Edition	.	.	1964
Reprinted	.	.	1966
Fourth Edition	.	.	1969
Reprinted	.	.	1972

PRINTED AND BOUND IN ENGLAND BY
HAZELL WATSON AND VINEY LTD
AYLESBURY, BUCKS

ISBN 0 85324 053 1

To all who have known doubt, perplexity and fear
as I have known them,

To all who have made mistakes as I have,

To all whose humility increases with their knowledge of this most fascinating subject,

THIS BOOK IS DEDICATED

PREFACE TO FOURTH EDITION

A millstone round the neck can carry its wearer into deep waters. Recurrent editions of a textbook seeking to keep up to date in the fast flood of modern obstetrical thinking can similarly affect the author whose life becomes more and more engulfed in the subject. In so far as it is possible to detect a major shift in current direction the emergence of fetal medicine, that is to say the study of intra-uterine development and well being of the fetus, is perhaps the most striking and allusions to this theme constantly recur throughout the pages that follow. Perinatal mortality studies, useful enough in themselves, contribute little to this wider understanding and our interest is more than ever focused upon the survivors, upon the living rather than the dead. Our limited knowledge, so far, recognises only some of the adverse influences which may handicap the child in later life and only a few of which are preventable, yet it is one of the ultimate objectives of our subject that no child of tomorrow may needlessly forfeit any of its natural endowment.

Since the last edition was completed, the new Queen Mother's Hospital has been commissioned and already more than 13,000 babies have been born in it. We seized the happy opportunity to cast aside much that was useless and traditional both in medical and in nursing care. Is your enema really necessary? Why not let small children visit their mothers? Are dressings a futile Crimean ritual and unabsorbable perineal sutures a sadistic abomination? With such questions as these in mind we were at least able to make something of a fresh start. This book now represents our current practice.

Alas, far more has had to be added to the text than subtracted, so that the net result is a regrettable increase in the size of the volume. The importance of chromosome abnormalities has been dealt with by Dr. Malcolm A. Ferguson Smith, who is in charge of our Cytogenetics Laboratory. Endotoxic shock is treated as an entity in its own right. Megablastic anaemia is described even more fully and the scale of immigration into the United Kingdom has made an account of the haemoglobinopathies a necessity. More is now known about rubella, and the means to forecast the likelihood of damage in a given pregnancy has come none too soon in view of the increasing number of requests for termination of pregnancy on this score. Blood clotting defects have come in for much more attention because of the rapid advances being made both in understanding and treatment. The biochemistry of fetal distress and its more rational management merit description too.

Sudden death in obstetrics is no longer acceptable and cardiac arrest calls nowadays for an intense therapeutic ritual rather than fatalism, however discouraging the ultimate outcome. The management of massive blood transfusion by central venous pressure monitoring is only another instance of more modern practice in a desperate emergency.

The battle against the indiscriminate use of powerful antibiotics without established indication has now been largely won and the chapter originally contributed by Dr. Stark and Dr. McAllister has been telescoped into the chapter on Puerperal Management and Complications; nevertheless the basic subject matter on the action and selection of antibiotics has been retained. Incidentally our hospital is fortunate in being able to welcome Dr. McAllister as Bacteriologist-in-Charge.

Not all units are blessed with the sort of paediatric service which the teaching hospital of today accepts as a matter of course. For this reason a fresh section is devoted to the full examination of the newborn baby and the detection of inborn errors of metabolism, deformity and such avoidable hazards to subsequent mental development as neonatal hypoglycaemia.

Dysmaturity has become in the last few years one of our greatest interests in conformity with the newer obstetrical philosophy.

As in previous editions a chapter is devoted entirely to the Rh factor and haemolytic disease. The exciting recent developments in this subject fully justify the space allocated.

Many reviewers and well-wishing critics of the previous edition expressed the hope that I would supply an intelligible account of the uses of sonar (ultrasonic echo sounding) in obstetrics. Such a demand in fact, was met earlier this year in an article which I published in the *British Medical Bulletin* (*Brit. med. Bull.*, 1968, **24**, No. 1, p. 71) and I am grateful to the Editor and to the British Council for permission to reproduce this article in full, because, at the moment, I cannot concisely better it.

These are some of the new matters which have been dealt with in this edition, although they are only a selection from the four and a half pages before me of listed material which I have noted.

It is with great sadness that I have to write of the tragic and untimely passing of my old friend Gordon Garland, who, nevertheless, completed the revision of his two chapters before his death. Our association goes back to the old St. Thomas's Hospital days of nearly twenty years ago. He was a true man of Norfolk with his penetrating wit and his utter reliability.

My friend and colleague here in Glasgow, Dr. Wallace Barr, has revised his contribution on Pregnancy Vomiting, while, from the other side of the world, an even older friend, Professor Harvey

Carey in Sydney, has completely rewritten his chapter on Pre-eclampsia.

I continue my happy association with Dr. Ellis Barnett, radiologist at the Western Infirmary, who has now entered the ultrasonic field with characteristic gusto.

It is with great pleasure that I welcome Dr. Alan Giles who has written an essay on Psychoprophylaxis.

My thanks and sympathy must go out as before to Mr. Douglas Luke, my publisher, the former for his industry and meticulous attention to detail and the latter for all that he has had to endure from an author who is involved in such a large number of competing interests. I have not even the excuse of illhealth to offer on this occasion, since, in spite of ignoring much professional advice I continue in better cardiac form than I deserve. His forebearance with me calls for gratitude indeed.

In Miss Adele Ure I continue to be blessed with the best secretary in Scotland. The rapidity and accuracy of her work never ceases to amaze me and without her industry and help I would have taken very much longer to complete this edition.

Doctors Zaheen, Akande and Chau Wing, from Pakistan, Nigeria and Hong Kong respectively, have helped me with the proof readings and drawn my attention to occasional mistakes in spelling and grammar.

Finally I must acknowledge with gratitude the help I have had from my junior colleagues at the Queen Mother's Hospital, whose outspoken criticisms I continue to enjoy and occasionally to accept. It is only right, of course, that their capacity for consecutive thinking and their clinical ability should exceed my own. After all, I have taught them most of what I know, which may be little enough, and their own individual knowledge and skill, by simple addition, should consequently endow them better than their chief. Ours is a happy and coherent unit continually divided in fascinating argument but always united in ultimate purpose. To one like myself, threatened with seniority and all its penalties, such a staff has brought great happiness and friendship.

Glasgow,   IAN DONALD
November 1968

PREFACE TO FIRST EDITION

THE art of teaching is the art of sharing enthusiasm. The teacher must, therefore, love what he teaches if he is not to become "as a tinkling cymbal". If, then, exuberance occasionally bubbles through the pages of this book, I know that my past students will understand, and I ask no forgiveness.

I have often wondered what drives men to write a textbook. In my case it was the persuasiveness of my publisher. He felt, and of course he is right, that there was a place for a book of a practical sort which would appeal to the clinician who lives in the rough and tumble of it all. as well as to aspirants for additional diplomas in the subject.

We agreed upon a strategic size, and therefore, we hope, upon a palatable price, but apart from that I was given a completely free hand. I gladly accepted the excuse to omit the inevitable dreary irrelevance of such matters as ovulation, menstruation, conception, infertility, diagnosis of pregnancy and the early development of the ovum, which can be found in most textbooks of midwifery, making them heavy upon the knee as well as upon the mental digestion of the reader. Having got rid of this burden, I found myself free to get down to the real business of midwifery. In doing so I may or may not have pleased my public (if any) but I certainly pleased myself. The would-be pianist does not struggle through his Beethoven because of the imagined needs of a hypothetical audience. His efforts are owed to the Master. It is in this spirit that I have written, and I can only hope that some will find it infectious.

The task of nearly two years has been made pleasurable by all the willing and at times argumentative help I have had from colleagues and friends, above all, Gordon Garland, who has scrutinised every sentence I have written and at times supplied sobering criticism. I owe much to his encouragement, though it would not be fair to hold him in any way responsible for my statements. In addition to writing two chapters on the malpresentations he has read the proofs and has provided many of the illustrations. The toxæmias of pregnancy are not easy to deal with in a modern way without becoming "woolly", and I am therefore very glad of Harvey Carey's chapter thereon with his uncompromising clarity. Hilda Roberts, besides giving most of my anæsthetics in the last two years, has devoted years of practical research to the relief of pain in labour and has very fittingly written this chapter.

My views upon the misuse of the antibiotics are so strong that I

thought it a good plan to seek the help of one whose views are even stronger and certainly more expert. I therefore asked William Hayes for a chapter on these lines before his recent visit to the U.S.A. The book is worth while if only for this authoritative piece of work, the like of which is not to be found in most other volumes.

Illustrations are often more of a problem to the author than the text itself, unless he happens to be a collector from lifelong habit. A great many are the work of the photographic and X-ray departments of the Postgraduate Medical School and Hammersmith Hospital, whose help is gratefully acknowledged. In other instances acknowledgements are made in the appropriate places. The line drawings are by Miss Pat Burrows who, besides her rapid skill, has the convenient property of being able to rise to the occasion demanded, regardless of the Sabbath.

One could not write a book, even of this modest size, in the midst of ordinary professional activity without the help of a good secretary, and I have been fortunate in Miss Joan Bush. She worked fast and well, and her cheerful composure helped to prevent things from getting out of hand when time appeared to be running short.

The Postgraduate Medical School library is a remarkable place, the more so because of the efficiency of the Librarian, Miss Atkins, for whose help I am much indebted.

I started this preface by alluding to the persuasiveness of my publisher, but Mr. Douglas Luke is more than that. He is a delightful slave driver, but he is also patient and meticulous, for all his enthusiasm. Our association has been a very happy one, although I will try to discourage him, for the present, from making me write another book.

It would not be fair, in all these acknowledgements, to omit mention of my long-suffering wife and family, who have put up with me and my book for so many months. Most of the time that I gave to the task was really their time and their contribution has been the calm with which they have managed to surround my domestic life and without which I would surely have failed.

In retrospect it has been worth while and if, in the pages that follow, I have at times provoked, instructed and amused, then I am content.

September 1954   IAN DONALD

CONTENTS

CHAPTER I

THE SCOPE OF ANTENATAL CARE

THE scope of antenatal care is now widening rapidly in two directions; the first, naturally enough, in the field of more sophisticated investigations which are bound to multiply as obstetrics becomes less of an art and more of a science and as it comes increasingly within our power to estimate the intra-uterine progress of the baby and its development, as well as the welfare of its mother. Such cases, of course, will provide a time-consuming minority only, but their proper selection must be the concern of all who practise modern obstetrics. The other direction, equally important, is the increasing degree to which antenatal care is being shared between the hospital clinic and the patient's own family doctor, who, if he is to be an effective member of such a team, must learn to think in the same intellectual language as the hospital staff with whom he co-operates.

The advantages are bilateral. In our own experience, which is steadily extending, we enjoy a welcome reduction in size and crowding of the clinics and have more time to give careful attention to detail in a smaller number of patients.

Working against the clock is bad in both hospital and general practice. To the family doctor the advantages are that he can maintain contact with his patient at this important time without the loss of useful hospital facilities but perhaps from the patient's point of view, since it is her welfare which is the whole object of the exercise, the strengthened bond between doctors working inside and outside hospital should mean that she is getting the best of both worlds. None of this, however, will be of any avail without an agreed and conscientiously administered system of referral and filtration with the mutual respect and consideration which such a scheme demands.

We all of us have our Liaison Committees and they do good work, but speaking personally I have always had less faith in committee decisions than personal agreements quickly arrived at between those concerned and have always found it more satisfactory to settle a point immediately with a family doctor by direct contact rather than by consulting committees. To have earned the reputation of being a bad committee man has proved of inestimable value and saved me many hours of boredom and loss of profitable time listening to others who cannot make up their minds.

The first requisite in establishing good liaison with doctors outside the hospital is a proper system of communication. This should apply

1

as much to antenatal consultations as reports following a patient's discharge from hospital. The latter should be brief, legible and easy to file. In obstetrics, consultation reports are best entered on forms already used by the practitioner outside and we are encouraging as much as possible the use of a Maternity Services record card such as Form EC 24 R/2 (card and envelope) Scotland, which the patient carries with her when she attends hospital. Unless the matter is one of some complexity requiring a full letter, it is very little extra work for the hospital doctor to enter his findings on this card alongside those of the patient's own doctor. The risk of the patient losing the card is trivial compared with the value of this rapid form of inter-communication and anyway the hospital, of course, has to keep its own fuller records which are always available.

Even with all this co-operation both within and without hospital we are only on the threshold of a new and far more important type of antenatal care than hitherto, and, inasmuch as prevention is always better than cure, it is the function of antenatal care to reduce the need for desperate measures at the time of delivery. Unfortunately the present situation leaves little room for more than "divine dis-content", since we cannot yet match the recent improvement in labour room tactics with those of antenatal care itself. Nevertheless, gone are the days, I hope, of the hospital "cram clinic" which treated its patients like machine parts on an assembly line, being mainly concerned with the prevention of eclampsia, the correction of mal-presentation and recognising disproportion, if it could. The ability to see 60 patients in 65 minutes is a type of pre-war insult—according to the patient little more recognition than the status of an appendage of her gravid uterus and its contents. To a woman who may have waited an hour or more in an unattractive waiting space in even less attrac-tive company, the rapid exposure of her bulging abdominal surface and the overhearing of a few muttered remarks to some assistant writing notes, followed by a hurried dismissal, must have seemed a travesty of medical care as indeed it was. Yet such tactics have not entirely died out.

If the survey of the present position is disquieting, at least a brief look back into history gives comfort for what has been done in a relatively short period of time.

History

Antenatal care began as a social service in Paris in 1788 for women who had committed the double inconvenience of being both pregnant and destitute (femmes abandonnées). These pitiable creatures were housed, sometimes two or three to a bed, in the Hotel Dieu and Hôpital Salpetrière from the thirty-sixth week of pregnancy onwards. For over a hundred more years the problem of disposal seems to have

been a more pressing objective than treatment or preventive care. To some extent this was due to a failure to recognise the importance of emergencies peculiar to the gravid state and illnesses occurring in pregnancy found their way to an unwelcome reception in general wards whose staff feared, with good reason, that the patient might do something awkward like going into labour and generally making a nuisance of herself in unsuitable surroundings.

It was in Edinburgh at the very end of the last century that the first effective medical and scientific interest was shown in the antenatal patient. In 1902 the first antenatal bed (all of one bed in fact) was endowed for the purpose. Admittedly Ballantyne's original concern was fœtal deformity and stillbirth but this soon came to embrace a wider interest in maternal well-being which, on more general adoption by the end of the 1914–18 war, had swamped concern for the unborn child. In fact until the period following the last war it was thoughtlessly assumed that antenatal care which was good enough for the mother was good enough to cover the needs of the baby as well.

A few heretics talked about "antenatal pædiatrics" but they were not taken very seriously. This complacency has been shaken first by the recognition of the possible effects of certain viruses upon the baby following Gregg's observations in 1941, in Australia, on the association between maternal rubella in early pregnancy and cataract; secondly by Dr. Alice Stewart's enquiry into the harmful effects of X-rays upon the foetus, increasing the hazard of leukaemia in later childhood and, finally at the end of 1961, came the terrible tragedy of thalidomide deformed babies, so promptly spotted, reported and acted upon [11, 12, 16, 17] after the association between this drug and limb and intestinal deformities was first suspected in Western Germany. The firm supplying thalidomide very rightly withdrew the drug from sale at the first suggestion of responsibility, but even so it was reckoned that not less than 800 babies in this country alone were likely to have been damaged. If such a catastrophe could follow the taking, in early pregnancy, of so apparently harmless a sedative and anti-emetic as thalidomide then what of the possible effects of all sorts of other agencies—drugs, poisons, radiations, metabolic diseases, even psychosomatic and stress disorders? The intra-uterine vulnerability of the baby is now in all our minds and congenital abnormalities can no longer be accepted with fatalism. And so the wheel has turned full circle and Ballantyne's original teratological interest is revived.

Perinatal Mortality

Obstetrical units throughout the country have been stimulated to a sort of self examination by the ever-increasing practice of studying

perinatal mortality statistics, which reached its most intensive peak in the nation-wide Perinatal Mortality Survey instituted by the National Birthday Trust[13]. Perinatal mortality is defined as the sum of still-births and deaths within the first week of life, because there is a good deal of overlap in the aetiology of both types of disaster. As people like Sir Dugald Baird have repeatedly pointed out, this rate depends a good deal upon the social standards of different areas and there is danger of comparing like with unlike. For example, in poor industrial areas like Glasgow and Dundee the rate is considerably worse than in the country as a whole (34·4 per thousand total births in Scotland in 1963)[7] and the rate improves in the more prosperous Southern parts of England. Even the best obstetrical care can to some extent be offset by bad social conditions, at least as far as perinatal and mortality statistics go.

Five social classes are conveniently recognised as follows:—
  I. Professional workers, directors and departmental managers. It includes all those whose incomes attract liability to surtax and those in jobs holding such eventual prospects, together with their families.
 II. So-called "white collared workers," small farmers, small shop-keepers, sales representatives and teachers.
III. Skilled artisans, foremen and clerical workers without administrative responsibility.
 IV. Semi-skilled workers, but in reasonably regular employment.
  V. Labourers—both employed and unemployed, the Epsilons of Aldous Huxley's *Brave New World*.
So much for our democratic society.

The perinatal mortality rate has been halved since 1939 and to medical science must go the major credit for this improvement which, almost as a corollary, is not matched by an alteration in the incidence of fœtal abnormality.

Adverse influences on fœtal development.—It is now clear that agents lightly tolerated by the mother can damage the rapidly growing tissues of her child. Here is fresh scope for antenatal care not only in a negative sense but positively as well to improve a child's endowment at birth.

Perinatal mortality is too loosely accepted these days as an index of the standard of obstetrical care, and one might go much further and ask, "What about the survivors?" After all, our interest is with the living and not the dead and the casual phrase, "Alive and Well" gives little indication how well in fact the baby has survived its antenatal hazards and those attending its birth.[4, 5] It would be surprising if influences, either chemical or physical, which reached the baby during the critical stages of its intra-uterine development did not have

possible far-reaching effects upon its intellectual and physical capacity, quite apart from the more obvious forms of handicap. Here lies one of the biggest gaps in obstetrical knowledge. Even so-called intra-uterine asphyxia can only be explained in a minority of cases, yet macerated stillbirth is simply the end-product of intra-uterine sub-nutrition and sub-oxygenation. The damaging effects of X-rays[18] and rubella virus[8] are among the few that are well known.

The tragedy of fresh stillbirth is becoming relatively uncommon in obstetrical units. Apart from unexplained macerated stillbirths, the large components of perinatal loss are represented by fœtal abnormalities, abruptio placentæ, pre-eclamptic toxæmia, while fresh obstetrical stillbirths commonly associated with cord accidents and postmaturity only come fifth down the list. In all this the association of prematurity stands out prominently in between two-thirds to three-quarters of the total, sometimes as cause and sometimes as effect.

In estimating these fœtal hazards present-day antenatal care still ranks little better than soothsaying. Behind the iron curtain of the maternal abdominal wall and uterus the baby's well-being defies accurate assessment by standard clinical means. I, myself, can easily be a kilogramme adrift in either direction in assessing a baby's weight, a figure far higher than that of any of my good midwifery Sisters. Maturity assessment either clinically or radiologically has an error of plus or minus three weeks and there is no reliable antenatal method yet of predicting a baby's endurance and capacity to withstand a difficult labour. Certain maternal complications like pre-eclamptic toxæmia, diabetes, renal disorders and, above all, a bad obstetric history are well known to be associated with greater fœtal hazard, but these adverse factors are no more than warning pointers.

In all this uncertainty in what is, after all, one of the most important potential aspects of antenatal care, only a few factors are proven and in spite of an intensive witch hunt for possibly teratogenic drugs, in addition to thalidomide, remarkably little has so far been substantiated. There are two reasons for this—firstly, the natural incidence of fœtal abnormality (namely 2–3 per cent of all babies, alive or dead) for which no explanation can be found, and, secondly, the matter of species difference which to some extent invalidates the observations made on experimental animals, such as rodents, which do not apply in the case of the human fœtus. Nevertheless there is every need for a large corporate effort to be made by all practitioners, as encouraged by the Royal College of General Practitioners, to report possible associations between fœtal abnormality and drugs given in early pregnancy. Any suspected association, even though remote, should be forwarded promptly in writing to the Medical Assessor, Committee on Safety of Drugs, Queen Anne's Chambers, 41 Tothill Street, London, S.W.1.

So far it is recognised that androgenic steroids may masculinise a female fœtus if used within the first trimester and there is a general belief that some of the synthetic progestational agents may likewise produce androgenic effects.

The cortico-steroids have from time to time been blamed for causing cleft palate, as is known to occur experimentally in mice and possibly other fusion failures as well, but the risk is not a large one and may certainly be less than that of withholding such drugs from a mother who very genuinely needs them. Nevertheless the matter deserves caution.

Because most hormones given therapeutically can cross the placenta their effect on the fœtal endocrine system should be anticipated. Anti-thyroid drugs may so depress the activity of an otherwise normal fœtal thyroid gland that the fœtal pituitary may endeavour to over-come the defect by increasing its output of thyroid stimulating hormone, the fœtus as a consequence developing a goitre. Fortunately the effect is reversible.

Oral hypoglycaemic agents used in the treatment of diabetics may have an undesirable effect on the fœtus inasmuch as they may cross the placenta and affect the baby who is by no means diabetic, and is vulnerable to prolonged hypoglycaemia.

Many drugs, including quinine, and, of course lead and ergot poisoning may cause fœtal death, but the pregnant patient of today does not encounter such hazards.

If anticoagulants have to be given during pregnancy, heparin, which does not affect the fœtus, is far safer than the "Coumadin" class of drugs, which may cause fœtal bleeding from coagulation defects. Quite apart from teratogenic effects many drugs which readily cross the placenta can adversely affect the child, such as, for example, hexamethonium bromide, once used to reduce blood pressure in pre-eclamptic toxaemia as a ganglionic blocking agent which had the disastrous effect of producing paralytic ileus in the baby.

Maternal addiction to narcotic drugs such as heroin can appear as a neonatal addiction too, with serious withdrawal symptoms after birth, of which there have been some sad instances recorded recently with this growing abuse in our society. Another addiction, though in this case less socially objectionable, namely cigarette smoking, has been shown in Aberdeen[19] to produce mild intra-uterine growth retardation and babies with significantly lower birth weights than in control cases. Even the vitamins are not without their potential harmful effects, particularly vitamin D, which if given in massive doses may produce hypercalcæmia and possibly adverse mental effects on the child. A maternal dose not exceeding 400 units a day, however, is safe. Large doses of vitamin K in the mother can produce hyper-bilirubinæmia and kernicterus in the baby.

Of the antibiotics, prolonged administration of streptomycin can be potentially ototoxic to the fœtus, but perhaps most striking of all is the danger of giving tetracyclines to the mother in pregnancy. The tetracycline molecule chelates very readily with metallic ions such as calcium so that it is deposited in bones and teeth. In the case of bones the drug is gradually eliminated in the course of the natural turnover of the chemical constituents, but not so with teeth which may be hideously discoloured. Fortunately it is the deciduous teeth which suffer more than the permanent teeth since it is they which undergo mineralisation *in utero* whereas the permanent front teeth do not start the process until a few months after birth. The discolouration of a young child's teeth so produced, besides being psychologically harmful because of the disfigurement, may, by this very fact, make the child less attractive to relatives whose affection might otherwise be lavished more generously upon it. This process in the deciduous teeth extends from the fourteenth week of gestation until after term and there is therefore good reason for not giving tetracyclines unless the mother is suffering from some infection for which no other anti-biotic is suitable, a most unlikely state of affairs. Tetracyclines have the further disadvantage that the blood levels may rise very high because of diminished excretion by diseased kidneys, for example, when treating pyelonephritis and the liver may consequently suffer toxic effects.

The suggestion has been made that thalidomide acted as a teratogen not by producing such abnormalities as phocomelia directly but by acting as an immuno-suppressive drug which prevented the alleged homograft rejection by the mother of a fœtus that was spontaneously deformed; in other words that it prevented the natural riddance through abortion of such biologically unacceptable offspring, but experimental work on the survival of skin homografts in rabbits has shown that thalidomide did not in any way prevent or postpone their rejection[1] and for the time being this ingenious explanation of the action of thalidomide cannot be accepted as a more likely alternative to the theory of direct teratogenicity.

Maternal Mortality

Midwifery has largely ceased to be the blood-and-thunder subject which it was less than thirty years ago. In terms of mater-nal mortality alone the improvement has been staggering, the national rate, excluding abortions, being 0·34 per 1,000 births in 1961 (0·37 per 1,000 in Scotland), whereas in 1928 just under three thousand women in England and Wales died as a result of pregnancy or associated complications, an incidence of one in 226. The figure is now getting very near to the irreducible minimum and has to include

coincident disasters and diseases. Nevertheless avoidable factors are present in no less than 38 per cent.[6, 14] The Ministry of Health figures in the latest available report covering the years 1961/63 show a slight change in the order of the major factors but basically not much difference from the previous report. During this three-year period deaths associated with abortion headed the list (139), followed closely by pulmonary embolism (129), of which, rather surprisingly, 36 were antepartum, while 66 followed vaginal delivery and 27 Cæsarean section.

Toxæmia of pregnancy came third in the list (104 deaths) and hæmorrhage accounted for 92 in the three-year period, a very creditable figure when one recalls that almost as many deaths from hæmorrhage occurred in the same period of time in one Glasgow hospital alone in the early 1930s.

Heart disease (81 deaths) heads the list of lethal associated diseases, particularly in older and multiparous women for whom better family planning might have been indicated. Deaths after Cæsarean section are a serious feature, even allowing for the abnormalities for which the operation was undertaken, and the hazards of general anæsthesia are also more widely recognised as causes of disaster.

The biggest drop has been shown in an analysis by Douglas (1955) to have occurred between 1942 and 1952. This period witnessed three very important events: firstly, the universal availability of banked blood throughout the country, introduced earlier under the stimulus of war; secondly, the introduction of antibiotics, starting with penicillin, to reinforce the control of sepsis already begun by the sulphonamides and, thirdly, the establishment of the National Health Service.

The full impact of this last-mentioned social reform will only be truly evaluated in years to come, but one of the more obvious benefits is the growth, in numbers and quality, of the hospital registrar class of practitioners who form the backbone of hospital midwifery today. This result may not have been intentional but the standards demanded by the Royal College of Obstetricians and Gynæcologists have seen to it that a good obstetric registrar is worth his weight in consultant gold.

The slow but steady improvement in anæsthetic services in maternity units is also a major contribution to maternal safety, although far too often emergency anæsthetics have still to be given by the inexperienced and the unskilled. The provision of antenatal beds in maternity units, although often abused inasmuch as many women have to spend needlessly long periods thus incarcerated because of the present inability to assess all risks accurately, has come hand-in-hand with the general recognition of the classes in whom booking for hospital delivery is positively indicated.

Domiciliary Delivery

Whatever the merits of this, and they are considerable, there is no doubt that domiciliary midwifery is dying in the more highly developed populations of the world socially, such as the white population of the United States, Sweden and Australia, much in the same way as traditional tonsillectomy on the kitchen table is more or less gone for good. This trend would have more to be said for it if many hospitals were not rather grisly, out-of-date places with out-of-date thinking, especially on matters like visiting and patient freedom, and occasionally run by a human species of dragon, and if only food in all hospitals could be treated with the dignity and intelligent artistry which cooking deserves and if private nursing homes were not often so ruinously expensive. Discipline in hospital which varies from the irksome to the terrifying can almost be reminiscent of one's days at boarding school in childhood. It is essential in all new hospital planning that these objections be vigorously and consciously overcome as they have been in our new Queen Mother's Hospital, where open visiting is allowed and where children are allowed to visit their mothers and "see the new baby". Irregular dismissals, against medical advice, are therefore unknown and we keep no such register; nor is any notice, other than a direction notice, allowed to be displayed for the instruction of patients, including futile restrictions on smoking; the latter only encourages secret smoking in lavatories and bathrooms to the detriment of the drains and the general hygiene of the place.

In opening the Queen Mother's Hospital we gave serious thought to this question of open visiting, with children coming into hospital and decided, as has been proved to be the case, that the advantages in patient morale far outweighed the risks, particularly in long-stay cases. A woman's chief reason for dismissing herself from hospital against advice is that she is worried about what is going on at home and nothing can more readily reassure her than the right of her other children to visit her. Apart from an occasional drunken husband late at night and the theft of a few ashtrays, we have had absolutely no trouble and working class women are just as capable of behaving like duchesses, if given a chance, as anybody else. We feared that swarms of children might turn the place into a sort of Red Indian camp on a Sunday afternoon, but their behaviour has been overawed and demure. Husband attendance has been noticeably at peak levels when there is a television broadcast in the day rooms of a celebrated prize fight. The one hazard which has worried us is not so much some exotic infection introduced from outside, because, after all, the mother and her baby are returning to home and shopping in crowded departmental stores, but the possibility that one woman's child incubating whooping cough may infect the baby of another patient. Children

are, therefore, not allowed to see the babies of other patients and, of course, the Paediatric Department with its vulnerable premature babies has to be out of bounds to the general public. The only other trouble we have run into is what we call "the Pied Piper phenomenon" where a husband, going to visit his wife, is asked by all the other women in the street to take their children along off their hands on a spree to the new hospital. I even found a whole crowd of them in my office one evening, but they were doing no harm and simply wanted to get a better view of the ships passing up and down the Clyde. We have therefore had to discourage neighbours' children in a gentle reminder in the brochure which is handed out to all patients on booking. This experiment in human kindness towards patients has paid enormous dividends in producing a really happy hospital, in which patients feel free to walk away into the main corridors of the hospital, furnished with tables and chairs, where family groups can sit and watch the world, at least within the hospital, go by, and are no longer under the eye of the Ward Sister. This policy has made it possible to combine high standards of medical care with simultaneous removal of so-called advantages of being at home within the bosom of the family, which, to a parous woman, simply means bondage to the sink and the kitchen stove from which she deserves a proper rest in the immediate postnatal period.

The case for hospitals, of course, has been stressed in their ability to provide everything from expert anaesthesia to massive blood transfusion and all the facilities which modern medical science can offer. The dangers of cross-infection are proportional to the overcrowding of the unit and the degree to which it is overworked. Recognising that hospitals have much to provide in safety and in coping with emergencies, there has been a natural attempt to extend the practice of 24 or 48 hour admissions just to cover labour. In other words to turn the hospital into a sort of public convenience, or sausage machine, where simply the mechanics of labour and its potential hazards are coped with. This doleful expedient can produce a good showing as far as the percentage of institutional deliveries and gives the bureaucrats in charge of taxpayers' money the very excuse they need for not building any new maternity units. In Bradford, however, be it remembered, the institution of this principle was done in order to provide antenatal beds which were badly needed and which could only be got at the expense of a longer lying-in period, and the object was not simply to stuff more patients through the labour wards per unit period of time. The argument uses a parous woman's homesickness and anxiety about her other children as an excuse for dumping her at 48 hours notice back into the midst of all her domestic cares and responsibilities and can be squashed simply by providing the type of hospital which treats her and her family as human beings.

In a semi-derisory way newspapers have referred to the Queen Mother's Hospital as a sort of holiday camp. This, in fact, is a compliment. The idea that the patient's family doctor can have much control over what she gets up to the minute he has turned his back is, of course, absurd. The parous woman who is most harassed and worried about getting home to resume her domestic responsibilities is the one who is most in need of T.L.C. (tender, loving care). As for the idea of simply using institutions as places where the patient, already in established labour, can be hurried into, there to complete her second and third stages before being wrapped up and sent home a few hours later, is in my opinion a travesty in human management; nor is the back seat of a taxi a suitable alternative to a Labour Ward bed.

The effect upon midwives and hospital staff, and their recruitment into obstetrics of this sordid, mechanistic approach to labour, hardly needs mentioning, although there is so much present talk of improving human relations in hospital. The country can't eat its cake and have it. Admittedly with slick organisation there may be few maternal disasters and only a few babies will escape the recognition of acute neonatal emergencies within the first few days of life, ranging from jaundice to attacks of sudden hypoglæcemia, to say nothing of some more obscure congenital handicaps, as has been pointed out in a hospital in a very poor Brooklyn district where I had the privilege of working for a month as Guest Professor.[9] It is agreed that a lying-in period of fourteen days is absurdly extravagant and even ten days, although desirable, is longer than absolutely necessary and we have compromised in Glasgow in the normal case at around a week. A woman who says she will only come into hospital for 48 hours and that those are her conditions is the case that requires urgent investigation by the Medical Social Service Department to estimate and eliminate the reasons; this form of blackmail, in fact, need not be a problem.

Fullblown, key obstetric units are, of course, expensive, both in equipment and staffing and here is where the General Practitioner Obstetrical Unit should fill the gap and in full co-operation between General Practitioner and Obstetrician these units should in the future undertake what hitherto has been carried out in domiciliary practice. Selection, screening and filtration should be, therefore, at a very high level, since the need for a flying squad simply condemns domiciliary and small unit obstetrical practice in retrospect.

INDICATIONS FOR SPECIALIST HOSPITAL DELIVERY

Bad social conditions alone due to overcrowding, lack of sanitation, or the presence of disease in the family are all too often indications enough, but many could be adequately dealt with in G.P.

obstetric units. The young girl with the illegitimate pregnancy, however, comes into a special category and often needs rather more than medical care because of her background problems. The illegitimacy rate in cities like Glasgow and Dundee, and curiously enough, in country districts like Wigtownshire in the extreme South West of Scotland, are much worse than for the country as a whole and the rate would appear to be rising in cities. Nevertheless while it has been obvious for generations to all the less youthful of our citizens that the country is steadily going to the dogs, it should be remembered that exactly 100 years ago the illegitimacy rate in the country was almost double what it is today and that our glorious island history furnishes instances of far worse periods of social and moral degradation than we face at present. The illegitimacy rate in the 1860s was approximately 10 per cent of all live births; the overall figure now is about 5.2 per cent,[7] but over 8 per cent in Glasgow. Under the modern National Health Service the Medical Social Services are reaching a high degree of efficiency, especially in aftercare. The following, however, are the chief medical and obstetrical indications for delivering in specialised hospital units which are, to our way of thinking, absolute.

1. *Grand Multipara*
   Chief hazards:
   Uterine Rupture.
   Cervix and vault rupture.
   Postpartum hæmorrhage.
   Shock and anæmia.
   Antepartum hæmorrhage (all varieties).
   Malpresentation.
   Prematurity.
   Hypertensive disease.
   Precipitate labour.

2. *Previous Third stage abnormality*
   especially hæmorrhage, retained placenta or previous manual removal.
   Hazard—repetition common even after an intervening normal third stage.

3. *All major medical disorders:*
   e.g. Cardiac disease, diabetes, tubercle, thyrotoxicosis, cardiovascular disorders, unresponding anæmia, etc.

4. *Twins or Triplets*
   Chief hazards:
   Postpartum hæmorrhage.
   Antepartum hæmorrhage.

Malpresentation.
Anæmia.
Difficulties or delay in delivering second twin.
Prematurity.
Pre-eclampsia and eclampsia.
Hydramnios.

5. All *malpresentations* including multiparous breech.
   Hazards:
   High operative delivery rate.
   Higher fœtal risks.

6. *B.O.H.* (bad obstetric history)
   especially in the "recurrent" group of calamity (see Chapter III):
   e.g. Postmature stillbirth.
   Intra-uterine death (I.U.D.).
   Fœtal abnormality (F.A.).

7. *Disproportion* actual or suspect.
   Hazards: obvious.
   All European women with height of less than five feet should be included.

8. *Previous Cæsarean section, myomectomy or hysterotomy.*
   Hazard: ruptured uterus.
   Increased incidence of unsatisfactory labour necessitating further Cæsarean section.

9. *All hypertensive states.*
   Hazards:
   I.U.D.
   Eclampsia.
   Cerebral vascular accident.
   Abruptio placentæ.

10. *Prematurity and history of repeated premature labour.*
    Best incubator for transport to hospital is mother's uterus.

11. *Rh-negative women with antibodies* and hitherto non-immunized patients with Rh +ve husbands who are ABO compatible (see Rh Chapter).
    Hazard: Fœtal or neonatal death from hæmolytic disease.

12. *Gynæcological abnormality*, including history of operation on cervix, or repair of prolapse, stress incontinence or fistula, or third degree perineal tear.
    Hazard: Cervix or vaginal vault may split suddenly. Pelvic tumours may complicate pregnancy, labour and/or puerperium.

13. *Primiparæ.*
    Age over 30 or where fœtal head is high at term.
    Hazards: Inertia and unforeseen dystocia—this may well be a "premium pregnancy".

14. *History of infertility.*

15. *Gross obesity* (see Chapter III).

16. *Age alone.* Regardless of parity, i.e. over 35 years.

The above list is given in order of priority yet it has taken a pædiatrician to point out our shortcomings even today in applying this standard of selection. Neville Butler, director of the National Birthday Trust Fund Survey of Perinatal Mortality[13] dispelled any complacency at a meeting at the Royal College of Obstetricians & Gynæcologists on October 18th, 1961, with figures that remind us that all was far from well, even in G.P. units where the same selection should apply as for domiciliary booking. He pointed out that some of these units were booking the same sort of cases as consultant units (*Lancet* 1961, **2**, p. 976) and that high risk mothers such as primiparæ over the age of 30, women over 35 and grand multiparæ formed 15 per cent of all cases booked in G.P. units. From these 15 per cent came a quarter of the 480 perinatal deaths in G.P. cases booked and delivered in these units in the period reviewed. This might have been partly "bad luck" (if such a thing exists in midwifery), but Butler criticised the standard of antenatal care in many instances, for example, the hæmoglobin was not estimated in 46 per cent of cases nor the rhesus group in 5 per cent, nor was the blood pressure taken at every visit in 16 per cent. Compared with these distressing intimations the organisation of the G.P. units in the Oxford region, as described by Stallworthy at the same meeting, shows what can be achieved by a high standard of selection and liaison with parent or key hospitals, namely a halving of perinatal mortality in 5,000 deliveries to the striking figure of 13 per thousand.

The state of affairs in domiciliary practice is even less reassuring. The first results of this same survey presented at the Royal Society of Medicine (Pædiatric section) on April 28th, 1961, showed that 20 per cent of primiparæ and 66 per cent of grand multiparæ were booked for domiciliary delivery and that nearly a fifth of these very women had to be admitted to hospital later as emergencies in pregnancy or labour. So much for the overall standard of selection, but the standard of care was unflatteringly revealed in the fact that the hæmoglobin was not estimated in 32 per cent of all cases and in 60 per cent of those receiving antenatal care solely under the domi-

ciliary service (*Brit. med. J.* 1961, **1,** p. 1313), nor, in one in six of all mothers, was the blood pressure taken at every visit.

The present scale of remuneration to general practitioners undertaking obstetrics under the National Health Service is £15, if approved or on the obstetric list, and £8. 15s. if not. These sums cover total obstetrical care both antenatal, intrapartum and postnatal. The fees for total antenatal care are £8. 15s. and £5. 2s. respectively but if shared, as is more commonly the practice, each antenatal visit earns 18s. for the approved or 10s. 6d. for those not approved up to a maximum of £6. 6s. and three and a half guineas respectively. These payments were agreed in 1966 and may easily be out of date in the near future.

Not least among the many benefits to womankind of this generation and the children of the next as a result of the ever-widening scope of modern antenatal care, is the fact that to many of the population it represents the first comprehensive health check up since leaving school, and its implications go far beyond immediate obstetrical considerations.

If a woman can reach delivery as fit as she was at the start of her pregnancy, then why not fitter? Notable examples are cases of nutritional anæmia diagnosed early in pregnancy and many cases of cardiac disability which are thoroughly supervised and treated throughout pregnancy.

It lies within the power of antenatal care to stamp out congenital syphilis utterly; the incidence of eclampsia can be lowered to an irreducible minimum; premature labour can to some extent be prevented; and many of the more dramatic disasters of labour itself forestalled by the early recognition of their causes. Above all, the patient's emotional reactions to her pregnancy and forthcoming labour are paramount and, by one means or another, it is one of the important functions of this work to engender confidence and to eliminate fear.

Antenatal classes

These vary widely in their scope and efficiency, but all have the primary objective of fighting ignorance and fear based on ignorance As far as hospital clinics go they provide a splendid opportunity for the patient to get to know more about the place where she is going to face her coming ordeal and about the people who are going to help her through it and what they do for her. The confidence and trust engendered and the personal contacts established make a great difference to morale. These classes, like so many booklets, devote the greater part of their effort to baby management thereby focusing the patient's mind less on labour and its difficulties and more on the goal to be achieved, namely a healthy baby. Our own hospital now offers

to every pregnant woman enrolling 8 classes in mothercraft, 8 in physiotherapy, including lessons in muscular relaxation in a gymnasium and talks on the physiology of pregnancy and labour. Between two to three times a month a film show is organised for patients, and husbands too, showing "To Janet a Son," always to very full houses in our main lecture theatre. There is also a course of what are called "adoptive" classes, numbering 3, which were pioneered by our midwifery staff for the benefit of women who, though not patients, are planning to adopt babies and require instruction and, above all, reassurance. A special Sister is appointed to look after those patients who have expressed a desire to breast feed. This wish is deliberately ascertained antenatally and without moral pressure and for those so choosing much can be done in the antenatal preparation of the breasts to ensure subsequent success. Questions and discussion are an important part of antenatal instruction in all its aspects and they help to make the patient feel that she is not on her own and unique in her problems but one of a helpful and interested community. Tours of the hospital are undertaken and the patients are given an opportunity to practise on self-administered anæsthetic machines.

All the above dedicated work is making a tremendous difference to the whole spirit of the hospital and the attitude of the patients and their friends and relatives, and could well be copied by units with a so-called stricter outlook. That this sort of attitude only works in a well-developed social community is not true because we have established an explant in Nairobi at the Kenyatta National Hospital, where a similar philosophy prevails.

ANTENATAL CLINICS

Since the 1914–18 war, the number of antenatal clinics which has sprung up all over the country has run into four figures. In certain quarters there is prejudice against this type of organisation on the grounds that the personal touch may be lacking, that it is desirable that the patient should be delivered by the same people who look after her during pregnancy and that doctors undertaking antenatal care should be able to follow cases right through for their own good also. Now these objections are not wholly valid. Firstly, in any large hospital department of obstetrics responsibility tends to become divided in a large majority of the patients. At best, a patient can be looked after by a team unless there is some special personal or medical reason for reserving the case for one member of it. The municipal clinics, situated, as they are usually, in the patient's home area, often exhibit more of the personal touch, based upon an intimate knowledge of the patient's circumstances, than a hospital department with its changing population of house surgeons and registrars. The teaching hospitals, of course, do most of their own ante-

natal work as a rule, but this is less from virtue than from the need to supply their students with instruction. But, for the majority of hospitals, the borough clinics help to distribute the load and to filter off the more complicated cases requiring expert hospital treatment.

It is essential, however, that very close liaison should be maintained between hospital and clinic, and this should be very much more on a personal than an official basis.

It is, of course, no use having fine clinics all over the country if there is not an adequate number of hospital beds to back them. Hitherto there has been a tendency to reserve special wards for antenatal cases and in many instances the number of beds so allocated has been far too few. We have now abandoned this practice and with a hospital made up almost entirely of single rooms and four-bedded wards, it is possible to interchange function between antenatal and lying-in care, using the same nursing staff for both, which gives some continuity of nursing care and interest, both for patient and nurse and, above all, allows a more efficient usage of beds.[3] So often in the past I have seen too much pressure on the antenatal wards and yet empty beds in the lying-in department and vice versa. This is very inefficient.

It is said that an occupancy rate of 85 per cent is an acceptable figure for the average maternity hospital approaching maximum turn-over, but largely thanks to the above principle our own average occupancy rate is running nearer to 90 per cent.

The municipal clinics are, of course, not only concerned with cases booked for delivery in hospital, but they undertake also the antenatal care of a very large part of the country's domiciliary practice. To district midwives the advantages are very great, and medical opinion is always available on the spot. Not least of the activities of such a clinic is the welfare side, and disparaging criticism is usually ill-informed.

The patient who is able to engage the private services of a doctor who will see her through pregnancy, delivery and beyond is in a different category, and usually in a higher income group, but to a large part of the population the clinics and the municipal and hospital maternity services must make up in efficiency what they lack in private individual care.

ROUTINE PROCEDURES

The following is a brief summary:

History-taking

This is quite an art and should not be left to members of the nursing staff, nor should it take the nature of form filling. It should be

dealt with under three headings—medical history, obstetrical and family history. Details of previous hospitalisation should be entered, and specific enquiry should be made into a history of rheumatism, chorea, fits, nervous breakdowns, pleurisy and urinary infections. The usual dreary negative list with which one is presented includes mumps, scarlet fever, a distant family history of twins and, oddly enough, diphtheria, and is obstetrically irrelevant.

The obstetric history should note the menstrual rhythm and any irregularities. This information may help later to settle a doubt about the maturity of the fœtus. Any period of antecedent involuntary sterility is also worth recording. Fully summarised details should be obtained of all previous deliveries and abortions; in each instance the complications of pregnancy, if any, should be listed; whether the labour was premature or overran the patient's dates, whether it was induced, and if so why; the nature and duration of the labour, the birth weight of the child, details of its survival or fate, puerperal complications and the duration of successful breast feeding.

The family history should take account of hypertension, diabetes, pulmonary tuberculosis and rheumatic heart disease, all of which may be of some relevance.

The present symptoms, if any are volunteered, are recorded, but it is doubtful if leading questions do not prove misleading. Most women reply in the affirmative if asked about headaches, backache or discharge, and almost half of them admit to constipation if questioned directly. There is not much point in making an impressive list of symptoms too irrelevant for the patient to bother to mention.

Booking Examination

The earlier the better. The patient should be weighed and a specimen of urine examined for albumin and sugar and, if vomiting has not yet ceased, for acetone. The examination of the urine simultaneously for protein and glucose has been enormously simplified by the introduction of reagent strips which will handle both tests at the same time, such as, for example, "Uristix", manufactured by Ames Co., a division of Miles Laboratories, Ltd. All that is required is to dip a strip impregnated with a double set of reagents into the urine and to read the results in accordance with the maker's colour chart. Provided the container in which the urine is supplied is clean and free from disinfectants, detergents and oxidising agents, this rapid method of urine screening is reliable and labour-saving. What is important above all is that false negative tests are much less likely to occur than false positives; in other words any failure due to carelessness is in the "fail safe" direction. The value of screening for bacilluria in hospital antenatal clinics is discussed more fully in a later chapter. The work and organisation thereof are by no means negligible, though the

results may yet prove to be far reaching. General medical examination should include the teeth and gums, and a search is made for signs of aural and nasopharyngeal sepsis. The thyroid is palpated and the triangles of the neck are examined for the presence of enlarged glands. While the patient is sitting up for this, the vertebral column should be looked at for any signs of deformity. There now follows an examination of the heart and chest and a detailed inspection of the nipples. Now, and not before, the blood pressure is taken, the patient having settled down so that a reliable reading can be obtained. With the sphygmomanometer cuff still applied, 10 ml. of blood are withdrawn by syringe and divided into three samples, one for Wassermann and Kahn reactions, another for blood group, Rh grouping and the estimation of antibody titre if present, and the third for hæmoglobin estimation, the latter must of course be collected in non-clotting specimen tubes. The abdomen is next examined, particular attention being paid to the size of the uterus, if palpable. The hands and nails are examined for evidence of tremor, œdema, nail biting, koilonychia and pallor of the nail beds. The legs are looked at for the presence of varicose veins and œdema, and the feet for serious degrees of deformity. The size of shoe is worth noting as an index of bony stature. External pelvimetry with callipers is a waste of time.

Provided there has been no recent bleeding, a vaginal examination is now made. Any discharge present is cultured, the position and size of the uterus is noted and pelvic tumours excluded. It is not often worth while attempting an assessment of the pelvic size or shape at this stage of pregnancy. This is better deferred until the softening and relaxation of the soft parts facilitate a more accurate assessment.

By now one should have a very fair estimate of the patient and her reactions. If pregnancy is normal, there should be no hesitation in telling her so and questions should be both encouraged and answered. Their very nature may indicate an important though unspoken fear that there may be something wrong with the baby.

Subsequent Visits

Provided pregnancy continues without complications, the patient should be seen at least every month until the 28th week, thereafter every fortnight until the 36th week, and then weekly until delivery. At each of these subsequent visits she is weighed, since any excessive gain often signifies undue water retention and the pre-eclamptic diathesis. The weight gain should not exceed 5 pounds in any one month or 2 pounds in a week. At each visit, of course, the urine is tested for protein and the blood pressure is recorded.

The maximum permissible weight gain throughout the whole of pregnancy is about 21 lb. although up to 28 lb. does not call for more

than vigilance. This figure of 21 lb. is made up of 7 lb. in the first 20 weeks, 7 lb. in the next ten weeks from the 20th to the 30th week and finally 7 lb. between the 30th week and term. Every encouragement should be given to the patient in the view that there is no need to put on weight permanently just because of having babies although this is often a very handy excuse.

The value of antenatal cervical cytology is far more debatable than that of postnatal cytology which should never be omitted. The chance of getting false positive results antenatally is not inconsiderable and it would be as well to repeat the smear test before rushing into cervical biopsy which may give the patient very real cause for alarm. While, of course, it is important never to miss a case of invasive cancer of the cervix in pregnancy, the results of antenatal cytology are not entirely an unmixed blessing and far more people suffer from the fear of cancer as a result than the disease itself. I cannot recall a single case of invasive cervical cancer in pregnancy that owed its detection to routine antenatal cervical smearing.

It is our practice to estimate the hæmoglobin at every antenatal visit and to record the result on the patient's notes before the doctor even sees the patient. This is a counsel of perfection and is paying enormous dividends in stamping out anæmia long before labour, in reducing the need for parenteral iron therapy by the detection of iron deficiencies early on, by spotting folic acid deficiencies earlier than they otherwise would be and in calling for a much earlier investigation of a patient's anæmia when it fails to respond to treatment. This is hardly possible in general practice but at least four readings should be obtained in pregnancy, namely at booking, at somewhere around 20 to 24 weeks gestation, at 32–34 weeks gestation and near term. Of all antenatal services the detection and correction of anaemia in good time is probably more important than all others.

Abdominal palpation of the uterus becomes increasingly important as pregnancy advances, but even in the early stages it should not be omitted, as, by this time, an assessment of the period of gestation in relation to uterine size is easier; also the sooner twins are diagnosed the kinder for the patient, who will have thereby more time for additional preparations. The patient should be instructed to note the first fœtal movements felt, as this, too, will help to pinpoint the period of gestation. An experienced multipara can recognise them at the sixteenth week but a primigravida will not be aware of them before the eighteenth and often the twentieth week.

At the 34th week, a further estimation of the hæmoglobin should be made in all cases, since iron deficiency anæmia can creep on very surreptitiously, but rapidly, in pregnancy and, if the patient happens to be Rh-negative, a further test for antibodies is worth doing, although it is very unusual for iso-immunisation to occur during the

first pregnancy without some placental accident. If, however, antibodies are detected in the booking blood specimen the test should be repeated at least monthly, since any rise in antibody titre may call for earlier investigation by amniocentesis and possibly elective treatment.

At the 36th week in primigravidæ, a full digital assessment of the pelvis is undertaken, as described in the chapter on disproportion. The information so obtained is of immense value. It is better not to leave this examination any later, because any vaginal interference during the last four weeks of pregnancy should be undertaken with full aseptic and antiseptic ritual. It is true that pathogenic microorganisms introduced by such an examination do not usually survive very long in the vagina, but one cannot be certain that labour may not supervene while the organisms still retain their potency if the examination is too long deferred.

The relationship of the fœtal head to the pelvic brim becomes more important as term approaches. The deeply engaged head can easily be mistaken for the engaged breech with extended legs and *vice versa*. A rectal examination often helps to settle the point, and at the same time the ripeness of the cervix can be assessed.

DIET

It is not so much what a woman eats that matters as what she fails to eat, and the deficiencies are more important than the excesses. One thing is certain, the baby will be the last to suffer in cases of malnutrition, for it is the complete parasite.

Although malnutrition in England and America is uncommon, the same cannot be said for subnutrition, and the subject still retains its importance. Since the baby will take the best of what is going, its size and development are only reduced materially in advanced malnutrition, but there is no doubt that the incidence of prematurity is influenced by the mother's diet and her social circumstances. The growth and development of the fœtus are more related to the social background in the patient's own childhood and to genetic factors than to the variations in maternal diet ordinarily encountered in the present pregnancy and, as a corollary, it is no longer reckoned that a woman can procure an easier delivery with a small baby by dietary restriction[19].

The first requisite is an adequate supply of fluid, and the patient should be advised to take two pints of fluid over and above her usual intake. It is the best and most natural defence against constipation and helps to tread down stasis in the urinary tract with its resultant liability to infection.

Constipation is very largely a neurosis, and its evils are much exaggerated, but nothing is to be gained by the passage of hard,

abrasive stools, and one's first attack on such a problem should be to ensure an adequate fluid intake, and secondly, to see that the diet contains enough cellulose-containing foods, commonly referred to as "roughage". Of these, fruits, vegetables and especially prunes are among the most important. The use of purgative drugs is often ill-advised and even more often unnecessary. Of all of them, paraffin is perhaps one of the most vicious because of its apparent and alleged harmlessness. By coating the villous crypts in the small intestine it must, to some extent, interfere with absorption from the gut. What the patient therefore gains in having loose, oily stools she loses in vitamin and mineral intake.

The normal quantitative requirements of a woman in pregnancy amount to about 2,800 to 3,000 calories a day. A hundred grammes of animal protein and 100 g. of fat per day are desirable levels of intake, but it is not much use telling a woman to eat 100 g. of protein a day if she does not know where it comes from nor how to measure it, and it is important, therefore, to give her only the plainest and most simple advice. The majority of patients are not very much interested in the subject of diet, and those that are have usually least reason to be so and often present a neurotic predisposition. Most well-to-do people eat a reasonably well-balanced diet, but it is among the poorer classes that mistakes are made. In the latter, carbohydrates, because of their cheapness, are relied upon largely to fill up the gaps. Unfortunately, they cannot replace the value of high-class protein supplying the three essential amino acids, trypto-phan, tyrosine and cysteine, and it is mainly in animal proteins that these necessary constituents are found.

Even the apparently well-nourished, however, are liable to a deficient intake of iron and vitamin D, and iron deficiency anæmia is still much too common. The daily requirements of iron are about 20 mg., and during the last three months of pregnancy the baby makes its greatest demands upon the available store. Liver, green vegetables and meat are natural sources of iron, but any case exhibiting a hæmoglobin less than 85 per cent (12·6 g.) should receive a supple-mentary supply for which the ferrous salts are eminently suitable. Proprietary preparations, such as "Fersolate", "Cerevon" and "Fersamal" are both effective and well tolerated. The dose ranges up to 6 tablets a day. As discussed later in the chapter on Anæmia, we have found that the dietary intake of both iron and folic acid is deficient in an industrial population such as we are dealing with in Glasgow and it is our present practice to prescribe, in addition to iron, a very small supplement of folic acid of 300 microgrammes a day ("Pregamal").

Two pints of milk a day would go very far towards meeting all the dietary demands of the pregnancy, but few women can bring them-

selves to drink that much. One pint a day at least should be insisted upon. The essential calcium requirements are thereby met, although other natural sources are fruits and vegetables.

Phosphorus, also necessary for skeletal growth, is supplied by eggs, cheese, milk, meat, liver and oatmeal. A diet deficient in either calcium or phosphorus predisposes the baby to the development of rickets or a latent tendency to this disease and the subsequent liability to dental caries. These propensities, engendered during intra-uterine life, persist into infancy and childhood, even though the diet after birth may be sound. Extreme cases of deficiency can provoke osteomalacia in the mother, but this disease is limited mainly to famine-stricken areas.

The role of vitamin D in the prevention of rickets is now universally appreciated. In areas where sunshine is short and eggs too expensive to buy and fresh milk taken in insufficient quantity, vitamin D deficiency is a very real danger. Two teaspoonfuls of cod liver oil a day will effectively protect the fœtus against this risk and should be prescribed. Alternatively, halibut liver oil may be taken. It is equally effective and, because of its greater potency, can be taken in small quantities in capsules.

The stress laid upon vitamin D should not detract from the importance of all the other vitamins, but the deficiency effects of these in pregnancy are less obvious. So far as we can tell at present, a normal middle-class diet reinforced as above, and with orange juice and at least a pint of milk, will meet the nutritional demands of normal pregnancy.

No pregnant woman in the United Kingdom need go short of these necessary supplements to diet since the National Assistance Board issues special tokens to enable necessitous families to obtain free supplies of milk, orange juice, cod liver oil and vitamin A and D tablets.

Since June, 1961, changes have been introduced to cover their cost to the Government as follows: Concentrated orange juice 1s. 6d., and cod liver oil 1s. per 6 oz. bottle, vitamin A and D tablets 6d. per packet of 45. These items are issued at maternity and child welfare centres. Tokens are issued by National Insurance Offices for the supply of milk at half price to expectant and nursing mothers and children under five years of age or National Dried Milk at 2s. 4d. a tin as an alternative to liquid milk.

As a matter of principle the imposition of these charges is deplored but I am reassured by our Mothercraft Sister that the trade in orange juice is brisk, though cod liver oil sales remain dull.

The enlightened policy of recent years officially adopted in regard to the nutrition of the poorer classes has practically stamped indigenous rickets out of existence, and dental health among the new generation

of children would have been even better had it not been for the sinister increase in juvenile addiction to sweet eating. The recent flood of immigrants particularly from Pakistan, has however, re-introduced this problem in the U.K.

Smoking, an expensive, useless and dirty habit at the best of times and one often betraying a neurotic predisposition, has even less to be said in its favour in pregnancy. To forbid it, of course, would set up more conflicts in the psychologically handicapped addict than she or her family would be likely to endure, but an Aberdeen enquiry[10] suggests that the mean birth weight of the babies of mothers who smoke is lower and the prematurity rate higher than in non-smokers and that the difference cannot be attributed to the fact that smoking is commoner amongst the lower social grades and higher degrees of parity.

REST

This is even more important than exercise. A minimum of nine hours in bed at night, preferably ten, is recommended, and during the afternoon the expectant mother should be encouraged to lie down or at least put her feet up for one hour. This is often very difficult, especially for the parous patient who is most in need of it. A system of home helps is available, but the scope is still too limited throughout the country; the scheme, however, is likely to develop.

EXERCISE

The mental effect of exercise upon the patient is perhaps even more important than the nature of the exercise itself and the muscles which it is designed to train. Speaking as a mere male, it can be admitted confidentially that housework is the most exhausting of all forms of exercise and easily the most distasteful, while the mental effect which it can produce is little short of deplorable. As a form of exercise, therefore, for the pregnant woman, it cannot be recommended on this count. Exercise, then, to be of much value, should provide a mental break from routine humdrum activity. This means getting out of the house into the open air. It might be added that shopping does not count as exercise—in fact, it is even more harassing than housework.

Of all types of exercise, walking, short of fatigue, is the most natural and suitable. Golf and bathing are admirable, although diving is obviously contra-indicated. Sports as energetic as tennis are not suitable after the first two months, and horse riding is positively foolhardy. The only objection to cycling is the danger of falling off. It is far better to allow an experienced cyclist to continue her activities for as long as she wishes than to encourage in her any idea of invalidism.

Exercises in pregnancy designed to promote relaxation in labour in the hope of expediting it and making it less painful are at present much in the news. The late Helen Heardman was a great protagonist of this type of treatment, although her book rather overstated the case. Physiotherapists, as a whole, are keen to co-operate in this type of antenatal treatment, and many hospitals hold classes in relaxation. The least that can be said for them is that they can do no harm and may indirectly benefit the patient by encouraging her in the view that she is thereby insuring herself against an unsatisfactory labour. Apart from these incidental and psychological effects, their value is by no means proven. A noteworthy contrast is the patient who spends the last few weeks of her pregnancy in hospital because of cardiac disease, and it is notorious how seldom inertia complicates labour in these cases. Relaxation classes provide good opportunities for instructing patients in the physiology of childbearing and in the hygiene of pregnancy and are of particular value in eliminating ignorance, which often lies at the root of many of the patient's unspoken fears. More than this, however, cannot be claimed for antenatal education and exercises, although an enlightened view would be that this is justification enough.

An interesting analysis[15] divided 2,700 primigravidæ into three groups, all matched in age. The first group consisted of 1,000 patients trained fully in relaxation exercises and techniques in addition to all the other incidental instruction on diet, hygiene and physiology. The second group received the instruction but not relaxation training, and the third, control group, had neither exercises nor lectures. The differences in the ensuing labours in respect of duration, need for forceps, analgesia and the incidence of postpartum hæmorrhage were negligible, while the perineal laceration rate in the exercise group was highest of all.

TRAVEL

For the patient who has a known tendency to abort, travel is contra-indicated during the early months of pregnancy, especially at what would have been periods of menstruation. In other respects, the chief thing against travel during pregnancy is the fatigue which it may involve and, towards the end of pregnancy, the possibility of labour supervening in inconvenient circumstances. Long car journeys should be interrupted about every two hours in order to allow a change of position and the re-establishment of healthy circulation. Travel by air has no risks peculiar to pregnancy and is particularly suitable for long journeys because of its alleged freedom from fatigue.

However, as an air traveller now of almost world-wide experience I am often forced to a contrary point of view and am reminded of the old saying, "Time to spare, go by Air."

Air travel, however, has made absolute the need for yellow fever inoculation which, astonishingly, has not yet reached India from Africa since the necessary mosquitoes are available in both countries under the most unfavourable circumstances. There would appear to be no contra-indication, however, because of pregnancy, to yellow fever inoculation.

A more common question posed is the desirability or otherwise of being vaccinated. The American Immigration Authorities are totally and intransigently opposed to the approach of anyone from anywhere who cannot produce a valid certificate of vaccination carried out within the last three years. A number of pregnant women prepared to face the financial expense of childbearing in the United States are very directly affected and they can be assured straight away that the danger attendant on revaccination is nil, but, where primary vaccination has to be undertaken, there has always been rather more doubt about the possible adverse effect upon the fœtus. A report from Dublin[2] concerns the successful vaccination of 112 pregnant women during a smallpox outbreak in 1960–1962. Three of the 113 viable children resulting from these pregnancies showed malformations but in only one of these had the mother been vaccinated in the earliest weeks of pregnancy and this child was born with spina bifida. The incidence of this condition, however, is common in Eire and was probably coincidental. Nevertheless fatal, generalised fœtal vaccinia has been reported from time to time. The risk, however, would appear to be entirely confined to primary vaccination in pregnancy, another good argument for getting this done in babyhood, as probably the commonest indication nowadays for vaccination is a trip abroad in later life, particularly to the New World.

COITUS

People vary very widely in their inclinations in this respect, and it is a good rule not to offer unsolicited advice unless there are very strong reasons for doing so, for example in cases of recurrent abortion. To the patient, however, who asks for advice on such a private matter, it should be stated that, ideally speaking, there should be abstinence between the 8th and 14th weeks of pregnancy and in the last four weeks as well. This advice should be given very gently, because one can never be wholly certain of the patient's marital background.

The use of the lateral position in coitus certainly prevents deeper penetration and possible hazard to the pregnancy and this is well worth remembering when counselling married women with mitral cardiac disease, where the combination of tachycardia and the supine position may sometimes occasion acute pulmonary distress.

DENTAL HYGIENE

Dental treatment is available free of charge throughout pregnancy and for one year after confinement but far too many women are more afraid of the dentist than they are of having a baby! It is commonly believed that dental caries is liable to progress rapidly because of the calcium demands of the fœtus, although this is not fully proven. The view, however, is too widely held to be erroneous and, quite apart from the question of progressive caries, oral sepsis may menace the safety of labour. Reparative dental work can safely be carried out at any stage of pregnancy, but dental extractions under a general anæsthetic are best undertaken in mid-pregnancy. The danger lies not so much in the extraction as in the anæsthetic, the risks being mainly those of asphyxia, which is particularly liable to occur in these cases when nitrous oxide is administered none too expertly.

CLOTHING

It is nowadays uncommon to see a woman so foolish as to wear garters during pregnancy, so no more need be said on this score. Shoes should have fairly low and broad heels, chiefly because a woman's balance in pregnancy is affected and she has to increase the extension of her lumbar spine to keep her centre of gravity over her feet. Above all, shoes should be comfortable. Abdominal belts are largely a matter of taste. The modern varieties are an enormous improvement upon the old corsets, and they are well designed with extensible panels to accommodate the enlarging uterus. To many women, especially the parous and the obese, they give a sense of comfort and security, but to the primigravid patient with a good abdominal wall they are by no means necessary.

Brassières should be chosen more for their functional efficiency than their cosmetic effect. They should lift the breast rather than flatten it and should be roomy enough at the apex to avoid depressing the nipples.

Maternity clothing provides less of a problem nowadays than it did, and there is no shortage of suitable and tasteful designs. The market is well catered for now that the hideous days have passed when pregnant women considered it was indelicate to be seen abroad.

BREASTS

Much can be done in pregnancy to prepare the breasts for successful lactation. The nipples can be trained in protraction by manipulation, and the wearing of Waller shells in the later weeks of pregnancy will often overcome apparently stubborn degrees of retraction.

The skin of the nipples requires no preparation other than ordin‹

ary washing with soap and water and careful drying. During the last few weeks of pregnancy the patient may, with advantage, be taught the art of manual expression of the breasts to encourage the early flow of colostrum and clearance of the ducts; the baby would otherwise have to perform the same task in the face of a possibly engorged and unyielding breast.

NOTIFICATION OF BIRTH

Under the Notification of Birth Acts of 1907, 1915 and 1965 notification has to be made of all births, alive or still, to the local Medical Officer of Health by whom notification forms are supplied. This responsibility lies upon the doctor or the midwife attending the patient at delivery and must be complied with within 21 days. At the same time the Registration Advice Card is given to the husband or next of kin of the mother advising him of where and how to register the birth, also within the period of 21 days. Neonatal deaths are registered on the usual type of Death Certificate.

BOOKLETS

Patients often ask for some advice on suitable literature to study during pregnancy. The choice will largely depend upon the patient's educational background. There are too many excellent publications to specify, and one would hesitate to proclaim an exclusive choice. An excellent booklet entitled *The Health of Mother and Child* is produced as a result of joint efforts on the part of the Department of Health for Scotland and the City of Glasgow Corporation and has been made available at special rates to all local authorities. The usual price is 9*d.* Applications for copies should be addressed to the Central Council for Health Education, Tavistock House, Tavistock Square, London, W.C.1. The book gives advice on hygiene in pregnancy, is well illustrated, and gives an excellent outline of the care, clothing and feeding of the baby. Another good little book is entitled *A Baby is Born*, by Dr. G. M. Kerr. *Baby and Child Care*, by Dr. Benjamin Spock (Pocket Books Inc., New York), gives an amusingly illustrated account of how to cope with the baby, while Dr. Lindsay Batten's *Single Handed Mother* (Allen & Unwin) is a masterpiece of comforting common sense.

The National Baby Welfare Council issues *Baby Book* (price 2*s.*) which is full of useful information about pregnancy, labour and baby management and the British Medical Association publishes a similar excellent booklet *You and Your Baby* composed of a number of short articles by eminent contributors, some of which have already appeared in *Family Doctor*. It is distributed through Maternity & Child Welfare Centres.

Many hospitals, including our own, issue their own booklet which is a mine of information about how to get an ambulance, whom to ring when labour supervenes and what to do if various complications occur, what to wear, what to eat, what to do and what not to do, what to bring into hospital and what the visiting arrangements are. A specimen is included at the end of this book as an appendix.

MONETARY BENEFITS AVAILABLE

In addition to the supply of cod liver oil, orange juice and vitamin tablets at cost price or free in necessitous cases, all pregnant women in the United Kingdom, regardless of their social position, are entitled to maternity benefits, provided at least 26 current health insurance contributions have been paid by the patient or her husband, or have been credited.

The details of these benefits have been clearly and fully set out in the Ministry of Pensions and National Insurance leaflet N.I. 17A. In brief summary, it can be stated that there are two types of benefit available.

Firstly, the maternity grant which is now raised to a lump sum of £22, doubled for surviving twins and trebled for triplets. The home confinement grant of £6 has been discontinued. These benefits may be claimed on form B.M. 4, obtainable from local Pensions and National Insurance Offices or Maternity and Child Welfare Clinics, and are disallowed if the claim is made later than three months after confinement. The second type is the maternity allowance of £4 a week payable for 18 weeks, starting 11 weeks before the expected date of confinement in the case of employed persons who have made the necessary number of current contributions. Again, failure to claim at the right time (and before delivery) may restrict payments to the seven weeks following and no more. Unmarried patients who are receiving the maternity allowance may also claim a dependant's allowance of 22s. 6d. per week in respect of the child and 14s. 6d. for every other dependent child during the six weeks following confinement. The maternity allowance is still payable to an unmarried mother even though the child is placed for adoption and the amount in any case continues to be payable even in the event of stillbirth or neonatal death. Total disqualification for allowances follows resumption of employment, emigration, death or, sad to relate, imprisonment.

REFERENCES

1. BORE, P. J., and SCOTHORNE, R. J. (1966). *Lancet*, **1**, 1240.
2. BOURKE, G. J., and WHITTY, R. J. (1964). *Brit. med. J.*, **1**, 1544.
3. DONALD, I. (1961). *Scot. med. J.*, **6**, 164.
4. DONALD, I. (1966). *J. Coll. gen. Practit.*, **13**, No. 60, Suppl. *1*, 40.

5. DONALD, I. (1966). *Proc. roy. Soc. Med.*, **59,** 184.
6. DOUGLAS, C. A. (1955). *J. Obstet. Gynaec. Brit. Emp.* **62,** 216.
7. DOUGLAS, C. A. (1966). Infant & Perinatal Mortality in Scotland & U.S. Public Health Service, No. 1000, Series 3, No. 5, Washington, D.C.
8. GREGG, H. M. (1941). *Trans. ophthal. Soc. Aust.*, **3,** 35.
9. HELLMAN, L. M., KOHL, S. G., and PALMER, J. (1962). *Lancet*, **1,** 228.
10. HERRIOT, A., BILLEWICZ, W. Z., and HYTTON, F. F. (1962). *Lancet*, **1,** 771.
11. LENZ, W. (1962). *Lancet*, **1,** 45.
12. MCBRIDE, W. G. (1961). *Lancet*, **2,** 1358.
13. Perinatal Mortality Survey (1958). National Birthday Trust Fund, by BUTLER, N. R. and BONHAM, D. G. Edinburgh: E. & S. Livingstone.
14. Ministry of Health (1963). Report on Confidential Enquiries into Maternal Deaths in England & Wales, 1961/63. London: H.M. Stationery Office.
15. RODWAY, H. E. (1957). *J. Obstet. Gynaec. Brit. Emp.*, **64,** 545.
16. SMITHELLS, R. W. (1962). *Lancet*, **1,** 1270.
17. SPEIRS, A. L. (1962). *Lancet*, **1,** 303.
18. STEWART, ALICE (1956). *Lancet*, **2,** 447.
19. THOMSON, A. M. (1951). *Brit. J. Nutr.*, **5,** 158.
20. WALSH, SADIE D., and CLARK, F. R. (1967). *Scot. med. J.*, **12,** 302.

CHAPTER II

ABORTION AND INTRA-UTERINE DEATH

MORE women die as a result of the methods used to procure abortion than from the abortion process itself, and, to most general practitioners, the subject will afford more anxiety than all the rest of gynæcology put together. It is a pity, therefore, that teaching hospitals admit cases of abortion far less readily than, for example, cases of prolapse, which are not in themselves dangerous.

It is not easy to assess accurately the percentage of pregnancies that end in abortion and it is harder still to do more than guess the incidence of interference, for even the illest patients will often go to their graves with their secrets. It has been estimated that one in every five or six pregnancies in the United States ends in criminal abortion, though this estimate cannot be much more than a rough guess.

The wildness of the existing guesswork has become particularly evident as a result of the British Parliament's interest in reforming the laws of abortion on grounds other than strictly medical. Estimates of criminal abortion in the United Kingdom[1] have varied between 25,000 and 100,000 a year and it is strange that Parliament can think of introducing legislation when so obviously short of factual information and not even prepared to accede to the request for the appointment of a Royal Commission to look into the whole matter and advise it.

The nearest estimates are only obtainable by inference from mortality figures assuming that the death rate from criminal abortion is higher than from therapeutic abortion carried out in hospital, for which the evidence from countries providing sound documentation, such as Denmark,[5] show a figure of 7 deaths per 10,000.

In our own experience the women most ready to confess to criminal abortion are those who have inflicted it themselves. The implication of third parties is unusual. It is terribly difficult therefore to separate the criminal from the spontaneous abortion rate, but it is interesting to observe that whereas in supposed spontaneous abortion the aborted material examined shows a chromosome abnormality in about 22 per cent,[9] no chromosomal abnormalities were found in the series of induced abortions, ectopic pregnancies and stillbirths at the same time. Furthermore, the iller the aborting patient on admission to hospital, the more likely is criminal interference to be suspected.

The incidence of abortion in cases attending an antenatal clinic is strikingly less than the usual 15–20 per cent abortion rate for the

31

population as a whole, and the difference is surely due to the fact that the patient who takes the trouble to book early at an antenatal clinic is presumably interested in the pregnancy, and it is from this group of patients that the incidence of abortion as a natural phenomenon should be calculated. The figure then would be found to be less than 5 per cent.

MORTALITY AND CAUSES OF DEATH

One of the chief causes of death, even nowadays, is sepsis, although antibiotics have made a great difference. The effects of sepsis are very often magnified by hæmorrhage, which ranks as the second factor in causing the patient's death. Thirdly, shock may kill the patient, but in these cases the shock is nearly always due to the method employed in interfering with the pregnancy. Lastly, anuria and uræmia may carry the patient off some days later following severe shock and hæmorrhage.

There has, in recent years, been a striking reduction in the number of women who died as a result of abortion (Table I), (Min. of Health,

TABLE I

DEATHS FROM ABORTION, ENGLAND AND WALES (REGISTRAR-GENERAL)

1942	.	.	313	1951	.	.	107	1960	.	.	62
1943	.	.	321	1952	.	.	90	1961	.	.	54
1944	.	.	313	1953	.	.	76	1962	.	.	57
1945	.	.	233	1954	.	.	76	1963	.	.	49
1946	.	.	157	1955	.	.	68	1964	.	.	50
1947	.	.	143	1956	.	.	72	1965	.	.	52
1948	.	.	125	1957	.	.	61	1966	.	.	53
1949	.	.	118	1958	.	.	63				
1950	.	.	103	1959	.	.	47				

Note the abrupt fall from 1944 onwards—presumably due to penicillin.

1960). Nearly all of these deaths are unnecessary. Hæmorrhage, after all, can be effectively controlled and treated, and most cases of sepsis are the result of local interference, for which the reasons will most often be found to lie in unsatisfactory domestic and housing conditions in the case of parous women, to whom the advent of another pregnancy comes as the "last straw". The issues, therefore, are as much sociological as medical.

SYMPTOMS AND SIGNS OF ABORTION

The first symptom is that of bleeding, which precedes the onset of pain. Any case, therefore, who presents with the symptom of pain before bleeding should be suspected of suffering from some other

condition, for example ectopic pregnancy. Where there has been interference, pain may also come first.

At this stage there should be no fever, and the aborting patient who has a temperature, while the cervical os is yet closed, is likely to be either a case of criminal interference or one suffering from some other febrile illness, for example poliomyelitis, pyelitis, an acute infectious fever or some such general disturbance which demands recognition and of which the threat to abort is an incidental result. Bearing these possibilities in mind, one should be ready to spot mischief farther afield before it is too late, and I can recall a sad instance of the recognition of poliomyelitis being put off, simply because septic abortion was diagnosed.

Following the onset of bleeding, intermittent uterine contractions occur which are painful and, after a variable interval, something more than blood clot is passed. If the patient's general condition is worse than can be accounted for by the estimate of the quantity of blood lost, other possibilities must be considered, particularly that of hæmoperitoneum. The diagnosis of abortion is not difficult, provided it is thought of. I know a colleague who, for example, divides all patients in the childbearing period of life into four categories: the married and pregnant, the married and not pregnant, the unmarried and not pregnant, and the unmarried and pregnant, and in all cases in this age group the evidences of pregnancy, recent or present, should be sought if one is to avoid being caught out.

The appearance of the blood lost *per vaginam* should also be noted, being, as a rule, brighter and more copious than in cases of ectopic gestation, though this is by no means invariable. In assessing the patient's general condition, the pulse, pallor and blood pressure are vital observations, but there is one sign of the utmost gravity which must here be noted and, if encountered in any case of genital hæmorrhage, provides a desperate warning of the patient's nearness to death. The sign is that of ballooning of the vagina, due to extreme atony of the vaginal musculature, so that on vaginal examination one gets the impression of a huge cavern filled with clots, whose walls seem to be almost out of reach and in which it is often quite difficult to reach the cervix. Such a case is in urgent need of resuscitation before any attempt is made to move her.

To decide whether an abortion is threatened or inevitable is often difficult, and in cases who are only bleeding slightly it is usually wise to defer the diagnosis for several days for fear of precipitating inevitable abortion by vaginal examination. Many "threatened" abortions are, in fact, inevitable due to the death of the fœtus, and it is often impossible before the process of cervical dilatation starts to decide whether the case is worth striving to save from aborting. Where products of conception are passed and recognised, or where

they can be felt projecting through the cervix and when the cervix itself is dilated, the inevitability of the abortion is obvious, and it only remains to be decided whether the ovum has been passed wholly, partly or not at all; in other words, whether the inevitable abortion is complete, incomplete or missed. As a general rule, the more severe the bleeding and the more definite the intermittent pains of uterine contraction, the more likely is the case to abort inevitably, although the accepted signs of inevitable abortion have yet to appear.

Any patient in whom early pregnancy is suspected, who is bleeding more than slightly or who has a temperature or in whom pain is a prominent feature, should be examined *per vaginam* on admission to hospital, not only to exclude other differential diagnoses, but also to decide what measures if any should be undertaken forthwith to expedite the abortion process and control the bleeding.

On vaginal examination in cases of inevitable abortion two types of findings are likely to be encountered. In the first, the uterine body is bulky and the cervix is open; and one may be aware of retained products and clot within the cavity of the uterus but not easily within reach. This situation is more dangerous from the probability of further hæmorrhage than the second group, in which a uterine fundus, only slightly enlarged, appears to be sitting on top of a widely dilated lower segment and cervical canal from which products of conception can be easily picked out. In this latter instance the abortion process is far more nearly complete and if the products of conception can be withdrawn easily by means of a sponge forceps, further bleeding may cease and it is even possible that little other than decidual remnants may be found on subsequent curettage. Vaginal examination is therefore very useful in distinguishing the two types of case and their urgency. These examinations should be carried out with at least some regard to asepsis and limiting the introduction of infection and it is our practice to cleanse the vulva with an antiseptic cream and to make the examination with dry, sterile gloves and wearing a mask but we do not usually regard a full scrub-up as necessary.

It is in the cases of mild bleeding that a conservative attitude is indicated. As already mentioned, a vaginal examination may turn a threatened abortion into an inevitable one, or so it is said, although I think that an examination of this vigour is neither indicated nor necessary. The more honest reason for deferring vaginal examination in these cases is that any severe bleeding which might presently arise cannot then be attributed to it. The case, then, is regarded as one of threatened abortion until the signs of abortion are manifest, even though in a number of cases optimism is not rewarded. Any cases, however, who continue to bleed, even though slightly, for more than four or five days must be examined vaginally and by speculum, as otherwise, from time to time, other pelvic pathological lesions will be

missed, for example carcinoma of the cervix, cervical erosion and polyp.

IMMUNOLOGICAL TESTS FOR PREGNANCY

These are absolutely invaluable because of the quick answers given and they are of particular help in deciding whether or not the patient may have a continuing pregnancy and one for which it is worth adopting a conservative attitude. The older methods of bio-assay usually prolonged doubt by a matter of days and afforded very little more accuracy. We have now practically discarded them. The immunological tests can be carried out as ward side-room procedure and fall into two groups: the single urine drop method, or the small test tube. The first is very rapid (e.g. "Gravindex") and may give an answer within a few minutes; the second, (e.g. "Pregnosticon" or "Prepuerin") take about two hours, and in our experience at least are a little more accurate, mainly because observer error is associated with naked eye observation of precipitation in the case of the drop test. This, however, can be overcome by using a microscope under low power.

The principle is the same in all of them. One of the ingredients is an anti-human chorionic gonadotrophic serum which, when added to a pregnant patient's urine, is neutralised by the chorionic gonadotrophins in it. The other reagent is a suspension or erythrocytes or latex particles which are coated or primed with human chorionic gonadotrophin. Normally these erythrocytes or latex particles inter-react with the anti-HCG serum and are precipitated either as visible granules in the case of the slide test or as a diffuse yellow-brown sediment in the test tube. This is a negative result but if the patient's urine contains free chorionic gonadotrophin because of the existence of pregnancy, this substance reacts first with the anti-HCG serum and provided sufficient HCG is present the primed erythrocytes or latex particles are not sedimented by the neutralized anti-HCG and settle in the test tube as a characteristic brown ring at the bottom. This indicates a positive result. In the case of the "Pregnosticon" test (Organon) which we chiefly use, a fresh suspension of erythrocytes primed with human chorionic gonadotrophin is made up with the suspension fluid provided. Meanwhile 0·1 ml. of urine, if necessary diluted to whatsoever titre is being estimated, is added to an ampoule of anti-HCG serum. The urine is best filtered first and the likelihood of false positives, particularly in women over 40 and who may be approaching the menopause, is reduced by diluting with an equal quantity of water. To the mixture of urine which has now had an opportunity to react with the anti-HCG serum, if any HCG is, in fact, present, is now added 0·4 ml. of the primed cell suspension. The triple mixture should then be shaken for about a minute and left to settle in a special rack for 2 hours without disturbance. A clear brown ring indicates a positive result (Plate 1). This test can be undertaken at room temperature and does not even require centrifugation and, as can be seen, the minimum of apparatus is needed. It is as well to set up a control tube at the same time to eliminate inaccuracies in reading and to check the

activity of the reagents which have a limited shelf life of not more than twelve months when stored at between 0° C. and 4° C. A made up suspension of primed erythrocytes and suspension fluid is not reliable after more than a week of storage.

These tests are extremely sensitive and false negatives are rare, but false positives are by no means infrequent especially if proper precautions are not taken. As Sharman has reported,[42] proteinuria may itself provide a false positive and he recommends separating it from the urine when present in more than trivial amount, by precipitation with an equal volume of saturated solution of ammonium sulphate followed by filtration. Alternatively, the urine may be acidified, drop by drop, with 33 per cent acetic acid until slightly acid to litmus, heated to about 70° C. and then filtered. Fortunately, boiling the urine does not affect the human chorionic gonadotrophin as far as this test is concerned. Any blood present in the urine, as may indeed occur in cases of abortion, should be filtered off or a catheter specimen used, because hæmoglobin itself is a protein and may tend to give false positives. Urine, also, which is excessively alkaline may give a false positive even in the absence of protein. False results can also be due to cleaning pipettes with detergents or soaps which should not be used, and for cleansing purposes a bichromate solution or plentiful distilled water is recommended.

These immunological tests by their accuracy and speed, commonly able to detect pregnancy within the first ten days after the first missed period, are much to be preferred to tablets combining progestational and œstrogenic hormones administered to the patient in the hope of inducing withdrawal bleeding and thereby satisfying her that she is not pregnant. Furthermore, the tablet test has the objection that the result is not known for a few days and is not reliable in women with abnormal bleeding patterns in whom a pregnancy diagnosis test is most urgently wanted. In the case of a continuing pregnancy a woman might be encouraged to blame the tablets for any abnormality of the fœtus which might subsequently appear, however unfounded her suspicions.[42] Since in any busy gynæcological unit the immunological tests are being done every day, often in considerable numbers, there would appear to be no point in using the hormone tablet test, although it might be useful in general practice.

Ultrasonography.—Even quicker and more useful is ultrasonography since we have the apparatus to hand and in daily use, and the first signs of an early gestation sac show up as a white ring within the uterus as early as five and a half weeks after the first day of the last period and with even more clarity by the sixth week;[18, 19] after which time the progressive growth of the gestation sac can be observed and the maturity estimated (Fig. 1). Even twin gestation sacs at seven-and-a-half weeks have been revealed (Fig. 2) indicating the earliest known diagnosis of multiple pregnancy. Furthermore, the level of gestation whether in the upper or lower uterine segment can also be seen and we have a strong suspicion, at present being followed up, that the likelihood of abortion is related in some measure to the level of implantation of the sac (Fig. 3). Finally in cases of blighted ovum, failure of development of a normal looking sac

PLATE I

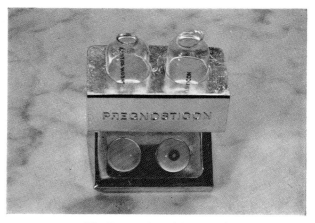

The Pregnosticon 2-Test Rack

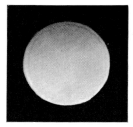
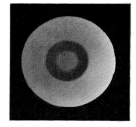

(a) Negative Result   (b) Positive Result

The Pregnosticon Test

(By courtesy of Organon Laboratories, Ltd.)

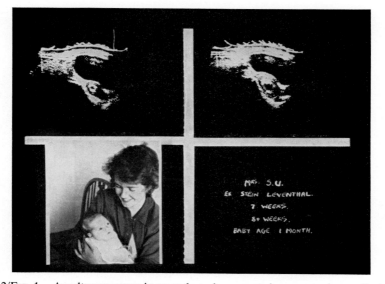

2/Fig. 1.—An ultrasonogram in an early and unexpected pregnancy in a patient previously operated on for Stein-Leventhal syndrome. Top left picture shows a longitudinal section, cranialwards to the left with the level of the symphysis pubis marked by a vertical line. Behind a distended bladder (black) there is seen a normal sized anteverted uterus containing a small, white ring representing a gestation sac of seven weeks. The ultrasonogram, top right, shows the same patient ten days later. Note how both the uterus and the gestation sac have grown. The bottom picture shows the same baby a few months old.

has been observed many weeks before abortion has ultimately taken place (Fig. 4 a–d).

DIFFERENTIAL DIAGNOSIS

The most important differential diagnosis is that of ectopic gestation, in which the clinical findings are by no means always characteristic. In this instance, however, the onset of pain tends to precede that of bleeding, a history of fainting attacks is characteristic, the patient's symptoms and general condition may be out of proportion to the amount of blood lost, vaginal tenderness and pain on moving the cervix gently are usually marked, a boggy indefinite mass may be felt either behind the uterus or to one side of it, and the vaginal loss often has a dark "prune-juice" appearance. Abdominal rigidity is very rare.

A prolonged clinical lifetime has not, however, reduced the number of mistakes which I (and incidentally my colleagues) from time to time make, resulting either in a missed diagnosis or occasionally in an

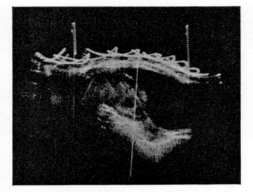

2/FIG. 2.—Twin gestation sacs (indicated by white intermediate vertical line) found at eight weeks' gestation although urine tests for pregnancy negative. L.S. behind moderately full bladder to the right.

(By courtesy of the Editor, *Brit. J. Radiol.*)

unnecessary laparotomy. Cases frequently present in altogether atypical fashion. Commonly, a persistently positive immunological urine test leads one to treat a case of continuing mild vaginal bleeding as one of threatened abortion, with only vague clinical signs within the pelvis. Ultimate curettage in such a case show only decidua and no villi, which should immediately alert one to the diagnosis of a pregnancy elsewhere. Even a negative urine test does not eliminate the possibility of a tubal mole with continuing invasive properties.

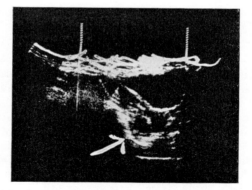

2/FIG. 3.—Low implantation of gestation sac in a case of recurrent abortion. An abnormally shaped uterus is visible behind a partially filled bladder in longitudinal section. The sac can be made out in the lower segment. The patient again, aborted four weeks later.

(By courtesy of the Editor, *Brit. J. Radiol.*)

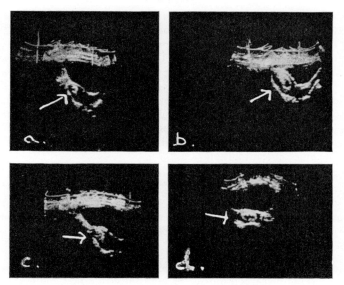

2/Fɪɢ. 4.—Blighted ovum in a case of recurrent abortion due to genetic defect
viz. translocation on chromosome III in husband.

(*a*) Shows apparently normal gestation sac at six seeks in upper segment of
uterus behind full bladder. L.S.

(*b*) At eight weeks, growth of gestation sac has clearly occured. L.S.

(*c*) At nine and a half weeks. No further growth, in fact shrinkage although
urine tests still positive. L.S.

(*d*) 10½ weeks—no further sign of growth, just a crenated sac. T.S. behind full
bladder.

Patient aborted for the fifth time ten days later. No foetus.

(By courtesy of the Editor, *Brit. J. Radiol.*)

Such a mistake once resulted in a massive hæmoperitoneum some
days after I had discharged the patient from hospital. This incident
was brought to our notice by the inevitable "chortle" letter which
one receives from time to time from rival hospitals, advising one of
errors committed and how the patient was snatched from the jaws of
death by their own superior clinical acumen. Perhaps the most
dangerous pitfall of all is to rely upon examination under anaesthesia.
A tubal pregnancy on the point of rupture can be so provoked the
minute the examining fingers approach it, with the result that nothing
is now felt and the patient may be returned to the ward where, if she
is not very closely watched, her collapse from hæmoperitoneum may
not be observed until too late. I know of two fatal instances of this
sort in other hospitals. Once when visiting one of the London Teaching Hospitals I noticed two cases who appeared to have been to the

operating theatre twice in the one day and to have had massive transfusions, and my inquiries prompted the confession that both had been examined under anaesthesia to exclude ectopic pregnancy and had been brought back to the theatre in a hurry later the same day. The dangers of examining the patient with an ectopic pregnancy in the anaesthetised and non-protesting state have led many clinicians to preach that if there is a suspicion from history or signs of ectopic pregnancy, laparotomy should be undertaken forthwith and that it is better to look inside unnecessarily than to miss the diagnosis. This was indeed my teaching until the new fibre optic peritoneoscopes came on the market.

Peritoneoscopy

Peritoneoscopy (or laparoscopy) now features very prominently in our gynæcological practice and we may undertake as many as four or five cases in a week. Among the indications for this simple and useful investigation are possible ectopic pregnancy. For the process we anæsthetise and catheterise the patient in the dorsal position, and then tilt her into the Trendelenburg position and induce a pneumoperitoneum with helium or carbon dioxide or both through a needle introduced a few centimetres below the umbilicus. A fibre optic peritoneoscope is then introduced, as described by Steptoe,[44] at the lower border of the umbilicus and an immediate view of the pelvic viscera from above is obtained often superior to that provided at laparotomy by some surgeons. If tubes and ovaries are normal and the pouch of Douglas clear of inflammatory disease or endometriosis, we take the opportunity of inspecting the appendix as well. We take a good deal of trouble at the end of the operation to evacuate as much gas as possible from the pneumoperitoneum and the patient suffers so little disturbance that she can be dismissed safely the next day. If, on the other hand, an ectopic pregnancy is seen it is a simple matter to proceed with the patient under the same anæsthetic to laparotomy. A considerable personal experience of posterior culdoscopy has now been discarded because of the inferior view obtained and all the palaver of having to turn the patient round into the Trendelenburg position from the genupectoral in order to proceed to operation in the positive case. Armed with facilities for laparoscopy it is now inexcusable to miss the diagnosis of ectopic pregnancy in either direction and, in fact, since adopting the technique in my department this mistake has been made only once, by a junior who happened to be on duty and who had not confidently mastered peritoneoscopic technique.

All types of functional uterine hæmorrhage may simulate abortion, particularly cases of metropathia hæmorrhagica, in which a period of amenorrhœa may have preceded the onset of the loss, but pain is never a feature of such bleeding apart from that due entirely to the passage of large clots.

Fibroids, likewise, may produce bleeding, together with signs of uterine enlargement, and occasionally there is associated pain due either to the attempt on the part of the uterus to extrude a fibroid polyp, or, occasionally, due to acute degeneration in the fibroid, but fibroids never, repeat never, produce amenorrhœa. Other pelvic lesions which may present as cases of apparent abortion include new-growths of the cervix and polyps.

Hydatidiform mole comes into the differential diagnosis of abortion and this is dealt with more fully later in the chapter.

Now and then the bleeding comes neither from uterus nor cervix, but from a torn vessel in a ruptured hymen from which, occasionally, hæmorrhage can be very profuse, to the point of exsanguination and vaginal ballooning as already described. Such a possibility was very sharply brought home to me on a Service Out-station during the war. The girl was pulseless, the vagina was ballooned with atony and full of a bewildering mass of clots, so that I had difficulty in identifying the cervix at first. There was so much blood and clot about that I did not at once recognise the source of the hæmorrhage, which was from a large hymeneal tear, and I assumed that she was aborting.

Lastly, a patient who has recently, secretly, delivered herself of a baby at term can easily be mistaken for a case of abortion if not very carefully examined, for the uterus is bulky and bleeding, and only careful examination of the cervix and perineum for tell-tale signs of laceration may prevent one from making a humiliating mistake. I have been caught out by just such a case seen for the first time, and it was the police who later dealt with the matter of a new-born strangled infant found within a cupboard in the patient's room. The placenta, incidentally, was never found!

Treatment of Threatened Abortion

Rest in bed with sedation is the keystone of treatment, and hormone therapy is of no more than very questionable value once the threat to abort is manifest. Morphine is not recommended. It often induces vomiting and even more often appears to expedite abortion. Sodium amytal, 0·2 g. (3 gr.) four hourly, is far more effective. At this stage, the use of progesterone often appears to act more as an abortifacient than as a remedy. Occasionally isoxuprine ("Duvadilan") may appear to damp down uterine activity but we have not yet had sufficient experience of the use of this drug to be able to assess its efficacy, especially when one bears in mind that with a normally implanted ovum or one known by sonar to be alive and growing and in which there is no cervical incompetence, the chances of pregnancy continuing successfully on its own are very high.

There is certainly nothing to commend the exhibition of progestational agents without evidence of deficiency and this is hard to
come by because even normal cases show wide variations in pregnanediol excretion. Although present day methods of assay are in
themselves becoming more accurate[12, 24], it has been suggested[40] that
24-hour outputs below 4 mg. are more likely to be associated with
abortion, but these may well include cases of missed abortion. It
is our experience that ultrasonography gives a far more reliable and
ready answer to whether or not pregnancy is continuing simply by
studying the appearance of intra-uterine growth which, as already
mentioned, can be carried out from the sixth week of pregnancy onwards (Fig. 1). After the eleventh week if should be possible to pick
up the fœtal heart by the ultrasonic Doppler effect, using some such
apparatus as the "Doptone".[23] Any pulsating structure and particularly, of course, the fœtal heart or cord, will modify the frequency of
an echo to an ultrasonic beam reflected towards it. It will thus give a
signal which, even in early pregnancy, has a recognisable rate of
around 140 beats per minute and is readily identified as fœtal in
origin. This proof of continuing intra-uterine life is as reassuring to
the patient who can hear it on the loud-speaker, as to the clinician
who may be in doubt that pregnancy is continuing and whether to
regard a case of continued bleeding as salvable.

Patients should be kept in bed until all signs of fresh bleeding have
ceased for at least forty-eight hours, and the bowels should be left
strictly alone. At the end of five days a vaginal examination is made
to ensure that all is well, a urinary pregnancy test is performed, and
the patient advised before discharge to avoid heavy lifting, sexual
intercourse and powerful purgation, at least until safely past the 16th
week.

A study of the changes in cervical mucus is often helpful and has
now become a routine test in our department. It is very simple to
carry out and involves the removal of a small quantity of mucus
from the cervical canal with a throat swab, after first mopping the
surface of the cervix. The specimen so obtained is spread fairly
thickly on a dry slide, without coverslip, and examined under low
power microscopy about twenty minutes later, after it has had time
to dry.

It has long been known that the quantity and appearance of this
mucus is related to œstrogen and progesterone activity and in 1946
Papanicolaou observed fern-like crystallisation in the first half of
the menstrual cycle which tended to disappear in the second half.
Furthermore, these crystals were absent in pregnancy and after the
menopause.

Typical fern-like crystals are seen in Fig. 5 and they are believed
to consist of sodium and potassium chloride bound with a small

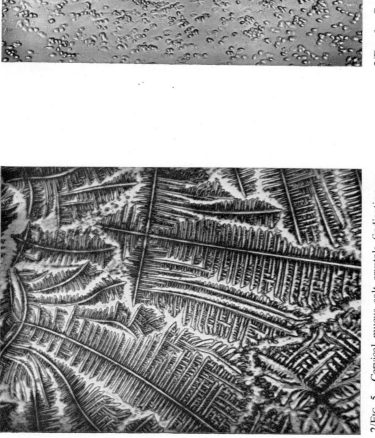

2/Fig. 5.—Cervical mucus salt crystals (indicating un-balanced estrogen activity and incompatible with pregnancy).

2/Fig. 6.—Cervical mucus. Premenstrual and normal pregnancy. (**Progesterone effect.**)

amount of organic material. Their presence is an indication of œstrogen activity, whereas their appearance can be modified or inhibited by progesterone (Fig. 6). This latter picture is characteristic of the premenstrual part of the cycle, indicating that ovulation has occurred. If there are endocervical cells only and no crystals after an expected period has been missed, this appearance suggests pregnancy, the phenomenon being believed due to œstrogen activity now balanced by progesterone.

By contrast the picture of ovarian inactivity, e.g. after the menopause, is shown in Fig. 7, which is lacking in both crystals and cells.

The presence of blood spoils the test so that it cannot be employed until bleeding has settled down, but in cases of repeated abortion, before a threat develops, complete absence of crystals and the presence of endocervical cells indicates a good prognosis. As a test for pregnancy it is only reliable in a negative sense, fern-like crystals excluding the diagnosis, whereas their absence might be due either to the premenstrual or the early gravid state. However, if an intramuscular injection of œstradiol, 10 mg., fails to produce the crystals four days later, pregnancy can be fairly reliably assumed. This test is not now used by us because of our ultrasonic and urine testing facilities.

Often, however, one gets an equivocal result with atypical ferning (Fig. 8). This appearance commonly indicates that all is not well with the pregnancy and precedes early abortion some days later. The injection of depot progesterone (125–250 mg.) can reverse this picture and abolish the ferns, but the pregnancy may already be past salvage and disappointments are common.

This simple test, therefore, can clearly exclude the diagnosis of pregnancy, e.g. at the menopause or in metropathia hæmorrhagica, can help to confirm that active pregnancy is continuing or can give warning to expect a threat to abort in the near future.

Incidentally crystals have been reported in the cervical mucus of cases of hydatidiform mole[28].

After the initial threat to abort has been controlled we are guided in whether or not to give progesterone by using the cervical mucus test. Where ferning appears (usually atypical) we inject depot progesterone (Primolut depot), usually 250 mg. weekly, until the crystals disappear and follow up in this fashion until the 18th week.

Ethisterone is too weak to be of any use and norethisterone preparations carry the risk of masculinising a female fœtus in utero.

The efficacy of all treatments, whether bizarre or rational, must be viewed against the natural recovery rate, for instance Perera (1961) treated 467 cases of threatened abortion with bed rest and barbiturates alone and 72 per cent of the pregnancies continued.

Even though threatened abortion may be successfully treated,

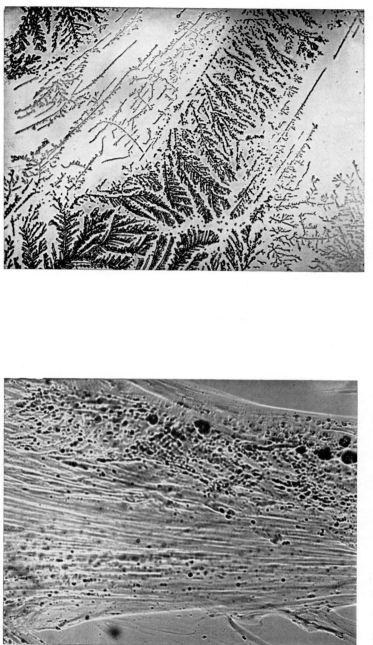

2/Fig. 7.—Post-menopausal cervical mucus. (Ovarian inactivity.)

2/Fig. 8.—Atypical crystals in cervical mucus.

(Figs. 6–9 by courtesy of Dr. R. R. Macdonald [29] and the Editor *J. Obstet. Gynaec. Brit. Cwlth.*)

the pregnancy continues at greater risk than normal, premature labour, intra-uterine fœtal death and antepartum hæmorrhage of both main varieties being about three times as common as usual. The evidence that threatened abortion increases the incidence of subsequent fœtal abnormality is less clear. Whereas Turnbull and Walker (1956) found it to be doubled, Thompson and Lein (1961), in a study of 404 cases, found that it was no higher than in all pregnancies and this too is our impression. Fœtal abnormality is far less likely to be the result of threatened abortion than the cause of abortion itself.

TREATMENT OF COMPLETE ABORTION

In the case of an abortion which is adjudged complete by inspection of the ovum which has been passed no local treatment is indicated, but any patient who bleeds more than enough to stain a pad every few hours should be suspected of still retaining products of conception. There is a general tendency in hospital practice to explore and curette the uterus in every case of abortion occurring in the first three months of pregnancy however completely the products of conception may appear to have been passed and however little postabortum bleeding there may be, on the ground that in about a quarter of these cases readmission would otherwise be necessary for persistent or recurring bleeding. This may be sound hospital economics but is not sufficient reason for unthinkingly subjecting a large number of women unnecessarily to an operation which yields only shreds of decidua. Ultrasonic examination of the post-abortum uterus[19] can reveal whether the uterine cavity contains a sufficient quantity of retained products to justify curettage (Fig. 9a and b). This operation after a recent abortion is not totally harmless, quite apart from the immediate risks of perforation or of disseminating infection. If, in a subsequent pregnancy, the placenta happens to be sited over an area of uterine damage caused by the curette there is great danger of uterine rupture. One of the most dramatic cases of hæmoperitoneum that I can recall concerned a young woman in her twenty-eighth week of pregnancy who was admitted on a Saturday afternoon so ill that the differential diagnosis ranged from abruptio placentæ to most other conceivable intra-abdominal surgical catastrophes. A diagnosis of acute hæmoperitoneum was established by needle aspiration and at laparotomy the placenta was found bulging through the uterine fundus, presumably at the site of an undiagnosed perforation some years earlier at the time of curettage, following a sixteen weeks abortion. She lost her uterus, her baby and very nearly her life, being saved only by very rapidly induced hypothermia on the operating table and the usual gamut of resuscitative measures. Another such instance is demonstrated in Plate II.

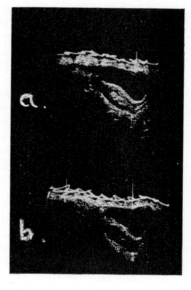

2/FIG. 9.—Retained products of conception. Bleeding eight weeks after delivery though uterus well involuted. (*a*) and (*b*) Before and after evacuation of uterus at which a piece of placental tissue was removed.

(By courtesy of the Editor, *Brit. J. Radiol.*)

The motto, "Is your curettage really necessary?" could well be applied to many aspects of gynaecology besides this one and I take great satisfaction in discharging a patient without routine curettage when neither her bleeding nor uterine size, nor ultrasonic findings indicate the need for it. The administration of ergot may assist involution, and retention of urine should be watched for. The patient, provided her general condition is good, can be allowed up as soon as she feels like it, and a sterile vaginal examination is made. If the cervix is by now closed and the uterus involuting well, the patient may be discharged home in a few days. A retroversion of the uterus, if present, is worth correcting and maintaining in correction with a Hodge pessary after the first post-abortum week because it is always possible that it may have been an ætiological factor in the abortion, and the chances of cure are better now than subsequently, after full involution of the uterus and its supports has taken place.

TREATMENT OF INCOMPLETE ABORTION

In these cases, the placenta or chorion is wholly or partly retained within the uterus, and as long as this is so the patient is liable to bleed. One's objective, therefore, is to encourage the uterus to complete the process and turn an incomplete abortion into a complete one. To this end, ergometrine 0·5 mg. intramuscularly is given and repeated, if necessary, in four hours. As an alternative, oxytocin in doses of 5 to 10 units may be given, coupled with morphine 15 mg.

(gr. ¼). A great favourite is what is called the "triple mixture" of an injection of all three as above simultaneously. Very often this will prevent further serious bleeding and will allow adequate time for restoring the patient's blood volume where necessary and preparing her properly for the operating theatre, including the passage of some hours since food was last taken. Under this scheme it is seldom that the patient has to be taken to the operating theatre in the middle of the night and she can await a safer operation and anaesthetic deliberately undertaken next morning. Only in the unlikely event of uncontrollable hæmorrhage or in cases of suspected uterine rupture is emergency operation immediately indicated, but such cases are often better treated by preliminary resuscitation. Rapid deterioration of the patient's condition meanwhile should alert one to some hideous associated catastrophe, such as a case I recall in which an abortionist had avulsed the whole of the patient's sigmoid colon through a rent in the uterus and, for a time, unbeknown to those in attendance on the patient, the torn end of the descending colon was discharging fæces copiously into the peritoneal cavity. Her life was eventually saved by total hysterectomy and terminal colostomy and the doctors were promptly threatened with legal proceedings for carrying out such an operation without the patient's written consent. The abortionist whose identity was known escaped prosecution.

The delivery of the placenta usually occurs within a few hours, but occasionally it is retained for longer. If it is not delivered within 12 hours, its spontaneous and complete expulsion becomes less likely, especially with the progressive tendency of the cervix to close, so that the patient continues at some risk of bleeding, and the placental mass may become infected *in utero*. One can usually wait safely up to 12 hours for the placenta in cases of abortion, but further delay is without profit, and it should then be removed by exploration of the uterine cavity under an anæsthetic. If the patient bleeds meanwhile, however, the situation is altogether different, and hæmorrhage demands intervention in its own right. Ergometrine should be given in the first instance and will, in the majority of cases, control bleeding at least for the time being. The necessary preparations for blood transfusion are made and a vaginal examination with full antiseptic precautions is undertaken. This can be done in the ward, but should be deferred preferably until the ergometrine has been given and taken effect. Often a mass of placental tissue will be found lying within the cervical canal, from which it can be quite simply picked out with the finger or sponge forceps without an anæsthetic, but if this fails or bleeding is provoked, the patient should be taken to the theatre forthwith, anæsthetised and the abortion completed by evacuation of the uterus.

Under no circumstances should operative intervention be under-

PLATE II

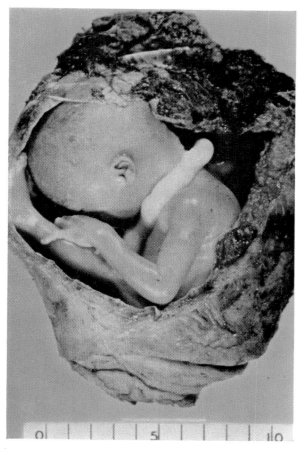

A case of spontaneous uterine rupture at twenty-three weeks due to placenta percreta involving the entire fundus and postero-lateral aspect of the uterus in a patient who had previously been curetted twice because of haemorrhage following a twin abortion complicated by coliform sepsis. The patient had no living children.

(By courtesy of Dr. A. Lobo, Nairobi)

taken without ensuring that the patient's general condition permits it. Some cases are already so exsanguinated and shocked that immediate attention must first be given to their resuscitation. Blood transfusion is the most important single measure, but very great care must be taken in cross-matching, not only because of the dangers of transfusion reactions immediately but also because of the great risk of subsequent anuria to which this particular type of patient is exposed. It is much safer to have a blood drip running before anæsthesia is induced so that any reaction can be noticed at once. Dextran infusions may provoke clotting defects and we never use them now. The intravenous injection of methedrine 20 mg. is often useful in desperate cases to produce an immediate rise in blood pressure, and the continuous administration of oxygen by mask is helpful in addition to other general measures, such as judicious warmth and the raising of the foot of the bed. Hydrocortisone added to the drip infusion or transfusion is of inestimable value in the really shocked case and has the additional advantage that it is very hard to produce overdosage. 500 mg. can be added to the half litre and up to a total of 2 g. may have to be given in desperate cases. In less serious cases 100 mg. may be added to the half litre. Treatment with hydrocortisone should thereafter be tapered over the course of the next few days.

As soon as the patient's systolic blood pressure begins to approach 100 mm. of mercury, the operation may be started under thiopentone anæsthesia. The vulva is shaved and painted with antiseptic and a catheter is passed. These measures are often better deferred until the patient is already on the operating table. The vagina is emptied of blood clot and, if bleeding threatens to start again, more ergometrine can be added to the intravenous drip. The cervix is usually already dilated sufficiently to admit a finger, but if not, it should be gently and slowly dilated to size 16 Hegar, in order to allow the passage of a finger. A half hand should be pushed into the vagina and either the index or middle finger, whichever is more convenient, is passed into the uterus. The internal finger cannot, as a rule, be inserted farther into the uterus than the proximal interphalangeal joint unless the cervix is well dilated and it is, therefore, difficult to obtain access to the whole of the internal uterine surface. It is now that the other hand, working through the abdominal wall, performs the most important function by pressing the uterus down over the internal finger, so that the whole of the uterine interior can be properly explored. This requires a good anæsthetic with adequate muscular relaxation. The gloved finger thus loosens up all the retained placental tissue and is the only really safe instrument for the purpose. Having loosened the tissue, the sponge forceps may now be used, and their function is simply to pick out the fragments from the

uterine cavity. This is far preferable to plunging about wildly inside the uterine cavity with sponge forceps, tearing out the placenta piece-meal. The best forceps to use are those having no ratchet, as one thereby retains a sense of feel of what is being grasped. The instru-ment should be inserted very gently until the top of the uterus is lightly felt, the blades are then opened, rotated through a right angle and closed on the material to be removed. The uterus can be per-forated with the greatest ease, but the preliminary exploration of its cavity with the finger will reduce the risk by appraising one of its dimensions, and the prior injection of ergometrine will harden its musculature and provide additional protection. Brisk bleeding demands further digital exploration rather than the blind use of metallic instruments. If the uterus is perforated in the course of this operation—and the first warning thereof may be the prolapse of omentum or bowel into the birth canal—the only safe measure is immediate laparotomy and repair of the rent. It will, therefore, be appreciated that the evacuation of the pregnant uterus demands the availability of proper theatre facilities.

Properly done, the whole placenta may be delivered in one piece. After its delivery, the uterus should be finally explored with the finger to make sure that no portion remains. If the uterus has been properly evacuated, there should be little more bleeding than follows dilatation and curettage in the non-gravid patient. Continued hæmorrhage almost certainly indicates incomplete removal of placenta and the need for further exploration. A breathing space for the surgeon can be obtained, in cases of profuse hæmorrhage requir-ing hastened blood transfusion, by digital compression of the uterus. For this at least two fingers are pressed up into the vaginal vault on either side of the cervix and the uterine body compressed through the abdominal wall against them. By this means also, the uterus can be rubbed up to contract after evacuation is completed in order to reduce the collection of clot within its cavity which, by its presence, may provoke yet more bleeding.

In less recent cases of incomplete abortion, curettage of the uterine wall may be necessary, and for this purpose there is no instrument more suitable than the spoon type of curette. The same precautions, as before, against perforating the uterus must, of course, be taken. The flushing curette is popular with many surgeons, but is seldom necessary. It often appears to start up unnecessary bleeding, it breaks down the natural defence barriers which are forming against infection, and injudicious use may force liquid up the Fallopian tubes. In any case, it makes a great mess.

The use of intra-uterine packing is debatable. Certainly plugging will effectively stop hæmorrhage, but the most efficient way of arresting bleeding is to empty the uterus properly, in which case the

plug is not necessary and serves to increase the risk of uterine sepsis.

The use of chemotherapy and antibiotics is clearly indicated as cover in cases known to be septic, but it is a mistake to use these substances simply as a protective umbrella under which to operate, for they may mask the true bacteriology of infection when it later reveals itself.

TREATMENT OF SEPTIC ABORTION

So far, the two indications given for surgical evacuation of the uterus are, firstly, hæmorrhage, and secondly, unduly long retention of placental tissue *in utero*. Nothing has yet been said of the place of evacuation in established sepsis, and here opinions vary.

As a general rule our preference is not to supervene surgically in the presence of uncontrolled uterine sepsis because of the danger of converting a local infection into a general one, which is infinitely more dangerous. When necrotic tissue is readily accessible and can be picked out, this, of course, should be done as before. Cultures, both aerobic and anaerobic should be obtained before any antiseptics are introduced into the genital tract and, pending the return of sensitivity reports from the bacteriologists, broad spectrum antibiotics should be exhibited in serious cases in massive dosage. This therapy should become more specific as soon as the bacteriologist's report is available. A continuing tachycardia indicates the need for blood culture as do rigors. Failure to respond within 48 hours suggests either the development of a pelvic abscess or some hitherto undiagnosed complication, such as uterine perforation or rupture in criminally induced cases, for which curettage would do nothing but harm.

The hazards of surgical evacuation of the uterus are greatly increased in septic abortion because the uterus is even more easily perforated and infected material can be readily disseminated. The need to perform laparotomy in such a case might well indicate hysterectomy as the safest course, a tragedy which might never have occurred if steps had been taken first to master the infection. If meanwhile, however, there is no response to treatment, an unlikely event, it may necessary to explore the uterus after 36 hours.

In cases developing septicæmia the responsible organism is most often the *Staphylococcus aureus*, the anærobic *Streptococcus* or *Clostridium welchii*. Hæmolytic streptococci usually yield very readily to antibiotics and are less often fatal today. *Escherichia coli* infections are commonly responsible and may be associated with bacteræmic shock.

Clostridium welchii is often cultured on routine examination of patients in whom there is no clinical evidence of gas infection; nevertheless, when this organism gains a foothold the case comes into a class of its own. The presence of damaged or devitalised tissue is

essential for its growth and, therefore, this type of sepsis is particularly favoured by criminal methods of interference, including the use of the syringe. The patient has a sub-normal temperature, a rapid, thready pulse, a very low blood pressure and oliguria. Consciousness is retained to the last, and X-rays may show the presence of gas. Anti-gas gangrene serum in doses of 100,000 units should be injected four hourly at first, penicillin should be massively prescribed, ileus is treated by gastric or duodenal suction and intravenous glucose saline, and very carefully matched blood should be given with judicious care. The patient undoubtedly needs the last, but the presence of oliguria allows of no more than a limited fluid intake (see section on anuria).

In summary, the presence of retained products in septic abortion is not in itself generally accepted by most of us as a primary reason for routine evacuation. The patient, if she is going to die, will do so because of a generalised infection rather than the local condition, and every effort must be made to attend to this first. In the wide choice of antibiotics now available, we can defy the basic principles of surgery with less penalty, but, even so, penicillin affords no justification for routine and ill-considered interference.

Endotoxic Shock

This is also sometimes referred to as "bacterǣmic shock" and is chiefly associated with infection by Gram-negative organisms, particularly *E. coli.* Whereas Gram-positive organisms produce exotoxins which can inflict their damage at a distance, the originating bacteria meanwhile multiplying, in the case of Gram-negative organisms endotoxins may be relased from the cell wall of the bacteria in the course of their death. The endotoxin so produced is not specific to any particular organism, although most commonly originating from the coliforms, and consists of a phospho-lipopolysaccharide which is closely linked to a protein and acts as a pyrogen and also destroys other living cells, particularly leucocytes, by increasing the permeability of the lysosomes within them. This accounts for the leucopenia so commonly associated with endotoxic shock. Hydrocortisone, apart from its other effects upon the vasomotor system, acts directly by countering this abnormal permeability.

Endotoxic shock differs very significantly from the other two types, namely the oligǣmic or hypovolǣmic and the cardiac type following infarction. The action of endotoxin is mainly peripheral and its chief effect is one of vasoconstriction so that there is a reduced venous return to the heart. Pyrexia may be a notable feature as, for example, after T.A.B. inoculation and there is an increase in the production of the catechol amines, adrenaline and noradrenaline, also histamine, and in experimental animals a fall in serotonin has

been noted. If in such an animal exposed to endotoxin the reticulo-endothelial system is blocked by thorotrast, then one tenth of the expected lethal dose of endotoxin will kill the animal, so the reticulo-endothelial system would appear to be protective.

Metabolic effects are profound with mounting acidosis due to tissue hypoxia and an initial hyperglycæmia giving place to hypo-glycæmia. Hypovolæmia is not normally a feature of the condition and therefore fluid replacement therapy, especially in the presence of oliguria, may be dangerous.

There are three main stages in the production of endotoxic shock. The first is one of vasoconstriction with ischæmic hypoxia and the release of catecholamines. The second is the stage of stagnant hypoxia with apparent oligæmia. In the third stage, acidosis becomes pro-found and cardiac failure supervenes. The mortality of the condition varies with the efficacy of treatment, but may be between 50 and 70 per cent.

The clinical features are of sudden and often unexpected collapse with rigors and pyrexia. The condition is not confined by any means to septic abortion and sometimes follows bladder instrumentation in males. Because of vasoconstriction there is marked peripheral cyanosis. The association of hypotension and rigors helps to dis-tinguish endotoxic shock from the other two main types, namely, cardiac and oligæmic in which there is usually no such association. The systolic blood pressure is often 60 mm. Hg or less and the patient is cold and clammy, becomes easily delirious and lapses into coma. Respiratory hyperventilation due to acidosis may be observed and, as already mentioned, there is initial leucopenia. Further examination of the blood shows a low Po_2 and a base deficit. The hæmatocrit reading will only be raised if there has been associated fluid loss; otherwise it is likely to be normal. Measurement of the central venuous pressure will, with most certainty however, indicate oligæmia if present, in which case it will be reduced, unlike myocardial or pulmonary infarction in which the C.V.P. is raised.

The treatment has to be prompt and courageous. Fluid loss must be replaced, preferably under direct monitoring of the central venous pressure, which will not only give guidance as to the adequacy of replacement but will give warning of overhydration and congestion. The fluid used may be blood in cases associated with hæmorrhage, 5 per cent intravenous glucose or a plasma volume expander such as "Rheomacrodex". A poor urine flow may indicate intravenous mannitol, as in the treatment of anuria. The need for hydrocortisone is urgent and in a severe case 1 g. should be given immediately intravenously, followed by doses ranging up to 500 mg. per half litre of intravenous fluid in the worst cases. Overdosage with hydro-cortisone is not to be feared and up to 3.5 g. can be administered in 24

hours. It produces peripheral vasodilatation which may call for more fluid replacement already being monitored. Vasopressor drugs are normally dangerous and should be given only if there is obvious cardiac failure. Metaraminol ("Aramine") is favoured by some because it increases renal blood flow and a dosage of up to 200 mg. in the hour in 5 per cent dextrose has been recommended, though I have no personal experience of doses exceeding half that amount.[10] In any case this drug is overshadowed in importance by hydrocortisone which may be life saving. Acidosis is corrected by sodium bicarbonate, starting with 100 mEq. and correcting according to blood examination. Meantime the infection must be vigorously countered and pending a bacteriologist's report, including blood culture, a wide spectrum but non-toxic antibiotic should be given in maximum dosage and for this purpose cephaloridine is the best yet available. It is non-toxic and avoids the great disadvantage of the tetracyclines of an uncontrollable build-up if there is any renal shut down. In using artificial plasma volume expanders a watch must be kept against the development of hypofibrinogenæmia. The value of isoprenaline as a dilator of peripheral vessels is somewhat debatable because of its associated hypotensive effect which must be watched for. The use of hyperbaric oxygen is much disputed because of the already existing vasoconstriction which is part of the pathology of the condition. However, one of our cases near to death with this condition revived so quickly in a hyperbaric pressure chamber that it was tempting not to regard her dramatic recovery as a coincidence; but it has to be admitted she was receiving the rest of the gamut of treatment at the same time, although our use of hydrocortisone in this case was timid by modern standards.

Oliguria in spite of all the above indicates a very bad prognosis, but once the infection is mastered and urine secretion is adequate, recovery is unbelievably fast and apparently complete. These cases can be amongst the most terrifying in clinical practice and a matter of a few hours only may determine the issue of life or death.

TREATMENT OF MISSED ABORTION

The greatest pitfall in this case is to diagnose missed abortion when, in fact, active pregnancy is continuing. To eliminate this mistake there is only one safe rule, namely, to wait and see, for there is no immediate need to intervene. Proof should be fully afforded before taking active steps; the urine pregnancy tests should be negative, the uterus after adequate observation should be seen not to enlarge, and all the signs of continuing pregnancy should have abated. Ultrasonic examination may clearly indicate the cessation of further growth, but of particular use is the ultrasonic Doppler effect using an

apparatus such as the "Doptone" or "Sonicaid" (British), which is capable of picking up the fœtal heart from the eleventh week onwards in many cases, and certainly by the twelfth or thirteenth week and thus immediately dispel the diagnosis of intra-uterine death.[23] After the sixteenth week X-rays may help (Fig. 10a and b). The patient will nearly always safely and spontaneously discharge the contents of her uterus in due course, certainly within the next nine months, though she may be irked by the delay and inconvenienced by a persistent dark vaginal loss. Our own record is a case which failed to deliver in spite of repeated attempts with oxytocin over the course of two years. There is however, a very real danger of a clotting defect, usually due to hypofibrinogenæmia, developing if a dead fœtus is retained *in utero* for more than a month.[3] Most of us nowadays therefore will intervene in the absence of spontaneous abortion by the end of a month. One method of playing for time is to attempt sensitisation of the uterus with doses of stilboestrol 5 mg. three times a day for up to a week, following this with quinine by mouth 5 gr. every three hours, up to four or five doses. If this does not work, one should proceed to an oxytocin drip in escalating dosage.[26] There is, of course, in such a case, no danger of uterine rupture and one can start straight off with 10 units of oxytocin in half a litre of intravenous dextrose or saline running at 25 drops a minute and increasing the concentration according to effect, if necessary up to 100 units of oxytocin to the half litre. Usually much less is effective, but the drip therapy may have to be repeated more than once with a day or two's rest in between. If hypofibrinogenæmia has developed before delivery, this must be corrected by fibrinogen replacement, but most instances of this ugly complication, however, are concerned with retained hydropic fœtuses due to Rh. hæmolytic disease.

Surgical interference is to be avoided because of the appalling risks of sepsis, particularly from anærobic organisms like *Cl. welchii*. Such attempts at uterine evacuation are often unpleasantly hæmorrhagic and the cervix may prove very unyielding. I have used laminaria tents in the past but only good luck, rather than good management, prevented catastrophe. A dead fœtus *in utero* provides an anærobe with the most perfect culture medium it could ever hope to encounter and the folly of surgical interference is likely to turn what is no more than a nuisance to the patient into a rapidly fatal infection.

In the unlikely event of really determined oxytocin drip therapy failing, recourse may be had to the intra-uterine injection of hypertonic saline introduced through the abdominal wall (see later), but this technique is only applicable in cases where the uterus is enlarged at least to the size of a 16-weeks pregnancy and readily accessible to an aspirating needle.

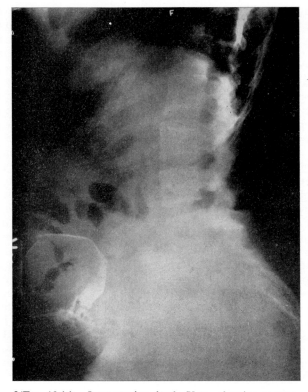

2/Fig. 10 (a).—Intra-uterine death. X-ray showing appearance of a skull in intra-uterine death of the fœtus. Note
overlap of the bones of the vault (Spalding's sign).

CAUSES OF ABORTION AND PROPHYLAXIS

The question of criminal interference and the degree to which it is
practised have already been discussed. The majority of cases of septic
abortion are so caused, likewise cases of severe uterine hæmorrhage
early in pregnancy with a tightly closed cervix. So far, no medicinal
method is reliably effective in a patient not naturally disposed to
abort. Of the local methods employed, crochet hooks and sticks of
slippery elm have tended to give place to the nowadays more common practice of violent syringing with Dettol or soap-and-water
solutions, and I remember a case who managed to fill her peritoneal
cavity, to the degree of shifting dullness, with a large quantity of
soap suds. It nearly killed her, and when, after her recovery, we commented upon her recklessness, she answered firmly that the adver-

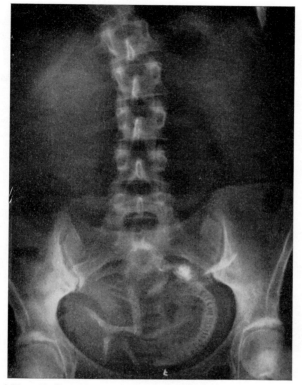

2/FIG. 10 (*b*).—Intra-uterine death. Note gross distortion of
fœtal spinal column.

(FIG. 10 *a* and *b* by courtesy of Dr. J. W. McLaren.)

tisements guaranteed the purity of the soap flakes! The modern fat
solvent detergent soaps are even more dangerous and we have had
a case in whom it is believed a considerable quantity of the substance
got into her central nervous system, which, besides nearly killing her,
produced practically a complete quadriplegia, and to this day she can
only move one arm slightly and continues a vegetative existence. Potassium permanganate crystals have also come into vogue. Besides being
ineffective they ulcerate the fornices and cervix, and may cause profuse
bleeding (Fig. 11).

Of spontaneous abortions, no cause either local or general can be
found in more than half. Many cases are due to faulty development
of the ovum, for which genetic factors may be to blame, and more
attention is now being paid to the minute examination of these
aborted fœtuses for evidences of early abnormality (Hertig and Rock,

P.O.P.—3*

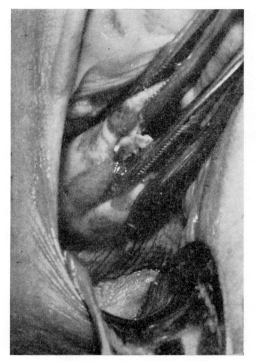

2/Fig. 11.—Potassium per-
manganate ulceration of
cervix and fornices caus-
ing repeated and profuse
hæmorrhage.

(By courtesy of the late Dr.
G. W. Garland.)

1949). The more carefully spontaneously aborted material is examined
the more often will there be found some chromosomal abnormality.
This involves immediate tissue culture of the material as soon as it is
passed and this is only possible if it is fresh enough to culture. The
material should be put in a sterile jar and taken immediately to the
cytogenetic laboratory. We are fortunate in having such facilities
and at the end of this chapter Dr. Malcolm Ferguson-Smith gives an
account of chromosome anomalies as a prominent cause of spontaneous abortion.

Of particular interest to us is the study of the process of ovum
blighting as it occurs in early pregnancy *in utero*. The characteristic
ring representing the gestation sac on ultrasonography of the uterus
through a full bladder has already been mentioned and the study of
its rate of growth on repeated examination. The blighted ovum
sometimes shows no such clean ring development and a speckled
mess is presently seen to occupy the uterus, which does not appreciably grow after about the 9th week in our limited experience so far
(Fig. 12). We have thus been able to foretell an inevitable abortion
often weeks before it occurred.[19]

If, for any reason, the fœtus dies *in utero*, abortion becomes inevitable, but this is only begging the question. General maternal diseases such as syphilis, nephritis, diabetes and infections associated with hyperpyrexia have long been accepted as causes, though nowadays they operate less commonly. Lead poisoning is now rare in England and is seldom a cause.

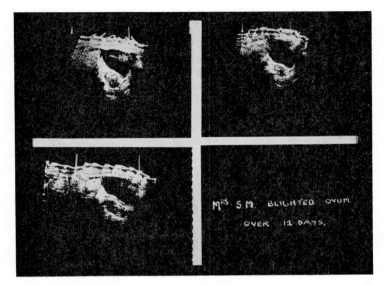

2/Fig. 12.—A case of blighted ovum. Ultrasonograms taken in longitudinal section (cranialwards to the left) over a period of twelve days. The distended bladder (large black area) permits a view of the uterus behind which is not appreciably enlarged and contains only a speckled and non-growing mass. The patient was a recurrent aborter and again passed a blighted ovum.

(By courtesy of Year Book Medical Publishers, Inc.)

Profound anæmia, malnutrition and hypothyroidism are all significant ætiological factors, and it will be seen that a search (if worth while) for the cause of abortion demands an examination of the patient in a wide sense, including Wassermann reaction, thyroid and renal function and hæmatological investigation.

Rh iso-immunisation is not now regarded as a significant cause, for the abortion rate is no higher in Rh-negative patients. Perhaps one of the most important single factors is the trauma of sexual intercourse which may easily provoke abortion in the early weeks of pregnancy in a woman whose hold on pregnancy is none too secure.

Emotional factors such as severe shock and great fatigue may also result in the interruption of pregnancy.

Examination of the pelvic organs may reveal local conditions which might reasonably be inculpated. The significance of retroversion, for example, in this respect is debated, as about 10 per cent of all women have a retroverted uterus which is without pathological significance. Nevertheless, such a uterus does in fact abort rather more easily than one in normal position, and when abortion is recurrent there is much to be said for correcting the retroversion between pregnancies. When a patient with a history of abortion is found to be pregnant again with a retroverted uterus, she should be warned of the dangers of intercourse in the early months of pregnancy and before the retroversion has corrected itself. The use of the lateral position in coitus is certainly safer than the dorsal because it prevents deeper penetration. The prognostic value of hormone estimations is dubious and low output levels may be the result of abortion rather than indicating a cause in cases where a pregnancy is already beyond salvage.[25] Consequently such measurements of œstriol and pregnanediol excretion are of little help in determining the management of recurrent abortion,[31] although they are thoroughly worth while obtaining in order to provide a useful yardstick much later in pregnancy when the problem of dysmaturity comes on the horizon.

If a retroverted uterus is found early in pregnancy, the patient should be advised to encourage its spontaneous correction by lying on her front as often and for as long as she can and by seeing to it that her bladder is never allowed to become overfilled.

Fibroids are frequently associated with infertility and are often blamed for abortion, though their role in this respect is by no means general. Myomectomy between pregnancies, however, often increases a patient's chances of conception and carrying her pregnancy to term.

Deep lacerations of the cervix and high cervical amputation undoubtedly favour abortion, and cases of cervical incompetence with membranes bulging through a partially dilated os, commonly abort in the second trimester. Dilation of the cervix, as a treatment for spasmodic dysmenorrhœa, may also render the cervix incompetent, especially when the operation has resulted in splitting of the internal os rather than a careful overall stretching.

The question of genital hypoplasia as a factor is worth discussing, and patients with maldevelopment of the uterus are particularly less likely to conceive or, having done so, to retain their pregnancies. The diagnosis of hypoplasia is often made on evidence which is too slender and should be based upon more than a clinical impression of uterine size. Measurement of the cavity by a sound and hysterography are frequently necessary to justify the diagnosis. This is an important matter, because patients are often treated with œstrogens in the hope of increasing genital development; but a woman who has passed puberty cannot, by taking thought, or stilbœstrol either,

for that matter, add one cubit to her uterine stature. Vitamin deficiency, particularly of alphatocopherol (vitamin E), has long been known to produce abortion in rats, but the evidence that this occurs in humans is too slender to justify further comment.

Certain prophylactic measures are well worth enjoining. The avoidance of undue fatigue, especially at period times, and the lifting of heavy weights, continence during the first 14 weeks, and a quiet existence will greatly reduce the likelihood of abortion. Very hot baths are said to be harmful, and spirituous liquor and other such dissipations should be eschewed. To a patient who has aborted before, or in whom the threat to abort has already developed and subsided, advice in these respects is essential.

Prophylactic progesterone injections are given far more often than evidence of progesterone deficiency, if any, is discovered to justify their use.

The indulgence in very active forms of sport, including horse-riding, is of course asking for trouble.

Advice is often sought on the question of travel. Journeys by air are not contra-indicated, especially in these days of pressurised cabins at high altitudes. Lengthy journeys by car should be punctuated by halts at frequent intervals to allow the patient to move about and change her position.

Another common query is the advisability of anæsthesia for minor operations, such as dental extraction. The main risk here is that of asphyxia due to some anæsthetic accident. For this reason, the use of nitrous oxide is somewhat undesirable. Most dentists prefer to postpone, if possible, such an operation until the second trimester, because there is always the possibility that the patient might abort anyway and be encouraged to blame the operation for it.

HABITUAL ABORTION

In defining habitual abortion most of us would accept an abortion sequence of not less than three, though patients are naturally anxious about their prospects after a sequence of two, in which case a recurrent factor can be less accurately inferred. Malpas[33] found that there was a recurrent factor in 1 per cent of women, whereas 17 per cent of women abort from random and accidental causes which are not recurrent. All the possible causes, both local and general, which have already been mentioned will have to be reviewed and excluded by examination. Nevertheless, causative factors in recurrent abortion are discernible in less than half the cases. Faulty early development of the embryo is an important recurrent factor, and ovum blighting as already described may be repeated in subsequent pregnancies.

Listeria monocytogenes, an organism little noticed hitherto because

of its resemblance to diphtheroids, is known to be a cause of abortion in certain animals and evidence is accumulating in Western Germany that in humans too such an infection may be a cause of habitual abortion as well as perinatal mortality[41].

Listeria can be found in the seminal fluid of husbands and in the cervical mucus of some women who habitually abort[38] but so far there has been little reported of the infection in this country and our own pathologists strongly deny any suggestion from me that they have been missing the characteristic granulomata over the last few years. Nevertheless, we may hear more of this matter and its importance lies in its easy curability with antibiotics, particularly demethyl-chlortetracycline (Ledermycin).

The majority of cases are unexplained, and treatment, therefore, becomes empirical. It might be pointed out here that any treatment has to be seen against the background of the spontaneous cure rate. Malpas found that following one previous abortion the spontaneous cure rate was between 50 and 78 per cent with the chances progressively diminishing with each successive abortion until, after a sequence of four, they had reached very slender proportions.

In patients who habitually abort during the second trimester it is occasionally found that the cervix is already partially dilated, allowing the membranes to bulge, often some weeks before abortion starts. Presently liquor starts to leak away, followed in a few days by abortion, or in some cases there is no such additional warning. It would appear that in these cases the mechanical factor of cervical incompetence might be responsible and a variety of operations have been designed, mainly modifications or simplifications of the Shirodkar type of operation. The membranes must first be reduced within the uterus and then, by one means or another, the cervical canal is reformed and practically closed by unabsorbable sutures. An impressive series was first reported from Melbourne.[27]

The modification of this operation which we now use is that devised by Gavin Boyd in Belfast and is simplicity itself. The cervix is gently drawn down with two sponge forceps applied to anterior and posterior lips of the cervix (preferable to vulsella which often tear the softened cervix) and a simple braided tantalum wire suture is inserted as a purse string round the outside of the cervix taking four "bites" at the level of the internal os and without displacing the bladder by dissection. The knot is carefully tightened, just enough to provide a slight resistance to the passage of a No. 6 Hegar dilator and not tight enough to endanger the blood supply of the cervix. A commonly employed alternative is nylon tape, but it does not tie so well as tantalum wire.

This operation probably works by interfering with uterine polarity by discouraging the internal os and neighbouring lower segment

from "taking up". If this is indeed the case it would be logical to extend the indications for the operation and not to await the gross signs of incompetence itself. The purpose after all is not to make the cervix apparently competent but to discourage uterine contractions which will dilate the cervix and so achieve abortion. On this basis it is our practice to use the operation in cases with a history of two previous abortions without apparent cause occurring after the first ten weeks and in whom there is no evidence of blood clotting defect nor of cervical mucus fern-like crystals indicating œstrogen/progesterone imbalance. There is always a disheartening risk that one may be trying by such a stitch to "lock up" a pregnancy already doomed and it is now our invariable practice to observe continuing intra-uterine growth over a period of some days by sonar before operating.

Such criteria may dilute some of the worst cases with others that might have been normal anyway, but my colleague Wallace Barr reports 96 successful pregnancies out of 114 cases selected as above, results surely good enough to quell criticism (although one of these cases started to abort some time after the operation and, on the wire suture being hurriedly removed, bleeding and contractions ceased and the pregnancy continued uninterrupted!).

A suitable time to operate is at the fourteenth week although we have no hesitation in doing so earlier, even the tenth week, where the history indicates it. If labour supervenes, the stitch, of course, should be removed. Sometimes the patient aborts in spite of the presence of the stitch and nearly always it will be found that the encircling stitch has cut out of the posterior lip of the cervix and the products of conception have been passed through the cervix behind what is left of the stitch. A deep bite posteriorly is therefore essential when inserting it.

The suture is removed at the onset of labour or at the 38th week, whichever is the sooner. The procedure is so simple and harmless that it has every right to take its place among all the more picturesque attacks upon the problem, none of which can be scientifically evaluated for want of suitable untreated controls. These patients are usually desperate women who would not take kindly to being an "untreated control".

We do not recommend operation between pregnancies. The non-pregnant cervix does not heal predictably after trachelorrhaphy and it is impossible to gauge the desired degree of closure until pregnancy is well established.

An extreme instance of this type of deformity as a cause of recurrent abortion was shown in a case of mine who, at her first labour elsewhere delivered the baby through the back of the lower uterine segment and through the posterior fornix, by-passing the cervix

entirely. The injury cannot have been noticed at the time, or repair there and then might have succeeded, but she was now left with a hole in the posterior fornix through which a finger could be poked into the uterus. Surprisingly she conceived, to her great distress, with monotonous regularity and had a series of abortions, each bloodier than the last. A diaphragm contraceptive was of course useless and her husband unco-operative. I tried to persuade her to accept an attempt at repair (offered without noticeable conviction) and finally yielded to her request for hysterectomy to prevent yet a fifth hæmorrhagic disaster. Today I would have offered her sterilisation by bilateral tubal diathermy through a peritoneoscope as described by Steptoe,[44] a method which is now in use more or less weekly in our department.

SEQUELÆ OF ABORTION

Many women suffer years of ill health following a serious abortion, and follow-up supervision is therefore important. The patient may have very great difficulty in restoring a normal hæmoglobin level; post-abortum anæmia may reduce her health and efficiency for years to come and may easily prejudice the outlook in a further pregnancy. The detection and correction of anæmia are, therefore, the most important items of aftercare.

Infection contracted at the time of abortion may persist in a chronic form, giving rise to continued ill health, pain, dysmenorrhœa, menorrhagia and dyspareunia, while tubal occlusion puts an end to the patient's reproductive career.

A uterus which was not previously retroverted may now be found so, and the malposition may become permanent. It is often associated with subinvolution, and the more chronic form of pelvic sepsis, and chronic cervicitis, with its associated symptom of vaginal discharge, may persist for years. A history of abortion in the first pregnancy is associated with a much higher incidence of threatened abortion and premature labour in the next[30] and the perinatal death rate is appreciably higher due to prematurity, fœtal abnormality or both.

It is likely that a common ætiological factor operates in this class of recurrent misfortune.

HYDATIDIFORM MOLE

The cause of this strange condition is unknown, but it must be due to a defect of the ovum, because it can co-exist with a healthy twin. Hydatidiform degeneration can also be partial without belonging to a separate twin and I have had a case in which normal villi were interspersed with gross hydatidiform change and a developing fœtus. So far we have twice demonstrated by sonar the co-existence of hydatidi-

form mole and a normal fœtus, and have had the courage to make the pre-operative diagnosis. The problem of what to do next was solved in both instances by either acute pre-eclampsia or hæmorrhage so that therapeutic abortion became not a matter of opinion but of necessity (Fig. 13). A change, partly degenerative and partly hyper-plastic, occurs in the chorionic villi, causing them to take the form of cysts which vary in size from a grape seed to a cherry. Most commonly

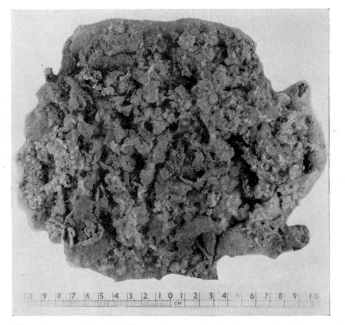

2/Fig. 13.—A case of hydatidiform degeneration interspersed with normal villi and an actively growing foetus within the sac. Fulminating pre-eclampsia necessitated therapeutic abortion.

the entire villous system undergoes vesicular change and no fœtus or normal placenta can be found within the uterus, but occasionally these changes may only partially affect an otherwise normal placenta. Both trophoblastic layers, namely syncitium and Langhan's layer, persist, but the mesodermal core of the villus undergoes a myxoma-tous change and its blood vessels disappear (Fig. 14). The vesicles, of course, draw their nourishment from the maternal blood supply. Because of the persistence of the trophoblastic elements, the power to invade the decidua persists, and may even cause penetration of the uterine wall. Maternal blood vessels encountered are easily entered,

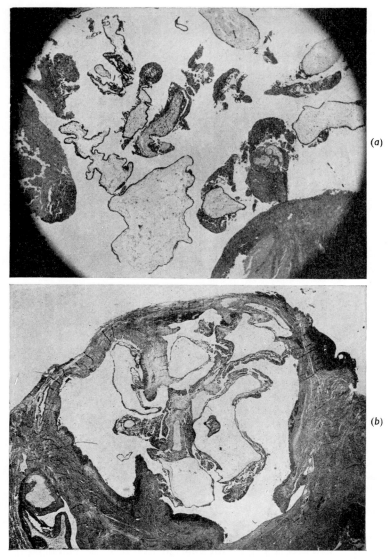

_(a)_

_(b)_

2/Fɪɢ. 14 (*a*).—Hydatidiform mole. Chorionic villi are enlarged by œdema, are devoid of blood vessels and some of them have hyperplastic trophoblast.

2/Fɪɢ. 14 (*b*).—"Malignant" hydatidiform mole. Mole removed 8 weeks previously. Friedman test became positive again. Hysterectomy specimen. Low-power magnification showing hydatidiform mole embedded in myometrium and deeper invasion by some hyperplastic trophoblast (bottom left corner). Patient recovered.

(By courtesy of Prof. C. V. Harrison.)

so that small trophoblastic elements may be swept into the general maternal circulation. The syncitium shows a marked tendency to budding, and the Langhan's layer shows proliferative activity, but it is difficult from histological examination to judge whether or not a particular hydatidiform mole is benign or malignant, the latter being much less common. Commonly there is enlargement of both ovaries due to multiple theca-lutein cysts. They are the result of the stimulus of high circulating chorionic gonadotrophin levels in the blood and after riddance of the mole they regress spontaneously.

The disease, though uncommon, is by no means rare, since many cases are not reported. A rough estimate of the incidence would be about 1 in 2,000 pregnancies. In China, and Malaysia where there is a large Chinese population, the disease is about four times as common.

Symptoms

The cardinal symptom is bleeding, though its presence is by no means invariable. It may be preceded by a sanious, watery discharge, most commonly between the 3rd and 4th month of pregnancy. It is usually unremittent and occasionally very profuse. All the usual symptoms of pregnancy are present in full measure, and vomiting, for example, may be exaggerated to the degree of hyperemesis. The patient is likely to become progressively more anæmic and nearly always looks far from well. Pain is not usually present, unless concealed bleeding within the uterus occurs to an appreciable degree or the mole becomes infected. Pre-eclamptic toxæmia is often superadded, and eclampsia may develop at an early stage of pregnancy.

Diagnosis

Examination of the patient reveals all the usual signs of early pregnancy, but the uterus is, more often than not, larger than the period of gestation would suggest. Occasionally the size of the uterus is normal, and uncommonly it may actually be smaller than normal. Brews found that the uterus was unduly enlarged five times as frequently as diminished. Palpation of the uterus gives an impression which is hard to describe but is not quite normal, and its consistency appears to the touch to be more doughy than cystic. On bimanual examination ballottement cannot be elicited, since the whole cavity of the uterus is filled with vesicles instead of fœtus and liquor amnii. A straight X-ray of the lower abdomen is often helpful in one sense, inasmuch as the radiographic evidences of fœtal parts rule out all major degrees of hydatidiform mole. As one is usually in doubt, however, long before the 16th week, the usefulness of radiological

examination is somewhat limited, since fœtal parts cannot be seen earlier than this.

Signs of pre-eclamptic toxæmia are occasionally present, being rare in early pregnancy except in cases of hydatidiform mole. The urine contains large quantities of chorionic gonadotrophin, so that a pregnancy test may be positive in one-in-a-hundred dilution; but this is not conclusive, because even normal pregnancies may give positive results in these dilutions within the first 100 days. I have even had cases where the pregnancy test on the urine was only positive undiluted and in one case the test was even negative, so too much reliance cannot be placed on gonadotrophin levels in the urine.

Occasionally ovarian theca-lutein cysts may be detected on careful vaginal examination. These cysts are often as large as tennis balls, although the size is variable.

It is very difficult to be certain of the diagnosis of hydatidiform mole before the spontaneous discharge of vesicles *per vaginam*, which may not be observed for some weeks. The most important and common differential diagnosis is that of threatened abortion in a pregnancy otherwise normal; therefore, an expectant line of treatment often has to be adopted for a long time. Serious mistakes in intervention are commonly made in the belief that a hydatidiform mole is present because of a positive pregnancy test in high dilution and because of errors in the patient's dates. My own researches in the diagnostic uses of ultrasonic echo sounding (sonar) have naturally extended to this problem and our apparatus[14, 15] can distinguish between early fœtal parts *in utero* and a mass of vesicles, by displaying the echoes from these structures on the face of a cathode ray tube, which is photographed. The dot-like echoes from clusters of vesicles (Fig. 15a) can be almost suppressed by reducing the amplification or "gain" of the apparatus (Fig. 15b) whereas fœtal echoes are not only demonstrable, strong and clear from the tenth week onwards, but cannot be suppressed by the same reduction in gain settings (Fig. 15c). Our positive identification of hydatidiform mole by this means now extends to many dozens of cases, while the method has proved equally valuable in excluding the diagnosis of hydatidiform mole by demonstrating fœtal echoes long before standard radiology would be of any help.[32]

A carneous mole or missed abortion may be confused with hydatidiform mole, but here the uterus ceases to enlarge, the symptoms of pregnancy regress, and the urine test usually becomes negative within about a fortnight. It was suggested as long ago as 1949[21] that a hydatidiform mole may in fact arise in the placental remnants of a missed abortion which has not died and we have from time to time demonstrated what would appear to be a small sac in the midst of the molar mass by sonar before abortion.[17, 18] The possibility is therefore

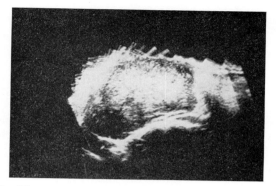

2/Fig. 15 (*a*).—Ultrasonogram in longitudinal section of uterus containing hydatidiform mole. High gain amplification.

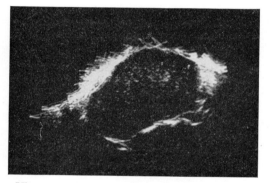

2/Fig. 15 (*b*).—Ultrasonogram. Same case as Fig. 8*a*. Reduced gain practically extinguishes echoes of hydatidiform mole, unlike fœtal echoes.

(Fig. 15 *a* and *b* by courtesy of the Editor *Brit. J. Radiol.*)

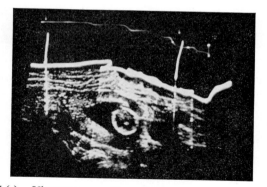

2/Fig. 15 (*c*).—Ultrasonogram. Normal pregnancy of 15-week gestation, showing foetal echoes. Note foetal head.

suggested that one of the hazards of a retained missed abortion is the subsequent development of hydatidiform change, particularly if the chorionic gonadotrophin tests remain positive.

A retroverted gravid uterus incarcerated within the pelvis and causing retention of urine is another diagnostic possibility, but vaginal examination should rule this out.

Fibroids in association with pregnancy may be accompanied by a threat to abort, and the uterine enlargement due to their presence may contribute to error.

Sometimes the uterus containing a hydatidiform mole may be so large that it reaches almost to the xiphisternum and hydramnios may be diagnosed, although there is no fluid thrill, no ballottement, and bleeding is the predominant symptom.

Needless to say, everything that is passed and all pads should be very carefully inspected, as otherwise the passage of a few tell-tale

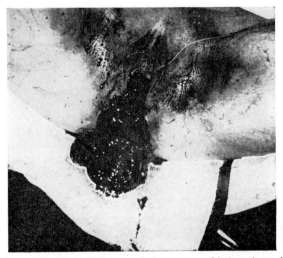

2/Fig. 16.—Hydatidiform mole in process of being aborted.

vesicles may be missed and the true diagnosis consequently put off, the patient meanwhile becoming steadily more anæmic and requiring treatment on that account. Often the first indication of the presence of hydatidiform mole is the onset of its spontaneous expulsion, which is frequently incomplete at first and accompanied by profuse hæmorrhage (Fig. 16).

Treatment

As soon as the condition is definitely diagnosed, steps should be taken to empty the uterus or to encourage it to empty itself, because

further delay will only increase the risks of hæmorrhage. In women in the younger age groups, spontaneous evacuation, encouraged, if necessary, by a full medical induction, including the use of quinine and a brisk oxytocin drip, is the most satisfactory outcome, but the risks of malignancy increase with the patient's age, so that over the age of 40 hysterectomy is undoubtedly the safest course. Recently we had a case of hydatidiform mole in a widow aged 53. The diagnosis was not made until after hysterectomy (no preliminary curettage) and to my even greater fury the specimen was not photographed!

An escalating oxytocin drip starting with 10 units to the half litre and rising, if necessary, to ten times that concentration is nowadays the most commonly used method of getting the patient to abort the mole. It is most likely to work if the abortion process has already started as demonstrated by the preliminary passage of some vesicles. The attempt can be repeated. Often, however, this meets with no success, and one is left with the alternatives of some type of surgical induction and evacuation or resorting to abdominal hysterotomy. When the mole is expelled, either spontaneously or as the result of drug induction, the uterus should always be explored with the gloved finger because expulsion is frequently incomplete. In other cases, the patient makes no attempt to get rid of her mole and the cervix remains tightly closed. Laminaria tents to dilate the cervix have been advocated in the past and I have used them (which dates me), but even these can fail to bring on abortion, and the dangers of infection are considerable, dangers which are enhanced by a state of anæmia and the presence of quantities of suitable culture material within the uterus. A single tent inserted within the cervix is seldom adequate, and, if possible, two or three should be inserted side by side. The resulting amount of dilatation of the cervix is then usually sufficient after 24 hours to allow the passage of a finger into the uterine cavity.

The alternative of dilating the cervix with metal dilators, although less likely to provoke sepsis, may result in considerable tearing of the cervix and lower segment, because sufficient dilatation must be achieved to allow a finger to be passed with ease. Digital exploration of the uterine cavity must not only be thorough but reasonably brisk, as great hæmorrhage can attend the manœuvre. One should always use a slow intravenous oxytocin drip, 10 units in 500 ml., during the operation to harden up the soft, atonic uterine wall. No instrument other than the gloved finger is safe for the purpose because of the exceptional ease with which the uterine wall can be perforated, especially if its integrity has been undermined by direct invasion by trophoblast. A blood transfusion already set up as a precautionary measure may be life saving. Ergometrine, likewise, should be at hand for intravenous use for the immediate control of any undue hæmorrhage. The size of the uterine cavity may be such as to

make it impossible to explore more than a fraction of its volume forthwith, and the procedure is to pass the half hand into the vagina and to loosen up as much of the mole as can be reached and to pick out the loosened fragments with ovum forceps, the other hand, meanwhile, being kept upon the body of the uterus through the abdominal wall, steering it towards the internal finger. As the uterus shuts down with the successive removal of each mass of tissue, more and more of the uterine cavity comes within digital reach until, by judicious bimanual manipulation, the entire internal surface can be thoroughly explored. Some surgeons favour the use of a flushing curette, but the weight of the water-filled rubber tubing on its handle makes delicate control difficult and increases the risk of perforation. Having emptied the uterus, more ergometrine is given to control bleeding, and it may be necessary for a couple of minutes to resort to bimanual compression. This can be a very messy and bloody operation, and it is necessary to get a move on if an undue quantity of blood is not to be lost. Curettage should be repeated 5 to 7 days later after delivery of the mole, whether spontaneous or assisted, in order to remove residual fragments.

For these reasons, there is much to be said for abdominal hysterotomy when the cervix is tightly closed, and when two or more escalating oxytocin drips have failed I have never yet regretted "chickening-out" and performing abdominal hysterectomy if vaginal abortion threatens to be difficult or dangerous. The lower segment approach can usually be made. It has, moreover, the advantage that the uterus can be inspected for the presence of the penetrating variety of mole which may justify proceeding to hysterectomy. Certainly less blood will be lost in evacuating the uterus by the abdominal route, and the situation is much more easily kept under control. At laparotomy, the presence of quite large lutein cysts may be observed, usually bilateral, and their sheer size may encourage one to resect them, but they should be left strictly alone, as they always absorb and disappear within the next few weeks.

In a more elderly patient in whom hysterectomy is indicated, it is a good plan to suture the cervix before proceeding, to prevent the dissemination of trophoblastic tissues.

As may be gathered, this is a dangerous condition. The immediate risks are those of hæmorrhage, shock and sepsis, yet in spite of these, mortality is not as high as one would expect. Further curettage, one to two weeks after the moles is aborted, is recommended as part of the routine follow-up in all cases delivered per vaginam.

Choriocarcinoma (chorion epithelioma).—Apart from the immediate risks, the remote danger of choriocarcinoma is a serious matter, and estimates of its likelihood vary around 10 per cent. This highly malignant condition may follow normal pregnancy, abortion or

tubal pregnancy, but the risk is immeasurably greater after hydatidiform mole. If choriocarcinoma is going to develop, it will almost certainly do so within two years, and seldom in under two months, although Fig. 17 shows a uterus originally evacuated for septic abortion, not once but twice within a fortnight because of continued bleeding and discharge and in which the curettings showed choriocarcinoma on the second occasion. The patient has remained well since. A close follow-up of the patient, therefore, is essential for two or three years. Urine pregnancy tests must be carried out at frequent

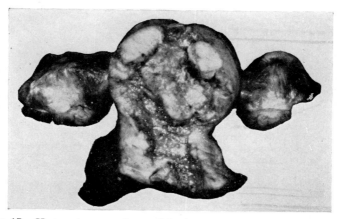

2/Fig. 17.—Hysterectomy specimen of choriocarcinoma. Presented as incomplete septic abortion. Satisfactory recovery.

intervals, certainly not exceeding two months, during the first year of observation and three-monthly during the second. Usually the test becomes negative within a few weeks of expulsion of a hydatidiform mole although I once had a case in which it remained positive in undiluted urine for just over a year. She subsequently had a normal pregnancy. What is particularly significant is a test which becomes positive after a period of being negative, and it may be very difficult to tell at first whether a patient has developed a choriocarcinoma or has started a fresh pregnancy. Ultrasonography may help, as already indicated. Positive results in dilutions of 500 or over are almost pathognomonic of choriocarcinoma and indicate the need for immediate panhysterectomy or chemotherapy. A diagnostic curettage may settle the point by yielding the necessary histological evidence, but it is by no means a certain method of excluding this dreadful complication, because the growth may be embedded within the uterine wall and may not be accessible to the exploring curette (Figs. 18 and 19).

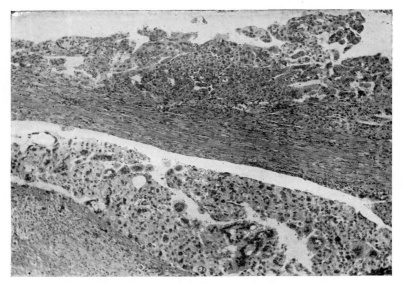

2/FIG. 18 (*a*).—Choriocarcinoma invading myometrium. In the upper parts of the field the Langhans cells and syncytium are present together; in the lower part, the tumour consists largely of syncytium. The myometrium is also infiltrated with neutrophils.

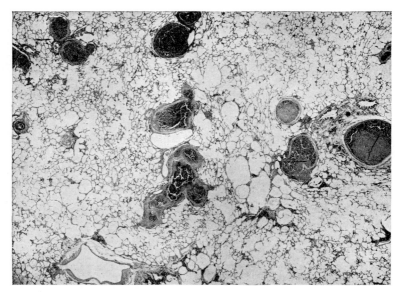

2/FIG. 18 (*b*).—Choriocarcinomatous metastases. Low-power view of lung showing pulmonary arteries distended by masses of tumour and thrombosis.

(By courtesy of Prof. C. V. Harrison.)

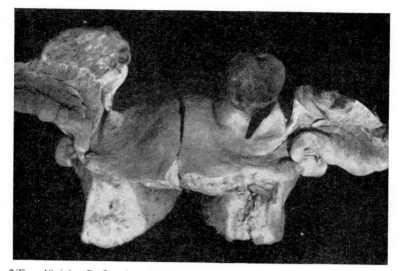

2/Fig. 19 (*a*).—Perforating choriocarcinoma. Patient continued bleeding after abortion at three months. Curetted twice—sections not conclusive. Admitted subsequently with acute hæmoperitoneum. Recovered.

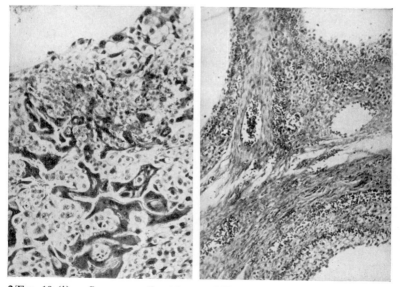

2/Fig. 19 (*b*).— Same case. Curettings. Choriocarcinoma.

2/Fig. 19 (*c*).—Same case. Theca lutein cysts.

(By courtesy of the late Dr. G. W. Garland.)

A discussion of the varying grades of malignancy of choriocar-cinoma would be out of place in this book, but the very serious prognosis is due to its rapid and widespread dissemination by the blood stream, even before warning signs of irregular vaginal bleeding occur, and the patient may present with hæmoptysis as the first sign. Other signs of developing choriocarcinoma are the appearance of metastatic deposits in the lower vagina and vulva, and uterine enlargement.

The serious outlook for these cases has been transformed by the use of amethopterin (methotrexate-Lederle). This substance (4-amino-N^{10}-methylpteroylglutamic acid) acts as a folic acid antagonist. Folic acid (pteroylglutamic acid) is prevented by methotrexate from conversion into folinic acid (citrovorum factor) which is essential for the synthesis of nucleic acid and hence the mitotic process. It would appear to be particularly applicable to this virulent type of tumour[34] Chan (1962) suggests that it should be given even before hysterectomy, especially where metastases are already evident, in the belief that surgical manipulation increases spread of the disease. This chemotherapy or nothing approach to treatment, however, has been more recently queried from Singapore[47] by Tow and Cheng, who have shown that timely hysterectomy in cases where the tumour is localised to the uterus is well worth carrying out and that chemotherapy has its major role in the management of metastatic choriocarcinoma. We ourselves have treated cases by chemotherapy using the dosage scheme of Bagshawe and McDonald. This takes the form of combined treatment using methotrexate and 6-mercaptopurine. Methotrexate is administered by mouth in divided doses totalling 25 mg. a day, usually for a five-day course provided the patient's general condition can stand it. More recently the intravenous route has been used. Likewise 6-mercaptopurine in divided doses totalling 600 mg. a day are given at the same time. This latter drug is toxic to fœtal tissues and is an antagonist to hypoxanthine and adenine. As soon as the white cell count starts to fall antibiotic cover is instituted. The patient is preferably nursed in isolation in an infection-free environment. The courses may have to be repeated especially if the gonadotrophin pregnancy tests become positive again suggesting recrudescence of the disease. Side-effects are severe but usually come at the end of or after a 5-day course, so that the damage is already done by then. They consist of stomatitis going on to ulceration, intense dysphagia, vomiting, diarrhœa, occasionally jaundice, great susceptibility to infections, skin pigmentation and loss of hair. Some of these are due to profound leukopenia and thrombocytopenia which result from the treatment. There may be proteinuria as well. Fortunately these signs are usually reversible after the cessation of treatment, even the hair growing again.

PLATE III

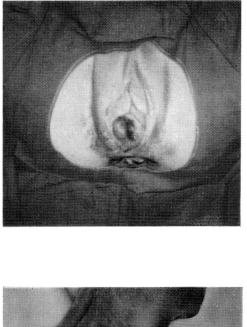

(a)

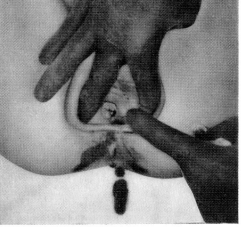

(b)

(a) Choriocarcinomatous deposit at vulva before treatment with methotrexate.

(b) Same case after treatment with methotrexate. Healed.

(By courtesy of Lederle Laboratories and John Wright and Sons, Ltd., Bristol.)

It has been suggested that the effect of this treatment may be mitigated by prior aspiration of bone marrow, its storage under powerful refrigeration and reinjection after the end of treatment, but we have no personal experience of this.

To some extent methotrexate has an antidote in the form of folinic acid (citrovorum factor).

In the first of our own cases there was no antecedent pregnancy, the origin being teratomatous, and antibodies to her husband's leucocytes could not be demonstrated as might have been expected if the growth had originated from a pregnancy for which her husband was responsible.[20] There was no response and she died rapidly.

Another of our cases had had a hydatidiform mole some months earlier and had recently undergone total hysterectomy elsewhere for histologically proven choriocarcinoma.[16] She was now referred to us within a few weeks with metastatic deposits in the vaginal vault and vulva (Plate III, *a*) the latter being excruciatingly tender. She had pulmonary metastases and a hæmoglobin level of 35 per cent. Her response to methotrexate was dramatic, so I rashly put her on as a case for the Glasgow Fellowship in which I was examining. To the candidate's horror he was greeted with torrential hæmorrhage due to separation and sloughing of the vaginal and vulval deposits. The examination was halted while my co-examiner and I dealt hurriedly with the situation. Ultimately packing under anæsthesia was of no avail (obviously arterial bleeding) and I had to ligate the anterior division of the left internal iliac artery with strong silk before peace was restored. (The candidate passed!) Following two courses there are no signs of the original metastases (Plate III, *b*) and her urine pregnancy tests remain negative (7 years) but at the time, as is usual with such treatment, she was reduced to a very wretched state with leucopenia, ulcerative stomatitis and dysphagia.

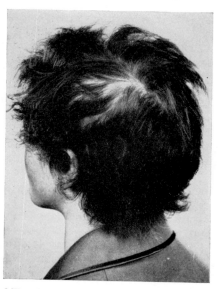

2/FIG. 20.—Loss of hair due to methotrexate.

Her hair, which threatened to fall out (Fig. 20), has since grown again and she now runs her farm and her husband as before.

Instances of recurrent hydatidiform mole are rare, much more so in fact than the development of choriocarcinoma. It has been customary to advise the patient to avoid a further pregnancy for two years while she is observed for signs of the gonadotrophin pregnancy test becoming positive again. The reason for this is the obvious clinical confusion which could immediately arise if the patient became pregnant with an enlarging uterus and then threatened to abort; one would be in acute doubt whether or not she had a recurrent choriocarcinoma instead. The need for such advice can now be questioned on two grounds; firstly, she would be unlikely to conceive if choriocarcinoma were still active, because of the high circulating chorionic gonadotrophins which would depress further ovulation, and, secondly, even a very early fœtus can now be picked out by sonar. We had such a case referred to us from Bristol, in whom we found an early pregnancy instead of tumour and she was successfully delivered of a healthy baby at term.[18]

INTRA-UTERINE FŒTAL DEATH

The term I.U.D. (preferably used thus in the patient's hearing) embraces cases before the 28th week of pregnancy (missed abortion) and those occurring later which result in macerated stillbirth.

A very slovenly practice has grown up of referring to the intra-uterine contraceptive device as an I.U.D. instead of an I.U.C.D. leaving out the "C". I well recall a case referred to my by an exasperated general practitioner, who had had one of his patients X-rayed for fœtal parts since he suspected a pregnancy in spite of the previous insertion (elsewhere) of an intra-uterine contraceptive device. The radiologist reported not only the fœtal parts, but that that "I.U.D." was present. The patient thus came to my clinic thoroughly alarmed that her baby had "died *in utero.*" Fortunately I was able to demonstrate to her an active fœtal heart beat.

Maceration is a destructive aseptic process which first reveals itself by blistering and peeling of the fœtal skin. This appears between 12 and 24 hours after fœtal death and in a case of stillbirth exculpates causes operating during labour except when labour is seriously prolonged.

The process, however, involves the whole body, giving rise to the characteristic radiological signs. The ligaments are softened and the vertebral column is liable to sag or collapse, especially with the patient in the erect posture. The ribs may concertina together and the skull bones, already loosened in their mutual attachments, overlap each other at the sutures because of the shrinkage of the brain (Spalding's sign, Fig. 10a).

It takes several days for Spalding's sign to appear after intra-

uterine death, usually a week or more. Of all the radiological signs it is the most definite but is disqualified if the membranes are already ruptured or if labour is in progress. Two X-rays taken within several hours with identical positioning may show total absence of fœtal movement if the pictures are viewed superimposed. This is highly suggestive of fœtal death.

Gas bubbles appear in the heart, aorta, vena cava, liver, cord and abdominal cavity[39] quite apart from infective putrefaction (Fig. 21 *a* and *b*). These signs are very reliable in the diagnosis of intra-uterine death and, appearing within the first few days, provide the first conclusive evidence.[45]

Macerated stillbirth nearly always indicates fœtal death in pregnancy and not in labour, and in most cases is caused by anoxia. By contrast, fresh stillbirth, i.e. non-macerated, usually indicates either death due to anoxia or trauma or both. The distinction is an important one in compiling a patient's past obstetric history or in attempting to pinpoint a cause for stillbirth. Unfortunately necropsy studies in macerated stillbirths are often unrewarding and except in cases of hæmolytic disease, syphilis and congenital malformation may show nothing more than signs of asphyxia and even more often the tissues may be too softened and necrotic to be examined properly.

CAUSES OF MACERATED STILLBIRTH

One of the commonest is pre-eclamptic toxæmia. Because of the hypertensive spasm of the vessels supplying the maternal placental site the blood flow is seriously reduced and likewise therefore the oxygen supply rate to the baby. The difference in blood flow rates through the maternal placenta has been first illustrated by Browne and Veall's isotope technique (1953) of measuring clearance rates of radiosodium from the choriodecidual space. It is the small baby who, by its unsatisfactory growth, proclaims the inadequacy of its own placenta and who is most likely to die *in utero* before labour. Infarction of the placenta makes the fœtal suboxygenation progressive and irreversible so that intra-uterine death is not far off. It would clearly be of the greatest importance to be able to foresee this disaster and to secure the baby's delivery before its unfavourable intra-uterine environment killed it. In this respect 24 hour œstriol excretion levels are of more use than pregnanediol and our practice is to average three consecutive days collections. Even so, mistakes are liable to be made and the whole specimen may not be forwarded to the laboratory. We therefore do a creatinine excretion rate as well. The latter is fairly constant and any discrepancy quickly indicates that the 24-hour specimen is not complete. There is unfortunately quite a wide variation in what may be regarded as normal œstriol

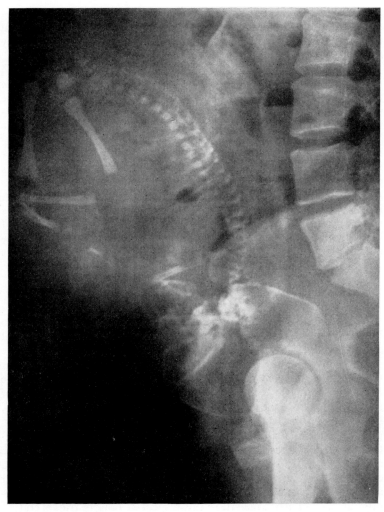

2/Fɪɢ. 21(*a*).—Intra-uterine death. Gas present in cardiac chambers, abdominal aorta and superior mesenteric artery. This early sign is diagnostic of intra-uterine death. Spalding's sign is not yet visible.

(By courtesy of Dr. Ellis Barnett.)

excretion, but the chart in Chapter XXV (25/Fig. 1)) shows the normally accepted ranges at different stages of pregancy. Of even greater
usefulness, if the apparatus is available, is the study of intra-uterine
growth by fœtal biparietal cephalometry.[15, 51] The growth rate here is
maximal between the 20th and 30th weeks, after which it tends to

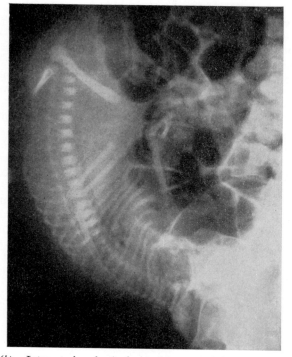

2/FIG. 21 (b).—Intra-uterine death during labour at 41½ weeks gestation. The
first stage was prolonged and the foetus died in slightly less than 24 hours before
this picture was taken. Note the gas shadows in the thoracic and abdominal aorta
and both common iliac vessels.

(By courtesy of Dr. E. Sweet.)

level off, but where growth apparently ceases death can be anticipated within a matter of ten days, especially if the evidence is reinforced by low œstriol levels. It is therefore our practice to carry out
these sonar measurements at least once a week and sometimes twice
a week in the cases obviously at risk.

Chronic hypertension operates in like fashion but the fœtal prognosis on the whole is somewhat better, provided pre-eclamptic
toxæmia does not supervene.

Chronic nephritis, fortunately an uncommon complication of pregnancy nowadays, has a very bad prognosis for the baby who frequently dies from placental infarction and anoxia before even the stage of viability is reached.

Hyperpyrexia, i.e. a body temperature over 103° F., can kill the fœtus directly.

Diabetic pregnancy as a cause of I.U.D. is dealt with in Chapter V and hæmolytic disease in Chapter XXVII.

Fœtal malformations may cause death before, during or after labour, according to their nature and extent.

Postmaturity, as a cause, is a disappointing matter since in such cases one is dealing with no particular disease in either mother or baby and one feels that had only labour been successfully induced a few days earlier the tragedy might have been prevented.

Syphilis, a traditional cause, has been practically eradicated from obstetric practice.

Placental insufficiency is commonly diagnosed in order to explain so-called idiopathic cases of intra-uterine death but this is begging the question. In about a fifth of cases of I.U.D. no more definite reason can be given.

It will be seen, therefore, that any hope of effectively reducing the incidence of macerated stillbirth will depend upon the early detection and treatment of pre-eclamptic toxæmia and hypertension, the careful management of diabetes, including opportune termination of pregnancy, the judicious use of induction of labour in cases of Rh isoimmunisation and in established postmaturity, and the elimination of syphilis.

Clearly then, sound antenatal care has much to offer but cannot prevent all cases of intra-uterine death.

MANAGEMENT

The diagnosis having been established beyond all shadow of doubt from the clinical evidences of absent fœtal heart sounds, absent movements, cessation of uterine growth and recession of all the other signs of continuing pregnancy and confirmed by the radiological signs mentioned above, one is faced with the choice of the following alternatives.

Firstly, a conservative attitude may be taken and spontaneous labour awaited. Secondly, attempts may be made to induce labour medically. Thirdly, surgical methods of interfering with the pregnancy may be employed. The third choice is thoroughly dangerous and usually unnecessary. No one, of course, would dream of evacuation of the uterus by the abdominal route, the fœtus is too large to remove from below and surgical induction of labour is all that is left to choose from.

Surgical induction by any of the traditional methods, usually artificial rupture of the membranes, may not only reap the fearful penalty of an intra-uterine infection with gas-forming anaerobes but may fail to bring on labour, leaving one with a thoroughly nasty problem on hand.

If the patient is left strictly alone, labour will start usually within a month although occasionally the case may hang fire until term would have been reached. Very exceptionally the delay may be even longer. There are very few women who could face such an unhappy wait with equanimity and such therapeutic purism would hardly be humane. It is now recognised, moreover, that the prolonged retention of a dead fœtus *in utero* may interfere with the coagulation mechanism in the blood. The defect is usually one of hypofibrinogenæmia. This was first noticed in the case of fœtal death due to Rh iso-immunisation of the mother but it can occur in other varieties of intra-uterine death as well.[3]

Fortunately the disorder does not develop in less than four weeks after the death of the fœtus, during which time the onset of labour, whether spontaneous or medically induced, is to be hoped for.

Intensive œstrogen therapy sometimes succeeds in supposedly sensitising the uterus. The technique is to give enormous doses, preferably in hospital so that the medication can be supervised. Stilbœstrol 5 mg. is given by mouth every half-hour until a total dose of 200–300 mg. has been reached. Surprisingly, such patients tolerate it without nausea or vomiting.

If this does not establish labour, a full medical induction, including the use of quinine (see Chapter XV), is given, followed by an intravenous oxytocin drip. If this does not work, the patient is rested for a full week and the process repeated. In fact it is worth going to great lengths to avoid the hazards of surgical interference which, it is felt, are still considerable in spite of the antibiotics.

Intra-amniotic injection of hypertonic solutions.—One is faced with a hard core of cases, especially in the middle trimester of pregnancy, who will not go into labour as a result of oxytocin drip induction, and the method of injecting hypertonic solutions into the amniotic cavity may have to be considered. This was originally devised some 30 years ago but not really exploited until the present decade.[4, 13, 52] The technique was developed primarily as an alternative to abdominal hysterotomy in so-called "therapeutic" abortion and has been widely used in Sweden, in certain centres in the United Kingdom and in the United States. The use of hypertonic glucose[52] has proved too dangerous and at least two cases in these islands have been reported of fatal *Cl. welchii* infection following such an injection.[37] In one of them the gas pressure within the uterus was so great as to cause an amniotic embolus.[35] Therefore 20 per cent sodium chloride is preferable. The

operation should not be performed on any uterus smaller than would apply to a 16-week gestation. After a preliminary infiltration of the area of the abdominal wall with local anaesthesia about midway between the umbilicus and the symphysis pubis in the midline, the patient is catheterised and then placed in a moderate Trendelenburg position to discourage bowel puncture. A spinal needle about 5 inches long may be used, or a fine trocar and cannula capable of carrying a polythene catheter is introduced into the amniotic cavity, which should be identified by the free withdrawal of liquor amnii and, above all, no blood. Sometimes with a dead fœtus this fluid cannot be withdrawn, in which case about 100 ml. of normal saline can be injected and then recovered. The attempt should be abandoned if there is any doubt about being in the amniotic cavity, because most of the fatalities and disasters are attributed to the intravascular injection of hypertonic saline. Having satisfied oneself that the end of the needle or the catheter is safely in the amniotic cavity, an additional precaution is to measure the intra-uterine pressure at the same time. In 50 millilitre steps liquor amnii is withdrawn and replaced by 20 per cent sodium chloride up to a maximum of 200 millilitres, observing throughout that the normal resting pressure of the uterus is maintained. Before removing the needle or cannula it should be rinsed with a little physiological saline.

The method though fairly simple is not without danger as may be expected and patients with cardiac or renal disease, also pre-eclampsia, are particularly at risk because, following this injection, the maternal serum shows an increased sodium concentration up to 160 mEq/L, increased volume and osmolality and on top of this an antidiuretic effect, so that cardiac patients may be precipitated into pulmonary œdema and the patients with renal disease may become anuric.[49] Three fatal cases of severe brain damage from intra-amniotic, hypertonic saline have been reported from the London hospital,[8] and an impressive series of fatalities reported from Japan[50] has been sufficient to discourage a wider adoption of the method. The reported disasters have all concerned the deliberate termination of pregnancy, which makes them all the more tragic. When dealing with an intra-uterine death, the situation might well be worse, especially because of the difficulty sometimes of identifying the cavity. It is far preferable therefore to deal with the problem of intra-uterine death by medical means.

REFERENCES

1. Family Planning Association (1966). *Abortion in Britain*. London: Pitman Medical.
2. BAGSHAWE, K. D., and McDONALD, J. M. (1960). *Brit. med. J.*, **2**, 426.

3. BARRY, A. P., GEOGHEGAN, F., and SHEA, S. M. (1955). *Brit. med. J.*, **2,** 287.
4. BENGSTSSON, L. and STORMBY, N. (1962). *Acta. obstet. gynec. scand.*, **41,** 115.
5. BERTHELSON, H. G., and OSTERGAARD, E. (1959). *Dan med. Bull.*, **6,** 105.
6. BREWS, A. (1939). *J. Obstet. Gynaec. Brit. Emp.*, **46,** 813.
7. BROWNE, J. C. M., and VEALL, N. (1953). *J. Obstet. Gynaec. Brit. Emp.*, **60,** 141.
8. CAMERON, J. M., and DAYAN, A. D. (1966). *Brit. med. J.*, **1,** 1010.
9. CARR, D. H. (1967). *Amer. J. Obstet. Gynec.*, **97,** 283.
10. CAVANAGH, D., and McLEOD, A. G. W. (1966). *Amer. J. Obstet. Gynec.*, **96,** 913.
11. CHAN, D. P. C. (1962). *Brit. med. J.*, **2,** 957.
12. COYLE, M. G., GREIG, M., and WALKER, J. (1962). *Lancet*, **2,** 275.
13. CSAPO, A. (1966). *Year Book of Obstetrics and Gynecology*, ed. J. P. Greenhill. Chicago: Year Book Med. Publications.
14. DONALD, I., MacVICAR, J. and BROWN, T. G. (1958). *Lancet*, **1,** 1188.
15. DONALD, I., and BROWN, T. G. (1961). *Brit. J. Radiol.*, Vol. xxxiv, No. 405, p. 539.
16. DONALD, I. (1962). *In Methotrexate in the Treatment of Cancer*, Bristol: John Wright & Sons.
17. DONALD, I. (1964). *Med. and Biol. Ill.*, **14,** 216.
18. DONALD, I. (1965). *Amer. J. Obstet. Gynec.*, **93,** 935.
19. DONALD, I., and ABDULLA, U. (1967). *Brit. J. Radiol.*, **40,** 604.
20. DONIACH, I., CROOKSTON, J. H., and COPE, T. I. (1958). *J. Obstet. Gynaec. Brit. Emp.*, **65,** 553.
21. HERTIG, A. T., and EDMUNDS, H. W. (1940). *Arch. Path.*, **30,** 260.
22. HERTIG, A. T., and ROCK, J. (1949). *Amer. J. Obstet. Gynec.*, **38,** 968.
23. JOHNSON, W. L., STEGALL, H. F., LEIN, J. N., and RUSHMER, R. F. (1965). *Obstet. and Gynec.*, **26,** 305.
24. KLOPPER, A., MICHIE, E. A., and BROWN, J. B. (1955). *J. Endocr.*, **12,** 209.
25. KLOPPER, A., and MACNAUGHTON, M. (1965). *J. Obst. Gynaec. Brit. Cwlth.*, **72,** 1022.
26. LOUDON, J. D. O. (1959). *J. Obstet. Gynaec. Brit. Emp.*, **66,** 277.
27. McDONALD, I. A. (1957). *J. Obstet. Gynaec. Brit. Emp.*, **64,** 346.
28. MACDONALD, R. R. (1960). M. D. Thesis, Univ. of Glasgow.
29. MACDONALD, R. R. (1963). *J. Obstet. Gynaec. Brit. Cwlth.*, **70,** 580.
30. MACNAUGHTON, M. C. (1961). *J. Obstet. Gynaec. Brit. Cwlth.*, **68,** 789.
31. MACNAUGHTON, M. (1966). *J. Obstet. Gynaec. Brit. Cwlth.*, **73,** 290.
32. MACVICAR, J., and DONALD, I. (1963). *J. Obstet. Gynaec. Brit. Cwlth.*, **70,** 387.
33. MALPAS, P. (1938). *J. Obstet. Gynaec. Brit. Emp.*, **45,** 932.
34. MANLY, G. A. (1961). *J. Obstet. Gynaec. Brit. Cwlth.*, 68, 277.
35. O'DRISCOLL, K., and GEOGHEGAN, F. (1964). *British. med. J.*, **1,** 1113.
36. PERERA, W. (1961). *Brit. med. J.*, **1,** 705.
37. PINKERTON, J. H. M. (1966). *Brit. med. J.*, **1,** 1049.
38. RAPPAPORT, F., RABINOVITZ, M., TOAFF, R., KROCHIK, N. (1960). *Lancet*, **1,** 1273.
39. ROBERTS, J. R. (1944). *Amer. J. Roentgenol.*, **51,** 631.

40. RUSSELL, C. S., PAINE, C. G., COYLE, M. G., and DEWHURST, C. J.(1957). *J. Obstet. Gynaec. Brit. Emp.*, **64,** 649.
41. SEELIGER, H. P. R. (1961). *Listeriosis.* Basle: S. Karger.
42. SHARMAN, A., and PEARSTON, T. (1964). *J. med. Lab. Technol.*, **21,** 271.
43. SHARMAN, A. (1967). *Lancet,* **1,** 1328.
44. STEPTOE, P. C. (1967). *Laparoscopy in Gynaecology*, Chapter XVI. Edinburgh: E. & S. Livingstone.
45. STEWART, A. M. (1957). *J. Obstet. Gynaec. Brit. Emp.*, **64,** 915.
46. THOMPSON, J. F., and LEIN, J. N., (1961). *Obstet. and Gynec.*, **18,** 40.
47. TOW, W. S. H., and CHENG, W. C. (1967). *Brit. med. J.*, **1,** 521.
48. TURNBULL, E. P. N., and WALKER, J. (1956). *J. Obstet. Gynaec. Brit. Emp.*, **63,** 553.
49. TURNBULL, A. C., and ANDERSON, A. B. M. (1966). *Brit. med. J.*, **1,** 672.
50. WAGATSUMA, T. (1965). *Amer. J. Obstet. Gynec.*, **93,** 743.
51. WILLOCKS, J., DONALD, I., DUGGAN, T. C., and DAY, N. (1964). *J. Obstet. Gynaec. Brit. Cwlth.*, **71,** 11.
52. WOOD, C., BOOTH, R. T., and PINKERTON, J. H. M. (1962). *Brit. med. J.*, **2,** 706.

ADDENDUM TO CHAPTER II

NOTES ON CHROMOSOMAL ABNORMALITIES IN OBSTETRICS

by DR. MALCOLM A. FERGUSON-SMITH

Senior Lecturer in Medical Genetics, University of Glasgow

Spontaneous Abortion

It has long been suspected that faulty development of the ovum is an important cause of spontaneous abortion, but the relative parts played by genetic and environmental factors were unknown. The early studies have concentrated mainly on the careful histological examination of aborted embryos (Hertig and Rock, 1949). During recent years chromosome analysis of aborted material has demonstrated dramatically how frequently one class of genetic disorder, the chromosome aberrations, accounts for spontaneous abortions. It is now clear that at least 20 per cent of all spontaneous abortions have gross chromosomal aberrations detectable under the laboratory microscope (Carr, 1967), and one suspects that genetic aberrations beyond the resolution of the microscope account for a significant proportion of the remainder. The types of chromosome abnormality present in these abortuses are in most instances similar to those found in liveborn infants with multiple developmental malformations. Thus the most frequent aberration is a missing sex chromosome, the 45, XO chromosome complement characteristic of most cases of Turner's syndrome, and caused by a disorder of meiosis whereby the sex chromosome fails to be included in either the sperm or egg. XO conceptions account for 21 per cent of chromosomally abnormal abortions or 4 per cent of all spontaneous abortions. As the XO state occurs in rather more than 1 in 5,000 liveborns, and assuming that 15 per cent of all pregnancies end in abortion, only 2.5 per cent of XO conceptions survive to term.

The second most frequent aberration found in spontaneous abortions seems to be triploidy, a situation where every chromosome is represented three times instead of twice in each cell in the embryo (Fig. 22) i.e. each cell has 69 instead of 46 chromosomes. This defect arises by the accident of double fertilization of the ovum or by failure of extrusion of the second polar body. It occurs in about 17 per cent of chromosomally abnormal abortions (i.e. 3 per cent of all spontaneous abortions). Various types of chromosomal trisomy (where one chromosome only is present in triplicate) account for the majority

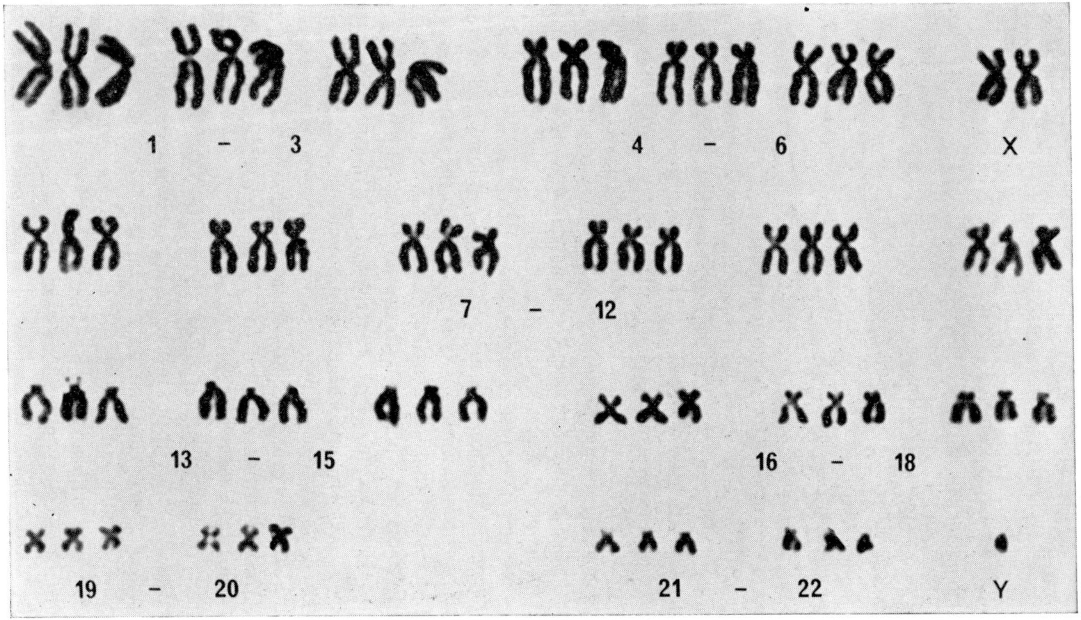

2/Fig. 22.—Chromosome analysis in a triploid cell cultured from an abortus of approximately 9 weeks gestation.

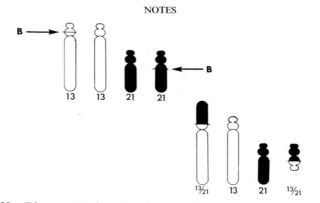

2/Fig. 23.—Diagram showing the origin of a translocation between two non-homologous chromosomes, numbers 13 and 21. Chromosome breakage had occured at B and, by chance, the normal process of repair had occurred between the wrong fragments. This particular aberration is a cause of familial mongolism.

of the remaining chromosomally abnormal abortions. These include the G(21–22) trisomy of mongolism as well as the D(13–15) and E(18) trisomes which are well known in the newborn. Trisomy 16, which has probably only once been described in the liveborn, proves to be the commonest single type of trisomy in abortions.

It has been found that almost all the chromosomally abnormal abortions occur between the 8–16th week of gestation. Calculated in another way, the frequency of chromosome aberrations in abortuses in the first and second trimesters is 30 per cent and 11 per cent respectively; in other words the the earlier the abortion, the greater the incidence of chromosomal abnormality. Pathological examination of these conceptions shows that the embryo is absent in about a third and grossly malformed in most of the remainder. The interesting exceptions are the triploid embryos which seem to have remarkably few malformations. Their abortion, typically around the sixth week, appears to be the result of defects of the placenta and fœtal membranes which, among other abnormalities, frequently show multiple amniotic polyps.

There is currently much interest in factors which might predispose to chromosome aberrations in abortuses and data on such agents as infections with viruses and mycoplasma, exposure to irradiation and radiomimetic drugs are being accumulated. So far, only increased maternal age has been found to be a significant factor, and this operates only in the case of the trisomic abortions.

Habitual Abortion

A history of recurrent abortion is frequently found in families in which a structural chromosome abnormality or translocation is be-

ing transmitted. A translocation arises by the exchange of chromosome fragments between two chromosomes of different pairs and is caused by agents such as irradiation which lead to chromosome breakage. When both products of the translocation are present the total complement of genes is unchanged (although abnormally distributed), the translocation is said to be "balanced," and development is normal. However, the offspring of the carrier of a "balanced" translocation may inherit only one of the products of the translocation, in which case the total complement of genes is "unbalanced," and embryonic development is defective. Thus, the usual finding in these families is that one parent has the "balanced" translocation and a varying proportion of the pregnancies result in normal offspring without the translocation, abnormal offspring with an "unbalanced" translocation, normal offspring carrying the "balanced" translocation like the parent, and miscarriages. These observations have prompted chromosome analysis in several series of patients and their husbands who have a history of recurrent abortion. Rather surprisingly, these studies have almost without exception failed to demonstrate a significant chromosome aberration, and it is now thought that the part played by gross transmissible chromosome aberrations in the ætiology of habitual abortion is small, possibly in the order of less than 1 per cent.

Investigation for chromosomal abnormalities in obstetrics (as distinct from gynæcology) is, however, indicated in dysmature babies, especially those with developmental abnormalities affecting more than one system because, in a proportion, a chromosomal aberration in the baby may point to a transmissible defect in one or other parent which may influence the prognosis of future pregnancies.

REFERENCES

1. CARR, D. H. (1967). *Amer. J. Obstet. Gynec.*, **97**, 283–293.
2. HERTIG, A. T. and ROCK, J. (1949). *Amer. J. Obstet. Gynec.*, **38**, 968.

CHAPTER III

SPECIAL CASES

FOUR special types of case are discussed in this chapter: the elderly primigravida, the grand multipara, the patient with the bad obstetric history and the grossly obese.

THE ELDERLY PRIMIGRAVIDA

There is a general tendency to include in this category all women going through their first pregnancy over the age of 35, but this is widening the definition too far and only confuses the issue by diluting results with large numbers of women who in no sense deserve to be classed as elderly and who run a perfectly normal obstetrical course. Earlier papers discuss only women over the age of 40.[10, 11] Their results, therefore, are the more worth while. Larger series more recently reported widen the definition to include age of 35 and over.[2]

Considering how common the problem is, it is surprising that the literature is not more replete with information on the subject, and it certainly deserves a review. There is no doubt that the elderly primigravida is somewhat more likely to encounter complications which are the result of the natural process of growing older, but even more important is the fact that her dwindling chances of further pregnancies put more of a premium on the present one. Furthermore, her endurance and her resistance to disease are not those of a woman in her early twenties, and she is therefore likely to require help earlier. A long history of antecedent infertility serves only to magnify this point. Notwithstanding all this, it must be emphasised that the majority of these patients, properly supervised, are capable of safe and successful pregnancy.

Complications of Pregnancy

A normal woman's fertility is at its maximum at about the age of 23, after which there is a gradual decline, so that by the age of 40 the chances of conception are greatly reduced. Having once conceived, the elderly primigravida has a greater predisposition to abort, and the usual precautions as outlined in the chapter on abortion should be advised.

Within the limitations of our knowledge of the ætiology of pre-eclamptic toxæmia, one is hardly surprised at an increased incidence

in the more elderly, because increasing age, of itself, favours hypertensive disease and reduces the resilience of the cardiovascular system as a whole.

Hyperemesis gravidarum is somewhat more common, but much of this can be accounted for by the patient's very natural anxiety. Placental abruption may be favoured by folic acid deficiency, hypertensive disease or both, but increasing age rather than primiparity is likely to be the more dominant cause.

Because a patient is getting older she naturally has more time to develop gynæcological abnormalities, of which fibroids are likely to be the most common, six out of Miller's 88 cases being thus recorded. In other respects pregnancy is not specifically complicated, although any general disease has added significance.

Complications of Labour

Premature labour is rather more likely; in fact, Nixon recorded an incidence of 10 per cent as against 3·8 per cent in young primigravidæ, but the later large series of Booth and Williams showed little difference in this respect, four-fifths of whom were below 40 but over 35 years of age.

The duration of labour tends to be increased by about 25 per cent on average. Much of this is due to the greater anxiety of the older woman facing labour for the first time, and some degree of inertia is common. Posterior positions of the occiput are very much more usual, while the effects are more troublesome, and in about a third of the cases labour is likely to be prolonged because of this malposition. Inertia is also particularly likely to complicate the case which has had labour induced, and the response to induction tends to be so unsatisfactory that one should have very good indications for embarking upon it. It is said that labour may be adversely influenced by the impaired joint mobility which comes with increasing years, but the significance of this is small compared with the functional activity of the uterus and the elasticity of the soft tissues of the birth canal.

Signs of maternal distress in labour, as might be expected, appear more readily in the older woman, so that delivery has to be more often assisted surgically; in fact, only 40 per cent of Miller's cases had spontaneous deliveries and 38 per cent required forceps. The Cæsarean section rate was increased fourfold. This situation has not changed much in modern times and certainly the forceps will be required about twice or three times as often as in younger women.

The perineum and lower vagina do not stretch so well, so that episiotomy is often indicated and should be unhesitatingly employed.

The inertia of the first and second stages of labour is likely to obtrude into the third stage. Manual removal of the placenta is re-

quired more frequently, and the co-existence of fibroids makes this operation more likely.

Barring the direct results of surgical intervention, the puerperium is not abnormal, but breast feeding is only satisfactorily established in a minority.

Maternal and Fœtal Mortality

The maternal mortality is only slightly higher, and this is in direct ratio to the appearance and nature of complications already described and the need for operative intervention. Under modern conditions this aspect of the problem has been reduced to very small proportions. The fœtal mortality, however, gives no grounds for complacency, although the appalling figure of 26 per cent given by Miller over 35 years ago, the majority dying of intracranial hæmorrhage after forceps delivery or breech extraction, has now been radically modified by the more ready use of Cæsarean section. Nowadays stillbirths are still more common with increasing maternal age, the rate being about three times as high in primigravidæ over 40 years of age as in young women in their teens or early twenties. Heady et al. (1955) furthermore noted an increase of 50 per cent in the neonatal death rate, and they observed that the stillbirth rate rises with maternal age for all parities. Prematurity accounts for some of the increased mortality, but it is particularly tragic that in these cases the chances of fœtal abnormality are unquestionably increased; moreover, the association of mongolism with elderly primiparity is well known although here, too, age is the more important factor.

Treatment

The elderly primigravida does not require any special surgical treatment on the grounds of age alone, but the need for detailed supervision both in pregnancy and labour is obvious. These patients should, therefore, be seen at more than usually frequent intervals throughout pregnancy and very early note taken of any signs of developing pre-eclamptic toxæmia.

The bony pelvis should be assessed and found to be above reproach before contemplating vaginal delivery, while the combination of malpresentation with elderly primiparity demands Cæsarean section as an elective procedure. There is no place for trial of labour in the elderly primigravida. The relative indications for Cæsarean section have to be extended, and for this reason an X-ray to exclude fœtal abnormality in all these cases is necessary, as such a discovery is likely to modify treatment.

As has been said elsewhere, Cæsarean section is no guarantee of live birth, and is not to be employed on grounds of elderly primiparity alone. The somewhat unsatisfactory response to induction of

labour has been commented upon already and the indications for it should be stringently met. If a patient's condition is bad enough to warrant induction at this age, there is a strong possibility that it warrants Cæsarean section instead. The elderly primigravida should not be allowed more than a week's postmaturity at the most and induction, if undertaken, should be followed by Cæsarean section within twenty-four hours if it misfires.

One fact needs stressing particularly. These patients are anxious and very unsure of their ability to deliver themselves safely. Sympathetic but firm, confident handling is therefore an essential part of treatment, and the patient should be encouraged to hope for normal delivery, and the attendant should conduct his vigilance without a trace of ceremony.

THE GRAND MULTIPARA

Nowadays grand multiparity is usually defined as applying to cases which have had five or more previous viable babies, although Barns (1953) and Feeney (1953) produced impressive papers restricted to women carrying their eighth pregnancy or over. Barns's cases numbered 306 and Feeney, at the Coombe Lying-in Hospital, in a two-year period, collected the astonishing number of 518 grand multiparæ, including two cases, one in her 20th and the other in her 21st pregnancy, out of a total of 4,115 deliveries, an incidence of grand multiparity of 12·6 per cent.

Ever since Solomons in 1934 drew attention to what he called "the dangerous multipara", increasing cognisance has been taken of grand multiparity as a clinical entity in its own right. These patients are liable to a series of dramatic complications, all the more dangerous because they are often unsuspected, and, as will be seen, it is foolhardy to expect a woman who has had a long series of previous uneventful deliveries to maintain her unblemished record indefinitely.

Solomons pointed out that in child bearing, practice does not make perfect and indeed was impressed with the increased maternal mortality associated with grand multiparity. Today the penalty of death has receded, but formidable risks remain of a similar nature as before. The pooled results of several institutions over a short period of time are now available for assessing hazards which no single unit can nowadays supply, because very high degrees of parity are becoming less common. A study of over 5,000 grand multiparæ has been made through the American Obstetrical Statistical Co-operative,[9] covering women at least para seven and upwards, amounting to 4·3 per cent of all patients delivered in these institutions over a 3-year period. Over 60 per cent of the series was white,

a fact which reduced the average age to under 35 in two-thirds. This increases the value of this report as it helps to reduce the adverse factor of age alone. In this series the incidence of anæmia was more than doubled, hypertensive disease, including pre-eclamptic toxæmia superimposed on chronic hypertension had an increased occurrence which could not be gainsaid, hæmorrhage of all varieties before, during and after delivery was mainly doubled, uterine rupture trebled and the primary Cæsarean section rate because of a wide variety of complications was as great as in less parous women.

Many factors operate to increase the hazards of high parity. For one thing the patient is getting older, and her cardiovascular system is consequently less resilient, so that hypertensive disease is more manifest. Other general conditions which are part of the normal process of ageing are liable likewise to intrude themselves upon the clinical picture. Obesity, which is often gross in these cases, increases the dangers of childbearing, as is well known, and not the least reason for this is the difficulty of making an accurate examination.

Sociological factors play a very important part, for the majority of these patients are poor, overworked and tired. Many of them have never fully regained a good blood picture, and anæmia may dog them from one pregnancy to the next without respite. They tend to feed their numerous children at the expense of their own nutrition, so that they are consequently often very short of vitamins and first-class protein. They are too busy to attend to their health, and in a rapid succession of pregnancies and periods of lactation they are likely to become seriously depleted of calcium. It is small wonder, then, that dental fitness is unusual and their mouths are often full of useless and infected stumps.

With increasing weight and lumbar lordosis, the abdominal wall gives up the unequal struggle, and we have, therefore, the picture of a harassed woman who stands badly, walks badly, eats indifferently and cannot get enough sleep.

Complications of Pregnancy

The abortion rate is increased, but it is difficult to say how much of this is spontaneous as, undoubtedly, these women are driven in many cases to seek interference. Anæmia is so common in multiparous pregnancy that it should always be looked for and treated energetically. It is usually of the iron deficiency type but megaloblastic anæmia may supervene very rapidly because folic acid reserves are often low before the next pregnancy even starts. Every effort should be made to see that the patient's hæmoglobin is at least 80 per cent before she approaches term. The method of achieving this will depend upon the time at one's disposal, and the choice lies between administering iron by mouth or by injection or, for those in

more urgent need, by transfusion of packed cells. The women who faces labour with a hæmoglobin of 65 per cent or less does so in real peril, and this matter is dealt with more fully elsewhere.

Hyperemesis is relatively uncommon in multiparous patients, but is far more significant and should always be taken seriously. It is so seldom neurotic that an organic origin must be diligently sought. Hiatus hernia is more common than generally recognised in multiparæ.

Hypertensive vascular disease comes increasingly into the picture with the patient's higher age group and, if present, necessitates prolonged periods of bed-rest during pregnancy. Termination of pregnancy in the worst cases is fairly widely practised in some centres; although we are of the opinion that with proper hospital supervision this should seldom be necessary. Nevertheless, the fœtal prognosis is adversely affected; premature induction of labour is often necessary and these cases should not be allowed to become postmature. Unfortunately it is in just such cases of grand multiparity that the dates are most often in doubt. In spite of the increased incidence of hypertensive disease, pre-eclamptic toxæmia and eclampsia are no more common in grand multiparæ, but the effects of eclampsia are more serious, and the mortality is raised because the patient is less well equipped than younger women to contend with them.

To the patient with a cardiac disability, high degrees of multiparity constitute a very definite additional risk. The patient, of course, is older, and therefore cardiac failure more likely. Although pregnancy may be regarded as only an incident in the progressive disease process, its advent may nevertheless be unwelcome.

As might be expected, any of the minor ailments of pregnancy are exaggerated, particularly such conditions as hæmorrhoids and varicose veins, which may be very troublesome indeed.

Twin pregnancy is about three times as common in grand multiparity, and this fact can be partly explained by the patient's high degree of fertility. Placenta prævia likewise is more common in direct proportion to the patient's parity, and antepartum hæmorrhage may be very sudden and profuse, so that its effects in the likely presence of iron deficiency anæmia are magnified.

Accidental antepartum hæmorrhage is largely a complication of multiparity, and in 148 of Solomon's cases at the Rotunda Hospital no less than 130 were multiparous. In grand multiparity placental abruption is far more likely to complicate pre-eclamptic toxæmia or folic acid deficiency. All four maternal deaths in Barns's series were associated with antepartum hæmorrhage, and this complication accounted for the greatest number of fœtal deaths.

Malpresentations are very much more common, and are favoured by a pendulous abdomen and lordosis of the lumbar spine, and in

any case it is usual for the head not to engage in the pelvis until the onset of labour.

Fortunately, fœtal abnormality is no more common in grand multiparity, but *erythroblastosis fœtalis* in the Rh iso-immunised case has an enhanced opportunity.

The onset of labour is commonly premature, and, for this, associated sociological factors are largely to blame.

Complications in Labour

It is when we come to labour that the grand multipara is capable of exhibiting the greatest treachery. Feeney gave a very revealing list of complications in his 518 cases:

Breech presentation	33
Oblique lie	14
Presentation and prolapse of cord . .	14
Disproportion	14
Postpartum hæmorrhage	71
Rupture of uterus	6
Obstetric shock	7
Precipitate labour	2

These observations deserve comment. Malpresentation, as already stated, is favoured by a pendulous abdomen together with the high angle of pelvic inclination resulting from associated lordosis of the spine. Even in cases in which the presentation is normal the head may remain free after the onset of labour, thereby favouring prolapse of the cord if the membranes rupture with a sudden gush of liquor. In many of these cases the lie is unstable, and treatment by external version and abdominal binder is ineffective. Transverse lie in Eastman's opinion (1940) becomes ten times as common as usual after the ninth pregnancy.

Feeney's finding of no less than 14 cases of disproportion may at first seem surprising, as one is tempted to regard the pelvis of a highly parous patient as beyond question. Nothing could be more dangerous than such a complacent attitude. In the first place babies tend to get larger with successive pregnancies, and may consequently give rise to cephalo-pelvic disproportion for the first time. It must not be forgotten also that occasionally contracted pelvis can secondarily occur in the adult quite apart from osteomalacia. In grand multiparity two things may reduce pelvic capacity: firstly, the increasing inclination of the pelvic brim already referred to, and, secondly, the occasional subluxation forwards of the sacrum upon the sacro-iliac joints so that the sacral promontory advances and the true conjugate is effectively reduced. Failure to recognise this condition may end in uterine rupture, especially in the presence of tumultuous pains.

Pendulous abdomen together with occipito-posterior position of the fœtus and undiagnosed brow presentation should always be kept in mind.

Uterine rupture constitutes one of the gravest risks of high parity, and it is important to realise that it may occur after only a short period of labour. Uterine contractions tend to be better co-ordinated and more forceful in multiparous labour, whereas the strength of the myometrium to resist rupture is by no means increased by successive pregnancies. The presence, moreover, of a larger size of baby than heretofore increases the strain, and the use of pituitary extracts is more than usually dangerous in this respect. An oxytocin drip is exceptionally dangerous in the grand multipara and even the closest supervision may not be able to prevent sudden and catastrophic uterine rupture.

The onset of uterine rupture does not always follow the classical textbook descriptions, and many cases are undoubtedly unrecognised and may be recorded as cases of postpartum hæmorrhage or so-called "obstetric shock". A fuller description of uterine rupture is given in another chapter.

Postpartum hæmorrhage is another real risk. This is an interesting matter, because the uterus seldom demonstrates an unwillingness to contract, and, in fact, hæmorrhage may follow precipitate labour. It is suggested that the essential difference between contraction and retraction operates here, and that only the latter will protect a woman against postpartum hæmorrhage. Now, where labour has been rapid, vigorous uterine contractions may cause early partial separation of the placenta, but the whole process has occurred too fast for retraction to catch up, so that bleeding may occur very early in the third stage. Furthermore, full retraction may be hampered by the increased quantities of elastic tissue in the myometrium, which is associated with high parity. Adherent placenta is also more common than in the primigravida. It follows, therefore, that the third stage is not to be lightly regarded, and unexplained bleeding or shock should always rouse a suspicion of spontaneous uterine rupture.

It is hardly surprising that Cæsarean section is not infrequently employed in grand multiparity, in fact, 21 out of 306 cases were so delivered in Barns's series. The complications enumerated above demand it from time to time.

The puerperal morbidity rate is not increased except in so far as major complications may have arisen during labour.

Mortality

Maternal mortality rises appreciably in the higher degrees of parity. In the years 1940–45 in England and Wales the maternal

mortality was 2·48 per thousand in primigravidæ, and then fell for the next three or four pregnancies. The curve, however, rose after the fifth, until at over ten pregnancies it reached the figure of 6·33 per thousand. Individual writers have given far more depressing figures; for instance, Eastman (1940) found that the mortality rose far more steeply from the ninth pregnancy onwards, and Solomons, 35 years ago, considered that the mortality rose progressively with each child after the fifth until by the tenth child the figure was five times the overall rate. In Eastman's series, rupture of the uterus accounted for a quarter of the deaths, chronic hypertensive disease for a fifth and placenta prævia for one-sixth. Parity of such degree is becoming less and less common even in Glasgow, so that it is hard to find comparable figures today.

The fœtal mortality shows a somewhat similar curve; for instance, in Barns's series it was 38·9 per thousand for primigravidæ, then fell for the next three pregnancies and rose thereafter progressively to 73·4 per thousand in pregnancies over the tenth. Eastman likewise found that the stillbirth rate was doubled after the ninth pregnancy. The neonatal death rate, however, is less markedly increased, and here the management of prematurity and better sociological conditions should improve the picture.

It goes without saying that in the light of the increased hazards to both mother and child, women who are expecting their fifth child or over must be delivered in hospital. It is agreed that this advice is not likely to be well received in all quarters, particularly by the patients, who are so tied up with their large families that they are unwilling to leave them even in the interests of personal safety. To many of them the advent of another confinement is no more serious apparently than an attack of toothache, but the doctor undertaking these cases in their own homes should critically review the facilities at his disposal for coping with the occasional and dramatic catastrophe. A compromise is often sought by promising the patient dismissal from hospital within the first 48 hours after delivery. While this is obviously better than flat refusal to come into hospital at all, it should only be reluctantly conceded since these are the women most in need of decent postnatal care such as a modern attractive hospital can give.

THE BAD OBSTETRIC HISTORY

RECURRENT *versus* NON-RECURRENT FACTORS

It is not uncommon for a particular case to be described as having a "bad obstetric history". The term requires clarifying, because it is often loosely used to signify that a woman has had previous disappointments in childbearing. In many cases there are no more than

compassionate aspects as distinct from factors which are obstetrically relevant to the present pregnancy. In other words, the term
ought really to be restricted to those patients in whom the obstetrical
future is likely to be modified by the nature of the previous disaster.
Certain factors may operate recurrently in successive pregnancies or
their threat may influence one's management, and these will be
considered in this section.

History-taking in obstetrics is every bit as important as in any
other branch of medicine, and the fullest information should always
be sought about previous deliveries and abortions. The parous
woman bears in her history more information than clinical examination is likely to provide.

Any history of stillbirth demands enquiry, if necessary from the
patient's previous attendant, as to whether it was a fresh case or
macerated, whether labour had followed intra-uterine death or the
baby had died in the process of delivery, whether the onset of labour
was spontaneous or induced, and if the latter for what reason, the
period of gestation, and the nature of any operative intervention.
Necropsy details, especially of intracranial hæmorrhage and tentorial tearing, are of the greatest importance, likewise the degree of
moulding at birth. The weight of the child should be ascertained and
the views of the patient's previous attendant obtained as to the cause
of death. Likewise, in the case of neonatal death the maturity and
weight should be known, the duration of life and the cause of death.
A history of fœtal deformity is significant.

The duration of previous labour should be ascertained. Very prolonged labours and precipitate deliveries are significant. With regard
to the former, reasons for the delay should be sought, and particular
note should be taken of a history of the hypertonic variety of inertia
which has a greater tendency to occur in subsequent deliveries than
where the uterus previously relaxed well between contractions.

The indications for Cæsarean section if done in the past are important; for example, if placenta prævia had been the reason, one
would be less concerned about vaginal delivery next time, whereas
disproportion or a failure of trial of labour makes the need for repeated sectioning more than probable. Above all, the integrity of the
uterine scar must be in doubt if there is any history of puerperal
sepsis. The standard of obstetrical notekeeping in this country has
so greatly improved in recent years that the fullest information can
nearly always be obtained on enquiry from sister hospitals, and registrars in answering these letters would do well to summarise all
the above facts.

The subject of intra-uterine death always raises the question
whether the same factors may not operate again. Where pre-eclamptic
toxæmia was associated previously it does not necessarily follow

that the patient will suffer a repetition, but the trickiest decisions are in those cases of recurrent intra-uterine death for no apparent cause shortly before term. For these the syndrome of "placental insufficiency" has been postulated. Every now and then one meets such a sequence, and it furnishes a very clear indication not only for a very general investigation but also for securing premature delivery before it is too late. Unfortunately reliable estimates of placental function still elude us. The clinical observation of "small for dates baby," namely, poor or absent maternal weight gain,[7] low œstriol excretion rates, vaginal cytological changes and poor growth curves as determined by sonar are all helpful indications but none, except perhaps the last (which is not yet generally available) is absolute. [4, 13, 14, 15]

In any case in which a previous disaster was associated with even so much as a suspicion of disproportion, it is worth while perusing the full notes of that labour and obtaining, if possible, the previous X-rays. It must be remembered that trials of labour fail more often because of uterine inertia than because of the dimensions of the bony pelvis, and the present pregnancy should be very critically considered in the light of this information before deciding as a matter of course that elective Cæsarean section will be necessary.

A history of third-stage accidents is always relevant, and adherent placenta particularly tends to be recurrent. It is now general practice to recommend hospital confinement in the case of any woman who has had a manual removal of the placenta or a postpartum hæmorrhage in any previous labour.

Postmaturity is significant in obstetric history. In many patients it recurs apparently as a natural phenomenon. The size of the babies and the nature of any dystocia will indicate whether the patient can be safely allowed to overrun her dates this time.

The incidence of fœtal abnormality climbs steeply with each instance. After one monster the chances next time are about six or eight times as great, and after two such consecutive disasters the chances of a third are in the region of 60 or 70 per cent. Any previous history, therefore, of fœtal abnormality indicates the need for the taking of a straight X-ray. It is certain that the patient herself, who very naturally fears a repetition, deserves this reassurance.

The previous appearance of pre-eclamptic toxæmia or any hypertensive disorder indicates a closer supervision in this pregnancy. In respect of recurrence it will often appear that the case who has had full-blown eclampsia is in less danger than one who has had a long low-grade pre-eclampsia which has niggled on for many weeks.

Nephritis is an uncommon complication of pregnancy, but a past history is highly significant, and where there is doubt that this disease is still operative it is worth admitting the patient to hospital early in pregnancy for thorough assessment. Urological disorders are

always noteworthy in the history. The more common types of urinary infection due to the *Bacillus coli* have a marked tendency to recur in the course of subsequent pregnancies, especially if the infection was not previously fully eradicated. More significant still is a history of genito-urinary tuberculosis. This is a matter which is dealt with more fully in the section on abnormalities of the urinary tract.

Previous injuries to the bladder, particularly vesico-vaginal fistula of obstetrical origin, which have been successfully treated, demand Cæsarean section rather than the risk of repeating this calamity, and a history of stress incontinence which has been successfully operated upon in most cases contra-indicates the local stresses of a subsequent vaginal delivery. Where, however, colporrhaphy has been performed for prolapse rather than for stress incontinence, the rules are less rigid, and the decision will depend largely upon one's assessment at term of the available capacity of the vaginal vault. This is often more important than the fact of previous amputation of the cervix.

Histories of third-degree tears and damage to the rectum are a sure indication for generous episiotomy as soon as the head gets anywhere near the pelvic floor. To allow the scar of a previous repair of this nature to give way would be wanton indeed, and on the second occasion one might be less lucky in curing the patient of the very terrible disability of rectal incontinence.

The fullest details should always be obtained of previous pregnancies and labours in cardiac cases. This will provide additional warning of the patient's liability to decompensate, and will to some extent determine the need for hospitalisation during the pregnancy.

The question of Rh iso-immunisation is dealt with elsewhere. The likelihood of the present fœtus being affected will be made almost certain if, on genotyping, the patient's husband is found to be homozygous. Nevertheless, the severity of the disease in previous babies does not necessarily indicate a hopeless outlook for the future, and the possibilities of salvage have so greatly increased within recent years that sterilization has ceased to feature as treatment in the worst affected cases.

Maternal syphilis as a cause of recurrent stillbirth hardly needs stressing these days when any doctor who omits a Wassermann reaction in pregnancy, whatever the social status of his patient, is almost guilty of culpable negligence. There can now be little excuse for this sort of disaster.

Lastly, a history of puerperal insanity raises a very difficult issue. The fear that this hideous complication of childbirth may recur is one that may well justify the termination of pregnancy, but the decision is essentially one for the expert psychiatrist. As a general rule psychiatric grounds for terminating pregnancy would be better met by admitting the patient to a mental institution and treating her

illness or preventing her suicide rather than taking the illogical step of destroying her pregnancy.

The above short list shows that there is much to reckon with in good history-taking in obstetrics, and in a busy antenatal clinic it is so often below standard that some vital and relevant detail is often missed. The practice of entrusting this task to nurses who are not fully aware of the significance of all these points, and who therefore omit to make specific enquiry, is to be deplored, and it is not difficult as a rule to catch out one's house surgeon on such points as these. It might also be added as a point of minor importance that candidates in examinations often make a very bad showing on this aspect of their presentation of a clinical case, and may reveal a lack of experience by their emphasis on a host of irrelevant details at the expense of a proper assessment of the facts which really matter. This may count far more than the correct elicitation of physical signs.

GROSS OBESITY

If there is one thing that a woman dislikes more than fatness it is the means by which it can be controlled. Pregnancy provides a moratorium and a vigorous policy of weight reduction is likely to be suspended for the time being. It is the purpose of this section to review the possible effects of obesity on pregnancy and vice versa. Starting with the latter it is unlikely that pregnancy will make a fat woman thin unless something is very radically wrong such as uncontrolled hyperemesis or extreme malnutrition. A weight gain of up to 24 lb. can be regarded as physiological in any pregnancy. Much of this can be accounted for straight away as follows:

Fœtus	7 lb.
Placenta	$1\frac{1}{4}$ lb.
Liquor, say	$1\frac{3}{4}$ lb.
Uterus	2 lb.
Breast hypertrophy	2 lb.
Physiological hydræmia, approx.	2 lb.
	16 lb.

The remainder is made up mostly of water and to a lesser extent of fat. Theoretically most of this is got rid of by delivery and the diuresis which follows it.

Pregnancy, *per se*, is therefore not fattening, except temporarily, yet there are many women who fail to regain their figures after it is all over. It is claimed, however, that they have largely failed to regain their original eating habits. This is altogether understandable since the harassments of a new baby in the house, the "weariness, the

fever and the fret" (Keats) may undermine resolve or interest in herself for the time being. What is likely to follow in the ensuing years of multiparous child rearing is a degradation in feeding standards for the mother with regard to protein because carbohydrates are so much cheaper and so much less trouble to prepare for the table. The role which child bearing and rearing has upon developing obesity therefore operates only indirectly by altering the circumstances and outlook of a considerable proportion of women.

The effects of obesity on the course and outcome of pregnancy may now be reviewed. The problem is such a common one that it is surprising that more has not been written about it since obstetricians do not regard it favourably. From the patient's own point of view pregnancy is likely to be a far more uncomfortable business than for a thinner woman and skin disorders, especially of the intertriginous variety, may be more troublesome. Œdema of the lower extremities is exaggerated which still further reduces comfortable mobility.

Dyspnœa on exertion or secondary to bronchitis has often more than nuisance value and the subjective effects of anæmia are magnified. But the most striking complicating factor in obese pregnancy is hypertension, both essential, so-called, and that due to superimposed pre-eclamptic toxæmia.

It is doubtful if obesity *per se* causes a high blood pressure but hypertension, overt or latent, is commonly associated with the obese type. To understand this association one would have to review the causes of obesity itself but apart from certain endocrine disorders such as pre-diabetes and pituitary dyscrasias which, in themselves, to some extent limit fertility, there is no doubt that to many otherwise healthy women obesity is a psychosomatic response to stress in life, as is hypertension too. The woman who finds little enough comfort in her husband may console herself with compulsive eating. This is what we call "eating for comfort". True, she will deny that she ever eats a proper meal, and the more the pity, but she does not admit to the constant nibbling throughout the day from her larder and kitchen shelves with an overwhelming taste for carbohydrates. The association between hypertension and obesity may therefore be based upon a common psychological background. To these people dietary restrictions are more in the nature of a spiritual exercise demanding default than a practical proposition.

In the series recorded by Emerson (1962) no less than one in five patients was overweight, yet the incidence of hypertension of 140/90 mm. Hg and above at the beginning of pregnancy was seven times as high as in women of normal build. Likewise, pre-eclamptic toxæmia supervened more than four times as commonly. A further corollary is the markedly increased incidence of antepartum hæmorrhage, especially the toxæmic accidental variety.

Malpresentation is, as might be expected, not only harder to detect but also harder to correct by external version and there is a greater need for antepartum radiology to exclude this and twins as well.

Labour is no better favoured by obesity. The need for surgical induction is commoner because of hypertension, pre-eclamptic toxæmia or postmaturity and labour is often tryingly inert and incoordinate. The babies are often much larger than clinical examination would lead one to expect and minor degrees of disproportion may only declare themselves by unsatisfactory labour. The need for operative delivery both by forceps and Cæsarean section is about doubled (Emerson) and in the case of the latter, the fatness of the abdominal wall may discourage healing by first intention and postoperative chest complications may not only be troublesome of themselves, but, because of poor ventilation, may encourage venous stasis and thrombosis.

Postpartum hæmorrhage is also more common (more than four times in Emerson's series) and veins are less accessible for transfusion. Lastly, obese women do not lactate as well as their thinner sisters. The babies of these patients have a higher perinatal mortality partly because of maternal hypertension and partly because of more difficult delivery.

For these reasons major degrees of obesity contribute an indication for hospital confinement. Increased vigilance for pre-eclamptic toxæmia is necessary and anæmia should be watched for at an early stage.

Appetite killing drugs and tranquillisers are not recommended but a high protein and fat and low carbohydrate diet should be resolutely encouraged, preferably with the expert help of a dietitian. Diuretics and salt restriction are relatively useless and only make the patient more miserable than she need be.

At the first and most minor signs of supervening pre-eclamptic toxæmia the patient should be admitted to hospital, not forgetting that thin eclamptics are much easier to nurse and pull through than fat ones.

The traditional idea that fatness and jollity are associated is certainly not true in pregnancy and these women need sympathy and help not only to forestall the complications which they face but to rehabilitate their morale and self-respect.

REFERENCES

1. BARNS, T. (1953). *Edinb. med. J.*, **60**, 28.
2. BOOTH, R. T., and WILLIAMS, G. L. (1964). *J. Obstet. Gynaec. Brit. Cwlth.*, **71**, 249.
3. BROWNE, J. C. M. (1963). *Scot. med. J.*, **8**, 459.

4. DONALD, I., and BROWN, T. G. (1961). *Brit. J. Radiol.*, **34,** 539.
5. EASTMAN, N. J. (1949). *N.Y. St. J. Med.*, **40,** 1708.
6. EMERSON, E. G. (1962). *Brit. med. J.*, **2,** 516.
7. FEENEY, J. R. (1953). *J. Irish med. Ass.*, **32,** 36.
8. HEADY, J. A., DALY, C., and MORRIS, J. N. (1955). *Lancet*, **1,** 395.
9. ISRAEL, L. S., and BLAZAR, A. J. (1965). *Amer. J. Obstet. Gynec.*, **91,** 326.
10. MILLER, D. (1931, 1932). *Trans. Edinb. obstet. Soc.*, **52,** 161.
11. NIXON, W. C. W. (1931). *J. Obstet. Gynaec. Brit. Emp.*, **38,** 821.
12. SOLOMONS, B. (1934). *Lancet*, **2,** 8.
13. Thompson, H. E., HOLMES, J. H., GOTTESFELD, K. A., and TAYLOR, E. S. (1965). *Amer. J. Obstet. Gynec.*, **92,** 44.
14. WILLOCKS, J., DONALD, I., DUGGAN, T. C., and DAY, N. (1964). *J. Obstet. Gynaec. Brit. Cwlth.*, **71,** 11.
15. WILLOCKS, J., DONALD, I., CAMPBELL, S., and DUNSMORE, I. R. (1967). *Ibid*, **74,** 639.

CHAPTER IV

THE CARDIAC CASE

In the eyes of the physician, pregnancy comes as a temporary complication in the disease process of the patient's cardiac lesion, a process which, in any case, is likely to shorten life. The question at issue is how to prevent, as far as possible, the additional burden of the pregnant state from accelerating the rate of the patient's decline.

Fortunately, under good supervision, provided that the extra demands of pregnancy are satisfactorily met at the time, it should generally be possible for the patient to emerge from the experience of childbirth without any degradation in her cardiac condition, and this should be the obstetrician's aim. Any complication, however, is likely to increase cardiac strain, quite apart from that of delivery, and in this subject particularly prevention is better than cure.

As a cause of maternal mortality a relatively greater part is now taken by cardiac disease, but this is only one side of the picture. Postpartum invalidism is almost as important.

Incidence of Cardiac Disease in Pregnancy

This varies from centre to centre and depends largely upon the degree to which minor cardiac lesions are sought out and registered and also upon the subjective interpretation on the part of the doctor of the minor types of symptoms and signs which may appear at antenatal examination. For instance, Bunim and Taube classified approximately 2 per cent of all patients attending at the antenatal clinics as having cardiac lesions, whereas MacRae, reviewing a total attendance of 29,713 patients at Queen Charlotte's Hospital, recorded the incidence as 0·8 per cent (225 cases). Of these, 13 had congenital lesions, and in the remainder a definite history of rheumatic disease was obtained in 91·1 per cent. In a more recent series of 500 cases in Glasgow in the years 1949–59 quoted by Sutherland and Bruce (1962) the incidence works out at 3·2 per cent of all pregnancies attending their unit. In more than a quarter of these cases no relevant rheumatic history was obtained.

Although the full-blown clinical picture of acute rheumatic fever in childhood is far less commonly seen nowadays, the incidence of rheumatic valvular disease of the heart shows no sign of lessening and it is clear that the milder clinical forms of rheumatic fever, which often go unrecognized in children, are just as capable as ever of damaging both the heart valves and the myocardium. For instance,

over 900 deaths from mitral stenosis and its complications occurred in the general population of Scotland alone in 1960 and the recent hope that within a generation cardiac disease would seldom complicate pregnancy seems unlikely to be realised. It would appear that the response in the form of rheumatic carditis to streptococcal infections in childhood is a family defect and all patients, pregnant or not, who have a significant family history should be very carefully scrutinised from this point of view. The diagnosis of mitral stenosis was missed repeatedly in my own case, for example, until incipient failure and atrial fibrillation brought the matter to a head and it now appears that three generations of my own family have not escaped. The point to be made is that family history of rheumatic heart disease is even more commonly significant than a history of rheumatic fever or chorea in the patient herself.

Types of Cardiac Lesions

Most authorities are agreed that well over 90 per cent are cases of rheumatic heart disease in one form or another, of which mitral stenosis is easily the commonest and accounts for more than three-quarters of all cases. When combined with other types of valvular lesion the figure for mitral stenosis is even higher, and Barry found it to be present in 247 out of his 266 cases. Aortic incompetence by itself is much less common and accounts for less than 10 per cent of the cases. Isolated aortic lesions are not in themselves worse than mitral lesions, and the nature of the valvular damage matters very much less than the state of the myocardium.

It is not surprising that rheumatic heart disease should form the main bulk of cases, considering the age of the patient and the point along the disease process at which the patient is likely to be fertile.

Bunim and Taube describe the *four phases* of rheumatic disease as follows:

1. An initial infection manifested by carditis, polyarthritis, chorea or muscle and joint pains.
2. Recrudescences, single or multiple, which, following on a hæmolytic streptococcal infection, resemble the primary episode.
3. A latent or inactive phase lasting from puberty until the fourth or fifth decade.
4. The stage of diminishing cardiac reserve leading progressively to congestive failure and death.

It will be seen, therefore, that a patient is most likely to be pregnant during the third phase.

Other types of heart disease, in addition to being in some instances less common, are found less often in pregnancy because of

the factor of age incidence. Many cases of congenital heart disease, for example, do not live long enough, or are not in sufficient health, to marry and become pregnant, while hypertensive heart disease and syphilitic heart disease tend to belong to a later period of life.

Apart from valvular disease, the list has to be completed by mentioning atrial flutter and paroxysmal tachycardia. Fortunately these do not increase the risks in childbearing. A certain number of cases can only be classed as suffering from a form of myocarditis without clinically demonstrable valvular lesions, and Haig and Gilchrist found that one in ten of their cases classed as suffering from heart disease showed no signs of an organic lesion several years after pregnancy. They suggested that in these cases the myocardium only was damaged. Many cases only come to light as a result of antenatal examination, and both Oram and Morgan Jones reported that approximately 40 per cent of their patients with cardiac lesions were symptom free before their pregnancies.

PHYSIOLOGY

While it should be one's endeavour to ensure that a patient's heart is no worse after pregnancy than it was before, there is no doubt that childbearing in no way confers any beneficial effect whatsoever upon a damaged heart. It would be as well, therefore, to review the nature of the additional temporary burden.

The circulatory strain is unpredictable, and during the long period over which it operates adjustment has to be made to certain basic physiological changes. Firstly, the heart has to deal with an increase in the volume of circulating blood. This increase is progressive, although it rises more steeply during the second half of pregnancy, and it is only reduced during the early part of the puerperium. The increase amounts to 25–30 per cent. The circulation of the enlarging and highly vascular uterus and placental site accounts only for some of this increase, and much of it is due to the fluid retention of pregnancy resulting in a hydræmic plethora.

There is a considerable increase in body weight which inevitably means more work for the heart. This increase is due chiefly to water retention, but is caused also by the weight of the fœtus, liquor and the enlarged uterus, and some increase in fat deposition is usual. Furthermore, the metabolic rate is increased out of proportion to the weight increase.

In the next place, the heart, in the latter half of pregnancy, has to operate against certain mechanical disadvantages due to the enlarging uterus. This causes displacement and rotation of the heart and, to some extent, splints the diaphragm. Respiration is embarrassed and, as a result, the venous return is slowed down to the detriment

of the heart's activity. In spite of the splinting of the diaphragm, however, the vital capacity is not decreased, because some compensation is provided by the increase in the diameter of the thoracic cage.

The above mechanical factors are probably the least important of all, because the changes so far recorded in cardiac activity appear at an earlier stage of pregnancy than could be accounted for by the factor of mechanical displacement by the uterus, and the cardiac output shows some increase even as early as the 12th week.

The extra demands of pregnancy have to be met by increase in cardiac minute volume. From a study of post-mortem material and from X-ray measurements of the heart in pregnancy it does not appear that the heart normally hypertrophies or dilates in any approximate ratio to the amount of work now demanded of it, and the question of existing cardiac reserve, therefore, is all-important (cf. Fig. 1).

The extra work which the heart has to do is partly compensated for by a lowering of blood viscosity, and which reaches its lowest level between the 33rd and the 36th week.[14] There is also some reduction in the rate of blood flow as measured by such tests as the fluorescin method (arm to eye), while, in the lower part of the body, it is well known that the circulation is more stagnant. Pulse-rate changes are not remarkable during pregnancy, although there is a slight tendency to quickening at the time of maximum cardiac output. The blood pressure alters only slightly, a small drop being characteristic during the middle of pregnancy.

In other words, in spite of some compensating factors, pregnancy inevitably involves the heart in increased effort. By means of cardiac catheterisation methods carried out under basal conditions Hamilton investigated cardiac output in pregnant and non-pregnant women. In the latter he found the average output is 4·5 litres per minute, but that in pregnancy the output increases rapidly during the 10th to the 13th week, reaching 5·14 litres per minute. Thereafter the increase is progressive though slower until the 21st week, when it reached 5·71 litres. The curve now flattens off until an output of 5·73 litres is reached between the 26th and the 29th week. This represents an increase of 27 per cent over the non-pregnant value. A gradual fall to 5·5 litres now occurs towards term, and during the last three weeks of pregnancy it starts to drop fairly rapidly to the non-pregnant level.

Many studies have been undertaken since that time and though all of them indicate an increased cardiac output, there has been considerable disagreement about the time of onset of rise in cardiac output, the time in pregnancy when peak levels are reached, the magnitude of the increase and what happens thereafter and how quickly. These discrepancies have been attributed[17] to the variety of experimental conditions and methods employed by different workers. Results can

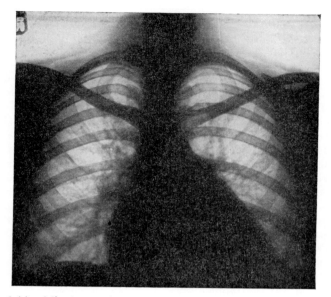

4/Fig. 1 (*a*).—Mitral stenosis and aortic incompetence at 36 weeks' gestation. Shows cardiac enlargement in the transverse diameter.

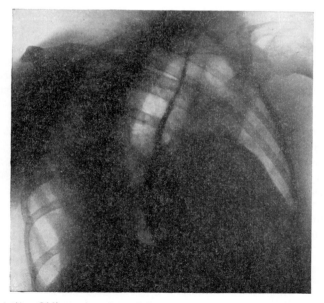

4/Fig. 1 (*b*).—Oblique view shows left atrium mainly involved. The pulmonary arteries are slightly prominent and so are the main pulmonary vessels.

be influenced by the patient's excitement, by respiration, by uterine contractions and by body movements, but most important of all are the effects of posture because, with the patient under test lying on her back, reduced venous return to the heart and therefore a reduced cardiac output can be caused by supine venacaval occlusion. Resting cardiac output may rise by 1·2 to 3·1 litres per minute; that is to say by about 30 to 40 per cent according to the latest work from Edinburgh,[17] but it is asserted from this source that most of the increase is established by the end of the first trimester and maintained until after term. Using a dye-dilution technique, cardiac output has been estimated at Hammersmith in 30 women at monthly intervals during pregnancy and the puerperium,[32] a massive work involving the recording and calculation of over 1,300 dye-dilution curves. This team has concluded that although cardiac output is increased in the first trimester, the maximum level is only reached between the 24th and 32nd week of pregnancy, thereafter declining to approach non-pregnant levels at term, with a further fall after delivery. As there is little increase in pulse rate, the increase in cardiac output is due to an increase in stroke volume. These findings are in agreement with what has been standard teaching for over a dozen years.

The arguments as to methodology may continue but meantime most present-day clinicians treat their patients in the belief that there is an early increase in cardiac output, that the strain is worst by about the 32nd week, if not earlier, and that barring complications such as infections of all types, particularly respiratory, embolic phenomena and obstetrical complications in late pregnancy, the patient can look forward to some shedding of her cardiac load towards the end of pregnancy. Therefore, if the cardiac state is carefully assessed between the 28th and the 32nd week, one is in a position, barring complications, to make a reasonable estimate of how the heart will behave during labour.

The onset of pre-eclamptic toxæmia puts an additional load upon the heart, although this is not so in a patient suffering from essential hypertension. If, by some mischance, intra-uterine death of the fœtus should occur, the heart is automatically relieved of some of its burden, even though the fœtus is retained *in utero*.

To sum up, as far as cardiac function is concerned, a pregnant woman at rest is in a position similar to a non-pregnant woman doing moderate work.

THE RISKS OF PREGNANCY WITH HEART DISEASE

In recent years there has been a great reduction in mortality. This is not due to any revolutionary change in treatment but to the increased care with which these cases are supervised. Antibiotics, too,

have played their part. Of all the medical complications of pregnancy cardiac disease heads the list as a cause of maternal mortality, but, even so, now occupies fifth place (84 cases, see Chapter I). Under present conditions the patient with heart disease is at five times the risk of the normal patient.

What is particularly striking is the enormous difference in the mortality rate between the unbooked and the antenatally supervised cases, the mortality of the former being at least three times as high. Atrial fibrillation complicating pregnancy still has a very high mortality, and Morgan Jones (1952) reported that 35 out of 85 such cases died. More recent figures given by Szekely and Snaith (1961) in Newcastle upon Tyne still demonstrate the gravity of atrial fibrillation. In their cases the incidence of frank heart failure developing during pregnancy or shortly thereafter rose from 25 per cent in cases fibrillating before their pregnancy began to over 70 per cent in those who developed their fibrillation during pregnancy or the puerperium.

Because of the considerable risk of embolism occurring shortly after its onset, atrial fibrillation should be treated as a medical emergency. As a means of restoring sinus rhythm quinidine is now regarded as a very dangerous drug, although it is not so long ago since I myself lived on it for over a year, and 2,000 volt cardioversion is the favoured treatment by physicians. This involves a high voltage shock applied externally to the chest wall using direct current, the shock being triggered by the Q.R.S. complex of the electro-cardiogram. I have personal experience of this on more than one occasion. The effects are by no means permanent. Unfortunately my experience does not extend to pregnant women. Undoubtedly the most immediate hazard associated with attempts to restore sinus rhythm is that of cerebral embolism and long term anticoagulant therapy is the only means of protection. It should be maintained until labour starts when it is withheld and its effects temporarily reversed by the injection of vitamin K_1. Mendelson (1956) also recommends that vitamin K_1 should also be given to the baby (dose 2 mg.). The patient should, of course, be adequately digitalised to prevent an uncontrollable tachycardia due to fibrillation which may precipitate her into cardiac failure.

Deaths are often due to acute pulmonary œdema, although right-sided heart failure is the chief cause of death in non-pregnant cases. Mitral stenosis, by far the commonest lesion, greatly raises the pulmonary venous pressure which tends to localise the œdema to the lungs; in fact, pulmonary œdema occurs as the commonest and most dramatic form of disaster, and may present as an acute emergency. Any cause of tachycardia, ranging from paroxysmal tachycardia to emotional or infective types of accelerated cardiac output,

can precipitate acute pulmonary œdema by piling up blood behind the mitral valve.

During pregnancy itself the onset of an attack of acute rheumatism is a very serious risk and, superimposed upon a damaged heart, is far more likely to cause death than myocardial stress due to the presence of the valve lesion. Death may rapidly follow delivery in cases of active rheumatic carditis, and clinically the patient behaves as though in a state of acute obstetric shock.

A freshly superimposed endocarditis is a very real risk, and is to be suspected when a patient shows tachycardia at rest, dyspnœa, fever, œdema, anæmia and occasionally proteinuria. Subacute bacterial endocarditis occurs in about 1 per cent of cases, and apart from a persistent pyrexia and anæmia, splenic enlargement may be demonstrated and embolic phenomena may occur. Blood culture may be positive. In fatal cases fresh, very mushy vegetations may be found on the heart valves.

The danger of pulmonary embolism is somewhat increased, particularly if there has been interference such as Cæsarean section.

It is interesting to note that death during the last eight weeks of pregnancy is uncommon. This is the period during which the load upon the heart is lightening. Death, too, during labour itself is uncommon, but it may occur suddenly during the next 24 hours or first few days of the puerperium. I often preach "the rule of fives" by which I mean that death may occur within 5 minutes, 5 hours, 5 days, 5 weeks and 5 months of delivery.

Causes of Death

Two-thirds of the deaths occur after delivery, and congestive cardiac failure and acute pulmonary œdema accounted for three-quarters of all cases in Haig and Gilchrist's series. Slightly more than half were found to have died within the first 24 hours after delivery and about one-third died within the next 4 days. Fortunately nowadays no single unit gets enough cases to produce more up-to-date statistics.

Bacterial endocarditis accounted for 15 per cent and peritonitis following Cæsarean section for 4 per cent. Of the remaining 7 per cent, one case was attributable to acute rheumatic fever, another to an anæsthetic accident during the repair of a perineal laceration, and one to a mismatched blood transfusion. In cases dying a few days after delivery, more often than not fresh vegetations can be found upon the heart valves.

The mortality of acute pulmonary œdema in pregnancy is ten times as high according to Gilchrist (1962) as in cases of congestive cardiac failure. This complication cannot be foreseen by studies of exercise tolerance nor from the history, but a small heart with

pulmonary hypertension and a tight mitral stenosis is the most dangerous in this respect.

PULMONARY CONGESTION AND ACUTE PULMONARY ŒDEMA

Right-sided heart failure usually comes on gradually and responds well to treatment in pregnancy, but acute pulmonary œdema is of rapid onset and is far more dramatically dangerous. It is particularly liable to occur suddenly a few hours or minutes after delivery, and is thought to be due to an overloading of the circulation with blood which would normally have been diverted through the placental site.

During pregnancy the signs of failure are often not to be found in engorgement of the neck veins, nor in ankle œdema of cardiac origin, but are demonstrated by increasing pulmonary congestion with attacks of paroxysmal dyspnœa. This last symptom usually accompanies acute exacerbations of pulmonary congestion. It is important therefore to watch the lung bases closely for evidences of pulmonary congestion, for this gives an index of the liability of the patient to develop acute pulmonary œdema which can be rapidly fatal. If moist sounds at the lung bases persist after coughing or deep breathing, they signify pulmonary congestion, confirmed by a typical "hilar moustache" on screening. This radiological appearance is due to increased pulmonary vascular markings. The following are the signs of increasing pulmonary congestion:

1. Dyspnœa. In severe cases paroxysmal attacks develop.
2. Persistent moist sounds at the lung bases.
3. Radiological signs of vascular congestion, especially in the hilar regions. Repeated screening of the chest for signs of early hilar congestion provides a good warning of failure (Fig. 2).
4. Hæmoptysis. This is usually a very serious sign.
5. A diminution in the vital capacity.

The onset of acute pulmonary œdema can be precipitated not only by an upper respiratory infection, which is perhaps the commonest mechanism in the antenatal period, but also by anything which increases the output of the heart, particularly the right ventricle, above the level at which the mitral valve can accept and pass the volume of blood returning from the lungs. If this level is exceeded, pulmonary congestion and then pulmonary œdema rapidly build up due to back pressure. Because the mitral valve cannot cope with greater volumes, it is imperative to reduce the right ventricular output to the pulmonary vascular bed in such cases, before the overloading becomes irreversible and the capillaries have been rendered permeable by anoxia.

This kind of heart attack can, therefore, be precipitated by excite-

ment or exertion or any other major cause of tachycardia in cases of "button-hole" mitral stenosis. Furthermore, tachycardia does not allow sufficient time for left ventricular filling. This mechanism is, in effect, not so very different from that which may obtain in the third stage of labour with the sudden shut-down of the uterine arterio-venous anastomosis although, in this case, a resultant increase in peripheral resistance has to be faced as well.

When acute pulmonary œdema occurs in the first half of pregnancy for no apparent reason apart from the known existence of mitral

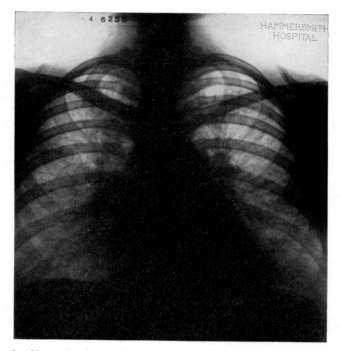

4/FIG. 2.—X-ray showing cardiac enlargement. Well-marked congestive changes showing incipient pulmonary œdema. Calcareous left hilar gland and cal-careous focus in left mid-zone. Mitral stenosis.

stenosis it is as well to consider coitus, in the usual dorsal position for the woman, as a possible cause. In a recent case of mine who twice had to be admitted for acute pulmonary œdema, and who for that reason was being considered for valvotomy, the true reason, as above, came to light and is obvious enough if one thinks of it. The use of the lateral position for coitus removes this hazard and in this case, after suitable advice, no further attacks occurred and she

completed her pregnancy without mishap and without the need for valvotomy.

Acute pulmonary œdema may also be triggered off by an initial small pulmonary embolus, and I have seen such a case who greeted me normally one morning but who, a few minutes later and before I had completed my round, was in desperate straits with lungs rapidly becoming more œdematous every minute. She was dangerously ill for many days thereafter but recovered in time to deliver herself several weeks later. It is believed that a pulmonary embolus started the emergency.

Treatment of Acute Pulmonary Œdema

Minutes often count. The patient should be propped up at once and morphine gr. ¼ (15 mg.) injected intravenously. Oxygen should be given, and in severe cases no time should be lost in carrying out venesection which can be dramatically life-saving if performed early enough and in time to relieve the overburdened pulmonary circulation. About 500–600 ml. of blood should be let off as quickly as possible. This treatment requires courage and also the certainty that the patient's collapse, especially in labour, is not due to other causes; nor can it be employed in the presence of severe anæmia. Hanging the legs down over the edge of the bed and before the application of venous tourniquets may suffice for the less desperate cases. Until recently it was recommended that Digoxin in large dosage of up to 1·5 mg. should be injected intravenously and repeated, 0·5 mg. six-hourly, until the patient was well digitalised, but a note of warning is necessary here. In so far as the condition may be entirely due to a button-hole mitral valve, such treatment could aggravate matters by increasing right ventricular output beyond the mitral valve's capacity, actually intensifying dyspnœa and pulmonary œdema (McMichael). In other cases, such as in "hypodynamic" ventricular states, Digoxin may produce benefit since an improved left ventricular performance may reduce the right ventricular load provided the mitral valve is adequate to handle the volume.

The extent, therefore, to which Digoxin may be prescribed is not easy to determine in any given case without the maximum fore-knowledge of the cardiac pathology which is often lacking and we are now more cautious in the use of this powerful drug, being guided mainly by the degree of tachycardia and the need to control it.

These cases are often complicated by bronchospasm which aggravates their dyspnœa, and intravenous aminophylline (250 mg.) may be of great help. We have also used amyl nitrite inhalations with short-lived but definite benefit.

As a temporary emergency measure, tourniquets can be applied to the limbs sufficiently tight to occlude venous return and therefore

reduce the output of the right heart. This constitutes, in effect, a type of venesection without costing the patient blood which, perhaps through trauma for example, she may none too readily afford. Antibiotic cover with penicillin is also advisable.

These are among the most worrying cases to be encountered in modern obstetrics and in no instance is the patient likely to be out of acute danger for many hours, usually three or four days at least, so that one is often left wondering what next to do. By now an oxygen tent will have been set up and it is important to secure adequate rest with sedatives, to maintain digitalisation as long as persisting tachycardia indicates it and to promote diuresis with frusemide (Lasix) 40–80 mg. which, by mouth, begins to be effective within two hours. Above all, respiratory tract infection is to be feared and we have, in this instance, one of the very few valid indications for prophylactic penicillin therapy.

DIFFERENTIAL DIAGNOSIS AND ASSESSMENT

It is easy to be mistaken, since even a healthy woman in pregnancy often produces symptoms and signs which are simply due to the physiological adjustments which the heart has to undertake to meet the new circulatory demands. The earlier in pregnancy that the diagnosis can be made the more likely is it to be accurate. Early diagnosis also makes for safe delivery. If one cannot be certain of the presence of a cardiac lesion in early pregnancy it is unlikely that the diagnosis will become any easier later on, because murmurs may become masked, and a rising diaphragm later confuses the clinical picture and assessment. Foreknowledge of the cardiac condition will enable one to decide whether later signs are due to cardiac disability or to exaggeration of the normal physiological changes of late pregnancy, and without it the assessment of right-sided heart failure becomes increasingly difficult as pregnancy advances.

A family history of rheumatic fever is very important. It is now recognised that this is a disease with a certain hereditary predisposition. I feel strongly about this because it has gone through three generations of my own family (predominantly redheads too) and in my own generation has affected three out of four siblings. Nowadays permanent cardiac damage can be prevented by daily prophylaxis with oral penicillin (125 mg. twice a day). It stops the ravages of yet another streptococcal infection in a patient already sensitised. The initial sensitising infection is caused by the Group A beta hæmolytic streptococcus and it is believed that it is subsequent infections which do the cardiac damage. Therefore infection is only one side of the ætiology, the patient's own sensitivity response being even more important. In deciding whether or not a patient has had rheumatic

fever, and is therefore at risk, account has to be taken of certain diagnostic criteria, such as carditis producing murmurs at the time of the infection, cardiac enlargement, pericarditis and occasionally congestive cardiac failure. An arthritis flitting from joint to joint is almost diagnostic, likewise a true history of chorea. Subcutaneous nodules felt particularly over the extensor surfaces of elbows, knees or wrists and in the occipital region, or spinous processes of the vertebræ may have been noted. Less conclusive criteria of rheumatic fever are painful joints without objective findings of tenderness or limitation of movement, a prolonged P-R interval in electrocardiogram, an increased erythrocyte sedimentation rate or unexplained leucocytosis. The child so affected may have loss of weight and fatigue easily, is liable to an elevated sleeping pulse rate, sweating, pallor, anæmia and general malaise. Unfortunately only in the few instances where a doctor has known his patient for many years is the diagnosis of past rheumatic fever easy to establish. Furthermore the severity of the original infection bears no relationship to the extent of subsequent cardiac damage. The important thing is to recognise the cases at risk as indicated by such a history, including the family history, and never to forget that a rheumatic cardiac lesion may become apparent for the first time after an obstetrical catastrophe and not before it.

The signs of mitral stenosis in early pregnancy often alter as pregnancy advances and, moreover, mitral stenosis may be wrongly diagnosed because a physiological third sound in diastole may mimic a pre-systolic murmur. The first sound may also be split and produce the same impression. Towards the end of pregnancy the pulmonary second sound is often increased without any cardiac pathology, and apical systolic murmurs of no significance are common.

Breathlessness on exertion and œdema of the ankles are so common in normal pregnancy, occurring in about 30 per cent of healthy women, that they should not be regarded as evidence of heart disease unless other cardiac signs are present. This source of confusion would have been avoided if the heart condition had been properly assessed at the beginning of pregnancy.

A significant history should put one on guard, and Barry recommends that the heart should be examined at every antenatal visit if this is the case. The importance of auscultating the heart with the patient half turned on to her left side cannot be overstressed if significant mitral pre-systolic murmurs are not to be missed. A large number of patients are referred from the antenatal clinic to the cardiologist with a provisional diagnosis of heart disease but are in fact found to be normal.

Effort syndrome has to be distinguished. In this condition there is often sub-mammary pain, dyspnœa, palpitations and premature

systoles. The dyspnœa is not related specifically to exertion, but may come on even at rest or when the patient is psychologically upset. Morgan Jones found premature systoles in 15 out of 100 pregnant patients with heart disease, but by themselves they are not significant. They only "appear to disappear" on exertion because of tachycardia. Sinus arrhythmia is another common source of pulse irregularity and is physiological. A pulse rate of over 100 with a patient completely at rest, however, suggests cardiac pathology, and fibrillation denotes a severe lesion. Heart block is rather uncommon, and doubtful cases should always be subjected to electrocardiography.

Angina of effort is very rare in pregnancy, mainly because of the factor of age incidence.

The assessment of cardiac enlargement in pregnancy is notoriously difficult, because in normal cases the apex beat is displaced upwards into the fourth space and as far out as the mid-clavicular line or farther. Mensuration of the heart, to be accurate, should be undertaken as early in pregnancy as possible for this reason. Radiology also provides additional useful evidences of atrial enlargement by means of a barium swallow. Pulmonary venous congestion is very significant.

Anæmia, especially if there is a history of rheumatic fever, frequently confuses the issue because of itself it can produce many of the symptoms and signs of cardiac disability. If present in association with a heart lesion, the signs are greatly exaggerated. The routine estimation of the hæmoglobin at the same time is essential. This is now standard practice with us in all patients and at every antenatal visit.

It is far more important to assess the heart's condition according to functional capacity than to the nature of the structural damage, and this grading is done according to the patient's tolerance to effort, the presence or history of atrial fibrillation and the existence of pulmonary venous congestion.

The procedure has now been almost universally adopted of grading cardiac disease in accordance with the New York Heart Association classification. This classification consists of four Grades, I, II, III and IV. This is preferable to the former, I, IIa, IIb and III. Grade I cases have no limitation of activity. Signs but not symptoms are present. In Grade II, the patient has slight limitation under conditions of moderate activity. In Grade III, there are signs of incipient failure. Under circumstances of ordinary activity the patient suffers definite limitation. In Grade IV, there is complete limitation and signs of heart failure are present even at rest. Also included in Grade IV are patients who have any past history of cardiac failure and all cases of atrial fibrillation past or present. Atrial fibrillation is not an absolute bar to pregnancy, provided it can be controlled by digitalis, but it constitutes one of the most serious signs.

PROGNOSIS

In the long run the nulliparous patient with heart disease fares no better in life than the parous woman, and the death rate, age for age, shows no difference between the two groups. To judge from statistics also, the death rate does not appear to be influenced by the number of pregnancies. There is, however, a fallacy in inferring too much from such figures, because the patient who manages to achieve a large number of pregnancies is likely to have a well compensated heart lesion, and this will weight the figures unduly in favour of parity.

The prognosis depends utterly upon the thoroughness of medical supervision throughout pregnancy, during labour and after. For example, O'Driscoll and colleagues in Dublin (1962) in a prospective study of rheumatic heart disease complicating pregnancy between the years 1948–56 reported the final outcome 5 to 13 years later of 385 mothers who achieved 539 pregnancies in this period. The only deaths in pregnancy or within a year afterwards occurred in patients who were admitted in cardiac failure having had no previous ante-natal care whatsoever (7 cases), and of those who were traced subsequently in 1961 at the end of the longer follow-up period (94 per cent) 86 per cent were still living with an average age of 40·7 years and an average parity as regards viable infants of four. In no instance was therapeutic abortion carried out since this is regarded as a dangerous substitute for adequate care. Early diagnosis and thorough supervision can practically eliminate the immediate disasters nor is the patient's life expectancy subsequently shortened, a point of view with which most of us would now agree.

In Sutherland and Bruce's series the immediate death rate was 1·4 per cent and of the survivors more than half had no alteration in cardiac grading. Only 6·8 per cent suffered a sustained deterioration and in 17 per cent the patient's cardiac state was actually better when she was dismissed than when she first attended. The remainder suffered a temporary deterioration only.

It is quite certain that pregnancy never conferred any benefit upon a damaged heart although, at best, it may be no more than a temporary threat. Provided pregnancy is safely survived, the patient is often none the worse for it and life is not necessarily shortened. One's most immediate concern therefore is the immediate progress in the course of the pregnancy under review, and this must take many factors into account. Above all, the functional capacity of the heart must head the list of prognostic criteria; in other words, the patient's cardiac grading. It will be remembered that these groups are related to the patient's response to normal activity. Exercise tolerance tests are not applicable, because the patient's apparent reactions are too

much influenced by age, habits and training. There is a tendency for the patient to drop one grade during the course of her pregnancy, in other words, a Grade I case may easily become a Grade II or a Grade II may turn into a Grade III, although any complication, particularly infection, may precipitate failure in any group. On the whole, Grades I and II are good risks and Grades III and IV are bad.

A history of failure before pregnancy started, even though apparent recovery may have taken place, is a bad prognostic sign, and atrial fibrillation, as already stated, is the most serious sign of all. The nature or even the extent of valvular damage is of far less prognostic significance than the patient's functional grading, and the prognosis does not differ much between cases of mitral stenosis, for example, and aortic incompetence.

Age must be taken into account, because increasing years will place the patient, whether pregnant or not, nearer to ultimate failure, and for this reason the risk would appear to be doubled in patients after the age of 35, but only because the patient, in getting older, tends to occupy a lower functional grade.

Some guidance may be obtained from the history of how a patient fared in previous pregnancies, and other factors are the willingness of a patient to co-operate in submitting to in-patient care if necessary. Any complication of pregnancy doubles its significance in the case of the cardiac patient.

If a patient starts her pregnancy with no signs whatever of failure, she is unlikely to fail later in the absence of other complications, provided her lesion is not so gross as to make failure rapidly possible whether pregnant or not.

The prognosis is most fully revealed between the 28th and the 32nd week when the heart is shouldering its greatest load, and if the patient's condition is satisfactory then, the outlook for labour is very good. The need for assessing cardiac enlargement earlier in pregnancy has already been mentioned, and in most cases in which it can be unquestionably proven it is a bad prognostic sign.

Repeated Pregnancies

In subsequent pregnancies there is often a tendency for the patient to fall into a lower grade than that in which she passed her first pregnancy, but this to a large extent depends upon the care she gets, and much of the deterioration is due to the work involved in looking after such children as have already arrived. When cardiac breakdown occurs in later pregnancies, it most commonly does so with the third.

Fœtal Prognosis

This is also influenced somewhat adversely, the neonatal death rate being slightly higher in patients with cardiac disease, mainly

because of prematurity. Postmaturity tends not to be very common in cardiac disease, so that, fortunately, induction of labour seldom has to be undertaken on that account, but prematurity is definitely more common. Some of this may be due to the lower social grading as a general rule of patients with rheumatic heart disease, but certainly any failure during pregnancy enormously increases the hazard of premature labour supervening at what is now a most dangerous time and great effort must be directed towards getting the patient out of failure as much as getting her out of labour if possible. The two are a deadly combination.

MANAGEMENT DURING PREGNANCY

The patient's cardiac grade should be decided during the first four months of pregnancy if possible, and management will depend upon the grade in which she is placed, but certain general principles are applicable to all of them. In the first place, ample rest should be secured and exertion permitted only to a degree which falls just short of producing dyspnœa. The lesser grades need only be seen monthly during the early part of pregnancy, but the more severe should preferably be seen every week, although the exertion of visits to the antenatal clinic must be taken into account. As far as possible steps should be taken to avoid infection, and any febrile illness should be taken seriously should it occur. There is much to be said for the prophylactic use of sulphonamides in small dosage, e.g. 0·5 g. daily. During pregnancy failure is not as a rule unheralded, and a vigilant watch should be kept for its earliest signs, paying particular attention to the lung bases.

Cases in Grades I and II should have 12 hours in bed at night and, if possible, 2 hours' rest during the middle of the day and a home-help service is of enormous value in enabling a patient to carry out these instructions conscientiously. The patient should go to bed even for a very mild cold, because respiratory tract infections are more likely to precipitate failure than labour itself.

The patient should, of course, be weighed at every antenatal examination, and excessive weight gain should be restricted as far as possible by diet and reduced salt intake. More severe degrees of fluid retention call for admission to hospital.

Anæmia is one of the most common complications, which should be diagnosed early and vigorously treated.

Re-assessment of the patient's grade is carried out between the 28th and 32nd week, and any deterioration should thereupon be reversed by complete bed rest before labour becomes imminent. Cases in Grade III already have some signs of failure, and should be in hospital if necessary throughout pregnancy, while cases in Grade

IV are in such peril that there should be no question of allowing them up and about.

It may seem curious that one advises admission to hospital during the last fortnight of pregnancy in cases in Grades I and II when this is the period when the heart is being gently but progressively relieved of some of its load, and it is popularly taught that one is aiming to rest the heart before labour starts. The chief reason, of course, is that the patient is far less likely to catch a respiratory tract infection if she is kept in hospital during that time, and if one should occur it can be spotted immediately and treated energetically. The standard practice of admission to hospital at or before the 38th week obviates the dangers of transporting such a case after labour has actually started. Certain types of influenza, e.g. Asian 'flu, of which there was an epidemic in West Scotland some years ago, proved very dangerous in pregnant patients with rheumatic heart disease and we had four maternal deaths from this ugly combination within the region over a short period of time.

The condition of the teeth should be attended to thoroughly, because there is some evidence that the risk of subacute bacterial endocarditis may thereby be reduced. If this dreaded complication occurs, it should be treated with massive doses of penicillin, and labour should be conducted under this protective "umbrella", which must be continued for at least two weeks into the puerperium.

Subacute bacterial endocarditis is due to the *Streptococcus viridans* and vegetations are liable to form on any valve which is deformed either congenitally or by disease. The infection may lie dormant in the genital tract, but a particularly dangerous source is provided by dental roots and areas of dental caries. A patient who has a proven or suspected bacterial endocarditis should be put on to large doses of penicillin at once, starting with a loading dose of two million units, and while blood cultures are obtained the dental roots should be X-rayed. Extraction should only be undertaken with full antibiotic cover, preferably as soon as possible after the antibiotic has been started because although resistance to penicillin is uncommon, provided adequate dosage is maintained, occasionally the *Str. viridans* may require another potent antibiotic. If the patient is already receiving penicillin at the time a dental extraction is contemplated, it is as well to switch to another antibiotic, for example, erythromycin 300 mg. by intramuscular injection about a quarter of an hour before the extraction is undertaken; an oral dose thereafter of 250 mg. being maintained six hourly for two or three days.

Cephaloridine (2 grams intramuscularly) is also a good alternative and must be given unhesitatingly and repeated in 1 gram injections 8 or 12 hourly (a) if penicillin resistance is suspected; (b) where major dental treatment is to be undertaken in a patient already on

prophylactic penicillin, and (c) when the membranes rupture in the case of a patient already receiving penicillin, the objective being as stated to prevent the emergence of penicillin-resistant strains.

Apart from attention to teeth and such potential sources of infection, the patient's general health as regards diet, rest and fresh air should receive careful attention. Vitamins are often prescribed particularly the vitamin B complex and an adequate intake of calcium through milk is desirable. Urinary infections should be spotted early and eliminated as far as possible. Next to anæmia, preventive medicine here will yield one of the really big dividends in antenatal care.

The onset of pre-eclamptic toxæmia should be taken even more seriously than usual, not only because of the increased burden on the heart from the hypertension but also because of the increased fluid retention which is a part of that disease. Proteinuria may be due to pre-eclamptic toxæmia, cardiac failure, or both, or may be the first indication of urinary infection.

Occasionally and coincidentally hydramnios may complicate the picture and embarrass the patient's cardiac condition still further. This should be treated by abdominal paracentesis.

Above all, failure must be controlled before labour starts, and in nearly every case this is possible. The instances of inability to do so are due to the onset of an unpredictable upper respiratory tract infection.

Recently, the question of surgical treatment of mitral stenosis by valvotomy has come under consideration, and in suitable cases the operation can be carried out at almost any stage of pregnancy; in fact, Brock has performed such an operation as late as the 36th week. and O'Connell and Mulcahy report a successful case at term. Certain criteria of suitability, however, have to be observed, and these, to some extent, restrict its application, namely mitral stenosis should be of a severe degree with only a minor degree of associated mitral incompetence, the other valves should be almost normal, nor should there be any marked left ventricular enlargement. The operation has a very definite place as an emergency procedure in cases who continue in failure in spite of a fair trial of medical treatment, and Marshall and Pantridge find the operation preferable to termination of pregnancy. In a similar and more recent series Wade *et al.* likewise find that operation is not made more dangerous by pregnancy and that the fœtal chances are not worsened as compared with medically treated cases (although they warn that the groups of cases are not strictly comparable). They too feel that valvotomy is to be preferred to termination.

In my own practice I have never yet seen fit to recommend a case for mitral valvotomy during pregnancy and my attitude has somewhat hardened by having personally to undergo this operation myself. I found it a very disagreeable experience and would think more than

twice before I subjected a pregnant woman to it. It would be far better to carry out valvotomy as an elective procedure between pregnancies, as Gilchrist recommends, so that the only cases in pregnancy which can fairly be considered are cases of emergency. Unfortunately the operation is likely to be disqualified or certainly made more dangerous by the very conditions most likely to give rise to the emergency, namely an acute respiratory infection or a pulmonary embolus.

It is worth considering the likely fate of patients who have had mitral valvotomy either before the current pregnancy or during it, and the study of 36 such patients has been made at Guy's Hospital.[9] There were 18 in the latter group, namely those who still had to face delivery after valvotomy while pregnant. In this group only 3 reached the period of alleged maximum cardiac output, some of them deteriorating in much earlier pregnancy. The results were encouraging and indicated that valvotomy, whether carried out in pregnancy or not, did not appear to hasten the subsequent deterioration of the patient. The factor of age is very important and the advice is given that patients should complete their reproductive careers while still young, rather than waiting a long time between pregnancies because such delay does not improve their fitness for the next pregnancy, but merely gives them more time in which to get older and to deteriorate in accordance with the natural history of the disease.

Onset of Failure

The patient should be admitted at once and kept in hospital for the rest of pregnancy. Bed rest must be absolute and fluid intake should be restricted. Sedatives should be liberally given and the patient should be digitalised, whether or not the heart is failing with irregular rhythm. It has to be remembered that to some extent digitalis is a cumulative drug, and overdosage can easily occur, the signs of which are nausea, vomiting, a tightness in the chest and a pulse rate lower than 60. In severe overdosage the beats may be coupled. Atrial fibrillation, of course, demands digitalis and anticoagulant therapy, preferably with warfarin, the dose being controlled by thrombotest, must be established, because of the risk of embolism.

Smoking enormously aggravates the symptoms of pulmonary congestion, namely, sputum and cough, which exhausts the patient and aggravates the failure. We had one such case in a young woman who smoked secretly and managed to aim the cigarette ends through the window; for a time it appeared as though all our treatment was of no avail, until a one-eyed Matron visiting the hospital noticed the enormous collection on the path outside and drew the attention of the nursing staff to it. The patient, who besides her cardiac lesion

REFERENCES

1. BARRY, A. (1952). *Irish J. med. Sci.*, 6th series, October, p. 398.
2. *British Medical Journal* (1961). Leading article **1**, 1520.
3. BUNIM, J. J., and APPEL, S. B. (1950). *J. Amer. med. Ass.*, **142**, 90.
4. BUNIM, J. J., and TAUBE, H. (1951). *Med. Clin. N. Amer.*, **35**, 667.
5. CLAYTON, S., and ORAM, S. (1951). *Medical Disorders in Pregnancy* London: J. & A. Churchill.
6. CROOKS, J. (1957). *Postgrad. med. J.*, **33**, 322.
7. CROOKS, J. (1962). Personal communication.
8. CROOKS, J., KHAIR, S. A., MACGREGOR, A. G., and Turnbull, A. C. (1962). *Brit. med. J.* **2**, 1259.
9. ELLIS, J. D. (1967). *J. Obstet. Gynaec. Brit. Cwlth.*, **74**, 24.
10. GILCHRIST, A. R. (1962). Lock Lecture, Royal Faculty of Physicians and Surgeons, Glasgow, "Cardiological Problems in Younger Women."
11. HAIG, D. C., and GILCHRIST, A. R. (1949). *Edinb. med. J.*, **56**, 55.
12. HAMILTON, H. F. H. (1950). *Edinb. med. J.*, **57**, 1.
13. HAWE, P., and FRANCIS, H. H. (1962). *Brit. med. J.*, **2**, 817.
14. KELLAR, R. J. (1950). *Edinb. med. J.*, **57**, 27.
15. KENMURE, A. C. F., and CAMERON, A. J. V. (1967). *Brit. Heart J.*, **29**, 910.
16. KERR, A., and SODEMAN, W. A. (1951). *Amer. Heart J.*, **42**, 436.
17. LEES, M. M., TAYLOR, S. H., SCOTT, D. B., and KERR, M. G. (1967). *J. Obstet. Gynaec. Brit. Cwlth.*, **74**, 319.
18. MCMICHAEL, J. (1952). *Brit. med. J.*, **2**, 525.
19. MACRAE, D. J. (1948). *J. Obstet. Gynaec. Brit. Emp.*, **55**, 184.
20. MARSHALL, R. J., and PANTRIDGE, J. F. (1957). *Brit. med. J.*, **1**, 1097.
21. MENDELSON, C. L. (1956). *Amer. J. Obstet. Gynec.*, **72**, 1268.
22. MORGAN JONES, A. (1944). *Postgrad. med. J.*, **20**, 176.
23. MORGAN JONES, A. (1952). *Practitioner*, **168**, 49.
24. O'CONNELL, T. C. J., and MULCAHY, R. (1955). *Brit. med. J.*, **1**, 1191.
25. O'DRISCOLL, K. M., COYLE, C. F. V., and DRURY, M. I. (1962). *Brit. med J.*, **2**, 767.
26. PRITCHARD, J. A. (1953). *Obstet. gynec. Surv.*, **8**, 775.
27. RIVLIN, R. S., MELMAN, K. L., and SJOERDSMA, A. (1965). *New Engl. J. Med.*, **272**, 1143.
28. ROSENTHAL, L. (1955). *Brit. med. J.*, **1**, 16.
29. STEPTOE, P. C. (1967). *Laparoscopy in Gynaecology*. Edinburgh: E. & S. Livingstone.
30. SUTHERLAND, A. M., and BRUCE, D. F. (1962). *J. Obstet. Gynaec. Brit. Cwlth.*, **69**, 99.
31. SZEKELY, P., and SNAITH, L. (1961). *Brit. med. J.*, **1**, 1407.
32. WALTERS, W. A. W., MACGREGOR, W. G., and HILLS, M. (1966). *Clin. Sci.* **30**, 1.
33. WILSON, G. M. (1967). *Prescribers' J.*, **7**, 1.

CHAPTER V

DIABETES MELLITUS

THE interest in this complication of pregnancy is now increasing, not only because of its serious fœtal prognosis, but because of the interesting speculations and experimental work which are coming to light in the field of endocrinology. Diabetes is not a common complication as yet, and occurs on average once in every 300 pregnancies, although in certain centres with large diabetic clinics, as for example at King's College Hospital, the incidence is one in 50 pregnancies.

The Effect of Diabetes upon Fertility

Before the discovery of insulin, and in the case of the uncontrolled diabetic, infertility was the rule. Many of these cases tend to have amenorrhœa and, in the pre-insulin era, only about 2 per cent of diabetic patients conceived. Increasing numbers of diabetics are now becoming pregnant, and the fertility rate is now 25–30 per cent. Therefore, testing the urine for sugar in the case of a woman complaining of sterility still remains an important part of the investigation.

Once a diabetic woman has become pregnant, her chances of aborting are generally agreed to be considerably increased, although concrete evidence for this is hard to find, because figures for the abortion rate of the population as a whole are, for a variety of reasons, unreliable. Peel and Oakley reckoned that the rate for abortion in diabetics was reduced by about a third as a result of insulin, but admitted that the figures were not entirely trustworthy. In the series quoted by Louw and Sinclair (1957) only 2 out of 127 pregnant diabetics aborted.

GLYCOSURIA

We are concerned here with the case of the woman who, at the antenatal clinic, presents with a reducing substance in her urine. This, if present, is nearly always glucose, and only on rare occasions is the reduction of Benedict's or Fehling's solution due to lactose, as may uncommonly occur towards the end of pregnancy, or other reducing substances. Nobody nowadays bothers to do osazone tests or fermentation reactions to clinch the diagnosis of glycosuria, because modern paper strip materials embedded with the necessary agents such as Tes-Tape and Klinistix have got rid of half the mess and bother of side-room urine testing. Both are specific for glucose

qualitatively when dipped in urine although neither is quantitatively accurate.[11] They are mainly useful in antenatal clinics for confirming glycosuria but not for determining its severity. The chief point to settle is whether or not the presence of glucose in the urine denotes the existence of diabetes. If acetone is also present, it makes the diagnosis of diabetes more than probable, but in the majority of cases this is not found.

Glycosuria is commoner at some time or other in pregnancy the more often one looks for it; for instance in a series reported from Newport, Monmouthshire, over 9 per cent of 1,500 cases showed glycosuria and when a series of 30 cases of pregnancy were tested round the clock, glycosuria was found in over 70 per cent, whereas the incidence in a control group was 13 per cent.[7] Certainly it would appear that unselected cases in pregnancy given a 50 g. oral dose of glucose show a 90 per cent incidence of glycosuria by Klinistix testing. It is suggested that it may be worth reviewing the usefulness of the standard glucose tolerance test in pregnancy. We ourselves are interested in a modified glucose tolerance test introduced by one of our members[10] which is very suitable for out-patient practice and involves simply the taking of a fasting venous blood specimen and a two-hour specimen following 50 g. of glucose orally, and dispensing with urine testing. Using this test the criteria of the fasting blood sugar in the normal case should be less than 110 mg. per cent and the two-hour specimen should not be more than 30 mg. above the fasting level. If either figure is abnormal, then a full glucose tolerance test curve is done. The convenience of such an arrangement is very obvious, without loss of diagnostic accuracy. It is suggested that such a test should be carried out in all cases in which glycosuria is found in small amounts on more than one occasion, or on any one occasion in quantities amounting to more than a trace.

The commonest cause of glycosuria in pregnancy is a lowered renal threshold. In these cases the sugar tolerance curve is perfectly normal. This lowering of the renal threshold is a common physiological occurrence in normal pregnancy, but it occurs also in diabetes, and may make the latter much more difficult to control. The renal threshold usually falls between the third and the fifth month of pregnancy, and may remain at this low level until after delivery. The condition is of no pathological significance and no treatment is indicated.

A less common type of physiological glycosuria is that referred to by some as alimentary. It is due to a rapid absorption of carbohydrate from the gut, which produces, temporarily, a level of blood sugar above the renal threshold before the mechanism of storage has had time to take effect. Glucose tolerance estimations show what is known as a lag storage curve, a term which explains itself.

A few cases may show a type of tolerance curve which has the sustained lag characteristic of diabetes, without necessarily being, in fact, diabetic in the full clinical sense. This type of mild diabetic curve may appear temporarily in the presence of sepsis, thyrotoxicosis, hyperpituitarism, and chromaffin suprarenal tumours. It is also characteristic of many so-called senile diabetics.

In any patient who exhibits even transient glycosuria, it is important to check back on any close family history of diabetes and to review once more any relevant obstetrical history from the patient such as unexplained stillbirth or previous baby of more than 9 lb. birthweight. A full glucose tolerance test should be undertaken in such a case without more ado. At this moment, as I write, I am smarting for my failure to take notice of mild and temporary glycosuria many weeks ago in early pregnancy of one of my patients whose father is a known diabetic. Her own past obstetric history is unblemished and her antenatal course uneventful, but she has just been delivered of a large, macerated stillborn baby at term. Only a fortnight ago (after the fœtal heart had stopped without warning) did I ascertain her glucose tolerance which showed a diabetic type of curve without frank diabetes. Had such a curve been demonstrated a few months ago premature induction might have saved the baby. Although not yet a diabetic she is likely to become so in a few years. This matter is discussed later.

In not a few cases the existence of diabetes only comes to light as a result of the patient's routine examination in pregnancy.

While it is important to diagnose diabetes if present as early as possible in pregnancy, for the positive reasons of being able to institute treatment early and to stave off some of the worst disasters, it is catastrophic to fail to make the diagnosis through omission to test the urine for sugar. A case so neglected may, a few weeks later, present in coma provoked by an acute infection or some other such complication.

MATERNAL MORTALITY

Before insulin was introduced there was an immediate maternal mortality of over 25 per cent of the cases who approached anywhere near term. A few of these died during pregnancy, but the majority in the puerperium. As many again died within the ensuing two years, so that the mortality, as the result of pregnancy in diabetes, was about 50 per cent. Although the risks of childbearing are still appreciably greater in diabetics than in normal women, this prohibitive mortality has now, thanks to proper control, been reduced so that Peel and Oakley at King's College Hospital gave a mortality of 1·4 per cent in 141 cases as far back as 1949. In a control series

collected from a variety of centres by questionnaire, the mortality was 2·8 per cent, eight out of thirteen cases dying in coma.

At about the same time White from the New England Deaconess Hospital reported a series of 439 diabetic pregnancies, in which only one patient died, and that was 50 days after delivery, giving the astonishing figure of 0.2 per cent. More than half of this series had had diabetes since before the age of 20. In all 439 cases hormone assays were carried out. This very satisfactory figure was achieved in spite of the increased incidence of complications during pregnancy which is inevitable in diabetes, and White remarked that almost half the cases had a raised blood pressure or albuminuria or both.

FŒTAL MORTALITY

Effect of Maternal Diabetes on the Baby

The longer a patient has suffered from diabetes the more hazardous does pregnancy become for both mother and child, particularly if the duration of the disease exceeds 25 years, and it depends to a large extent upon the pre-existence of vascular disease. Peel and Oakley, however, did not consider that fœtal mortality is appreciably influenced by the duration of diabetes. White has drawn attention to the condition of the blood vessels of the mother in fœtal prognosis, and reports that, where radiological evidence of calcification of blood vessels within the pelvis exists, the chances of fœtal survival are no more than 10 per cent.

Unfortunately, the introduction of insulin has not conferred the same benefits upon the baby as it has upon the mother, and the fœtal loss, due to intra-uterine and neonatal death, still ranges in some centres from 40 per cent to 55 per cent. This is no improvement upon the 41 per cent loss which Whitridge Williams noted in 1909, although the comparison is not entirely fair since only the mildest cases of diabetes at that time became pregnant.

This depressing level refers to the country as a whole, but Peel up to the end of 1957 reported a total fœtal mortality of 24 per cent as compared with 40 per cent in a control questionnaire series (his later fœtal loss figures have now been reduced to 13 per cent). He states that intra-uterine fœtal death is particularly liable to occur in cases where the diabetes is inadequately controlled, where hydramnios is marked, when the baby's size is clearly excessive, in hypertension and in the pre-diabetic state. One-third of his cases died *in utero* and well over half of them died shortly after birth. This was in marked contrast to the number of babies dying in the control series, in which almost half died *in utero*, a quarter died during labour, and a further quarter died in the neonatal period. It would appear, therefore, that treatment not only influences the gross fœtal survival

rate, but the period at which death occurs, and, in this matter, earlier termination of pregnancy has had a considerable effect. It is now generally agreed that the intra-uterine death rate rises progressively during the last six weeks of pregnancy.

White's series was so large that an extensive and an accumulated experience must have contributed in no small measure to her success. In my own unit in Glasgow in four years we delivered thirty diabetic mothers with only two neonatal deaths and no stillbirths, a perinatal mortality of 6·7 per cent, and in both of these serious complicating factors operated, namely severe pre-eclamptic toxæmia in one and Rh hæmolytic disease in the other. The following factors influence the baby's chance of survival:

1. *Proper control of the maternal diabetes.* Although brief ketosis or hypoglycæmia seldom cause the death of the baby, diabetic coma is unquestionably dangerous.

2. *Pre-eclamptic toxæmia.* The occurrence of this complication more than doubles the fœtal mortality in the case of diabetic pregnancy as compared with non-diabetic, and although it is only one of the causes of intra-uterine death, it is associated with a fœtal loss of about 45 per cent.

3. *Essential hypertension.*

4. *Fœtal abnormality.* The incidence here is very much higher and ranges from 4 to 6 per cent in different centres.

5. *Prematurity.* In a large number of cases labour is deliberately induced or Cæsarean section performed some weeks before term, but in a significant number the spontaneous onset of premature labour also occurs.

6. *The existence of hydramnios.* Although frequently associated with fœtal abnormality, it is present, to some degree, in all diabetic pregnancies. If severe, it may precipitate spontaneous premature labour, or it may call for treatment which incidentally brings pregnancy to an end. It is often to be regarded as a sinister sign and betokens a higher risk of fœtal death.[4]

7. *The age of onset of the diabetes and the duration of the disease before pregnancy.* On the whole the younger the onset the worse the outlook.

8. *Hormone imbalance during pregnancy.* This matter is dealt with later.

9. *Dystocia.* This may occur during labour because the baby is unusually large. With proper obstetric supervision this factor should not operate.

10. *Asphyxia at birth.* These babies, especially after Cæsarean section, may be very difficult to resuscitate. (See chapter on resuscitation of the newborn.)

11. *Fœtal hypoglycæmia immediately after birth.* The blood sugar

in normal babies is about 40 to 50 mg. per cent during the first 24 hours of life, but in diabetic babies the level is often lower and may reach 25 mg. per cent, which accentuates the tremendous difference from the conditions obtaining while still *in utero*. Before birth, the fœtus tends to have a very high blood sugar comparable with that of its mother. Although it very quickly adjusts itself to its new environment, some degree of hyperinsulinism immediately after birth is likely to make itself felt.

12. *Atelectasis*. This is very common, and, as discussed in the chapter on resuscitation of the newborn, it may have something to do with the large quantities of fluid present in the stomach at birth, especially after Cæsarean section. The fluid is regurgitated and aspirated, and whereas the child begins by breathing fairly well, it develops cyanotic attacks a few hours afterwards and dies with atelectasis.

13. *Jaundice*. Jaundice may retard the child's progress from the second day onwards until it fades.

Most of the neonatal deaths occur within the first 48 hours, by far the larger number occurring within the first 12.

Lastly, there is an increased risk of neonatal infection, especially after vaginal delivery. Considering this formidable list of hazards, it is remarkable that the results are not worse.

The babies are so large for the period of gestation that they have in the past frequently been wrongly classed as postmature. The excessive birth weight is to some extent related to the degree of hydramnios present, Peel and Oakley reporting that 70 per cent of babies weighing more than 7 pounds at 36 weeks' gestation were associated with marked hydramnios. In appearance, these babies at birth often look as fat as butter, for they are bloated and œdematous. Their behaviour is lethargic, and cyanotic attacks appear to occur with a sort of indolent ease. Both spleen and liver are usually enlarged, and in both these organs there is excessive hæmopoiesis. The heart is also somewhat enlarged, and in the pancreas there is islet hyperplasia. Placental insufficiency is often postulated to account for these overgrown babies who die so readily *in utero* but this is almost impossible to establish from examination and histology of the placenta. Endometritis may be seen in biopsies of the placental bed but only in those diabetic cases complicated by pre-eclampsia or hypertension (Peel).

White distinguished fœtal prognosis in cases in which the mother showed no hormonal imbalance during pregnancy from those in which such was present, and she stated that where the balance is normal the fœtal survival is approximately 96 per cent, but that where imbalance is present the fœtal survival is only 50 per cent. By substitution therapy in the cases of hormonal imbalance, she managed to

improve fœtal survival from 50 per cent to 90 per cent and, in so doing, lowered the incidence of complicating pre-eclamptic toxæmia from 50 per cent to 5 per cent. These findings have not been supported on this side of the Atlantic.

The very wide variation in fœtal prospects shown by different workers only serves to emphasise the need for very close co-operation between physician, obstetrician, and pædiatrician, and this factor, more than any other, must influence the results.

THE PRE-DIABETIC STATE

Much interest has been focused upon the association of large babies and mothers who subsequently develop diabetes mellitus. While it has long been known that diabetic women tended to have large babies, it is only more recently that the association has been noticed in cases exhibiting a latent interval, often amounting to many years, before developing the disease. Kriss and Futcher noted that 77 per cent of 144 babies whose birth weights exceeded 10 pounds were born to women who subsequently developed diabetes, and, where a family history of diabetes existed, they noted too that the babies tended to be larger. They regard birth weights of over 10 pounds as significant, and it would appear that the average birth weight was greater in pre-diabetic cases than in those who had actually developed the disease.

The latent interval between the birth of such a child and the development of clinical diabetes may range up to 40 years, and Kriss and Futcher give the average as 24 years. What is even more important is that there is a higher fœtal mortality during the maternal pre-diabetic state than normal, although the onset of true diabetes worsens the fœtal outlook still further. Peel and Oakley quote a fœtal loss of 23 per cent in pre-diabetic pregnancies, and Gilbert and Dunlop found that the over-all pre-diabetic fœtal loss rate was twice as high as in non-diabetic pregnancy and three times as high in cases developing diabetes before the age of 45.

It also appears that the fœtal mortality rate increases the nearer the mother is to developing the full-blown disease, and the loss is at its highest in the two years before its appearance, reaching a figure which is not worsened during the period of established diabetes. The pre-diabetic loss rate, however, gives no indication of the severity of the diabetes to follow.

At a superficial glance it would appear that the babies of pre-diabetic mothers have a higher birth weight than those born to frank diabetics, but it is not nowadays possible to make a comparison, since pregnancy is so commonly interrupted prematurely when the diagnosis is established.

Considering the high perinatal death rate in the phase of maternal

pre-diabetes it would be useful if the diagnosis could be reliably established before catastrophe overtook the baby. To this end glucose tolerance curves are none too helpful although a tendency to the "lag" type of curve is often seen. Cortisone has a known diabetogenic activity and Fajans and Conn (1954) used this in developing the cortisone stressed glucose tolerance test in the hope of unmasking the potential diabetic whose carbohydrate tolerance was still normal by ordinary standards. The technique which they devised was to carry out first a normal glucose tolerance test after a standard 300 g. daily diet of carbohydrate for 3 days and then to repeat the test next day following a priming with 50 to 62·5 mg. of cortisone orally administered 8½ and 2 hours before the same glucose load as before. They found not only a number of hitherto undiagnosed diabetics among the relatives of known diabetics, but also found a positive result to the cortisone stressed tolerance test in no less than 24 per cent of these relatives of diabetics whose own diabetes had not yet declared itself.

Obstetricians as a whole, however, have not taken up the cortisone stressed glucose tolerance test and Peel, for example, frankly regards it as unreliable and misleading. Certainly a family history and a history of large stillborn babies is far more significant.

Because a pre-diabetic pregnant patient may give a normal glucose tolerance curve and yet her pre-diabetic state may cause abnormal deliveries, or presage, less commonly, acromegaly or Cushing's syndrome, a search for some test as sensitive and yet less misleading would be thoroughly worth while. Furthermore the glucose tolerance curve can be abnormal in pregnancy and yet return to normal in the puerperium (latent diabetes), only for such cases to become frankly diabetic in a few years' time.[5] One of the weaknesses of the standard glucose tolerance curve is that the oral administration of glucose may give variable results because of a variable absorption rate, hence the prednisone-glycosuria test was evolved.[12] In this test, glucose tolerance curve is first carried out to exclude genuine diabetes. Following this, 20 mg. of prednisone are given four hourly for three doses associated with fasting. Urine is collected over the next ten hours and the amount of glucose passed is estimated. If there is glycosuria blood samples are taken four and five hours after the last prednisone dose. Sugar in the urine is estimated by the copper thiosulphate titration method. In normal cases, whether pregnant or not, the glucose titration in the urine does not exceed 60 mg. per hour, whereas in pre-diabetes, in cases of mild diabetes and in all cases of renal glycosuria, much higher figures are given. Cases of renal glycosuria, of course, have already been identified by the simpler tests already enumerated.

Although diabetes, as already mentioned, is a cause of infertility,

this would not appear to be the case while the woman is still in the pre-diabetic state. It is now recognised as almost certain that excessive secretion of the growth factor by the anterior lobe of the pituitary is responsible for the combination of progressive maternal obesity, large babies, and the subsequent onset of diabetes. Certainly if women who have had babies weighing more than 10½ lb. are followed up for a number of years diabetes is likely to declare itself in a significant number.

Fitzgerald *et al.* (1961) in Birmingham studied 61 such cases and 20 were already diabetic within thirteen years and more than half those whose ages at the follow-up examination were over 45 years had abnormal glucose tolerance curves.

HORMONE IMBALANCE IN DIABETIC PREGNANCY

The role of the pituitary growth hormone has been studied by Young in relation to experimental diabetes. This worker, in the experimental extracts used, has not been able to demonstrate the separate existence of growth hormone, diabetogenic hormone, and pancreatotrophic hormone, and it seems that these three separate effects are merely related facets of the same substance.

The large size of the baby is not due to postmaturity, because, contrary to traditional belief, diabetic pregnancy is not often abnormally prolonged. Young has pointed out that for the growth hormone to operate, additional insulin together with an adequate blood sugar range must be produced by the pancreatic islets. This is produced either by the direct effect of the growth hormone upon the pancreas, thus increasing the production of insulin, or, he suggests, the growth hormone may antagonise the peripheral action of insulin and may cause it to be utilised in the tissues at such a high rate that the level of insulin in the blood falls, and as a result the islets may be stimulated to produce even more.

The known hypertrophy of the fœtal pancreatic islets in cases of maternal diabetes is due to hyperplasia of the beta cells and insulin is therefore more copiously produced in response to the high blood sugar levels obtaining both in mother and fœtus *in utero,* so that carbohydrate utilisation and storage as fat leads to the characteristic fat overgrown baby of such a pregnancy. This hypothesis has been soundly confirmed by Baird and Farquhar (1962) who demonstrated the rise in neonatal plasma insulin-like activity (P.I.A.) in response to a glucose load administered via the umbilical vein.

Now the rat's epiphyses do not fuse throughout life, and if given growth hormone it does not develop diabetes but grows larger. The same effect has been found in puppies and kittens, but if adult dogs and cats are given enough growth hormone for a long enough period

of time, the rate of growth declines and diabetes makes its appearance. If, however, sufficient insulin is now given at the same time, the diabetes is controlled and the rate of growth is resumed. It is only when the pancreas is called upon to produce more insulin than it can achieve that diabetes occurs. So long as an animal is capable of continuing its growth under the stimulus of the growth hormone, diabetes does not develop, but if further growth, for example in the adult whose epiphyses are already fused, cannot continue beyond a certain point, then diabetes follows.

In other words, the growth hormone in the young animal produces growth and not diabetes, and Young was not able to induce diabetes by this method in pregnant animals, because the alternative result of extra growth was reflected in the development of the fœtus. A small but continuous over-production of growth hormone, therefore, over a number of years demonstrates itself preferentially in the production of large babies and only later in the overt development of the diabetic state.

During pregnancy itself the hormones connected with placental function, namely œstrogen, progesterone, and chorionic gonadotrophin, were studied by Priscilla White, and Smith and Smith, but Peel suggested that any hormone imbalance is the result of failing placental function and not the cause of it.

An enquiry conducted by the Medical Research Council (1955) found that the perinatal mortality was practically the same whether stilbœstrol and ethisterone were given or not and that there was very little difference in the other complications.

Maternal Complications

Pregnancy is liable to aggravate the diabetic condition, and it may bring it out of latency, since many cases do not declare themselves until pregnancy occurs. In diabetes, the patient is prematurely aged both physically and gynæcologically by vascular disease and threatened ovarian failure respectively. It is small wonder, therefore, that certain complications, notably pre-eclamptic toxæmia, are prone to occur.

As pregnancy advances, carbohydrate tolerance is reduced and insulin requirements usually tend to rise, especially after the sixth month until shortly before term, although in a few cases the reverse may obtain. The renal threshold is very often reduced, and the patient loses sugar through her urine in even greater quantities than before, with the result that acidosis more easily occurs. Under these circumstances, in combating acidosis with insulin, hypoglycæmia is very easily provoked, so that the patient becomes more and more difficult to stabilise. Any diabetic patient, therefore, who is likely to

get hypoglycæmic reactions when not pregnant will now become much more vulnerable in this respect. Another feature of diabetic pregnancy is the increased liability to undue water retention, which is often associated with pre-eclamptic toxæmia and with the appearance of hydramnios.

Hydramnios, as previously stated, is almost invariably present in some degree, and is marked in about a quarter of the cases.

Pre-eclamptic toxæmia supervenes in about one case in every five and very greatly worsens the fœtal prognosis. In a large proportion of cases it is a terminal event, and its incidence in diabetic pregnancy is inevitably reduced somewhat in those centres where pregnancy is deliberately interrupted at the 36th week. Frequently hydramnios and pre-eclamptic toxæmia are co-existent. The amniotic sugar level is always raised, although the level is not related directly to the amount of excess fluid. The reason for hydramnios is not certain, but it is possible that the baby, as a result of its own hyperglycæmia, passes more urine than usual, and the presence of the sugar within the amniotic fluid may irritate the amnion to produce increased amounts of liquor, quite apart from the factor of increased osmosis. Because of hydramnios, malpresentations are naturally more common, and likewise premature labour more readily occurs. As already stated, intra-uterine death becomes increasingly likely during the last four or five weeks of pregnancy.

Any acute intercurrent infection, notably pyelitis, in the course of pregnancy may have far-reaching consequences. Not only is the patient's resistance lower than that of the non-diabetic, but the control of her diabetes is immediately undermined, and she may get out of control and go into coma.

The onset of labour is rarely postmature, and inertia frequently complicates its course. Difficulties may arise during labour due to the large size of the baby, and disproportion may prejudice the issue. Even after successful delivery of the head, large shoulders may obstruct safe delivery.

In the puerperium infection, too, may take a serious course, and full lactation is hard to achieve.

MANAGEMENT IN PREGNANCY

Provided that the patient is well controlled throughout pregnancy, the diabetic state is not permanently worsened. Unfortunately, many of these cases are hard to stabilise and constant supervision is necessary. It is often not possible to get the urine sugar free, and in many cases it is undesirable, because hypoglycæmia readily occurs as a result of the associated lowering during pregnancy of the renal threshold to glucose, and the help of an experienced physician is in-

valuable in deciding not only the optimum dosage of insulin but the spacing of the injections. Because of the patient's instability, protamine zinc insulin alone is seldom satisfactory and usually has to be combined with more frequent injections of the shorter-acting insulin. For the same reason the more modern oral diabetic drugs are even less satisfactory in pregnancy. These oral diabetic drugs can be divided into two main groups, namely, the sulphonylureas and the diguanides. Two commonly used examples of the former are tolbutamide and chlorpropamide and their main action is to stimulate the release of endogenous insulin with possibly an increase in the viable beta cells of the pancreatic islets, hence the hypoglycæmic action. It also appears that the liver may be inhibited in its output of glucose. Clearly the sulphonylureas will only be useful in cases capable of producing insulin under the stimulus of such drugs and therefore the sulphonylureas are to some extent restricted to the middle aged with diabetes of relatively recent onset. Diabetic patients with a history of ketosis do not respond well. The drugs of the sulphonylurea class vary in their biological half-life, from a few hours in the case of tolbutamide to about a couple of days in the case of chlorpropamide and the latter may accumulate dangerously if there is any element of renal failure. In addition to this there are toxic effects, mainly of a dyspeptic nature; very rarely marrow aplasia and intra-canalicular biliary stasis has been attributed to them. The diguanides work in a totally different manner by stimulating the uptake of glucose in muscle, rather than in fat, and there is increased production and accumulation of lactate and pyruvate. The blood sugar may be brought down but without preventing diabetic ketosis and again toxic dyspeptic side-effects may be caused. The main use of the diguanides (phenformin and metformin) is to supplement the action of the sulphonylureas and to assist in weight loss in the obese diabetic. Quite apart from their failure, even in combination, to prevent ketosis in diabetic patients who are already insulin deficient, which is what we are commonly facing in obstetrics, control is very difficult to maintain and toxicity is readily incurred. Consequently our own view is that the oral hypoglycæmic drugs are far better replaced by proper insulin control during pregnancy.

The importance of diabetic control increases as pregnancy advances and beyond the 30th week it must be rigorous indeed to reduce the hyperglycæmia which stimulates fœtal hyperinsulinism and so increases the fœtal growth beyond the limits of placental reserve.

We now prefer to admit our diabetic mothers at the 30th week and certainly no later than the 32nd week so that this control can be maintained from day to day from then onwards; this is also made easier by securing more rest for the patient. Yet another advantage

is the earlier detection of any rise of blood pressure. The aim of insulin control should be to maintain a blood sugar at least below 180 mg. per cent.

Infections, so far as possible, should be avoided, and when they occur should be treated seriously and energetically.

The diet should be generous and should provide 30 calories per kilogramme of body weight a day, and the daily protein intake should not be less than 2 g. per kilogramme of body weight. The total daily intake of carbohydrate should not be less than 200 g., allowance being made for the needs of the baby's growth. It is often advisable to restrict sodium intake, especially in those cases in which the weight is rising unduly rapidly. Where there is evidence of undue water retention, chlorothiazide (1–2 g. daily) can be given to counteract it or frusemide 40 mg. on alternate days.

The patient should be seen at frequent intervals throughout pregnancy until admission at the 30th week, and the blood pressure and urine should be examined at each visit. In every case an X-ray of the fœtus should be taken, because the discovery of a fœtal abnormality will influence the method of delivery. In cases allowed to proceed to spontaneous labour it is often found that insulin requirement falls a day or two before delivery.

INTERRUPTION OF PREGNANCY

There is practically no indication for therapeutic abortion, however severe the condition or however bad the past obstetric history, as skilful management should nowadays be fully effective. Sterilisation after delivery is seldom indicated except in cases demonstrating a permanently raised blood pressure.

After the 36th week of pregnancy the risk of intra-uterine death of the fœtus overtakes that of neonatal death, and one has to strike a balance between leaving a baby in its unhealthy environment or challenging it to cope with prematurity, which it is ill-equipped to fight. Any set rule for determining when to deliver the child is to be deplored, although the majority of obstetricians favour interrupting the pregnancy at the end of the 36th week. A mistake about dates may involve risk of a disastrous degree of prematurity. In deciding the optimum time one should take into account the presence or absence of pre-eclamptic toxæmia, the degree of hydramnios, the severity of the diabetes, the facilities for coping with prematurity, the patient's age and her obstetric history; therefore, it will be seen that there is no rule-of-thumb method. Our present technique is to study the continuing rate of fœtal growth by repeated biparietal cephalometry by sonar, which is carried out every few days. As long as there is continuing fœtal growth we feel it can safely be assumed that intra-

uterine fœtal death is not likely to occur in the immediate future, but that as soon as the growth curve flattens off delivery should be effected within the next seven to ten days in order to forestall such a disaster. In this way we are able to avoid unnecessary premature delivery, so often the result of rule-of-thumb practice, and obtain the maximum degree of maturity consistent with intra-uterine survival.

The practice of early termination tends to transfer one's fœtal deaths from the column of stillbirth to neonatal death, but nearly two-thirds of the intra-uterine deaths occur during the last four weeks of pregnancy, and this must weight one's decision. There is an increasing tendency to reserve surgical induction for multiparous patients who have previously delivered themselves satisfactorily by the vaginal route. In the primigravida the induction-delivery interval is often prolonged at this stage of pregnancy with its increased hazards both maternal and particularly fœtal, and, even when labour starts, it is frequently inert. In all severe diabetics, therefore, and in primigravidæ and elderly patients, Cæsarean section is being increasingly favoured as an elective procedure. Our own policy is to rupture the membranes and induce labour surgically, even in primigravidæ, with the reservation that if labour is not well established within 12 to 18 hours Cæsarean section will be undertaken without more ado.

As a result of this policy more than half our diabetics are now delivered vaginally and the section rate has been reduced to 46 per cent. Two recent cases thus achieved vaginal deliveries who had been delivered before by Cæsarean section by more timid obstetricians elsewhere and we feel that, given very through supervision, the risks of a "trial of induction" are insignificant and the advantages of an expeditious labour to mother and child are well worth the attempt.

LABOUR

When the fœtus is normal, vaginal delivery is only permissible if there is no obstetrical abnormality apart from the diabetes, and any case of suspected cephalopelvic disproportion should be delivered by Cæsarean section. Trial of labour has no place in the management of the diabetic patient. Where there is fœtal abnormality, vaginal delivery should, of course, be sought if possible. The above categorical statement about disproportion is occasioned by the fear of a prolonged labour. This complication, from whatever cause, is very dangerous to both mother and child. In any labour lasting more than 24 hours, diabetes becomes increasingly difficult to control because of poor carbohydrate intake, vomiting and dehydration, with the result that the patient may easily develop ketosis. In addition to this

risk, hypoglycæmia becomes a constant and recurring nuisance, and during labour the carbohydrate intake should be maintained by intravenous drip therapy, up to 10 g. of glucose per hour. The insulin dosage is split up into small injections given every four hours. One should aim to keep some glucose present at all times in the urine, but not ketone bodies. Where the patient threatens to become unstable, 20 units of insulin may be injected and covered by 40 g. of glucose. If the patient does develop diabetic ketosis it may be observed that her low pH may be associated with a low Pco_2 due to hyperpnoea. If this is the case 200 to 500 milliequivalents of sodium bicarbonate may be required by intravenous infusion (1 ml. of 8·4 per cent sodium bicarbonate equals 1 mEq.)

Since the patient's stabilisation can be so easily undermined by infection, there is something to be said for the use of prophylactic chemotherapy unless labour shows signs of being fairly rapid. These cases are very worrying in labour and require unremitting supervision.

The baby at birth must be very competently handled, for it is œdematous, lethargic, premature, prone to atelectasis and usually has a full stomach. Mucus must be very thoroughly aspirated by a tube passed into the stomach, in order to remove its contents before they are regurgitated and aspirated. An incubator should be immediately available, and the baby should be carefully supervised, even though apparently normal, for the first 48 hours, because it is very liable to develop a cyanotic attack and die without warning, even though its initial condition appears good. A rapid weight loss in the first 2 days is a very welcome sign.

PUERPERIUM

There is a sharp fall in the patient's insulin requirements immediately after delivery, and she is very liable to hypoglycæmia at first. The insulin dosage will therefore have to be re-adjusted, and it will be found that very much less is required during the first 24 hours. Thereafter, the patient must be restabilised.

The morbidity rate is not directly increased, but the effects of infection are more serious when they occur.

It is usually hard to establish satisfactory lactation, and the majority of diabetic mothers fail within a few days. The baby also, because of its lethargy and prematurity, is less efficient at sucking, and this contributes to the disappointing result. The baby also suffers from an initial, although usually short-lived, hypoglycæmia although after the first few hours of life it comes to better terms with its new blood sugar level. Feeding within the first 2 days is far more dangerous than not feeding it, and we have now abandoned the

routine use of glucose in the early days since it would appear to make little difference to survival chances. Above all, the baby has fluid to get rid of and it would be wanton to replace it at this stage.

Respiratory failure associated with atelectasis with hyaline membrane still represents a formidable hazard and at the first sign of a cyanotic attack the pharynx, œsophagus and stomach should be aspirated by mechanical suction and in any case every few hours for the first 2 days.

The remarkably low fœtal mortality rate of 10 per cent quoted by Nelson, Gillespie and White is lower than most series. Losses can, however, be kept down to between 20–25 per cent given good team work between physician, obstetrician and pædiatrician.

REFERENCES

1. BAIRD, J. D., and FARQUHAR, J. W. (1962). *Lancet*, **1**, 71.
2. BARNES, H. H. F., and MORGANS, M. E. (1949). *Brit. med. J.*, **1**, 51.
3. BARNES, H. H. F., and MORGANS, M. E. (1952). *Brit. med. J.*, **2**, 1058.
4. CLAYTON, S. G. (1956). *J. Obstet. Gynaec. Brit. Emp.*, **63**, 532.
5. DAVEY, D. A., JOPLIN, G. F., and SANTANDER, R. (1961). *Lancet*, **1**, 71.
6. FAJANS, S. S., and CONN, J. W. (1954). *Diabetes*, **3**, 296.
7. FINE, J. (1967). *Brit. med. J.*, **1**, 205.
8. FITZGERALD, M. G., MALINS, J. M., and O'SULLIVAN, D. J. (1961). *Lancet*, **1**, 1250.
9. GILBERT, J. A. L., and DUNLOP, D. M. (1949). *Brit. med. J.*, **1**, 48.
10. HOWIE, P. (1967). Personal communication.
11. HUNT, J. A., GRAY, C. H., and THOROGOOD, D. E. (1956). *Brit. med. J.*, **2**, 586.
12. JOPLIN, G. F., FRASER, R., and KEELEY, K. J. (1961). *Lancet*, **1**, 67.
13. KRISS, J. P., and FUTCHER, P. H. (1948). *J. clin. Endocr.*, **8**, 380.
14. LOUW, J. T., and SINCLAIR, R. ST. C. (1957). *S. Afr. med. J.*, **31**, 28.
15. Medical Research Council on Diabetes and Pregnancy (1955). *Lancet*, **2**, 833.
16. NELSON, H. B., GILLESPIE, L., and WHITE, P. (1953). *Obstet. and Gynec.*, **1**, 219.
17. PEEL, J., and OAKLEY, W. (1949). *Trans. 12th Brit. Congr. Obs. Gyn.*
18. PEEL, J. (1955). *Brit. med. J.*, **2**, 870.
19. PEEL, J. (1961). *Proc. roy. Soc. Med.*, **54**, 745.
20. SMITH, O. W. (1948). *Amer. J. Obstet. Gynec.*, **56**, 821.
21. SMITH, O. W., and SMITH, G. V. S. (1949). *Amer. J. Obstet. Gynec.*, **58**, 994.
22. TUNBRIDGE, R. E., PALEY, R. G., and COULSON, D. (1956). *Brit. med. J.*, **2**, 588.
23. WHITE, P. (1945). *J. Amer. med. Ass.*, **128**, 181.
24. WHITE, P. (1947). *Med. Clin. N. Amer.*, **31**, 395.
25. WHITE, P. (1949). *Amer. J. Med.*, **7**, 609.
26. YOUNG, F. G. (1951). *J. clin. Endocr.*, **11**, 531.

CHAPTER VI

ANÆMIA AND PULMONARY
TUBERCULOSIS

ANÆMIA

ANÆMIA may antedate conception; it is often aggravated by pregnancy, and the accidents of labour may perpetuate it. It is one of the prime concerns of antenatal care to forestall it, for the safety of labour and the puerperal state, to say nothing of future health, in very large measure depend upon the state of the patient's blood. So much importance, in fact, do we now attach to this matter that it is the practice in our hospital to estimate the hæmoglobin at every antenatal visit which the patient makes throughout pregnancy. In this way the early signs of incipient anæmia and failure to respond to medication are picked up at a very early stage, leaving plenty of time to evaluate and correct any deficiency. This is a counsel of perfection and where it is not possible to have a technician from the hæmatology department in attendance at every clinic, as we have, at least four hæmoglobin estimations should be carried out in pregnancy, namely, at first booking, then at about 24 to 26 weeks' gestation, then between the 32nd and 34th and finally just before term. It is not many patients who get even that much surveillance and the more is the pity, since megaloblastic anæmia particularly can become very rapidly manifest and leave inadequate time to correct it, as will presently be discussed. It often takes almost as long to identify the nature of a given anæmia as it takes to correct it, yet there can be no more important aspect of antenatal care. The patient who has been in a chronic state of sub-health from anæmia has a poor myocardium to match and it is a dangerous form of optimism to reckon that the immediate correction of anæmia is going to be followed by an immediate increase in the resilience of the patient to withstand a traumatic or infected labour, for which adequate preparation should have been instituted long before.

Physiology

Pregnancy causes a state of hydræmic plethora; in other words, the total volume of blood is increased partly by dilution, and the hæmoglobin is consequently reduced to a varying extent, occasion-

ally as far as 80 per cent (approximately 12 g. per 100 ml.). Levels below this are pathological, and one should aim at raising the hæmoglobin to 80 per cent or more if possible before delivery. The dilution picture is, however, normochromic and normocytic.

This phenomenon is commonly regarded as physiological, which is not the same thing as saying that it is either beneficial or even necessary. It can, in fact, be a positive danger by increasing the circulatory burden, for example, in cases of cardiac disease, and, because of the reduced oxygen-carrying power of diluted blood the fœtus may be less efficiently oxygenated. Nor is hydræmia an invariable accompaniment of pregnancy and most of us would agree that the term "physiological anæmia of pregnancy" were better dropped in recognising that in nearly all women the condition can be corrected before term.[5, 15] In round figures the pregnancy demands for iron come to a total of about 900 mg. of which about 500 to 600 mg. go to the uterus and its contents. Somewhere between 150 and 200 mg. are accounted for in an average blood loss at delivery and a similar amount is expended in lactation. On top of this there is an increased maternal hæmoglobin mass of about 500 mg., the iron of which is returned to store after delivery. On the credit side, however, there is an average saving of about 225mg. as a result of the amenorrhœa throughout pregnancy, but this still leaves a total likely ultimate iron deficit of about 600 or 700 mg. It will be seen, therefore, that time is required for a reasonable diet to make good the iron overdraft of pregnancy and consequently if pregnancies succeed each other rapidly the patient is unlikely to "get out of the red".

Just how common iron deficiency is amongst the women of the United Kingdom has been reviewed in an average housing estate practice on the West side of Glasgow, which also included some suburban communities and some of the poorer industrial districts. In this practice frank iron deficiency anæmia was present in over 8 per cent of cases, but latent iron deficiency without anæmia was found in at least three times as many of the female population of all ages.[33] These figures were obtained in women who were not pregnant, but serve to show that a large proportion of the population start their pregnancies short of iron. The term "latent iron deficiency" (i.e. tissue depletion of iron without anæmia) is defined as a state in which the saturation of the total iron binding capacity is below 16 per cent, but in which the hæmoglobin level is above 12g. per 100 ml., as stainable marrow-iron will not be found in cases in which the TIBC is below 16 per cent. To what extent latent iron deficiency is important in producing some of the alleged symptoms such as irritability and ready fatigue is not certain and not relevant to the present subject, but in pregnancy at least its importance lies in the fact that a patient may start her pregnancy without overt anæmia and yet have so little

iron to fall back upon that a serious drop in hæmoglobin may occur a few weeks later which may be missed for an unnecessarily long time unless the blood is frequently examined, as is our practice.

The commonest source of trouble in anæmic pregnancy is in-adequate absorption of iron. The normal daily requirement for the gravid woman is about 20 mg. of iron, even in cases in which the iron stores have not suffered depletion prior to pregnancy. The baby, especially in the later months of pregnancy, makes heavy de-mands upon maternal iron, and the average fœtal requirements amount to about 375 mg. Unfortunately, the margin between the patient's requirements and the quantity of iron normally available in a reasonably good diet is a very narrow one, in fact, the average diet seldom contains more than about 15 mg. a day. Of the total amount of iron in food, only a fraction (about 10 per cent) is available for absorption. Natural foods, such as liver, meat, peas, eggs and certain dried fruits, for example apricots, are good sources of iron. Phytic acid, present in brown bread, which also contains iron, tends to inter-fere with iron absorption by combining with iron to form insoluble salts. The presence of calcium in the diet, however, tends to divert some of this phytic acid effect. Iron absorption is favourably influ-enced by the presence of hydrochloric acid in the stomach; conversely, the absence of hydrochloric acid or the copious intake of alkaline powders tends to reduce it. Intestinal disorders, for example chronic diarrhœa, naturally interfere with iron absorption. The ferrous salts, as is well known, are far more readily absorbed than the ferric, and Vitamin C, amongst other properties, has the power of reducing ferric to ferrous iron, hence the dietary value of fresh grown vegetables. The therapeutic implications are therefore obvious.

In the formation of red cells an active bone marrow requires not only iron and incidental traces of copper for hæmoglobin formation, but also folic acid and vitamin B_{12}, vitamin C and nucleoprotein. The further role of vitamin C is to assist in the conversion of folic acid, derived from the vitamin B complex, into folinic acid, which is necessary for the synthesis of purines and pyrimidines which ultim-ately take part, with vitamin B_{12} (the hæmopoietic principle), in the synthesis of nucleic acid and hence of nucleoprotein. The following diagram illustrates the level in hæmopoiesis at which these dietetic factors operate.

Therefore it will be seen that a lack of folic acid gives rise to macro-cytic or, as is now more usually described, "megaloblastic" anæmia. True pernicious anæmia is due to a lack of vitamin B_{12}.

After about four months the normal red cell disintegrates and the hæmoglobin is broken down into hæmosiderin and bile pig-ments.

Hæmatocytoblast

Erythroblast   Myeloblast → W.B.C. stages

Abnormally ————————————— *Normally*

with folinic acid or Vit. B_{12} Pronormoblasts
deficiency   (no hæmoglobin)

Megaloblasts   Basophilic normoblasts

Large reticulocytes   Iron→

Macrocytes   Polychromatic normoblasts

Pyknotic normoblasts

Reticulocytes

Mature erythrocytes

Definitions

The following are some definitions:

The packed red cell volume (P.C.V.) is the number of cubic centimetres of packed red cells per 100 ml. of blood.

The mean corpuscular volume (M.C.V.) is the average volume of one red cell in cubic microns.

The mean corpuscular hæmoglobin (M.C.H.) is the average hæmoglobin content of one red cell in micromicrogrammes.

The mean corpuscular hæmoglobin concentration (M.C.H.C.) is the mean or average hæmoglobin concentration in percentage per unit volume of cells.

The difference between mean corpuscular hæmoglobin (M.C.H.) and mean corpuscular hæmoglobin concentration (M.C.H.C.) should be clearly understood. The former measures the weight of hæmoglobin in the average red corpuscle and expresses the result in parts of a gramme (micromicrogramme); the latter (M.C.H.C.) indicates the concentration of hæmoglobin in the average red cell, the ratio of weight of hæmoglobin to the volume in which it is contained and the result expressed in percentage. The distinction is an important one. In most types of anæmia, increases or decreases in the average size of the red corpuscles (M.C.V.) are associated with corresponding increases or decreases in the weight of hæmoglobin

(M.C.H.) carried in the corpuscles. The ratio of these to one another is indicated by the mean corpuscular hæmoglobin concentration (M.C.H.C.).

EXAMPLES

Calculation of Mean Cell Volume (M.C.V.)

P.C.V. ÷ R.B.C.

E.g., if the P.C.V. is 45 per cent, in 1 c.mm. of blood there are 0·45 c.mm. of cells.

Therefore, if there are 5,000,000 R.B.C.s per c.mm., they occupy a volume of 0·45 c.mm.

The volume of 1 cell in cubic microns (M.C.V.)

$$= \frac{0.45 \times 1{,}000 \times 1{,}000 \times 1{,}000}{5{,}000{,}000}$$

$$= 90 \text{ cubic microns.}$$

N.B. 1 mm. = 1,000 microns. 1 cubic mm. = 1,000 × 1,000 × 1,000 cubic microns.

Calculation of Mean Corpuscular Hæmoglobin (M.C.H.)

Hb. in G. ÷ R.B.C.

E.g., if there are 15 g. of Hb. per 100 ml. of blood, there is 15 ÷ 100 in 1 ml.

Therefore, in 1 c.mm. there is $\dfrac{15 \text{ g.}}{100 \times 1{,}000}$.

If there are 5,000,000 R.B.C.s per c.mm., the mean (or 1 cell) would contain $\dfrac{15 \text{ g.}}{100 \times 1{,}000 \times 5{,}000{,}000}$.

The formula has been calculated so that the result may be given in micromicrogrammes (millionth of a millionth of a gramme or $(g. \times 10^{-12})$).

The mean corpuscular hæmoglobin is therefore:

$$\frac{15 \times 1{,}000{,}000{,}000{,}000{,}000}{100 \times 1{,}000 \times 5{,}000{,}000} = 30 \text{ micromicrogrammes.}$$

Calculation of Mean Corpuscular Hæmoglobin Concentration (M.C.H.C.)

Hb. in g. ÷ P.C.V.

E.g., if there are 15 g. Hb. per 100 ml. of blood and if there are 45 per cent of packed red cells, the Hb. concentration would be 15 ÷ 45.

The result is expressed in per cent, so $\dfrac{15 \times 100}{45} = 33.3$ per cent.

Normal Values

R.B.C. 5 million/c.mm.
Hb. 14·8 G./100 ml.
Reticulocytes 0·2 per cent.
P.C.V. (hæmatocrit) 39–42 per cent.
M.C.V. 78–94 cμ
M.C.H. 27–32 μμg.
. M.C.H.C. 30 per cent (28–34 per cent).

Examples.—In iron deficiency anæmia (hypochromic microcytic) the reduction in red cell volume and hæmoglobin content are characteristically more marked than reduction in the number of red cells. M.C.H.C. is reduced.

In megaloblastic anæmia (macrocytic) the red cells are increased in volume, the mean corpuscular hæmoglobin is proportionally increased, and there is an increase in the size and hæmoglobin content of the red cells roughly inversely proportional to the number of cells. The mean corpuscular hæmoglobin concentration remains fairly normal throughout or may be slightly reduced.

In normocytic anæmia the number of red cells is reduced without any or at most a slight increase in M.C.V., and the M.C.H. and M.C.H.C. are normal throughout.

Table of Equivalents

Hb. per cent	Hb. g./100 ml.	Hb. per cent	Hb. g./100 ml.
10	1·5	70	10·3
15	2·2	75	11·1
20	3·0	80	11·8
25	3·7	85	12·6
30	4·4	90	13·3
35	5·2	95	14·1
40	5·9	100	14·8
45	6·6	105	15·5
50	7·4	110	16·3
55	8·1	115	17·0
60	8·9	120	17·8
65	9·6		

Clinically one may classify the anæmias associated with pregnancy as:

    (1) **Iron deficiency**
    (2) **Megaloblastic**

(3) **Hæmolytic**
(4) **Secondary**, for example to repeated bleeding, chronic infection, Hodgkin's disease, etc.
(5) **Aplastic varieties**

IRON DEFICIENCY ANÆMIA

This is the commonest type and, depending upon the social grades of patients, may be found in up to nearly a quarter of all pregnancies. Multiparity, previous menorrhagia and subnutrition favour its origin. It may be due to dietary insufficiency or to interferences with iron absorption. In the latter respect the digestive upsets which are common in pregnancy frequently operate adversely. Achlorhydria, too, if present, discourages absorption.

The importance of chronic infection in the ætiology of iron deficiency anæmia must not be overlooked and this is particularly true of chronic and apparently latent pyelonephritis. In fact a urinary infection may present as a case of apparently refractory anæmia and is more than twice as common in anæmic patients as in controls in spite of administering prophylactic iron and folic acid routinely in pregnancy.[22] In such cases appropriate antibacterial therapy is first necessary before a response to hæmatinics can be expected. The mechanism for this is not clear, but it must be a clinical observation common to all of us. One should not be put off by the absence of urinary symptoms as this type of infection is asymptomatic in about 90 per cent of cases.

More than one of the above types of anæmia may co-exist and, of course, their effects are additive.

In iron deficiency anæmia the blood picture shows both a low hæmoglobin and a reduced packed cell volume, the colour index is less than unity, and the M.C.V. and M.C.H.C. are both reduced. In other words, the picture is characteristically microcytic and hypochromic. New cells are being generated at the normal rate, and the reticulocyte count shows little deviation from normal. The cells, besides being smaller than usual, are of unequal sizes and staining (anisocytosis and polychromasia). There is no undue hæmolysis, and the serum bilirubin is not increased. The bone marrow is normoblastic in character.

In our clinic in Glasgow less than 50 per cent of patients come to the antenatal clinic with a hæmoglobin over 10 g. per 100 ml.[42] It is our practice to divide our antenatal cases from the point of view of anæmia into three groups—(1) those with hæmoglobin levels above 12 g. who, in our experience, have usually maintained their hæmatological wellbeing on a rechecking at the 34th to 36th week of preg-

nancy; (2) those with hæmoglobin levels between 10 and 12 g. (about 30 per cent of patients). These require routine iron by mouth and re-checking throughout pregnancy to make sure that they are not losing ground or failing to take their pills; (3) those who present with levels below 10 g. per cent. These are referred to a special hæmatological clinic for intensive therapy and supervision. It would appear that the second group with levels between 10 and 12 g. are cases who, though not yet ill, are of the low iron reserve group and who will almost certainly deteriorate under the demands of pregnancy unless pro-phylactic measures are taken forthwith to stop the drift.

The symptoms are often not very pronounced, but when present consist of fatigue, dyspnœa, palpitations, loss of appetite and diges-tive upset, and the patient usually demonstrates pallor of the mucous membranes and, in severe cases, a considerable degree of œdema, mainly of the lower extremities.

The treatment consists in making good the iron which the patient lacks, and the method will depend upon the time available before delivery. Provided one has at least ten weeks' grace and the anæmia is not severe, a satisfactory result can be obtained by oral medica-tion, and there are many satisfactory preparations of ferrous salts now available. Ferrous sulphate (0·2 g. tablets) is the cheapest of these and is suitable for most patients, but the more expensive ferrous gluconate, fumarate and succinate may produce less epigastric dis-comfort, nausea, vomiting and constipation in the minority who cannot tolerate ferrous sulphate. Where there is achlorhydria, 15 minims of acid hydrochlor. dil. three times a day may help. Prepara-tions of ferrous succinate to which succinic acid has been added are absorbed better than others it is believed, because the transport of iron across the mucosal cells is facilitated by the addition of succinic acid. Most symptoms of intolerance to iron are more related to the dose of elemental iron itself than the actual preparation and there-fore the daily dose of ferrous sulphate, for example, should not exceed three 200 mg. tablets, taken during or after a meal. Increasing the dosage does not improve the hæmatological response and adverse side-effects may well demand a reduction. Ferrous fumarate being a rather drably coloured brown tablet is less dangerous if it gets into the hands of small children, as it is not so likely to be mistaken for a sweet. If acute iron poisoning occurs in a child who has got hold of iron tablets the danger is very real and calls for immediate treatment with desferrioxamine mesylate (Desforal) which as a powerful iron chelator may be life-saving. An intravenous infusion of this sub-stance should be given at once in a dose of 20 millilitres in saline per Kg. every six hours for the next 24 to 48 hours; if for any reason such an infusion cannot be given immediately, an intramuscular injection of 1 g. of desferrioxamine mesylate should be given meanwhile, the

stomach should be washed out and 5 to 12 g. of the same substance in half a litre of saline should be left in the stomach.

For cases in which the need for iron in pregnancy is more pressing saccharated iron oxide preparations were introduced a few years ago for intravenous injection. This was a very important step forward in the treatment of iron deficiency states but these substances are not without their risks. For example, a test dose is always necessary first since alarming collapse and other sensitivity reactions such as dizziness, dyspnœa, vomiting and backache occur in about 5 per cent of cases even with careful selection.[41] Furthermore, the darkness of these solutions makes it difficult to check that the point of the syringe needle is in the lumen of the vein and a perivenous injection is very irritant to the tissues. For these reasons a solution suitable for intramuscular injection was gladly welcomed when it first appeared in the form of iron dextran complex (Imferon). It had hitherto been impossible to administer iron parenterally without the penalty of toxicity from the ionised metal and this difficulty was first overcome by binding ferric hydroxide to carbohydrates to form substances of a high molecular weight. This is rather similar to what happens in the physiological carriage of iron in circulation by bonding it for the time being with a beta globulin ("Transferrin"). Intramuscular iron dextran came in for extensive and enthusiastic use at the hands of all of us, since very favourable results were reported with an incidence of reactions in less than 0·5 per cent in some hundreds of cases.[43] A serious disadvantage, however, was the discoloration of the overlying skin so that the patient looked as though she had been beaten black and blue. This staining lasted a very long time, usually some years, although it was possible to reduce it by skilful technique such as the Z-technique which involves pulling the tissues laterally while the needle is being inserted so that the needle track, and therefore the track of back leakage, is zig-zagged. A further refinement is to inject a small quantity of saline down the needle before withdrawing it.

The enthusiasm for parenteral iron however is steadily diminishing as it is fairly widely recognised that the increase in hæmoglobin concentration is only marginally accelerated as compared with oral medication. One of the commonest troubles is that the patient is not taking her iron and the easiest way to find out is to inquire of her about the colour of her stools. If she reports that they are normal instead of black, one can be certain that she is not, in fact, taking her iron tablets.

Intramuscular iron therapy received a setback in popularity with reports that sarcoma could be induced at the site of intramuscular injection in rats subjected to massive doses of iron dextran complex (Imferon),[40] a finding confirmed in both rats and mice a year later.[24] The reaction was clearly a local one stimulated by the presence of very

do. Incidence figures of one in two thousand pregnancies have often been quoted, but in recent years the incidence works out in Glasgow for example at between 2 to 4 per cent of all pregnancies. The figure is considerably higher in parts of the world where nutrition is worse and especially where hæmolytic factors either congenital or parasitic operate. It is particularly common in West Africa and Fullerton and Watson-Williams (1962) found megaloblastic erythropoiesis in the majority of patients whose initial hæmoglobin in pregnancy was less than 7 g. per 100 ml. The association of hæmolysis due to malaria with megaloblastic anæmia is well known, but these workers have drawn attention to other types of hæmolysis as being likewise responsible particularly, for example, hæmoglobin SC disease. Although this variety of sickle-cell anæmia accounted for less than 10 per cent of their cases in Ibadan they hoped by this study to explain the development of megaloblastic anæmia in all patients who suffer from hæmolytic conditions as a primary cause of their anæmia. They found that folic acid clearance was very rapid even before megaloblastic anæmia appeared and they reckoned that when the rate of red cell destruction is about twice normal, the compensatory marrow hyperplasia, together with the demands of the fœtus, rapidly exhaust the available supplies of folic acid whereupon erythropoiesis becomes megaloblastic. Once this develops, anæmia rapidly progresses thereafter. The more usual causes, however, are a deficient supply of folic acid in the diet or defective absorption as in cases of tropical sprue.

The increased demands of pregnancy and particularly of twin pregnancy are well demonstrated by the more rapid clearance of injected folic acid from the plasma in pregnancy.[6] This has nothing to do with the absorption of vitamin B_{12}, which is usually normal in pregnancy.

Addisonian anæmia is therefore very uncommon in pregnancy. There are two reasons for this; firstly, it is rare at the age of child-bearing and, secondly, such cases are usually infertile.

What is astonishing is the infrequency of cases of megaloblastic anæmia reported from the United States. In Brooklyn, for example, it has been reckoned that folic acid deficiency is frequent during the last trimester of pregnancy amongst the lower social groups, yet megaloblastic anæmia of pregnancy remains exceedingly rare and it is suggested that there must be additional factors operating.[45] One wonders whether American views on the incidence will change in time as our own have recently.

A megaloblastic form of erythropoiesis is one thing (and marrow samples taken from an unselected group of pregnant patients show an incidence of this of about 25 per cent[46]), but a true megaloblastic anæmia of clinical significance is about one-tenth of that figure; in

other words most laboratory tests will reveal the tendency long before it becomes clinically significant. There is accumulating evidence to indicate that the average British diet is not equal to the demands of pregnancy, which are considerably in excess of the generally recognised 50 micrograms per day required in the non-pregnant state. A good deal of work has therefore been done to arrive at some sensible estimate of how much extra folic acid should be supplied in pregnancy. The picture is further complicated by the fact that diagnostic criteria are uncertain, hence there is very marked variation in the accepted incidence of the condition and we cannot do more than supply our own standards which, over the last few years, have served us so well. There can be no doubt that iron deficiency itself may conceal the morphological evidence of megaloblastic anæmia and may of itself be a factor in the ætiology of the folic acid deficiency state.[7] It is thus that the correction of the iron deficiency only at this point brings to light the underlying associated folic acid deficiency as well. An extensive trial was therefore undertaken at the Queen Mother's Hospital to find the optimum folic acid supplement which would effectively eliminate folic acid deficiency later on in pregnancy. The technique employed in this review was to investigate the fasting serum folate levels in the second and fourth day postpartum in a consecutive series of 350 patients from groups who had been allocated at random to different supplementary doses of folic acid. A dietary assessment was also undertaken at the same time. The method of assay was the *Lactobacillus casei* standard technique. The results were compared with an accepted normal range in the non-pregnant, namely 2·8 to 8 millimicrograms/ml. Marrow biopsy has now been given up except in the most inexplicable cases. For one thing the results are little better than an observation of the criteria presently to be described and, secondly, the process itself is inconvenient and often very painful to the patient. Marrow biopsy from the iliac crest is considerably better in this respect than from the sternum where pain can be very severe and one of my residents once had the shattering experience of going straight through into the heart. She withdrew the needle in a hurry and fortunately all was well.

In the survey referred to, the postpartum period was chosen for measuring the serum folate because the lowest levels associated with pregnancy are demonstrated at this time due to the combined demands of the fœtus and blood loss at delivery; also, as is well known, many cases of latent megaloblastic anæmia are first manifested after delivery in the immediate puerperium and not before it. Now, while, as already mentioned, the lowest non-pregnant adult serum folate value is 2·8 millimicrograms/ml., 75 per cent of the patients who fitted our criteria for the diagnosis of megaloblastic anæmia had levels below 2·5 m μg./ml. It appeared from this survey of an average

Glasgow population, with a diet which is clearly inadequate in all but the most favoured social classes, that a supplement of approximately 300 μg. a day is necessary to prevent a major fall in postpartum serum folate level and it is now our practice to prescribe this supplement in all cases, on the argument that it is insufficient to be wasteful and not a big enough dose to mask a vitamin B_{12} deficiency.[48]

If, for example, in a woman over 35 there is any element of doubt that one may be missing a case of Addisonian pernicious anæmia, one can be reasonably certain of excluding the condition by finding free gastric hydrochloric acid, but quite a number of pregnant women, especially those who are folic acid deficient and anæmic in any case, have an incidental gastric achlorhydria although this is not histamine fast and furthermore tends not to persist after delivery.

Criteria for the Diagnosis of Macrocytic or Megaloblastic Anæmia[48]

The hæmoglobin level must be below 10 g. per cent, and at least two of the following features, sought for in films of the buffy coat layer, must be present:

(a) More than 4 per cent of the neutrophil polymorphs must have 5 or more lobes.

(b) Orthochromatic macrocytes must be present with diameters exceeding 12 μ.

(c) Howell-Jolly bodies (which are residual nuclear inclusion bodies within the erythrocytes) are demonstrable (Fig. 1).

(d) Nucleated red cells, that is to say normoblasts showing premature hæmoglobinisation for their stage of nuclear development are found.

(e) Macropolycytes may be present. These are giant polymorphs within the buffy coat layer.

These findings have been supported by the study of a thousand serum folate estimations. Results from Montreal are similar, where a good correlation between the appearance of segmentation of the neutrophils in peripheral blood has been confirmed by marrow examination where, of course, the very earliest changes might be expected. Marrow biopsy is therefore now a rare operation in our hospital and reserved for the determination of other types of anæmia.

The clinical picture is that of a woman, usually in the later part of pregnancy, who demonstrates a fairly severe anæmia which has failed to respond to a genuine intake of iron, including parenteral therapy. Twins may be present and clearly here the increased demands of folic acid for such a pregnancy are responsible. What is less easy to explain is the common association of hydramnios with megaloblastic anæmia as well. Signs of pre-eclamptic toxæmia may often be present; in fact in one reported series[21] all three signs of

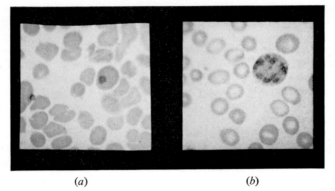

(a)   (b)

6/Fig. 1.—Megaloblastic anaemia—blood film.

(a) Howell-Jolly residual nuclear inclusion bodies within erythrocytes.
(b) Hypersegmented neutrophil.

(By courtesy of Dr. M. L. N. Willoughby.)

hypertension, albuminuria and œdema were found in 14 per cent of cases with megaloblastic anæmia, as against an overall incidence of 6 per cent of cases of pre-eclamptic toxæmia in Dublin.

Because of the key role of folic acid in D.N.A. synthesis, so readily demonstrable within the marrow, it is interesting to consider other parts of the body where rapidly proliferating cells might show the effects of such deficiency and for this reason cervical epithelial cells have been studied with this mechanism in view.[35] In fact a number of characteristic cytological changes have been thus described, which reverted to normal when the patient was successfully treated with folic acid. Since other cells within the body are also in the process of active proliferation and equally dependent upon D.N.A. synthesis, an observation of this sort sets one thinking about possible wider effects elsewhere, but, so far, experimental evidences are lacking.

In severe cases the spleen and occasionally the liver may be enlarged and there may be purpuric spots. Signs of congestive cardiac failure may be present and I, myself, have seen more than one case of jaundice, which was probably a contributory factor. The severity of the disease may vary from the apparently iron resistant case to a woman acutely ill in whom the differential diagnosis may be quite difficult. There may be a misleading history of pernicious anæmia in other members of the family. There is often atrophic glossitis but neurological lesions never.

Of one practical point one can be reasonably certain, namely, if the hæmoglobin drops sharply after a normal delivery, in which the blood loss has been minimal, the case is almost certain to prove on

proper examination to be one of folic acid deficiency. This must be put right over the next three months by iron and folic acid.

DIAGNOSIS OF ACHLORHYDRIA

A particularly useful ward procedure is the Azuresin diagnostic test (Squibb) better known as "Diagnex Blue". This test determines the presence or absence of free hydrochloric acid in the stomach without any special equipment. It depends upon the liberation of an indicator material (azure A) from a cation exchange resin, by the action of free gastric hydrochloric acid. This indicator is then absorbed from the stomach and excreted in the urine two hours later where its blueness can be seen and compared with a colour comparator supplied in each box of the test material. The test is valid except in cases of pyloric obstruction, severe hepatic or renal disease, in severe vomiting or marked dehydration or after partial or total gastrectomy, for obvious reasons.

The exclusion of achlorhydria, besides ruling out a diagnosis of pernicious anæmia, puts carcinoma of the stomach out of the differential diagnosis as well. These conditions are admittedly very rare in pregnancy but that fact would not diminish the catastrophe of missing them.

FIGLU test.—This test was all the rage and an enormous amount of unnecessary work was undertaken in carrying it out in the early 1960s. The enthusiasm for the test has now almost totally evaporated, and we seldom employ it. Nevertheless it is based upon a very important recognition of the biochemical pathways in the conversion of folic acid to folinic acid which is the really active principle, a deficiency which is revealed in the faulty metabolism of histidine to the end product glutamic acid. For this reason the mechanism is worth explaining. The term "FIGLU" is short for Formimino glutamic acid.

Histidine normally breaks down to FIGLU which is converted to glutamic acid only if sufficient folic acid is present. Folic acid is pteroylglutamic acid and picks up a formyl group from formiminoglutamic acid to form folinic acid which is N.5-formyl-tetra-hydropteroylglutamic acid. There is thus a metabolic relationship between histidine and folic acid, the former proceeding to glutamic acid through the stage of FIGLU and the latter proceeding to folinic acid.

Now, in pregnancy, there is an increased histidine breakdown load which may reveal a latent folic acid deficiency. This same deficiency by failure to make possible the full conversion of FIGLU to glutamic acid is thus revealed by a persistence of FIGLU excreted in the urine. The commonly used test is based on that described by Knowles et al. (1960). To make the test sure it is the common practice to give an additional histidine load of 15 g. crystals in water by mouth to the fasting patient at 0700 hours. The maximum histidine output in the urine appears within the next five hours, so, three hours later, at 1000 hours, the patient micturates and the specimen of urine is discarded. Thereafter all urine is collected until 1500 hours when the final specimen is passed. The urine is kept in a large Winchester bottle containing 2 ml. of concentrated hydrochloric acid to maintain an acid reaction since alkaline ammonia converts FIGLU to glutamic acid. Some thymol crystals are also placed in the bottle to dis-

courage bacterial growth. The specimen is then subjected to electrophoresis. The FIGLU runs at a different rate from glutamic acid and can be revealed by drying and staining the electrophoretic strip with ninhydrin.

The FIGLU excretion test provides an indirect means of demonstrating folic acid deficiency but does not indicate whether the deficiency is due to a dietary lack, malabsorption, increased utilisation, for example in twins, disorders of fat absorption with associated steatorrhœa in which absorption of vitamin B_{12} may also be unsatisfactory, or the increased demands of a marrow having to cope with pathological degrees of hæmolysis. Hibbard (1962) found that twenty out of seventy-four patients with a positive FIGLU test had normoblastic marrows, yet when they were given folic acid therapy their anæmia resolved and the FIGLU test became negative. It would appear that the FIGLU test had anticipated the marrow changes. Fifty-eight per cent of her seventy-four positive cases had previously received folic acid therapy, a fact which was confirmed by close questioning, the more readily since many of them were in-patients and these showed a satisfactory reticulocyte and hæmoglobin response when the folic acid was given parenterally and FIGLU disappeared from the urine. She suggests that in these cases the folic acid deficiency arose as a result of malabsorption rather than lack of dietary intake. This would indicate that giving folic acid by mouth routinely to anæmic patients may fail to correct those due to malabsorption.

One of the disadvantages of the FIGLU test is that it is too often positive without clinically significant degrees of megaloblastic anæmia in pregnancy. In other words it would appear too sensitive. The probable reasons are that there is a different type of absorption of folic acid in pregnancy and there is increased utilisation of histidine in pregnancy which makes it so much less useful than in the non-pregnant state, and a growing number of reports regard an estimate of serum folic acid levels as a better guide to the type of erythropoiesis.[8] In fact there now seems fairly general agreement that the urinary excretion of formimino glutamic acid is not only unsatisfactory as a test for folic acid deficiency in pregnancy but is within normal limits in half the patients who, in fact, have the actual disease, which puts the error in the opposite direction. In fact it has been found that there is a steady decline in the amount of formimino glutamic acid excreted in the urine throughout pregnancy, believed due to the increased utilisation of histidine for protein synthesis in the later weeks of pregnancy.[3]

Prophylactic Folic Acid Therapy

This is much debated. There are many units which give folic acid treatment in addition to iron as a blind routine, on the argument that it cannot do harm and that pernicious anæmia and carcinoma of the stomach are unlikely to be missed and are too rare anyway in

pregnancy to bother about. In parts of the world where megalo-blastic anæmia is very prevalent and the consequences acute and where laboratory facilities are limited there may be something to be said for this view, but there is no excuse for it in this country and least of all in teaching units. On general principles all routine treatment, as a substitute for intelligent investigation and thought, is to be condemned. Such a process can only lead to slovenly thinking in the first instance and presently to no thinking at all and we would end up knowing even less then we did before about folic acid metabolism and no one would suggest that there is not a great deal still to learn. Unnecessary treatment also involves unnecessary expense and some patients may not wholly escape the implication that there is something abnormal to treat. Finally there is a danger that we may be treating laboratory data rather than patients (Witts, 1962).

Notwithstanding all this there is much to be said for treating any acute anæmia presenting in the last month of pregnancy with empirical folic acid as well as with iron sorbitol while awaiting results of investigations, since time is short. The same argument applies in all cases of twins since time may be shorter than one thinks due to the possible onset of premature labour.[21] No case of megalo-blastic anæmia, however, should be put on to folic acid therapy without at least the Diagnex Blue test to exclude achlorhydria. Any case in whom the reticulocyte response and rise in hæmoglobin level is not apparent within ten days should have a full hæmatological investigation.

There would appear to be more than a possible relationship between folic acid deficiency and abruptio[27] placentæ and that such a deficiency may be an aetiological factor in foetal malformation and recurrent abortion, [28, 34] although there is still room for debate on these subjects.

The decision to use a dietary supplement of folic acid in pregnancy depends upon the type of population with which one is dealing and at least in Glasgow, as in other centres, an attempt has been made to assess the deficit. In our own practice we have found that in a survey of over three and a half thousand patients, randomly allocated to different supplementation groups treated with differing doses of folic acid supplements and checked by the post-partum serum folate level, a minimum daily requirement of 300 μg./day was sufficient to protect the vast majority of the patients.[49] For this reason we now prescribe in all our antenatal clinics 3 tablets a day of Pregamal, which contains 100 micrograms of folic acid and 200 mg. of ferrous fumarate, yielding approximately 65 mg. of ferrous iron in every tablet. A more recent alternative is one tablet only each day of "Ferrograd-Folic" which contains 105 mg. of elemental iron plus 350 micrograms of folic acid. Gastric irritation is minimal with this

preparation, thanks to its slow release of iron. These supplementary requirements might vary with different types of population and in different parts of the world and would be well worth estimating before prescribing on a large scale.

Megaloblastic anæmia of pregnancy may continue for up to five months into the postnatal period and occasionally may only first come to light in the puerperium often provoked out of latency by hæmorrhage at delivery. The usual time of onset, however, is between the fifth and seventh months of pregnancy. Anorexia and vomiting may confuse the differential diagnosis which includes leukæmic states.

Most types of clinically full-blown megaloblastic anæmia can cause the patient's death far more readily than is the case with iron deficiency anæmia, and treatment should be energetic. This consists of a liberal diet, folic acid in daily doses ranging from 15 to 30 mg. by mouth and, of course, parenteral iron, for example iron sorbitol, in cases seriously deficient in iron as well. Folic acid treatment should be maintained for four weeks after delivery.

This treatment can restore a normal blood picture within five weeks but the danger of even a small antepartum hæmorrhage in the uncorrected state should be keenly recognised and treated by transfusion. In fact hæmorrhage is the main if not the only indication for transfusion in this type of anæmia.[17] Transfusion given before investigation may wreck the chances of accurate diagnosis.

Thrombocytopenic purpura is an uncommon complication of pregnancy, but an impressive series of 44 pregnancies in cases of the idiopathic form of the disease have been reported from Manchester[25] without maternal fatality. Thirty-eight of the pregnancies were in women who had undergone previous splenectomy. In one, the operation was undertaken in pregnancy and in another during the puerperium; in the remaining four the operation was not carried out either before or after delivery and it would appear that the maternal risk is not great if splenectomy has already been carried out before pregnancy. The danger is greater in women still with their spleens *in situ*, and the operation itself in the course of pregnancy is hazardous and should not be considered in any case unless adrenal cortical steroid therapy has already failed. The expulsive efforts of the second stage may encourage purpuric hæmorrhages which may also involve the brain and should, therefore, be eliminated by the timely application of forceps. As might be expected, hæmorrhage at Cæsarean section or from genital tract lacerations, occurred in a quarter of the cases in this series. About 18 per cent of the live born babies showed purpuric manifestations with thrombocytopenia lasting up to twelve weeks, even in mothers who had apparently been cured by previous splenectomy. If, in fact, the thrombocytopenia is due to the destruction of platelets by circulating autoimmune antibodies, which may be

capable of crossing the placenta, this curious neonatal liability to the disease, thus passively acquired, seems understandable in a baby, which, unlike its mother, has a normally functioning spleen. A platelet count should therefore be done on all infants of mothers with a history of thrombocytopenic purpura, even though previously cured by splenectomy.

The other varieties of anæmia, such as the aplastic varieties and the hæmolytic anæmias, will not be discussed further in this chapter, as they are in no way peculiar to pregnancy, but the role of sepsis in favouring anæmia should not be overlooked, and its proper control is essential for healthy hæmopoiesis. The transfusion of packed cells, besides helping the patient to cope with her sepsis, will often permanently benefit her anæmic state.

EFFECTS OF ANÆMIA ON PREGNANCY AND LABOUR

The abortion and prematurity rates are somewhat increased, but it is nevertheless surprising how well the majority of fœtuses manage to survive in cases of quite considerable anæmia. Practically all the complications of pregnancy are aggravated quantitatively by anæmia, and, in particular, the patient with a cardiac lesion suffers from greatly increased dyspnœa.

Labour is not materially influenced by anæmia, and inertia is no more common, but the accidents of labour, especially those involving hæmorrhage or shock, are rendered correspondingly more serious, and the patient who comes into labour with a hæmoglobin level of less than 9·6 g. (65%) is at serious risk in this respect. Her ability to cope with infection in the puerperium is much undermined by anæmia, and her recovery in the postnatal period will be greatly retarded to the extent that she may now face years of chronic sub-health.

HAEMOGLOBINOPATHIES

There are a large number of variants of the hæmoglobin molecule, some of which are particularly common in certain populations such as West Africans and Mediterranean seaboard races. Hæmoglobin itself is a conjugated protein with a molecular weight of about 68 thousand, which contains a globin fraction bound to 4 hæm molecules. Abnormalities affecting the synthesis of the hæm part of the molecule are responsible for the porphyrias which need not concern us further here. The hæmoglobinopathies are concerned with disorders within the polypeptide chains which comprise the globin fraction. There are four possible chains, namely alpha, beta, gamma and delta, but most hæmoglobin in normal adult blood has, within the globin molecule, a pair of alpha and a pair of beta chains and is called Hb. A $(\alpha_2\beta_2)$.

This applies to over 90 per cent of the hæmoglobin and up to 3 per cent has two delta chains instead of the two beta chains and is known as Hb. A_2 ($\alpha_2\delta_2$).

Fœtal hæmoglobin (Hb. F) has a globin portion consisting of 2 alpha and 2 gamma chains ($\alpha_2\gamma_2$). This accounts for about 80 per cent of the hæmoglobin in cord blood at term. This fœtal hæmoglobin is gradually replaced by the normal adult hæmoglobin (Hb. A) over the first year of life.

Two classes of abnormality can result in a decreased proportion of the normal adult hæmoglobin A in later life; the thalassæmia syndromes and the hæmoglobinopathies. In beta thalassæmia there is an impaired synthesis of beta chains, resulting in a low concentration of normal Hb. A ($\alpha_2\beta_2$) with a compensatory increase in Hb. F ($\alpha_2\gamma_2$) and/or Hb. A_2 ($\alpha_2\delta_2$). A rare form of alpha-thalassæmia also exists, where there is impairment of alpha chains. This form affects the newborn, unlike beta-thalassæmia, since alpha but not beta chains are present in Hb. F. On the other hand when the Hb. A molecule is replaced in whole or in part by a pathological hæmoglobin because of abnormal polypeptide chains not to be found in normal globin, one is faced with a hæmoglobinopathy, viz. a qualitative rather than quantitative abnormality of Hb. A synthesis. These pathological polypeptide changes are, in fact, due to substitution alterations in the aminoacid residue; for example substitution of the aminoacid valine for glutamic acid results in the structural difference between sickle cell and normal hæmoglobin and because glutamic acid has a different electrical charge from valine, starch-gel electrophoresis is capable of separating and distinguishing the two. Sickle cell hæmoglobin also crystallises out readily in blood which is reduced after giving up its oxygen and the red cell envelope is consequently distorted, hence the term "sickling". Blood viscosity increases at the same time and vessels may become blocked with thrombosis and likewise hæmolysis may occur.

These abnormal hæmoglobins are also genetically determined and the blood of an individual may be either heterozygous or homozygous. For instance if the sickle cell gene is inherited from both parents, the child has the full-blown sickle cell disease, (SS) whereas, in the heterozygous, sickling does not normally occur because there is enough normal hæmoglobin in each red cell to prevent it. The heterozygous state produces what is called the sickle cell trait.

The heterozygotes with the sickle cell trait are said to have considerable resistance to malaria and therefore the trait is common in parts of the world where malaria has been traditionally rife.

There are quantitative variations in the amounts of abnormal hæmoglobin in any given case and in the case of sickle cell anæmia about three-quarters of the hæmoglobin is made up of the S-type,

namely homozygous (SS), whereas in the sickle cell trait more than half the hæmoglobin may be of the Hb. A variety. The laws of Mendelian inheritance apply.

The most commonly encountered abnormal hæmoglobins are S, C, D and E. These abnormalities reside in the beta-chain and, therefore, do not become manifest in the neonatal period. They may also exist in a variety of combinations including mixed syndromes with the thalassæmias. The anæmia in non-sickling hæmoglobinopathies (i.e. C, D, E) is usually very mild unless in combinations with thalassæmia.

The thalassæmias are a somewhat different class as already explained because here there is an abnormal quantitative relationship between the different types of hæmoglobin which can be found in normal blood, namely Hb. A, Hb. A_2, Hb. F. In thalassæmia minor (heterozygous form) the disease is not normally severe. In thalassæmia major (homozygous form) the disease is much more severe.

Until recently the hæmoglobinopathies were no more than a hæmatological curiosity in British obstetric practice but with the enormous influx of immigrants, especially from West Africa and the West Indies, they demand more recognition, and any case of refractory anæmia in a patient coming from these parts of the world and also from races on the Mediterranean seaboard should be investigated. Furthermore thalassæmia is being more frequently found amongst patients of apparently British stock. Thalassæmia and most hæmoglobinopathies are likely to present as refractory hypochronic anæmias during pregnancy, with target cells in the blood film, a constant reticulocytosis and a fasting serum iron level higher than the degree of hychromia would suggest. In the more severe forms they may present as a hæmolytic or aplastic crisis or, in the case of Hb. S, manifest thrombotic incidents.

The hæmatological features of the anæmia should raise the possibility of thalassæmia or hæmoglobinopathy the precise variety of which may require family studies and the application of techniques only available in specialised centres. Demonstration of the presence of Hb. S, however, is a simpler matter, depending upon its unusual physical characteristics already mentioned. By mixing a drop of blood with a reducing agent such as sodium dithionite and sealing the coverslip, sickling may be seen under the microscope in 20 minutes if the test is positive.[1] The major method, however, of identifying abnormal hæmoglobins is by starch-gel electrophoresis. Fresh heparinised blood (10–20 ml.) is required for this type of investigation.

The clinical effects of the hæmoglobinopathies are first of all to reduce fertility. In fact the death rate amongst children in severe cases is high and abortion is said to be more common. In sickle cell

disease (hæmoglobin SS) the patient is recurrently affected in two very damaging ways, namely hæmolytic crises and crises of infarction, and in between these crises she continues with chronic hæmolytic anæmia with some degree of jaundice and miserable health. The bone marrow endeavours to compensate by increased erythropoiesis and there is usually reticulocytosis. Stores of folic acid may, therefore, be exhausted and the patient never really becomes well between one crisis and the next. Infarction may strike in any part of the body and produce pain anywhere and even intracranial catastrophes, whereas the hæmolytic crises produce jaundice and fever. Infection may precipitate hæmolysis and infarction may be encouraged by circulatory stasis and local acidosis. Sickle cell hæmoglobin C. disease (SC) is less severe than full blown sickle cell (SS). In fact the SC case may suffer no more than moderate illhealth until pregnancy precipitates hæmolytic or infarctive crises, particularly in the last trimester or in the postpartum period.

The picture is a dismal one inasmuch as there is clearly no specific treatment; but transfusion may tide a patient over a crisis and a higher than usual dose of prophylactic folic acid should be given to meet increased requirements. Delivery should be covered by antibiotics to prevent triggering off a further hæmolytic crisis. These patients therefore call for what Bannerman and White have described as "maximal obstetric care".

PULMONARY TUBERCULOSIS

Patients with active pulmonary tuberculosis often appear to be perversely fertile, and the problem is certainly common enough to merit a consideration of the modern point of view regarding the effects of pregnancy upon the disease and vice versa. In recent years our attitude has changed from that which regarded pregnancy as a disaster in the course of the disease. This, however, does not mean that the complication is less important. On the contrary, the more hopeful attitude depends absolutely upon adequate supervision being available.

Routine chest radiography in pregnancy is less popular now because of radiation hazards, but mass miniature radiography is, in fact, not contra-indicated and full chest radiography should not be denied the patient whose history or contact demands it.

Effects of Pregnancy on the Disease

Edge (1952) from the Brompton Hospital concluded that pregnancy in general had no dramatic effect upon the course of the disease. Cohen (1946) also reported on 177 cases of pulmonary tuberculosis in pregnancy with a long follow-up of 120, and he likewise concluded

that pregnancy and labour rarely harm the pulmonary disease and pregnancy is no more than an incident in the disease process. The proviso is always made, however, that adequate treatment and supervision are instituted, not only through pregnancy and labour but in the even more important postnatal period. It is in the latter that mischief is most often evident, and the added work and fatigue of looking after a fretful baby can be more serious than the effects of pregnancy and labour added together.

It might be expected that the rise in the level of the diaphragm in pregnancy would be bound to affect the pulmonary lesion in one direction or another by reducing lung capacity, but this is compensated for by the increased width which occurs in the thoracic dimensions. The increased metabolic effort on the part of the patient should be offset by greater periods of rest. The outlook, of course, is immeasurably worse when there is associated tuberculous laryngitis, but this would apply whether the patient was pregnant or not.

A death rate of up to 30 per cent in five years was not unusual in former years in women of childbearing age who were sputum positive, whether pregnancy supervened or not. Modern antituberculous chemotherapy has transformed what was once a gloomy, long-term outlook.

What has been said above is all very well provided pregnancy itself is normal in other respects and there are no obstetrical complications, but when these are present the tuberculous patient is clearly at greater risk. Hyperemesis is indeed a serious complication and requires very urgent and energetic treatment. Trial of labour has only a limited place, anæsthesia must be judiciously selected and administered to prevent additional chest complications, and blood conservation is doubly important. The accidents of labour may make a terrible difference.

Major thoracic surgery is now taking a more prominent place in the treatment of tuberculosis, and here, too, it would appear that pregnancy does not materially alter the prognosis. Folsome and Kuntze (1953) have reviewed 25 cases subjected to major thoracic surgery for tuberculosis, including 14 cases of pneumonectomy, performed before and during pregnancy. There were 37 pregnancies with 4 maternal deaths (16 per cent), all of which occurred several months after delivery.

Conversely, the presence of pulmonary tuberculosis has, on the whole, little effect on pregnancy itself, although if the disease is active there is a slight tendency for the patient to go into premature labour.

The modern outlook for the patient has been summarised on a question and answer basis in a report of the Joint Pædiatrics & Obstetrics Committee of the Joint Tuberculosis Council (1958) and

confirms the above reassuring change of outlook, even breast feeding being encouraged in non-infective cases.

Management

The problem is primarily sociological. Overwork, overcrowding, fatigue and malnutrition are far greater enemies of the patient's chances than her pregnancy. Her medical treatment should follow the same lines as would have been adopted were she not pregnant, with rather more emphasis on necessary periods of hospitalisation. The corner stone of treatment, of course, is antituberculous chemotherapy. Although streptomycin crosses the placenta ototoxic effects have not yet been reported in the babies. Major surgery is preferably confined at present to the first half of pregnancy. Antenatal supervision should be as thorough as it is for the patient with a cardiac lesion, and periods of hospitalisation during pregnancy should be unhesitatingly recommended on even minor obstetrical indications. In any case, it is wise, as in the cardiac case, to admit the patient to hospital for 10 to 14 days before delivery. This not only improves supervision but guarantees adequate rest.

Treatment in labour largely follows the same lines as in cases of cardiac disease, with the same attention to the patient's general condition. Cæsarean section should only be employed where there are obstetrical indications, and its use is not to be recommended simply as a means of furnishing an opportunity to sterilise the patient at the same time. The second stage should not be allowed to be strenuous, and the forceps should be used whenever it appears that spontaneous delivery cannot take place without effort, but it has to be remembered that a normal delivery, with possibly the help of an episiotomy, is less of a strain on the patient as a whole than a forceps operation under general anæsthesia. Local anæsthesia for forceps is preferable.

It used to be thought that the changes in abdominal anatomy following delivery would have a deleterious effect upon the pulmonary lesion as a result of the sudden lowering of the diaphragm. As it so happens, however, there is no immediate diaphragmatic descent, and the old idea of inducing a pneumoperitoneum immediately after delivery, in order to keep the diaphragm up, has now been abandoned. Without paralysis of the phrenic nerve it is quite difficult anyway to alter the level of the diaphragm, and filling the peritoneal cavity with air simply bulges the flabby abdominal wall and, at the very least, merely increases the patient's discomfort.

Care of the Baby

Congenital tuberculosis in the baby is extremely rare, but the chances that it will contract the infection during the first few months

of life are very great. To separate the mother from her child may be theoretically desirable but is often not feasible. Nevertheless, until recently there was no other method of protecting a child from this deadly hazard, since a baby has no natural immunity to tuberculosis. In underdeveloped countries where artificial feeding is dangerous because of gastroenteritis and where neglect of the young in any hands other than the mother's is by no means uncommon, segregation of the babies from their mothers has its own peculiar dangers. Dormer and colleagues (1959) working in a Bantu tuberculosis unit of 1,000 beds in Durban found the mortality of babies born there to be appallingly high as a consequence of separation from their mothers— for example, in one year 15 out of 17 died. They therefore decided to keep the mothers and babies together and to protect the babies with isoniazid meanwhile, even though some of the mothers were sputum positive and all were nursed together in thirty-bedded wards. The dosage they gave was 25 mg. of isoniazid in syrup twice a day by mouth, increasing after 6 months to 50 mg. twice a day. There were no adverse effects and the babies remained Mantoux negative. Unfortunately the babies had still to face their primary infection as soon as the isoniazid prophylaxis was stopped after discharge home and these workers suggested the possibility of immunising the babies with isoniazid-resistant BCG vaccine, but gave no record of having done so. This has since been carried out by Gaisford and Griffiths in Manchester. Here, separation of mother and baby has been dispensed with, provided the mother does not suffer from isoniazid-resistant tuberculosis, and the baby is protected with isoniazid and at the same time immunized with an isoniazid-resistant BCG vaccine. It would not be rational to give the normal freeze-dried BCG vaccine as the concurrent isoniazid would ruin the effect, but it was found that the isoniazid-resistant vaccine was just as potent, and produced satisfactory tuberculin conversion without complications. Isoniazid prophylaxis is, of course, maintained until the tuberculin test becomes positive.

Breast feeding is definitely contra-indicated in all cases of activity of the tuberculosis process. Recently achieved quiescence of the lesion is also a contra-indication.

In the soundly healed case there is no objection on pulmonary grounds to breast feeding. Indeed, the labour involved in preparing artificial feeds can often be more tiresome than breast feeding. Artificial feeding for the single-handed mother can be a real strain, but if adequate help in the home is available the advantages are considerable.

These patients are far more likely to break down as a result of overwork and fatigue while the baby is still very young than because of the alleged strain of pregnancy, labour and lactation, and it is an

essential part of postnatal treatment to ensure that the patient receives all the domestic help that her condition demands. As in the cardiac case, the home-help service can be of great value.

Therapeutic Abortion

The more carefully pregnant patients with pulmonary tuberculosis are reviewed, and the more thoroughly they are treated, the less often will termination of pregnancy be called for. The indications for this type of intervention are mainly sociological, and, medically speaking, they cannot for that reason be regarded as wholly genuine. The ideal answer to the problem is to attend to the patient's social circumstances rather than to destroy a potentially healthy baby. Unfortunately this is a counsel of perfection, like ridding the world of slums and poverty. The highly multiparous patient suffering from the disease may often be found to be living in conditions of such irredeemable squalor that one may occasionally be forced, in the interests of expedition, to terminate and sterilise simply to preserve the patient as a functioning social unit for the sake of her numerous existing children.

The risks of therapeutic abortion, whether by the vaginal or by the abdominal route, are every bit as great as the risks of a continuing pregnancy, and the prognosis in either instance has to be viewed against the general five-year mortality in all patients, whether pregnant or not. Termination does not appear to influence the outlook significantly, nor is the course of the disease appreciably altered.

The patient with quiescent and arrested disease is only at slight risk in any case, and where the disease is active the only indication for termination is gross inadequacy of available supervision, a state of affairs which should not be admitted in any civilised community.

If the patient is well enough to benefit hypothetically from termination, she does not need it, and if her condition is so bad that she apparently requires abortion, she is too ill to recover after it.

FUTURE PREGNANCIES

It is generally held that it is better for the patient to avoid pregnancy until quiescence is assured for about two years, in order to obviate the possible risks of subsequent breakdown inherent in the rigours of infant rearing. In the past, victims of this disease have been traditionally advised to postpone marriage and pregnancy, but pregnancy should be discouraged only after very careful consideration, and only in cases where there would appear to be a reasonable prospect of arresting the disease in the very near future. Much will depend upon the social and domestic circumstances of the girl and her husband and the availability of additional help in the home.

In general it has to be admitted that the graver the patient's condition and the more acute the illness, the harder does differential diagnosis become.

JAUNDICE

Jaundice in pregnancy may be due to any of the following:

(1) Virus hepatitis
    (*a*) Infectious hepatitis, and
    (*b*) Homologous serum jaundice
(2) Drugs
(3) Pre-eclamptic toxæmia and eclampsia
(4) Acholuric jaundice
(5) Gallstones
(6) Infective mononucleosis
(7) "Recurrent jaundice of pregnancy"
(8) Acute fatty atrophy
(9) Neglected hyperemesis
(10) Weil's disease
(11) Cirrhosis
(12) Carcinoma of the head of the pancreas
The last three are very rare in pregnancy.

Jaundice in pregnancy is a very disturbing symptom or sign because of the ugly possibilities which it may indicate and the differential diagnosis is by no means easy. The following tests are now regarded as the most useful in helping one to arrive at the correct differential diagnosis which, nevertheless, can often only be made in retrospect.

	Normal ranges
Serum bilirubin	0·2–1·2 mg./100 ml.
Serum glutamic oxaloacetic transaminase (SGOT)	
also named	
Aspartate transaminase (AsT)	5–17 i.u./1
Serum glutamic pyruvic transaminase (SGPT)	
also named	
Alanine transaminase (AlT)	4–13 i.u./1
Alkaline phosphatase	3–13 King-Armstrong units/100 ml.
Prothrombin (Quick one stage)	10–14 seconds
Owren thrombotest	70–100% of standard normal
Serum albumin/globulin ratio	1·5-2

Other tests, though less useful.

Thymol turbidity	0–4 units
Flocculation	0
Urobilinogen in urine	0–4 mg./24 hrs.
Isocitrate dehydrogenase	1–3·5 i.u./1
Serum iron	80–160 μg/100 ml.

The transaminases (SGOT and SGPT or AsT and AlT) are likely to be as high as 250–1,000 i.u./1 in viral hepatitis. They are also raised in drug necrosis, congestive cardiac failure and shock, sometimes with infective mononucleosis complicated by jaundice and rarely with gallstones. Isocitrate dehydrogenase, however, is normal in the latter. Alkaline phosphatase is raised in extrahepatic obstructive jaundice but is very much lower in most viral types of hepatitis and in cirrhosis.

Virus Hepatitis

The transaminase is very high because this is an acute disease, although the degree of jaundice is not proportional to the transaminase levels. Of the two, SGPT is usually higher than SGOT and is the more indicative of viral hepatitis. The serum levels of these enzymes may reach 250–1,000 i.u./1. Cirrhosis has much lower levels being a chronic disease.

Obstructive jaundice can be ruled out if the alkaline phosphatase level is not greatly raised because this enzyme is excreted in the bile.

The erythrocyte sedimentation rate is lower than 10 mm. in the first hour in about a quarter of the patients whereas most other causes of jaundice produce a high sedimentation rate. Thymol turbidity level is not particularly raised.

The clinical picture is more or less the same as in the non-pregnant case, but the differential diagnosis is, of course, harder, especially in the presence of albuminuria which is common also to the pre-eclamptic state. The urine darkens first and the bilirubin rises before clinical jaundice is evident. The stools become pale and the duration of the disease is longer in the older patients. The sources of infection are believed to be by droplet and food. In cases of marked malnutrition the disease is likely to run a more vicious course and the worst cases may be associated with acute yellow atrophy. The mortality, however, is the same as in the non-pregnant woman and is very low indeed and there is no indication for terminating the pregnancy, in fact the operation may be dangerous at such a time. A temporary passive immunity may be obtained by giving gamma globulin but considering the favourable prognosis there is very little need for it.

As in any severe infectious illness during pregnancy, abortion or premature labour may ensue. In a series of 34 cases in which 30 were followed up[1] there was one maternal death, one case of residual cirrhosis of the liver and in 28 recovery was complete, but labour was premature in no less than 8, with two neonatal deaths and spontaneous abortion occurred in another two. Being a virus infection, the question naturally arises of the possible effect upon fœtal development and it is generally considered that the baby is not affected,[41]

although in one of my own cases, in which the infection occurred in early pregnancy, the baby showed a mild degree of hemi-hypertrophy, a rare condition. The question is by no means settled.

Homologous serum jaundice.—This may be contracted from blood or from plasma transfusion or by direct inoculation of the virus with syringes and needles used for venopuncture, even for finger or ear pricking in order to obtain small samples of blood, and it is now the practice in antenatal clinics to use disposable materials entirely. The disease is not the same as virus hepatitis because it differs immuno-logically. Also the incubation period is very much longer and the virus is not found in the stools of the patient. It is a complication of pregnancy much to be feared and we have had one maternal death in our practice which was probably due to this disease contracted in the above manner. This was before the institution of disposable materials in collecting blood samples. Hitherto syringes and needles had been boiled or autoclaved, but neither of these procedures may be suffi-cient to render the instruments safe.

It is surprising that more diseases are not transmitted by blood transfusion; in fact the four principal instances are:

Hepatitis
Syphilis
Malaria
and Brucellosis

Hepatitis is the most important and common, and it is reckoned that a patient receiving two units of blood is exposed to a risk of about 0·8 per cent.[10]

Large pool plasma puts the risk up to nearly 12 per cent but with small pool plasma, prepared from less than 10 bottles, the figure is 1·3 per cent. Massive blood transfusion therefore carries a distinct hazard. By no means are all cases due to a previous transfusion traced, because of the long incubation period which varies up to 160 days before the appearance of jaundice. When homologous serum jaundice does occur, however, the disease runs a fiercer course than the ordinary viral hepatitis referred to earlier, and apart from nausea, vomiting and anorexia, there may be joint pains and skin rashes. In favourable cases the illness may burn itself out in about 30 days but there is an appreciable mortality, seven deaths being reported in a series of 134 cases.[30] In blood donation centres a history of jaundice is a reason for rejecting the donor, but even this precaution does not eliminate the risk because about one in 200 healthy donors harbours the virus in his blood stream. The risks of malaria and syphilis trans-mission can be forestalled by examination of the blood and serology of the potential donor, although in the case of syphilis it is very un-

likely that active spirochætes would survive for more than two or three days in stored blood.

Drugs

Until chloroform became taboo as an anæsthetic in pregnancy and labour many cases of jaundice were often attributed, probably correctly, to this agent. The danger was greatest when the anæsthetic had to be repeatedly induced in the course of a complicated labour. Personally I have not seen such a case now for over thirty years. There are two main groups of drugs which are now regarded as causes of jaundice:

(a) those which mimic hepatitis, e.g. P.A.S. and Isoniazid
(SGOT levels start to rise above 20 i.u./l. and before jaundice)
and
(b) those that produce an intrahepatic obstruction,
e.g. the phenothiazines, the promazines, diabenase.
Methyl testosterone and anabolic agents.
Lastly, arsenic—an unlikely medicament these days.

The alkaline phosphatase level is raised and transaminase too, and isocitrate dehydrogenase (ICD) is a very sensitive index of drug damage to liver cells.

Pre-eclamptic Toxæmia and Eclampsia

Jaundice may appear as a manifestation of the pre-eclamptic state and some cases of severe eclampsia may indeed become jaundiced. Jaundice may also appear terminally in severe and neglected cases of hyperemesis.

Acholuric Jaundice

Acholuric jaundice may complicate pregnancy; the disease is familial and there is abnormal fragility of the red cells.

Gallstones

These are not common as causes of pregnant jaundice in this country, but in the better-fed parts of the world on the other side of the Atlantic the condition is very much more common. Parity is a factor in the ætiology of gallstones, and less than 10 per cent of sufferers have not borne children. A raised blood cholesterol is often associated with gallstones, and it has to be remembered that figures of 300 to 400 mg. per cent are not uncommon in pregnancy. The pressure in the gall-bladder area of the fœtal head in breech presentation may stimulate the pain of gall-stones, but when jaundice is also present it is worth remembering the possibility of cholelithiasis. The alkaline phosphatase levels are usually very high.

TABLE II
JAUNDICE IN PREGNANCY

	Transaminase	Iso-citrate dehydrogenase	Alkaline Phosphatase	Thymol turbidity	Prothrombin Time	E.S.R.	W.B.C.
Virus and Serum Jaundice	+++	+++	± (<30)	+	Prolonged	Low	Normal
Drugs, e.g. Chlorpromazine	++	++	++ (>30)	Normal	Normal	Normal	Often low
Pre-Eclampsia	Normal	Normal	Normal or slightly raised	±	Normal	Normal	Normal
Acholuric (congenital spherocytosis)	Normal or slightly raised	Normal or slightly raised	Normal	±	Normal	Normal	Normal
Gallstones and Obstructive Jaundice	Normal Rarely raised	Normal	+++ (>30)	Normal	Normal	Slightly raised	Slightly raised
Infective Mononucleosis	++	++	+	+	±	+	Normal
Recurrent jaundice of pregnancy	Normal	Normal	++	Normal	Prolonged	+	
Acute fatty degeneration	Low	Low	±	+	Prolonged	Low	++
Cirrhosis	+	+	+ (<30)	++	++	++	Normal or Low

Infective Mononucleosis

In these cases jaundice is not usually severe. The alkaline-phosphatase level is moderately raised, and the transaminase levels are unlikely to rise above 150 i.u./l. The diagnosis is made on other grounds.

"Recurrent Jaundice of Pregnancy"

I have not encountered such a case myself but in 33 patients with jaundice during pregnancy seen at the Rotunda Hospital over a 9-year period 3 were in this category[36] and the pathological condition appeared to be one of intra-hepatic cholestasis. The urine is dark and the stools are pale. The disease is usually at its worst during the last 4 months of pregnancy and the jaundice and pruritus may for a time be actually worse in the immediate puerperium before recovery. Premature labour and postpartum hæmorrhage due to vitamin K deficiency are possible complications. There is usually no maternal or fœtal mortality. The condition recurs in each succeeding pregnancy and is obstructive in type. It is a familial condition and generalised pruritus is a prominent clinical feature and may appear two or three weeks before jaundice. The transaminase levels are normal and the disease clears up after each pregnancy with normal cholangiographic appearances. It is thought to be due to a latent enzymatic defect.

Acute Fatty Atrophy

This has a very high mortality, usually well over 80 per cent. Ninety per cent of the cases occur during the last trimester and a few in the postpartum period. The patients present with vomiting and hæmatemesis and in two-thirds there is severe epigastric pain. Headache is severe in about half the cases and jaundice and coma supervene within a fortnight. The condition would appear to be a separate clinical entity in its own right and Sheehan (1940) described six cases in four hundred maternal deaths. The cause is not known but very severe shrinkage of the liver occurs without histological evidence of inflammatory reaction or necrosis, yet only the cells around the portal tracts remain normal in appearance. The white cell count is raised to about 18,000 to 20,000 per cubic mm., bilirubin, of course, is raised, but, unlike virus hepatitis, there is only a slight rise in transaminase levels. If these levels are reduced one can assume that the liver is incapable of producing them, which is a further bad prognostic sign. The prothrombin time is prolonged, the serum albumin levels are low and there is reduced erythrocyte sedimentation rate. The liver shows a massive, fatty necrosis and may weigh only about 800 to 850 g. (normal 1,200 to 1,500 g.). It is red and mushy. Fat is laid down both in the centrilobular areas and between

the cells. The cytoplasm of the liver cells is foamy in appearance and replaced with fat in multiple small droplets involving all the parenchymatous cells. There is an increase in Kupffer cells. With the condition there is often an associated low nephron necrosis, the renal tubular cells being replaced with fat and renal failure supervenes, with rising creatinine and blood urea levels. Pancreatitis is often associated. Sometimes fat emboli appear in the lungs and the ovaries contain hæmorrhagic cysts. The postpartum milder cases may survive and, in those that do, recovery of hepatic function is complete.

The treatment of jaundice in pregnancy, apart from dealing with any specific cause, is on general lines. The patient's appetite is at first impaired, but as soon as possible a diet rich in carbohydrate and later in protein and vitamin B complex is necessary, with the exclusion, as far as possible, of fat. It is also worth administering vitamin K because of the likely association of hypoprothrombinæmia. This may be particularly important from the baby's point of view should premature labour ensue.

CHOREA GRAVIDARUM

Fortunately, this is not a common complication of pregnancy. Beresford and Graham (1950) reviewed the subject fully, having collected details of 127 hitherto unpublished cases from British hospitals and added 3 more of their own. They estimated the incidence at approximately 1 in 3,000.

The clinical picture may vary from the very mild to the manic, and is characterised by restlessness and incoordinate, non-purposive and non-repetitive movements. Grimacing is noteworthy, and the jack-in-the-box tongue sign characteristic. General hypotonia and emotional lability are also features.

The majority of cases give a history of previous attacks of chorea or rheumatism, and the former may have appeared in earlier pregnancies, since the gravid state seems to favour recrudescences. The main precipitating causes of the present attack are worry and, occasionally, intercurrent infection.

Approximately one in three of the patients have clinical evidence of a cardiac lesion, and of those who die and come to necropsy carditis is found in the great majority.

About a third of the cases, however, give no history of either previous chorea or rheumatism. As a rule the disease subsides fairly soon after delivery and can often be controlled meanwhile by adequate rest, isolation and supervision.

The maternal mortality naturally varies with the severity of the case, but is influenced by the co-existence of a cardiac lesion and the tendency to develop bronchopneumonia. Neglected cases of the manic type may die of exhaustion. The fœtal mortality is mainly

influenced by the possibility of premature labour or the need to intervene and terminate the pregnancy.

The differential diagnosis rests between Huntingdon's chorea and hysteria. In the former there is a later age incidence and usually a family history, while in the latter other stigmata of hysteria are usually present.

The main complications are the development of an acute psychosis, which takes the form either of profound confusion or of mania, and may even necessitate supervision in a padded cell. Secondly, acute carditis and pericarditis may supervene and prove fatal.

The treatment consists in hospitalisation and the enforcement of absolute rest in isolation. Sedatives should be given liberally, and in the manic varieties it may be necessary to administer paraldehyde 5 ml. intramuscularly. Hyoscine 0·5 mg. has also been used with varying success. Promazine, by mouth, 50 mg., 8 hourly, in the severe and uncontrollable case can be of dramatic benefit.[11] The diet should be liberal and a watch maintained for the development of an active cardiac lesion. With good nursing and supervision it is often possible to bring the case under control, but in severe cases the question of terminating pregnancy arises. This is a serious step, because the patient is already ill enough as it is; nevertheless, occasionally it may be the only course to adopt. There is much to be said for sterilising the patient at the same time because of her proneness to suffer a recurrence of the disease in subsequent pregnancies.

VIRUS DISEASES IN PREGNANCY

The extent to which virus diseases contracted in pregnancy may damage the unborn fœtus varies from the trivial to the ultra severe. It was Gregg (1941) who first noted an association between congenital cataract and a history of rubella in early pregnancy. Many of these cases had also congenital cardiac lesions. The epidemic of rubella in question, which had taken place in Australia, was of a very severe variety. Nevertheless, since attention was first directed towards this complication of pregnancy, more cases of associated fœtal defect have come to light.

Retrospective analysis is difficult, because the diagnosis of rubella, made many months later after delivery, is often open to question. In Gregg's series of cases in Australia the position was more clear cut. He described 78 cases of congenital cataract which was obvious from birth and as a rule bilateral; two-thirds of the cases had microphthalmia. All but 10 of the mothers of these affected infants had a definite history of rubella, usually within the first or second month of pregnancy.

Prospective studies are now available on which to assess the risks

and it is quite clear that the likelihood of major congenital abnormality in the fœtus depends upon the time of attack by the rubella virus. For instance, in one large analysis[44] involving 222 live births in patients contracting rubella in the first trimester of pregnancy, major abnormalities were found in 61 per cent, in the case of the first four weeks, in 26 per cent in the second four weeks and in only 8 per cent in the third. In other words, the earlier in pregnancy, the worse the damage. Mental deficiency and deafness are not usually immediately obvious at birth, so that a longer follow up is necessary to assess the true hazard and as spontaneous abortion and stillbirth are also common complications, especially in mothers developing rubella within the first eight weeks, the chances of a healthy infant, completely undamaged, are about 35 per cent. If the children of such affected pregnancies are followed up to the tenth year of life and over, the findings in surviving children at this age indicate major abnormalities in about 15 per cent, in more than half of whom there is more than one abnormality, and minor abnormalities in a further 16 per cent, with again more than half with more than one defect.[48] Ninety-two per cent of this later series, however, were attending ordinary schools, even though some required hearing aids, or speech therapy.

It is clear that much so-called mental backwardness may be more apparent than real and related to some handicapping lesion such as deaf mutism which, even in educated households, may not be recognised for the first few years of the child's life.

The rubella virus can be isolated from placenta and fœtal tissues many weeks after the initial attack and would appear to act by a direct destructive effect upon dividing tissue cells rather than by producing chromosome abnormalities. It is even possible for the nursing staff to be infected by the congenital presence and excretion of rubella virus in babies surviving birth after a pregnancy infected much earlier, in fact it has been found up to eight months later in urine and stools and from throat washings, and may be isolated from many tissues at autopsy.[6] The case has even been described of virus being still present in the lens of a child, almost three years old, operated on for congenital cataract.[34]

Inquiry has naturally extended to the other virus infections in pregnancy, and Kaye and his colleagues, reviewing 273 congenital abnormalities of the grosser kind, for example cardiac lesions, mongolism, cataract, hydrocephalus, pyloric stenosis, cleft palate, atresia of the bowel and spina bifida, found an incidence of 21 per cent of fœtal abnormalities in virus diseases other than rubella, contracted within the first three months. Nevertheless, pregnant women do not contract these infections more commonly than anyone else, so that, taking fœtal abnormality as a whole, virus diseases make only a small, though serious, contribution to the problem.

Swan and Tostevin (1946) had also noted cases of fœtal abnormality following maternal measles, mumps, chickenpox and herpes zoster.

The Survey instituted by the Ministry of Health covered a very large, nation-wide survey, conducted prospectively into the possible effects of not only rubella but other virus infections during pregnancy.[32] In the case of rubella, records were available for an analysis of 578 pregnancies so complicated, in 202 of which the disease had occurred during the first twelve weeks. There were also 103 pregnancies complicated by measles, 298 by chickenpox, 501 by mumps, 33 by poliomyelitis and 166 by influenza. These were matched against a control series of 5,700 selected on the basis of all babies born on a certain date. This enquiry extended throughout England, Scotland and Wales during 1950 to 1957 and the results are nothing like as depressing as previous accounts would have suggested. In the first place it would appear that infection after the 16th week certainly (and probably after the 12th week) does not affect the fœtus, but the death rate *in utero* and up to two years of age is more than doubled when rubella is contracted within the first trimester. Furthermore, the abnormality rate is very much worse, the incidence of congenital heart disease being 4·7 per cent, as against 0·2 per cent in the control series, cataract 4·7, against 0·04 per cent, deafness 3 per cent (0·08) with probable deafness in a slightly greater number. The incidence of mental deficiency was about quadrupled to the figure of 1·8 per cent, as against 0·4 per cent. There was also an increased incidence of pyloric stenosis. Of the children who lived beyond the age of three years nearly 20 per cent had impaired hearing.

In a similar, but smaller series, quoted from Australia[38] the total incidence of all malformations added up to 26 per cent and one child in fifty was severely retarded mentally.

Although there was a suggestion that measles might raise the incidence of infant deaths and malformations the figures were not very conclusive. The other virus infections appeared to be very much less important as causes of abnormality although there was a higher death rate in cases of maternal influenza and poliomyelitis.

The importance of influenza is less easy to assess because of inaccuracies in diagnosis, but in the year 1957 to 1958 there was an epidemic of Asian influenza in Dublin of some severity in which 663 pregnant women contracting the disease were analysed.[12] The congenital deformity rate was about two and a half times that of the control group and the abnormalities were noted to be mainly of the central nervous system, particularly anencephaly.

As vaccination against smallpox involves inflicting the patient with a virus disease deliberately, there has naturally been some debate about the advisability of undertaking this in the early months. The general concensus of opinion is that the procedure is safe. On the

other hand MacArthur (1952) in a prospective study found that 16 (i.e. 47 per cent) of 34 women vaccinated in the second and third months of pregnancy failed to give birth to healthy children, mainly because of miscarriage (10), stillbirth (5) and congenital abnormality (1). The risks both to the mother and the baby of the patient contracting smallpox, however, are so horrifying that there should be no hesitation in advising vaccination even in the earliest months of pregnancy in the case of a patient who has been actually exposed. Acting on general principles, therefore, one would be inclined to recommend that vaccination be postponed, especially if it is primary, to the second and third trimesters, unless there are special reasons. The dangers from secondary vaccination must be minimal and the most pressing indication nowadays is in order to obtain one's visa to enter the United States.

In the present state of our knowledge, therefore, it would appear that the rubella virus stands out as the principal if not quite the main offender; the teratogenic effects of other viruses are still not widely recognised and a confidently reassuring attitude should be taken with the patient exposed to the other exanthemata.

There is a correlation between the time of onset of the infection in pregnancy and the period of gestation at which embryonic development is most rapid and, therefore, presumably most vulnerable, and this too selects the particular structure most likely to suffer damage. Once differentiation has taken place a particular organ ceases to be susceptible to rubella. Furthermore, rubella might so damage the embryo as to reduce its chances of being born alive. The following abnormalities are likely to be encountered either singly or in combination:

Deaf mutism.
Mental deficiency.
Microcephaly.
Congenital cardiac lesions.
Cataract.
Mongolism.
Cleft palate.
Spina bifida, etc. (Fig. 1).
Pyloric stenosis.

The cardiac lesions encountered include patent ductus, patent foramen ovale and interventricular septal defect. In the ears of deaf mutes the organ of Corti is absent. Kirman (1955) found a history of rubella in early pregnancy in the mothers of 0·9 per cent of 791 mental defectives reviewed.

A very severe epidemic of rubella swept the United States in 1964 with a noticeable increase in the type and extent of damage done to

unborn babies, and as a result of this epidemic there has been described the "expanded rubella syndrome".

Expanded rubella syndrome·—The following further clinical features may be encountered:[42]

Thrombocytopenia (100 per cent of cases).
Purpuric lesions.
Growth retardation (78 per cent).
Hepato-splenomegaly.

Central nervous system changes, including increased CSF protein, full fontanelle and osseous manifestations (84 per cent).

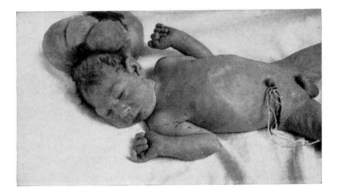

7/Fig. 1.—Large meningocele.

The osseous manifestations as demonstrated on X-ray consist of a large anterior fontanelle and in the metaphyses of the femora and tibiæ near the knee joint there is an altered trabecular pattern with linear areas of longitudinal radio-translucency, contrasted with areas of increased bone density. There may also be radio-translucency parallel to the growth plate. These lesions are said to be reversible.

Another report quotes a 33 per cent incidence of long bone X-ray changes as described above and, furthermore, over half the babies were of retarded development, weighing less than 2,500 g. at birth.[39]

This is a formidable list of possible misfortunes, and the patient who contracts a virus infection, particularly rubella, within the first three months of pregnancy is undoubtedly exposed to the risk of tragedy.

It goes without saying that women in early pregnancy should avoid, as far as possible, contact with virus infections, and the compulsory notification of cases of rubella would make a difference. Strangely enough the severity of fœtal malformation is not directly related to the severity of the clinical disease in the mother and quite

minor infections might pass unnoticed. To the woman who believes she has been exposed to the risk of rubella and who has no idea of whether or not she is susceptible, the mental anguish can be very great and various methods have been tried serologically to assess whether the patient has an immunity to the disease or whether, in fact, the disease has been recently contracted. It looks as though this problem may be solved on a fairly widespread scale, however, by demonstrating a rise in neutralising and hæmagglutination inhibiting antibodies whose level alters sharply early in the disease. It is this rise in antibody which helps to distinguish the patient already immune from rubella from one who has been recently infected and from such a calculation it should be possible to assess the risk to this particular pregnancy. Unfortunately, even so, because of the variable time and extent of this alteration in antibody level, doubt may remain. However the earliest immuno-globulins (IgM) to be found after the primary stimulus have a very high molecular weight, but these immuno-globulins are replaced within a few weeks by those of a lower molecular weight (IgG and IgA). New methods are described from St. Thomas's Hospital[2] which have been devised for distinguishing the two by hæmagglutination inhibition tests, titrating early and late convalescent sera before and after treating the sera with 2-mercaptoethanol, which is a sulphydryl-reducing compound that breaks down the IgM immuno-globulins. The amount of IgM immuno-globulin is therefore revealed by the difference between the level found in a control specimen from the patient compared with another treated with 2-mercaptoethanol. The discrepancy would appear to be most marked during the first few days of the illness, thereby proving beyond doubt the existence of a very recent infection. Clearly the test should be carried out at an early stage of infection, but may help to confirm or allay fears that pregnancy may be adversely affected. The test is claimed to be both simple and rapid and may determine treatment. Certainly it is hoped that no policy of terminating pregnancy will presently be carried out on any evidence less precise. Occasionally, one gets requests for termination of a given pregnancy simply because there is a story that a child of a woman further down the street has developed German measles, hardly a reason for liquidation of a pregnancy which may be perfectly normal however real the maternal anxiety. Fortunately the majority of women in the population have immunity to the disease already without being aware of having had it before. In the patient who is known to have been exposed to risk of infection with rubella and in whom it is certain, as far as this is possible, that she has not previously contracted the disease, and therefore obtained her own active immunity, attempts may be made to confer a temporary passive immunity by the use of gamma globulin.

In the absence of a policy of active immunisation of young girls before marriage, there would certainly appear to be a strong case for attempting to confer a passive immunity on the mother genuinely exposed, but limited to such cases if valuable material is not to be wasted, as indicated in the previous paragraphs. It is generally reckoned that 12 ml. of convalescent gamma globulin or double that amount, i.e. 24 ml. (2·9 g.) of pooled gamma globulin in one injection should suffice to protect a patient against an attack of rubella. The debatable value of this prophylaxis has to be weighed against the known risk. The truthful evaluation of gamma globulin prophylaxis will only be settled when serological studies proving the existence of a recent attack of virus can become more generally employed, but to the practitioner who has no access to such scientific proof it would require a certain boldness to deny the patient a request for protection. The protection afforded by 24 ml. (2·9 g. gamma globulin) lasts about three weeks, after which the passive immunity begins to wear off and it may in the case of renewed exposure be necessary to repeat it. Needless to say, an injection given too late after the patient is on the point of developing the disease will be of little benefit and if, in fact, the mother does develop unquestionable rubella the chances of fœtal abnormality have to be seriously considered and, as stated before, the nature of the abnormality will be related to the period of gestation at which the invasive period of the disease strikes. It is in such cases that the very difficult decision of whether or not to terminate the pregnancy has to be taken, remembering that the later in pregnancy, the less the risk, and the more amenable it may be to treatment in infancy and childhood. Likewise, the intravenous injection of 30 ml. of serum from patients convalescing from rubella has been tried, but the efficacy of this type of prophylaxis is not yet fully proven. It is a small but definite comfort, however, that the majority of cases developing German measles will bear children who have escaped harmful effects, and the outcome in future pregnancies is in no wise prejudiced.

The new Abortion Law in the United Kingdom which legalises the termination of pregnancy when there is a "substantial" risk of "serious" handicap to the child does not, in fact, define the level at which action should be taken and is therefore really of very little help to the patient or the clinician whose individual conscience alone can guide them, bearing in mind always that the policy of termination, on the offchance of fœtal abnormality, means that many a potentially normal baby will have to be sacrificed.

HERPES GESTATIONIS

This curious condition has a tendency to recur in subsequent pregnancies at an earlier stage each time. Fortunately with modern

corticosteroid therapy the patient can usually be kept under control and neither she nor the fœtus may come to permanent harm.[43, 52]

High doses of prednisone, for example, may be required, and the patient is liable to collapse under the stress of labour unless adequate corticosteroid therapy is maintained. She must, of course, be delivered in hospital under full specialist care, both obstetrical and dermatological. With these provisos there is no need to terminate pregnancy nor to advise the patient against further child-bearing.

ANTENATAL THROMBOSIS

The commonest variety of this complication of pregnancy is in veins already varicose. The condition can produce a great deal of discomfort and misery in pregnancy and seldom gets the treatment it deserves. Varicose veins themselves nearly always get worse, usually because of neglect to a large extent. Any varicosities in the legs noted at first booking should receive attention before and not after worsening. The best way to prevent aggravation of the condition is to make sure that the patient gets adequate rest during the day, with her feet up; but this is impossible for most women, therefore she must be advised against prolonged periods of standing, especially in the second half of pregnancy. Support from outside, in mild cases, can be obtained by rolling several pairs of stockings, one on top of top of the other, onto the legs and for this stockings which have already got holes and are not worth repairing are admirable. In more severe cases elastic stockings coming well up the thigh should be obtained at an early stage. Needless to say these supports should be applied while the patient is still in bed and before her feet are put to the ground; in other words before swelling has had time to occur and not after.

In spite of all these precautions, however, the condition may deteriorate surprisingly. The reluctance of surgeons to operate or to inject these veins with sclerosing fluids is due to the high rate of failure in pregnancy and the comforting reflection (at least comforting to the surgeon) that the condition will improve after pregnancy is all over; but it may well be necessary to treat by the injection of sclerosing agents, using the empty vein technique. Operations undertaken for the relief of varicose veins are likely to produce their biggest benefit by the necessary rest entailed post-operatively and are therefore seldom performed.

Commonly, however, an area of varicose vein undergoes superficial thrombophlebitis which can be very painful and disabling. The risk of embolism is by no means absent and the case should be treated with vigour. Firstly, bed rest with elevation of the foot, to improve the venous return, is essential. A period of pain and disability can unquestionably be shortened by intravenous heparin maintained in

standard dosage over a period of at least three days, by which time the danger of embolism or of further spread of the condition should have passed. Bandaging with ichthyol solutions is a time-honoured ritual which is more impressive in the picturesque mess it produces than actually beneficial. Heparin is recommended as the drug of choice for several reasons; firstly its action is immediate; secondly, with its molecular weight of 16 thousand it does not cross the placenta and therefore is perfectly safe for the fœtus; and thirdly, its effects are short-lived and can be quickly countered should the patient go into labour. Admittedly the more superficial the affected vein, the less likely is thrombo-embolism to occur, but this does not justify a casual attitude. With adequate treatment starting with 20,000 units, for example, followed by about 10,000 every six hours intravenously, or, maintained, better still, by intravenous drip, so as to prolong the clotting time to 20 minutes, it will be found that the thrombotic process does not extend and the pain disappears very quickly.[19]

The slower acting anticoagulants given orally, namely warfarin and phenindione, are less suitable because their effect is slow and because they cross the placenta and may produce or aggravate fœtal hypoprothrombinæmia with a dangerous tendency to hæmorrhagic disease should labour ensue while the fœtus is still affected by the drug.[26] The danger can be minimised by the timely injection of vitamin K_1 (Konakion) 10–20 mg. slowly to the mother by the intravenous route and before delivery actually takes place.

Fatal pulmonary embolism, which may occur antenatally and is becoming a more prominent cause of maternal death nowadays, can thus be prevented by anticoagulants. Therefore, thrombosis superficial or deep should not go untreated.

VOMITING, HIATUS HERNIA AND HEARTBURN

by WALLACE BARR, M.B., B.Sc., F.R.C.S. (Glas.), F.R.C.O.G., *Gynæcologist, Western Infirmary, Glasgow*

VOMITING

This is one of the most common of all the tribulations of the first trimester and in a survey by Diggory and Tomkinson (1962), no fewer than 88 out of a random series of 100 pregnant women experienced this symptom. It generally occurs during the early part of pregnancy and in many instances precedes the first missed menstrual period. For many, it is a minor complaint to which they are resigned but to others the anticipation of an uneventful pregnancy may be rudely shattered by weeks of intense discomfort with associated domestic upheaval and inconvenience.

The evidence of uncontrollable vomiting has shown a remarkable decline over the past three decades and in the adjoining table are shown the figures obtained from the records of the Glasgow Royal Maternity Hospital for three comparable five-year periods since 1936.

	1936–40	1946–50	1956–60
Total Births in Hospital	16,532	16,326	17,759
Admissions for Hyperemesis Gravidarum	396 (2·4%)	168 (1·0%)	97 (0·6%)
Termination of Pregnancy	33	4	nil
Maternal Deaths	15 (12 after termination)	nil	nil

It will be seen from this table that, although the total number of births in the hospital does not show much alteration, the number of cases of hyperemesis gravidarum requiring admission to hospital is dramatically reduced. It will also be seen that, although fifteen women perished from this cause between the years 1936 and 1940, there were no maternal deaths in the subsequent five-year periods reviewed and in the last of these there were no cases considered severe enough even to warrant termination.

It is difficult to explain this diminishing incidence of severe hyperemesis gravidarum but some at least of the credit must be given to the newer drugs which have recently become available, and many patients now seek advice earlier in the pregnancy.

Ætiology

Our ignorance of the cause is almost as striking as the success which nearly always attends treatment. The condition is commoner in first than in subsequent pregnancies and it has also been found that women who have nausea and vomiting in their first pregnancy are more likely to have symptoms again in later pregnancies: there is no relationship between maternal age and the incidence of hyperemesis gravidarum. It is safer to classify cases according to the severity of the vomiting than to use the old division into toxic and neurotic varieties. This is not only obsolete but dangerous too, as the diagnosis of neurosis may engender a regrettable complacency regarding the outcome of the condition.

In all cases and especially those of acute onset it is essential to exclude organic disease of extra-uterine origin such as appendicitis, gastroenteritis, intestinal obstruction, peptic ulcer, twisted ovarian

cyst, cerebral tumour, fulminating pre-eclamptic toxæmia, pyelitis and uræmia. Hydatidiform mole should also be excluded.

Only when these have been excluded, and not before, may one contemplate the many nebulous and ill-substantiated theories which have been conjured up to explain this curious condition. There are many who consider that hyperemesis is a manifestation of allergy. Kapeller Adler (1949) found large quantities of histamine in the urine of such patients, and according to Youssef and Barsoum (1953) adrenocortical insufficiency causes hypersensitivity to histamine and favours the development of allergic manifestations. Excessive supply of gonadotrophins has also been suggested as the cause of hyperemesis but this now seems unlikely since an investigation by Fairweather and Loraine (1962) showed that from the 7th to the 15th weeks of pregnancy the mean human chorionic gonadotrophin excretion in hyperemesis patients was significantly lower than in normally pregnant women. There are still those who think that the vomiting may be reflexly engendered by some pelvic abnormality, such as retroversion of the gravid uterus. The anatomy of the reflex arc is of doubtful authenticity, however, and the cures obtained by correcting the malposition are just as likely to be due to suggestion. Vitamin deficiency states and carbohydrate deficiencies have also been put forward as possible ætiological factors, but they are more likely to be effects than causes.

Fitzgerald (1956) in a discussion on the epidemiology of hyperemesis gravidarum points out that its incidence and severity in Aberdeen and North-east Scotland was significantly diminished during the last war and immediate post-war years, the assumption being that the major problems engendered by war conditions allowed the patient less time to worry about personal affairs. Few will deny that the psychogenic factor is of prime importance and it is probable that the many adjustments demanded by the newly-pregnant woman impose a mild condition of stress coupled with an irrationally exaggerated fear of the obstetric hazards confronting her, especially that of producing an abnormal child. These factors, superimposed upon the subtle physiological accompaniments of reduced gastric secretion and motility, provide a much more likely cause for the condition than the hitherto fashionable explanation that vomiting constitutes a symbolic rejection by the mother of her pregnancy.

Attempts have been made to establish a relationship between the incidence of abortion and the vomiting of early pregnancy. Semmens (1957) found vomiting twice as common in those who aborted, while Medalie (1957) showed from his figures that the more a patient vomited the *less* likelihood there was of abortion. This provides an interesting comment on the fallibility of statistical evidence and suggests that there is no relationship between the two.

Pathology and Biochemical Changes

There are no specific morbid anatomical findings and the changes described by Sheehan (1939) in the liver, heart, kidneys and central nervous system are common to all cases of severe malnutrition whatever the cause. They were frequently observed by us during World War II when we had the sad and unenviable task of dealing with some of the victims of political persecution in Germany and Holland. The lesions in the brain stem resembling Wernicke's encephalopathy are probably due to vitamin B_1 deficiency.

The biochemical changes which occur can also be attributed to chronic starvation and are not specific to hyperemesis. There is a loss of water and salt with consequent hæmoconcentration and reduction of urinary chlorides. Extracellular fluid is diminished and plasma, sodium and chloride are reduced. Ketosis occurs and the blood urea is elevated as a result of the disturbance in nitrogen metabolism. Potassium deficiency soon follows, as potassium is not stored by the normal adult and rapid loss occurs in the vomit and in the increased renal excretion. This hypokalæmia may cause further vomiting, which, together with liver damage, sets up a vicious circle difficult or impossible to break.

Clinical Features

The insidious change from the mild to the severe state has constantly to be watched for. So long as she is not losing weight appreciably, has a clean, moist tongue and no acetone in her urine, there is little cause for concern even if she protests that she vomits every morsel of food swallowed. As her condition deteriorates, the pulse rate starts to rise and blood pressure falls, the tongue becomes dry and furred while the breath smells strongly of acetone. Emaciation supervenes with dramatic speed, the urine becomes concentrated and in addition to acetone may contain albumin and bile with chlorides greatly diminished or absent. Epigastric tenderness is frequently noted. In the later stages the temperature starts to rise, jaundice supervenes and hæmatemesis may occur. She becomes apathetic and drowsy or confused and euphoric. Squint, diplopia and nystagmus may be noted and retinal hæmorrhages appear. Various palsies develop and there may be great tenderness in the legs together with other signs of peripheral neuritis. Ultimately Wernicke's encephalopathy becomes fully established and the patient usually dies in coma.

Treatment

In early cases, simple dietetic measures will often be effective and should be given a trial before resorting to the countless proprietary and often expensive remedies advertised by the drug manufacturers.

Constipation should be corrected and small carbohydrate meals taken frequently, while all greasy foods should be avoided. When the sickness has a well-defined morning incidence the time-honoured piece of toast or cream cracker taken before rising is often helpful.

Of the drugs to be employed, the antihistamines and vitamin B_6 preparations are often of value. Since Dougray (1949) first recommended the use of pyranisamine maleate (Anthisan) and promethaline hydrochloride (Phenergan), many other antihistamines have appeared of which dimenhydrinase (Dramamine) and promethazine-8-chlorotheophyllinate (Avomine) are among the most effective. Meclozine di-hydrochloride (Ancolan), also an antihistamine, was investigated in a double blind trial by Diggory and Tomkinson (1962) who reported it to be therapeutically effective to a high degree of statistical significance. The addition of pyridoxine (Ancoloxin) did not improve the results in their patients but it has long been considered, rightly or wrongly, that pyridoxine deficiency may occur in hyperemesis gravidarum. Wachstein and Gudaitis (1953) and we ourselves have found that pyridoxine hydrochloride combined with benzocaine and pentobarbital in the form of Nidoxital is often effective where other remedies have failed. Much has been written about cortisone preparations but in our opinion there is at present no very convincing evidence to justify their employment in vomiting of pregnancy.

Because the thalidomide disaster focused attention on the possible dangers of prescribing, during early pregnancy, drugs whose exact action on the developing foetus is not known, some evidence has been produced to suggest that certain anti-emetic drugs may possibly have teratogenic effects. The matter remains *sub judice* and until the issue has been finally resolved, it is suggested that the greatest discrimination is employed in the exhibition of any drug prescribed during the early stages of pregnancy (Barr, 1963). For the severe case the only place for the patient is a hospital bed where, out of the range of all visitors including her husband, she very often recovers abruptly without further treatment. The attitude of the nurse in attendance is important and the ideal approach is one of firm competence allied with tactful understanding. A fluid balance chart is kept and the blood pressure recorded at least twice daily.

If the vomiting does not immediately cease, all feeding by mouth is stopped, the lost fluids and chlorides are made good by intravenous infusion and ketosis is combated with glucose. Glucose 4·3 per cent in 0·18 per cent saline should be used and one should aim to administer at least 3 litres in 24 hours. Ten units of insulin may with advantage be added to each half-litre of glucose solution to encourage the intracellular shift of potassium ions and to increase glycogen storage. In addition, adequate sedation is obtained, usually with barbiturates,

for example sodium gardenal, gr. 3, by injection or Sparine 50 mg. by injection. Oral hygiene is attended to with mouth washes, and only when ketosis and dehydration have been overcome, and the patient has stopped vomiting, are fluids given by mouth in small and often repeated quantities. The patient then gradually proceeds to solids, and it is indeed unusual for this treatment not to succeed within a very few days. To prevent neuropathy, injections of vitamin B_1 (aneurine) and B_6 (pyridoxine hydrochloride) 100 mg. are given daily.

Therapeutic Abortion

If the patient fails to respond to the above energetic treatment therapeutic abortion has to be considered, especially in multiparæ, in whom vomiting often has a more sinister significance. The decision to operate is easily too long delayed, in which case death may be precipitated rather than prevented. It will be seen from the table given earlier that during the years 1936–40 there were 15 maternal deaths, 12 of which occurred after termination of pregnancy and in the series described by Bandstrup (1939) 17 out of the 40 deaths which were reported occurred in patients whose pregnancy was terminated, presumably too late. The following, then, are the indications for therapeutic abortion:

1. Jaundice.
2. Persistent albuminuria.
3. Polyneuritis and neurological signs.
4. Temperature consistently above 100·4 and a pulse remaining above 100.
5. The onset of psychosis, although Sheehan rather hints that abortion precipitates death in these cases.

It is nowadays so rarely that pregnancy has to be interrupted that one is very naturally reluctant to take such drastic action, but to operate too late is just as bad as not operating at all. The method of termination will vary according to circumstances but there is much to be said for abdominal hysterotomy, possibly under local anæsthesia.

Vomiting in Late Pregnancy

No case of vomiting occurring during the later weeks of pregnancy should be disregarded and a full investigation should always be undertaken as it may be a symptom of sinister import. We have recently seen a case of acute liver failure present only with retching and occasional vomiting followed rapidly by jaundice, severe hypotension, coma and death within 48 hours. Urinary infection is the most common cause of vomiting in late pregnancy and a clean speci-

men of urine should be examined in all cases for the presence of pus cells and organisms. Other causes are pre-eclamptic toxæmia, and occasionally acute hydramnios. Extraneous causes such as intestinal obstruction, gastroenteritis, cholecystitis, appendicitis and red degeneration in a fibroid should also be excluded.

HIATUS HERNIA

Hiatus hernia is a well recognised cause of gastro-intestinal upset during pregnancy and it is quite remarkable how published figures have shown that this condition, which was thought to be a rare one, is nowadays almost commonplace. Gorbach and Reid (1956), in reviewing 50 cases with persistent gastro-intestinal symptoms during the latter half of pregnancy found that no fewer than 62 per cent had some degree of hiatus hernia, while Mixson and Woloshin (1953) found 31 cases in 360 pregnancies selected at random.

We ourselves found a low incidence and in 85 patients with heartburn and nausea during pregnancy only 4 showed hiatus hernia on X-ray examination with barium.

It appears to be much commoner in multiparæ, presumably due to the increasing size of the diaphragmatic gap. Rigler and Eneboe (1935) report an incidence of 18·1 per cent in multiparæ against 5·1 per cent in primiparous patients.

Many cases go through pregnancy and labour uneventfully and many more are never diagnosed, but occasionally symptoms are severe. In most cases the chief complaint is intractable heartburn, unrelieved by alkalis or other medication and aggravated by the recumbent posture. In others vomiting is the main feature and a few of these go on to hæmatemesis as described by Egerton and Ruark (1955). In the third and by far the smallest group, the clinical picture is one of severe and sudden onset, epigastric pain being associated with shock, dyspnœa and often cyanosis. This may be due to "spillover" disease of the lung—the result of aspiration of material from the hernia itself or from an œsophagus obstructed by stricture. These are the cases in which sudden death may occur (Dupont, 1956) and it is suggested by Gorbach and Reid (1956) that they have a large foramen of Bochdalek in the left leaf of the diaphragm, the milder cases being those of so-called œsophageal hiatus hernia with congenitally short œsophagus or enlarged normal œsophageal opening in the diaphragm, so that during pregnancy the upper part of the stomach comes to lie above it.

Treatment in the vast majority of cases is conservative and consists of frequent small meals, sleeping in a propped-up position, sedation as required and the use of alkalis if they provide any relief. Mucaine (*vide infra*) may also be of value in this condition. Powerful

bearing down during the second stage tends to aggravate the condition and should be avoided by the timely application of forceps.

After delivery, although the symptoms usually clear up within a few days, Sutherland *et al.* (1956) reported that the hernia persists in 36 per cent of cases.

Heartburn

This is one of the minor disorders of pregnancy and its unfortunate victims seldom get much sympathy, but frequently, by disturbing sleep and appetite, it lowers morale and promotes a chronic depression out of all proportion to its severity. Moreover, it is extremely common and in our experience nearly 45 per cent of patients suffer from heartburn during pregnancy severely enough to compel them to seek relief.

As suggested by Lawler and McCreath (1951), it is almost certainly due to regurgitation of gastric content on lying down or stooping, and by screening patients with barium in the stomach we have been able to demonstrate such regurgitation in 64 of 85 patients with heartburn. In an overall analysis of 624 cases (Barr, 1958) it was found to bear little relationship to gastric acidity and hiatus hernia accounted for only 6 per cent of the cases X-rayed. Age and parity were not significant ætiological factors, nor was there any apparent association with nausea and vomiting of pregnancy, constipation or previous digestive disorders, and since it usually comes on during the first trimester encroachment upon the abdominal cavity by the enlarging uterus is not likely to be a factor. There was however a striking relationship to posture and no fewer than 92·3 per cent of cases found that lying down, bending or stooping, initiated an attack.

Using an inflated balloon in the stomach attached to tambour and recording drum, gastric motility during pregnancy was investigated and it was found in patients with heartburn that there is a significant reduction in gastric tonus rhythm, although peristaltic activity and emptying time remain unaltered. This reduced tone which is shared by the muscle of the lower œsophagus is probably responsible for regurgitation.

Treatment in the first instance is by alkalies which give relief in about half of all cases, especially if combined with a sensible dietary regime. Mucaine (oxethazine, a topical anæsthetic agent, in combination with aluminium hydroxide gel and magnesium hydroxide) has been recommended (Traherne, 1962), and we have employed it with considerable success in severe cases. The recommended dose is 1 or 2 teaspoonfuls 15 minutes before meals. It should not be washed down straightaway with a drink as this may diminish the effect. In those which do not respond to such simple measures, the value of Prostigmin, first suggested by Williams (1941), is beyond doubt and

Bower (1961) found that 76 per cent of patients unrelieved by alkalies obtained relief for an average period of about five days from an injection of Prostigmin. In about half these cases the effect was thought to be due to a genuine pharmacological action and in the remainder, to suggestion. In our opinion it is not necessary to administer it by injection and we have been obtaining a cure rate of more than 80 per cent with pyridostigmine (Mestinon) in a dosage of 15 mg. given by mouth four times daily. It is somewhat slower in onset than Prostigmin but longer acting.

REFERENCES

1. ADAMS, R. A., and COOMBES, B. (1965). *J. Amer. med. Ass.*, **192**, 195.
2. BANATVALA, J. E., BEST, JENNIFER, M., KENNEDY, E. A., SMITH, ELIZABETH A., and SPENCE, MARJORIE, E. (1967). *Brit. med. J.*, **2**, 285.
3. BANDSTRUP, E. (1939). *J. Obstet. Gynaec. Brit. Emp.*, **46**, 700.
4. BARR, W. (1958). *J. Obstet. Gynaec. Brit. Emp.*, **65**, 1019.
5. BARR, W. (1963). *Prescribers Jl.*, **3**, 3.
6. BELLANTI, J. A., ARTENSTEIN, M. S., OLSON, L. S., BENSCHER, E. L., LUERS, C. E., and MILSTEAD, K. S. (1965). *Amer. J. Dis. Child.*, **110**, 464.
7. BERESFORD, O. D., and GRAHAM, A. M. (1950). *J. Obstet. Gynaec. Brit. Emp.*, **57**, 616.
8. BLACK, W. P. (1960). *Brit. med. J.*, **1**, 1938.
9. BOWER, D. (1961). *J. Obstet. Gynaec. Brit. Cwlth.*, **68**, 846.
10. *British Medical Journal* (1966). Editorial. **2**, 426.
11. CAMPBELL, A. J. M., and HENDERSON, J. (1959). *Scot. med. J.*, **4**, 128.
12. COFFEY, V. P., and JESSOP, W. J. E. (1959). *Lancet*, **2**, 935.
13. DIGGORY, P. L. C., and TOMKINSON, J. S. (1962). *Lancet*, **2**, 370.
14. DOUGRAY, T. (1949). *Brit. med. J.*, **2**, 1081.
15. DUPONT, M. (1956). *Obstet. and Gynec.*, **55**, 505.
16. EGERTON, C. D., and RUARK, R. S. (1955). *Amer. J. Obstet. Gynec.*, **70**, 1245.
17. FAIRWEATHER, D. V. I., and LORAINE, J. A. (1962). *Brit. med. J.*, **1**, 666.
18. FITZGERALD, J. P. B. (1956). *Lancet*, **1**, 660.
19. FLESSA, H. C., KAPSTROM, A. B., GLUECK, HELEN, I., and WILL, J. J. (1965). *Amer. J. Obstet. Gynec.*, **93**, 570.
20. GORBACH, A. C., and REID, D. E. (1956). *New Engl. J. Med.*, **255**, 517.
21. GREGG, H. M. (1941). *Trans. ophthal. Soc. Aust.*, **3**, 35.
22. HUGHES, I. (1951). *Postgrad. med. J.*, **27**, 595.
23. KAPELLER-ADLER, R. (1949). *Lancet*, **2**, 745.
24. KAYE, B. M., ROSNER, D. C., and STEIN, I. F. (1953). *Amer. J. Obstet. Gynec.*, **65**, 109.
25. KIRMAN, B. H. (1955). *Lancet*, **2**, 113.
26. KRAUS, A. P., PERLOW, S., and SINGER, K. (1949). *J. Amer. med. Ass.*, **139**, 758.
27. *Lancet* (1953). Annotation. **2**, 330.
28. LASK, S. (1953). *Brit. med. J.*, **1**, 652.
29. LAWLER, N. A., and McCREATH, N. D. (1951). *Lancet*, **2**, 369.

30. LEHANE, D., KWANTES, C. M. S., UPWARD, M. G., and THOMSON, D. R. (1949). *Brit. med. J.*, **2**, 572.
31. MACARTHUR, P. (1952). *Lancet*, **2**, 1104.
32. MANSON, M. M., LOGAN, W. P. D., and LUZ, R. M. (1960). *Rubella and other Virus Infections in Pregnancy*. Min. of Health Reports on Public Health and Medical Subjects No. 101.
33. MEDALIE, J. H. (1957). *Lancet*, **2**, 117.
34. MENSER, MARGARET A., HARLEY, J. D., HERTZBERG, R., DORMAN, D. C., and MURPHY, A. M. (1967). *Lancet*, **2**, 387.
35. MIXSON, W. T., and WOLOSHIN, H. S. (1956). *Obstet. and Gynec.*, **8**, 249.
36. MOORE, H. C. (1963). *Lancet*, **2**, 57.
37. MURLESS, B. C. (1947). *Brit. med. J.*, **2**, 251.
38. PITT, D. B. (1961). *Med. J. Aust.*, **1**, 881.
39. PLOTKIN, S. A., OSKI, F. A., HARTNETT, E. M., HERVADA, A. R., FRIEDMAN, S., and GOWING, JEAN (1965). *Pediatrics*, **67**, 182.
40. RIGLER, L. G., and ENEBOE, J. B. (1935). *J. thorac. Surg.*, **4**, 262.
41. ROTH, L. G. (1953). *Amer. J. med. Sci.*, **225**, 139.
42. RUDOLPH, A. J., SINGLETON, E. B., ROSENBERG, H. S., SINGER, D. B., and PHILLIPS, C. A. (1965). *Amer. J. Dis. Child.*, **110**, 428.
43. RUSSELL, B., and THORNE, N. A. (1957). *Brit. J. Derm.*, **69**, 339.
44. SALLOMI, S. J. (1966). *Obstet. and Gynec.*, **27**, 252.
45. SEMMENS, J. P. (1957). *Obstet. and Gynec.*, **9**, 586.
46. SHEEHAN, H. L. (1939). *J. Obstet. Gynaec. Brit. Emp.*, **46**, 681.
47. SHEEHAN, H. L. (1940). *J. Obstet. Gynaec. Brit. Emp.*, **47**, 49.
48. SHERIDAN, MARY D. (1964). *Brit. med. J.*, **2**, 536.
49. SUTHERLAND, C. G., ATKINSON, J. C., BROGDON, B. G., CROW, N. E., and BROWN, W. E. (1956). *Obstet. and Gynec.*, **8**, 261.
50. SWAN, C., and TOSTEVIN, A. L. (1946). *Med. J. Aust.*, **1**, 465.
51. TRAHERNE, J. B. (1962). *Brit. med. J.*, **1**, 1415.
52. VICKERS, H. R. (1964). *Practitioner*, **192**, 639.
53. WACHSTEIN, M., and GUDAITIS, A. (1953). *Amer. J. Obstet. Gynec.*, **66** 1207.
54. WILLIAMS, N. H. (1941). *Amer. J. Obstet. Gynec.*, **42**, 814.
55. YOUSSEF, A. F., and BARSOUM, G. S. (1953). *J. Obstet. Gynaec. Brit. Emp.*, **60**, 388.

CHAPTER VIII

LOCAL ABNORMALITIES

In this chapter a variety of conditions occurring in the pelvic viscera is dealt with, as it affects the practising obstetrician.

CONGENITAL UTERINE ABNORMALITIES

The many different degrees of imperfect Mullerian development, fusion or canalisation, seldom trouble the practitioner because the grosser forms of uterine maldevelopment prevent pregnancy in the first place, and of the cases who conceive the majority run an un-eventful course and deliver themselves without undue difficulty. It is reckoned that two out of every thousand women have a suffici-ently severe degree of congenital uterine deformity to interfere with pregnancy.[18] From the practical point of view there is little point in describing all the varieties of uterine abnormality, which are of more anatomical than obstetrical interest, but if one appreciates how the Mullerian ducts from each side fuse together and become canalised it will at once be seen that a particular structural abnormality is simply a matter of degree in the embryological process. All degrees may be encountered, from the subseptate uterus at one end of the scale to the completely double uterus and cervix at the other (Fig. 1). Neither of these two extremes gives any trouble as a rule, but inter-mediate stages may do so. Where there is a full septum in the uterus the fœtus must perforce lie in the uterine axis longitudinally, but lesser degrees favour a transverse lie, so that one pole of the fœtus lies in each half of the uterus. The incomplete septum also prevents version. About 12 per cent of cases of transverse lie are reckoned to be associated with a subseptate uterus[10] and they are even more liable to inertia in labour. It would appear that the lower uterine segment may resist expansion. Retention of the placenta and atonic postpartum hæmorrhage are also more likely to occur. The bi-cornuate uterus with the single cervix is by no means uncommon, and occasionally the placenta may occupy one chamber and the fœtus the other, an arrangement which prejudices the safety of the third stage of labour, inasmuch as a placenta so situated is liable to be re-tained and may be difficult to remove.

One tends to think of a bicornuate uterus with its two horns stick-ing symmetrically upwards and outwards like a donkey's ears, but usually there is a good deal of inequality and asymmetry and a tend-ency for one of the horns to flop backwards, in which case it may

become trapped below the pelvic brim and prevent the engagement of the presenting part or even obstruct labour. In this position it is of course very vulnerable, and lochial drainage is likely to be inadequate. It is easy to see how torsion of the whole uterus may be favoured by the presence of a sizable non-gravid horn.

In the occasional case which gives trouble the clinical diagnosis is by no means easy unless hysterography has provided foreknowledge of the condition. Other pelvic tumours have to be distinguished, and, earlier in pregnancy of course, the question of ectopic pregnancy enters into the differential diagnosis.

It is often a more serious matter when one of the horns of a bicornuate uterus happens to be rudimentary. This may become the

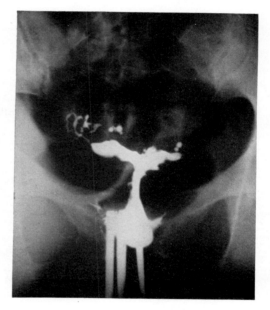

8/Fig. 1.—Double uterus. Hysterosalpingogram.

(By courtesy of Dr. Pecker, Lambeth Hospital.)

site of a pregnancy, and its walls are in no condition to withstand its growth, so that acute rupture with intra-peritoneal bleeding is very likely. In other cases the rudimentary horn has only a very narrow connection with the cervical canal or perhaps none at all, so that blood collecting within its lumen cannot be discharged and an acute hæmatometra develops. There is a fairly common association of congenital uterine abnormalities with other urogenital defects. In other words, the discovery of one freak indicates a search for others.

As already hinted, many of these cases go through their obstetrical careers sometimes undiagnosed and often without trouble, and pro-

vided a woman proves herself capable of conceiving, an optimistic prognosis can usually be given. When seen for the first time in pregnancy, in the absence of a double cervix, which can be ascertained with certainty, one should be very cautious of diagnosing congenital uterine abnormality because of apparent uterine asymmetry, which is common in the early months of pregnancy. The diagnosis is usually made between pregnancies, and hysterography is invaluable; but it should be pointed out that the case who delivers herself without any trouble should not be subjected to such an investigation purely to satisfy a point of academic interest.

Certain adverse effects upon pregnancy are well recognised. In reviewing a series of 42 pregnancies occurring in association with congenital uterine abnormalities MacGregor (1957) observed that 19 ended in abortion, and of the remaining 23 pregnancies premature labour occurred in 5 and the presentation was unstable in 8. In 5 instances manual removal of the placenta was necessary. Out of the 23 pregnancies reaching the stage of viability 4 babies were lost. Although the maternal and fœtal accident rate is high, especially from cord prolapse and placenta prævia, it will depend upon the completeness or otherwise of congenital abnormality, thus illustrating the paradox that the more trivial anatomical abnormalities are, for that very reason, the more treacherous.

CONGENITAL VAGINAL ABNORMALITIES

A completely double vagina with a longitudinal septum may occur and seldom gives any trouble; in fact, Munro Kerr and Chassar Moir stated that the more complete the malformation the less likely is dystocia. A septate vagina, however, may hold up delivery, but the amount of birth canal room can only be properly assessed towards term after the distensibility of the soft parts has had full time to develop.

Congenital strictures of the vagina are far more serious and may occur at any level in the Mullerian system, in other words in the upper three-quarters of the vagina. This abnormality again is due to imperfect canalisation. Occasionally the vaginal vault may be perfectly patent and the stricture may occur at the junction of the upper third and lower two-thirds. I once had a case with such a stricture which was barely adequate to allow the discharge of menstrual blood and caused an obstructive type of dysmenorrhœa, yet the passage of a spermatozoon must have been possible, for she became pregnant. The condition was not recognised until she went into labour at another hospital. She was delivered by Cæsarean section and the true state of affairs assessed at the time. I then did a modified McIndoe type of operation with Thiersch graft which relieved her dys-

menorrhœa and was structurally fairly satisfactory, although some vaginal narrowing was still palpable on follow-up examination. She again became pregnant and I delivered her by Cæsarean section as I was doubtful of the capacity of the vagina to allow the passage of the fœtus. However, in her third pregnancy she was delivered *per vias naturales*. It is impossible to assess the obstetrical importance of these strictures early in pregnancy, as the ensuing months may produce a remarkable change, so that with the softening up of the vagina the stricture may be no longer palpable. In the case of traumatic strictures, for example after plastic repair operations for prolapse, a vaginal or cervical stricture tends to be more dangerous; in fact, it is the narrowing of the vaginal vault that often occurs which is of even more importance than the actual state of the cervix, so that obstruction to delivery occurs at a particularly dangerous point with regard to the safety of the bladder.

Less common vaginal abnormalities in obstetrical practice are recto-vaginal and vesico-vaginal fistulæ. Their mere presence, after all, discourages the opportunity for conception; nevertheless, should the patient conceive, normal delivery commonly occurs, although in the case of recto-vaginal fistulæ the danger of complete perineal rupture is very great.

RETROVERSION

The importance of retroversion has, in the past, been greatly overestimated, for about one in every ten women has a retroverted uterus which is not necessarily of any pathological significance. Its discovery on routine examination in an otherwise normal patient, therefore, calls for no active measures. Retroversion has been found in 5·5 per cent of all primigravidæ before the 12th week of pregnancy and in 6·5 per cent of multiparæ.[2] Provided the retroverted uterus is both mobile and not tender on palpation, the likelihood is that no obstetrical trouble will ensue, and that, as the uterus enlarges, the malposition will naturally correct itself. It has been said that retroversion aggravates the severity of hyperemesis if present, but it is probable that the psychological effect of its manipulative correction does more to cure the patient of this symptom than the correction itself. There is no doubt, however, that women with retroversion conceive a little less easily than when the uterus is in the normal position, mainly because after coitus the cervix points away from the seminal pool in the posterior fornix, and all of us can recall instances in which conception has followed correction or advice to adopt a different position during coitus or immediately after. Symptoms from retroversion in pregnancy do not normally arise until incarceration within the pelvis threatens.

Retroversion is also regarded as being a possible ætiological factor

in early abortion, although there is little convincing statistical evidence of this; but coitus, in the early months of pregnancy, may, by direct trauma, precipitate miscarriage in a retroverted uterus predisposed to abort. Where the patient has already had one or two previous abortions and is now found to be pregnant again with retroversion, it is naturally prudent to advise her to abstain, at least until pregnancy has safely reached the 16th week.

Incarceration of the gravid uterus does not occur until after the third month, when the uterus has become large enough to fill the pelvic cavity. Normally by the 12th week the uterus should have already risen so that the fundus is palpable *per abdomen*, but where this has not occurred it is as well to see the patient at more frequent intervals and to be on the lookout for incarceration, which may produce symptoms as early as the 13th week. The symptoms of incarceration are mainly due to effects upon the bladder. A short period of frequency gives way to dysuria and finally to acute retention of urine. Œdema in the region of the bladder neck adds its effects to those of mechanical compression and neuromuscular incoordination from the great elongation of the anterior vaginal wall and the structures that lead to it, so that the onset of retention is usually sudden and is followed by overflow incontinence.

Fortunately this dangerous mishap is rather uncommon. Decompression of the bladder by catheterisation is an urgent necessity if it is to be saved from the risks of rupture, sloughing and almost ineradicable infection. For the time being the pregnancy is ignored and all attention is given to the bladder, which must be kept empty. In the majority of cases the uterus undergoes spontaneous correction within the course of 48 hours. To encourage this correction the patient should be told to lie as much as possible semi-prone or in an exaggerated Sims' position.

The problem arises when spontaneous correction does not occur. With the uterus continually enlarging, one of two things must happen: either the anterior wall will sacculate, thus permitting the pregnancy to enlarge into the abdomen, or the patient will abort, the bladder meanwhile continuing at risk until either of these solutions has occurred. Since neither is desirable, intervention is indicated after two days of catheter drainage of the bladder. An attempt is made, therefore, by manipulation, to correct the retroversion, and for this the genupectoral position of the patient is ideal but complicates the giving of an anæsthetic should it be necessary. It will often be found easier to push up the fundus by steering it to one side or other of the sacral promontory. The cervix should not be pulled upon with a vulsellum because it tears very easily in the gravid state and is often quite difficult to expose owing to its very displaced position. A finger in the rectum will often succeed where vaginal manipulation

fails. This operation should be done under the influence of morphia at least, and it carries with it a fairly high risk of provoking abortion. It is for this reason that 48 hours is allowed to elapse initially in the hope of spontaneous correction.

Very rarely, the uterus remains incarcerated because of the presence of adhesions in the depths of the pelvis. The combination of circumstances is rare, because such cases are usually infertile. Nevertheless, when all attempts at correction have failed and the bladder has remained for many days on continuous or regular catheter regime, the question of laparotomy and division of adhesions will arise. This will ultimately succeed in dealing with the condition except in the rarest instances, where abdominal hysterotomy is necessary.

The diagnosis of retroversion in pregnancy is not usually difficult. The soft, boggy, pulsatile body of the uterus is easily felt through the posterior fornix on bimanual examination; however, it may be mistaken for an ovarian cyst and vice versa. This is an important matter, because, as mentioned later, ovarian cysts demand surgical removal. Careful palpation, if necessary under an anæsthetic, will distinguish uterine body from ovarian tumour. An even more serious mistake is to diagnose the tense, hard, over-distended bladder in incarcerated retroversion as a uterine swelling and to ignore the true state of affairs. These patients in their acute illness are often at the same time threatening to abort and are bleeding *per vaginam.*

A posterior wall fibroid may be confused with a retroverted gravid uterus, and in fact it may be difficult to decide in pregnancy which swelling is fundus and which fibroid. Provided no urinary symptoms are developing, however, the case calls only for observation.

The most important differential diagnosis is that of pelvic hæmatocele due to ectopic pregnancy, and tenderness may prevent adequate clinical examination. The confusion will only arise in the case of the retroverted gravid uterus which is threatening to abort or is already the seat of infection as a result of abortion.

The treatment of gravid retroversion, in the absence of symptoms due to incarceration, is much debated, but the modern tendency is, if possible, not to interfere. Postural treatment by the use of the exaggerated Sims' position is worth encouraging; the patient should be advised against allowing her bladder to become over-filled, and abstinence from intercourse will reduce the risks of miscarriage. Cases in which manipulation is successful would probably have corrected themselves later spontaneously, and those in which it is difficult carry a high abortion risk. Some favour the use of a rubber-ring pessary, which is supposed, by its constant pressure upon the retroverted uterine body, to encourage correction, but it is probable

that these cases, too, owe their cure to Nature rather than to the treatment. Barnes found the results were very little different whatever treatment was, in fact, employed.

PENDULOUS BELLY

Acute anteversion of the gravid uterus occurs with pendulous belly. The condition is usually due to a weak abdominal wall, with wide divarication of the recti between which the uterus herniates. A marked lordosis of the spine is usually associated, and, in fact, is necessary if the patient is going to maintain her balance. In a few cases the distance between xiphisternum and symphysis pubis may be so greatly reduced by kyphosis of the thoracic spine that the pregnant uterus can find room for itself only in extreme forward displacement. If the uterus is grossly over-distended, for example by twins or hydramnios, gravity too plays a part in accentuating pendulous belly. Malpresentations are naturally more common in these cases, but since most of the patients owe their poor abdominal walls to high degrees of parity, the reason for malpresentation will be seen to lie as much in parity as in abnormal uterine position.

The condition has considerable nuisance value and makes the patient extremely uncomfortable, puts additional stresses upon her back and sacro-iliac joints and greatly increases her fatigue during pregnancy. The remedy is to supply a properly designed corset.

PROLAPSE IN PREGNANCY

Minor degrees of this are fairly common and may be associated with stress incontinence, but severe degrees seldom complicate pregnancy. The worst forms are those of acute onset following some sudden rise in intra-abdominal pressure. The trouble and inconvenience which a patient may experience are fortunately short-lived and limited to the earlier weeks of pregnancy since, as soon as the volume of the uterus exceeds that of the pelvic cavity, prolapse becomes impossible. Palliative treatment only is necessary, therefore, and a ring pessary usually suffices to supply the necessary support below; but where the perineum is markedly deficient the patient may have trouble in retaining it, in which case rest in bed is the only alternative.

TORSION OF UTERUS

Minor degrees of rotation of the uterus about its longitudinal axis are physiological, but acute torsion is an uncommon accident and does not occur in the case of an anatomically normal uterus. It is favoured by associated mechanical factors such as the presence of

fibroids or a bicornuate condition of the uterus. The case presents as an acute abdomen, and in many respects the symptoms resemble those of ectopic gestation if the accident occurs in early pregnancy, while in the later months the condition resembles concealed antepartum hæmorrhage with severe pain, shock and a hard and very tender uterus. The decision to open the abdomen is more likely to be made on the grounds of a misdiagnosis than because one recognises the condition clinically, and in any case the diagnosis will not be confirmed until laparotomy. Without operation the case may well deliver herself of a dead fœtus and continue to be classified as a case of concealed antepartum hæmorrhage.

FIBROIDS AND PREGNANCY

Although fibroids are found in about 20 per cent of all women who come to necropsy, their association with pregnancy is very much less common, and in hospital practice occurs in somewhere between 0·5 per cent and 1 per cent of cases. The reason for this is that the majority of pregnancies occur within age groups below that of the development of fibroids. Fibroids, particularly if submucous, may cause infertility. Alternatively, the very conditions which give rise to fibroids, which are as yet not fully understood, may in themselves be the primary cause of the patient's failure to conceive. It is, nevertheless, reasonable to perform myomectomy in a patient complaining of infertility.

In the majority of cases the presence of fibroids does not complicate pregnancy, but in others there is an increased tendency to abort. Much depends upon the mechanical influence of the position of the fibroid. If it is placed posteriorly and of a size sufficient to catch below the sacral promontory, incarceration may occur within the pelvis.

The commonest complication is the onset of acute degeneration, usually of the red variety, which may occur either in the second half of pregnancy or during the puerperium. It is only the larger fibroids, with their precarious blood supply, that are liable to degenerate acutely. Cystic degeneration of a fibroid is less common. The condition is characterised by the onset of abdominal pain of all grades of severity. Vomiting is frequently associated, and both temperature and pulse are likely to be raised. The tongue is often dirty and the patient looks ill. On examination, the most characteristic feature is the localisation of maximal tenderness to the actual site of the fibroid. The diagnosis of acute degeneration in a fibroid in pregnancy is enormously assisted by foreknowledge of the tumour's existence. In mild cases the symptoms subside after a few days, but in severe cases the patient may present the features of an acute abdominal

emergency, and may require morphia to control her pain. Provided one can be certain of the diagnosis, a conservative attitude is nearly always worth while, and treatment consists of the use of pain-relieving drugs, a light or fluid diet and good nursing. Usually within ten days the patient's condition has improved out of all recognition and only in exceptional instances is it necessary to operate.

Uterine torsion may be provoked by a fibroid, as has already been mentioned.

Accidental hæmorrhage is more common in association with fibroids, and occasionally it may be difficult to be certain how much of a patient's symptoms are due to abruptio placentæ and how much to degeneration in a fibroid.

Malpresentations and all their associated complications may be caused by fibroids situated below the presenting part. When seeing a patient early in pregnancy it may appear that a fibroid is bound to give trouble, and yet, as the weeks go by, most of the tumours rise safely into the abdomen and one may often have difficulty in identifying them by palpation later on. This is because fibroids are often much softened in the course of pregnancy and tend to become more discoid and flattened in shape.

Cervical fibroids, or fibroids very low in the uterine wall, may, however, remain below the presenting part as pregnancy advances and may threaten to obstruct labour. Now there is a great difference between such a fibroid anteriorly placed and one situated behind the uterine canal. The former has a far better opportunity of being drawn up out of the pelvis after the onset of labour than a posterior tumour which tends to get trapped within the pelvis. It is, therefore, usually possible to make a shrewd guess about the likelihood of a fibroid obstructing labour before its onset, by observing whether the fibroid is posterior or not, and in the case of the anterior tumour still within the pelvis at the end of pregnancy it is often worth while, other circumstances being favourable, to give labour a chance under close observation.

The onset of premature labour is a not uncommon risk, especially in cases of large multiple fibroids in which the sheer size of the uterus makes it mechanically difficult for the patient to hold her pregnancy until term.

In labour itself, provided no fibroid continues to occupy the pelvis and provided there is no malpresentation, progress is usually unhindered. Nevertheless, the incidence of inertia is higher, especially if any appreciable proportion of the uterine wall is occupied by fibroid and therefore unable to contribute to the expulsive efforts of the rest of the uterus.

More commonly, troubles are encountered in the third stage with a definitely increased incidence of postpartum hæmorrhage, partly

due to interference with the retractile power of the uterus. When the placenta happens to be sited over a fibroid, there is often a defective decidual reaction so that it is liable to be, partially at least, morbidly adherent, thus necessitating manual removal. Very rarely a fibroid situated at the fundus of the uterus may, for mechanical reasons, precipitate uterine inversion.

During the puerperium involution is retarded by fibroids, the lochial loss tends to be greater, and secondary postpartum hæmorrhage may occur in a few cases. For a variety of reasons, including degeneration of the fibroid, a possibly associated anæmia, a prolonged and inert labour, or because of the need for intra-uterine interference, the puerperium is more likely to be morbid.

Quite often during the puerperium a persistent low-grade pyrexia is attributable to degeneration in a fibroid, and I recall one case in which fever continued for some weeks until I removed a large necrotic fibroid by myomectomy, after which the patient's fever subsided.

So far we have mainly considered the manner in which fibroids may affect pregnancy, delivery and thereafter; but pregnancy is not without its effect upon fibroids. On the whole these effects tend to be beneficial inasmuch as they discourage growth, and simple atrophy commonly occurs postpartum, so that a fibroid which, earlier on, was felt with ease may be quite hard to find a few weeks after delivery. Red degeneration has already been mentioned, but this is a much more acute process than simple atrophy. A subserous pedunculated fibroid may become twisted and give rise to acute symptoms. Less commonly a fibroid becomes infected.

DIAGNOSIS

The diagnosis of fibroids in pregnancy is by no means always easy unless the tumour is discrete. Apparent asymmetry in early pregnancy has already been mentioned, and for this reason fibroids are quite often diagnosed when they do not exist. Fibroids never cause amenorrhœa, and any woman who has come to hospital for myomectomy or hysterectomy and whose period is only a few days overdue should be suspected of having become pregnant if disaster is to be avoided. The consistency of a fibroid is, of course, much harder than that of the gravid uterus, but even so one can be misled. I well recall a young patient in my wards who was admitted for myomectomy for a mass of fibroids the size of a 32-weeks pregnancy, one of which was degenerating. Her expected period was overdue on admission so we awaited confirmation of the diagnosis of pregnancy. She thereupon started to bleed intermittently and the urinary pregnancy tests remained equivocal. Ultrasonography, how-

ever, presently showed fœtal echoes at the top of the tumour mass and was therefore discredited—unjustly. After a few demoralising weeks the body, but not the head or the placenta of a 14-weeks fœtus was passed through an invisible cervix so high up in the left antero-lateral fornix that two attempts at exploration of the cavity (whose whereabouts could not be foretold) had to be abandoned. There followed a period of sepsis and fortunately only minor bleedings while the situation was got under control with antibiotics, after which I gave up the unequal struggle to preserve her reproductive function and performed hysterectomy. The head was never found but numerous submucous fibroids were clustered around above the internal os, any one of which might have tempted a convincing pull with ovum forceps had I been able to introduce such an instrument. Having preached for years that any non-malignant uterus capable of implanting a pregnancy deserves conservation I had to eat my words—not for the first time.

A retroverted gravid uterus has to be distinguished from a fibroid situated posteriorly. The size of the uterus may make one suspect a fibroid when in actual fact the case is one of twin pregnancy, and vice versa. An ectopic pregnancy with pelvic hæmatocele is less likely to be confused with a fibroid if one bears in mind that the margins of a hæmatocele are usually not very discrete. An ovarian tumour must be distinguished from a fibroid in the differential diagnosis because the treatment of the former is laparotomy and removal, while with the latter conservative measures are indicated. Lastly, the non-gravid half of a variety of double uterus may be clinically indistinguishable from a fibroid.

TREATMENT

In the non-pregnant state any fibroid exceeding in size that of a tennis ball is usually worth removing in order to forestall further growth or possible acute degeneration, unless the patient is already proceeding without trouble through the menopause. Cases of infertility and recurrent abortion indicate removal of the fibroid by myomectomy. One need have little fear of myomectomy scar rupture in subsequent pregnancy and labour, even though it has been necessary to open the cavity of the uterus, and Gemmell (1936) reported no case of such rupture in his own series, and observed that a study of the literature furnished rather few instances.

When fibroids are diagnosed for the first time in pregnancy, the indications for their removal are infrequent. Firstly, the operation is seldom necessary because the uterus has demonstrated its functional ability by conception; secondly, the operation is extremely bloody because of the great vascularity of the uterus and

thirdly, it is quite liable to be followed by abortion. One may have fears for the integrity of the scar in labour within the next few months, although these are usually groundless, but one of the chief difficulties is to procure satisfactory hæmostasis in the course of the operation, so that one may be faced with the choice of two unpleasant alternatives, namely to close the abdomen in the presence of a persistent ooze, or to proceed to hysterectomy. In either case one would wish never to have started the operation. Only acute torsion and the rarest and most refractory varieties of acute degeneration, or impaction of a fibroid in the pelvis, causing acute retenticn of urine, are likely to provide sufficient grounds for undertaking myomectomy in pregnancy.

There are other less cast-iron indications, such as the presence of fibroids so large that it is reckoned that the patient's only hope of prolonging pregnancy to the point of viability lies in myomectomy. Nevertheless, the operation is frequently performed, and 80 per cent of Gemmell's cases had living children. The safest time for operating is between the 16th and 20th weeks, as abortion is less likely to complicate convalescence at this time. It might be added here that abortion shortly after myomectomy is fraught with danger, especially if the products of conception are retained, because sepsis is thereby enhanced and magnified. Blood loss in the course of the operation can be very brisk and cannot be in any way minimised by the use of a myomectomy clamp, for obvious reasons, so that a supply of blood for transfusion should be at hand. Another technical difficulty is provided by the softness of the tissues, which may cause the sutures to cut out. One is further handicapped by trying throughout to handle the uterus as little as possible for fear of provoking abortion. It will, therefore, be clear that the indications for myomectomy in pregnancy must be overwhelming before one embarks on what may prove a very dangerous operation.

In the course of performing Cæsarean section it is naturally tempting to avail oneself of the opportunity of removing a fibroid at the same time. Cæsarean myomectomy, however, is an indefensible operation, and I have seen near disasters follow it both from hæmorrhage and from severe puerperal peritonitis. The only possible exception is the case of a subserous pedunculated fibroid with a stalk so narrow as to be capable of direct ligation with one stitch. Even though the fibroid presents directly in the line of the uterine incision, the temptation should be resisted and the uterus should be entered at a safer point. Cæsarean hysterectomy is vastly preferable to Cæsarean myomectomy, but fibroids do not often provide a satisfactory excuse for such radical surgery because the uterus, which has proved itself capable of carrying a pregnancy so far, is a uterus worth conserving. If, however, Cæsarean hysterectomy is necessary, and such cases are

indeed few, the total operation is preferable to the subtotal on general gynæcological principles. Nevertheless, it is often surprising how much of the cervix manages to get left behind, as revealed at postnatal examination.

During the puerperium, myomectomy may be indicated because of persistent illness from degeneration, or, for example, from torsion, but in any case it is better to put off the operation as long as possible in order to minimize the risks of sepsis. It goes without saying, therefore, that the best time to remove fibroids is some months after delivery, when involution is complete. The exercise of this forbearance will, in many instances, abolish the need for operating at all.

CARCINOMA OF THE CERVIX

Carcinoma of the cervix is by no means rare in pregnancy, although its incidence is reduced by the discouragement which its presence offers to conception. Munro Kerr many years ago reported an incidence of 1 in 2,000 pregnancies at the Glasgow Royal Maternity Hospital, but this figure is on the pessimistic side for the country as a whole. Most people are agreed that the presence of pregnancy worsens the prognosis, and that the growth develops more rapidly as a result of the increased blood supply. Furthermore, blood-borne metastasis is encouraged, thereby making the case less amenable to irradiation and surgery. These impressions, based usually upon a too limited personal experience, are not borne out by Kinch (1961) who reviewed 705 cases followed up over a five-year period and compared with a series of non-pregnant women matched for age. Kinch found in fact that the overall 5-year prognosis was the same in both groups but he noted a greater liability to rapid dissemination in Stage I cases in pregnancy for which he largely blamed the disturbance of vaginal delivery which he does not favour. The outlook is further worsened by the likelihood of severe hæmorrhage accompanying abortion or delivery, and the opportunities for post-abortum and puerperal sepsis are multiplied by the presence of a growth which is inevitably somewhat necrotic and infected.

The patient presents with bleeding which may be profuse and, to a lesser extent, with discharge, and for this reason a diagnosis of threatened abortion is likely to be made in the first instance. The importance, therefore, of making a pelvic examination if bleeding persists for more than five to seven days and inspecting the cervix is obvious. In the later trimester of pregnancy the examination should, of course, be restricted as far as possible to inspecting the cervix by speculum for fear that the case may be one of placenta prævia.

There may be some difficulty in deciding that a lesion on the cervix is a carcinoma. Hardness of the suspected portion is very characteristic, because in pregnancy no area of the cervix should demonstrate

hardness. Cervical biopsy is essential if there is the slightest doubt. Bleeding may be rather free as a result of this, and it should, therefore, only be carried out after admission to hospital. Even after biopsy the diagnosis may be uncertain, since the pregnant cervix can play some very dangerous histological tricks, encouraging a false positive diagnosis, particularly in the case of columnar cell tissue. One of our cases at Hammersmith Hospital proved to be of extraordinary interest and doubt.[14] The patient in question demonstrated apparent adenocarcinoma of the cervix in two successive pregnancies, in a cervix which was normal in the intervening months. I myself saw this case some years later, when frank invasive malignancy had developed in the vaginal vault long after hysterectomy. The services of a very experienced pathologist should always be sought before committing oneself to this diagnosis and the very radical treatment necessarily involved, and I bitterly remember performing Wertheim's hysterectomy on a case so diagnosed on cervical biopsy in a pregnant patient in whom the diagnosis was not substantiated by full histological examination of the excised uterus.

Lastly, carcinoma of the cervix occurring late in pregnancy may present as a case of apparent placenta prævia, and for this reason, amongst others, whenever possible an examination under anæsthesia should be performed before carrying out Cæsarean section, as otherwise the true diagnosis may be overlooked until routine examination of the pelvic organs is made much later (Fig. 2).

Carcinoma *in situ* of Cervix

The development of pre-invasive malignant change in cervical epithelium (carcinoma *in situ*) in pregnancy is a matter of great interest and controversy and it is not yet certain to what extent such lesions regress between pregnancies, but Kinch refers to the rapidly dying impression that the stage O lesion as diagnosed during pregnancy is an "evanescent situation".

The practice of taking routine Papanicolaou smears in early pregnancy is growing faster than its demonstrable value. Its main use is to exclude invasive cancer of the cervix which can usually be spotted on proper clinical examination. The diagnosis of pre-invasive carcinoma of the cervix at this stage in pregnancy is both worrying and to some extent futile as the management of the pregnancy should not be altered thereby. There is a tendency here for the tail to wag the dog and a positive or suspicious smear should not be acted upon surgically at once, but a repeat smear should be taken. Better still is the method devised by Faulds in Carlisle[5] of taking a sponge biopsy as is now our practice in our gynæcology department. This technique has replaced the use of the Ayre spatula, is very simple and merely involves the use of small chopped up pieces of polythene

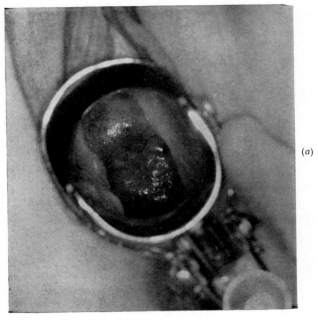

(a)

8/Fig. 2

(a) Carcinoma *in situ* in pregnancy. Aborted spontaneously. Papanicolaou smears positive. Extended hysterectomy with removal of appendages. Has since done well.

(b) (*opposite*). Showing dedifferentiation and mitoses (H. and E. × 346).

(c) (*opposite*). Shows carcinoma *in situ*, same case. The underlying cervical stroma shows a marked inflammatory infiltrate with lymphoid hyperplasia (H. and E. × 136).

sponge bought from Woolworths and allowed to dry hard. The little chunk of sponge is held in a vulsellum and after exposure of the cervix with a speculum, a corner of the sponge is pushed into the external os and rotated through 360°. With this sponge a cytological smear can be made and the sponge itself dropped into a bottle of fixative. The whole piece can now be paraffin blocked and sectioned, providing a very useful microhistological specimen, which enormously reduces the incidence of equivocal smear results which may easily cause unnecessary alarm and despondency. If the result of such a test is still positive or equivocal, one has no option but to undertake a proper cone biopsy of the cervix. Thus must be done in hospital because of the danger of bleeding due to the associated pregnancy for which the standard methods of electro-coagulation or packing

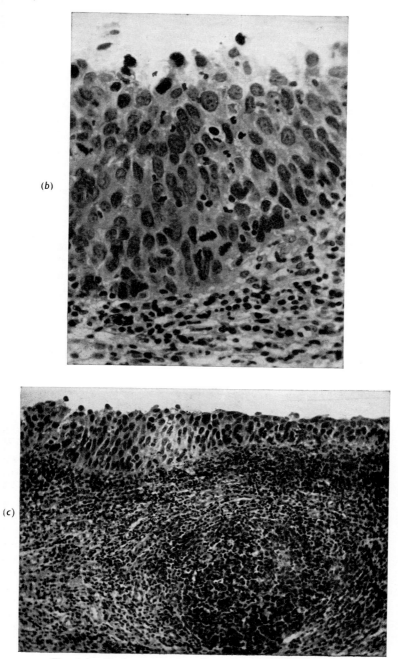

(b)

(c)

(FIG. 2 *b* and *c* by courtesy of Dr. J. E. Duncan Taylor)

tightly, particularly the latter, are likely to be rewarded by the onset of abortion. I have attempted to minimise blood loss by trying to tighten a soft rubber catheter round the cervix, gripped between the jaws of an artery forceps, rather like a venous tourniquet, but it is difficult to get the catheter applied high enough unless the cervix can be pulled well down, and furthermore the cervix itself "crinkles" (as after a Shirodkar suture) making it difficult to perform a neat biopsy. It is far better, in fact, to make the cone biopsy with a fistula-type knife blade starting from behind and working forwards, and ignoring the bleeding until the specimen has been fully obtained. I am not very fond of under-running sutures in the pregnant cervix and sometimes the number of bleeding points is too numerous to control by this means. Faced with this situation the best method of arresting the bleeding is to apply sponge forceps, commonly two pairs, from outside the cervix over both anterior and posterior lips, so that the raw bleeding surfaces are compressed together. A few minutes of this will usually stop the bleeding but, if not, the forceps can be reapplied and the patient sent back to the ward with them still on the cervix, to be removed an hour or so later. This is a simple method which does not expose the patient to the same risk of abortion. There is a growing opinion that far too much radical treatment is employed in cases of cervical carcinoma *in situ* and as many of the women are nowhere near the end of their reproductive lives a conservative attitude towards the type of surgical attack, if any, is well worth considering in the interests of future pregnancies.

Green, in fact, who has long pleaded for moderation in this respect has reported a series of 60 pregnancies in New Zealand occurring in patients previously treated, some by ring biopsy, that is to say less than 2 cm., and a larger number by cone biopsy, namely of more than 2 cm. It would appear that the more radical cone biopsy influences the course of subsequent pregnancy because out of 30 patients so treated no less than eight aborted, five had premature labours and all three term labours with cervical dystocia were in patients who had had cone biopsy. Thus with 16 out of 30 patients previously coned the incidence of complication was more than 50 per cent as compared with 2 out of 17 ring biopsy cases. This is a big penalty to pay for what should be really a diagnostic procedure. This is bad enough, but when one considers how often hysterectomy is undertaken for what is, after all, a pre-cancerous lesion in a young woman, the picture is even worse, and demonstrates how often in modern medicine the investigation and treatment are worse than the original disease. This is not to deny the importance of watching these cases closely, but is a plea for staving off the more radical forms of surgical attack, at least until the young woman has completed her childbearing. In McLaren's series of 141 patients treated by conisation and follow up

for carcinoma *in situ* or marked basal cell dysplasia, the procedure was reckoned adequate for both diagnosis and treatment in all but 14, but even so it is recommended that the patient must be followed up indefinitely, both clinically and cytologically. Sooner or later the patient begins to realise what she is being watched for, of course, and will not be happy until the uterus has been removed, and one cannot help feeling that she might have been lucky had the diagnosis been made just a little later in her life. In this last-mentioned series there were 39 pregnancies in 25 of the patients, with 3 abortions, one case of premature rupture of the membranes and one case of cervical stenosis.

In my own view a case so diagnosed and treated should be encouraged to complete her desired score in childbearing before the age of 35, after which her hysterectomy may be the only means of peace of mind for both her and her doctor and perhaps, most definitely of all, her husband. Needless to say, all such deliveries, after these operations on the cervix, must be undertaken in hospital because of the risk of cervical stenosis or damage in labour, and postnatal follow up must be thorough.

Treatment of carcinoma of the cervix.—This involves one of the most difficult decisions in all obstetrics. The case for Wertheim's hysterectomy is a strong one in gravid carcinoma of the cervix. The operation is likely to cause considerable blood loss, but is facilitated technically by the great ease with which the tissues can be stripped. Because the growth is likely to declare itself fairly early the chances of encountering an operable stage are correspondingly greater. The case first diagnosed late in pregnancy may with some justification be denied treatment for a short while in the hope of securing a viable child, but except in these borderline instances the pregnancy will have to be disregarded and treatment started with the minimum of delay. Late in pregnancy the alternatives are to perform Cæsarean section followed within ten days by irradiation or, preferably, Wertheim's Cæsarean hysterectomy. The latter is preferred, because the puerperium may be infected after Cæsarean section, and the presence of sepsis may delay the start of radium treatment. The employment of sub-total hysterectomy at the time of Cæsarean section has been advocated by some in order to reduce the hazard of infection and to ensure the prompt institution of radium treatment, but this is not recommended, because stump irradiation is very much less satisfactory than when proper cavitary application can be included, as in the usual techniques.

In the earlier part of pregnancy the choice lies between Wertheim's hysterectomy, abdominal hysterotomy followed by irradiation, or irradiation given first. The first method is preferred, the second involves delay in treatment and has the same objections as Cæsarean

section followed by irradiation mentioned above. The application of radium in the first instance with the pregnancy still *in situ* has much to recommend it, but it carries with it a very great danger of precipitating abortion at a most disadvantageous time. The technique of applying the radium should be very cautious, only the vaginal vault being packed, and the gauze plugging to hold the radium in place must be most gently inserted to prevent this complication. I once had to perform an emergency Wertheim's hysterectomy in the middle of the night on a patient four and a half months pregnant, who had started to abort and exsanguinate herself rapidly as a result of radium applied the previous day. She made a good recovery, but died about fifteen months later from multiple blood-borne metastases. Many would nowadays prefer to treat with supervoltage X-rays first. This will be followed by intra-uterine foetal death and abortion after which radium can be applied. This is a sound alternative to radical surgery.

Attempts are sometimes made to leave the pregnancy undisturbed and to confine treatment to radium. The effects of this on the foetus are difficult to forecast, but are likely to be very damaging, especially in the early months of pregnancy, and may result in such conditions as microcephaly. In the later months the effects are less obvious, but at the very least an area of baldness is probable.

OTHER LESIONS OF THE CERVIX

The most important of these, from the obstetrical point of view, is the scarring of the cervix which may follow previous amputation, for example in the course of a Manchester repair for prolapse and after deep cauterisation of the cervix for cervicitis. The latter is a notorious offender in this respect, and is far more likely to interfere with dilatation in labour than the operation of diathermy conisation. I recall having to perform Cæsarean section on a para 4 with an unblemished obstetrical record but who had had cervical cautery. There was cross-union between anterior and posterior lips of the cervix together with scarring and no dilatation took place in spite of three weeks postmaturity with several abortive attempts at labour, a hindwater induction carried out "blind" and with great difficulty two and a half days earlier and a fairly determined oxytocin drip. In fairness to myself I should point out that I only saw her a short time before her section! The cervix felt even worse from above at operation than from below and scissors were used from above to divide the band, followed by dilatation to secure lochial drainage. It is useless to assess the ability of the cervix to dilate until it has been put to the test of labour, but the possibility of cervical dystocia should be borne in mind in any patient with a history of these operations. Labour, following a previous Manchester repair, is far more likely to be

obstructed by scarring of the vagina in the vault than by cicatricial rigidity of the cervix. Needless to say, all patients who have had previous operations on the cervix or repairs of prolapse should be delivered in hospital. The Cæsarean section rate thereafter is likely to be high (18 out of 100 cases reviewed by Hunter and 23 per cent in the series of 156 cases reviewed by Averill). If the previous operation had been undertaken for stress incontinence, the case for Cæsarean section is even stronger since none would gladly risk a recurrence. Nevertheless, the physiological effects of pregnancy without those of labour can undermine the result of a previous repair and elective section is no guarantee against recurrent loss of urinary control or prolapse.

Labour should be conducted with great vigilance. Any reluctance on the part of the cervix to dilate or any palpable rigidity of the cervix found on vaginal examination is warning enough of an impending split to justify Cæsarean section. If vaginal delivery takes place, prophylactic episiotomy is obligatory.

Previous high amputation of the cervix or deep cervical laceration, as mentioned in the chapter on abortion, are causes of recurrent miscarriage.

Cervicitis, so common in gynæcological practice, gives surprisingly little trouble in obstetrics. Discharge is seldom troublesome, but there is the possibility of slight bleeding, especially after intercourse, so that the patient may be admitted for observation for either threatened abortion or for undiagnosed antepartum hæmorrhage. The routine inspection of the cervix by speculum should clarify the diagnosis, but there may be doubt about the possibility of carcinoma, in which case biopsy of the cervix is essential. Cervicitis is preferably not treated during pregnancy; for one thing it is seldom necessary. There is no serious objection to superficial cautery of a cervical erosion, but the case likely to benefit from such trivial treatment is unlikely to need it anyway. It is always worth doing bacterial cultures of the cervical secretions in cases of obvious cervicitis, if only to indicate the appropriate chemotherapy following labour.

Cervical polyps can cause intermittent bleeding during pregnancy, and for this reason their removal may be advisable. Avulsion of a polyp may be followed by persistent bleeding, and it is, therefore, better to admit the patient before twisting it off. The bleeding will stop readily with the use of styptics and gentle local pressure with gauze, coupled with an injection of morphia.

DISCHARGE IN PREGNANCY

This is a fairly common symptom, and an increase in vaginal transudate is physiological in pregnancy. In these cases microscopic

examination of the wet specimen will reveal large numbers of well-cornified squames and very few pus cells. For this no treatment is indicated. A purulent discharge, however, may be due to gonorrhœa, which calls for proper bacteriological confirmation before smothering the diagnosis with antibiotics.

Trichomonas vaginitis is not uncommon in pregnancy, but fortunately it responds, in most cases, to the usual proprietary pessary treatments rather more readily than in the non-pregnant state. Elsewhere (1952) I have drawn attention to the improved prognosis for *trichomonas vaginitis*, both in pregnancy and after the menopause, and have attributed this to the absence of recurrent menstruation in both these states as a factor favouring the more rapid elimination of the parasite. Occasionally it causes a bloodstained discharge in later pregnancy and may, in fact, present as a case of mild antepartum hæmorrhage. The diagnosis should be apparent, however, on routine speculum examination and microscopy of a wet smear.

Metronidazole (Flagyl) is amazingly effective in stamping out this very recurrent and occasionally persistent infection. Given by mouth in 200 mg. tablets three times a day for seven to ten days it succeeds at the first attempt in over 80 per cent of cases (and, in fact, has enabled us to close down our leucorrhœa clinic in my gynæcological unit and to absorb the work in other more general clinics). The persistent and recurrent cases are usually due to reinfection by coitus from the male partner unless he is treated at the same time and the use of a condom insisted upon for at least a month.

Local treatment with the usual proprietary pessaries such as Stovarsol usually suffices and is preferred by us in pregnancy before resorting to metronidazole, especially in early pregnancy. Although reports so far indicate no harmful effect on pregnant women or their babies one is reminded by the thalidomide disaster to think twice before prescribing systemic drugs which are even remotely capable of causing a drop in polymorph count, and 3 out of 41 of the cases (non-pregnant) investigated by Rodin *et al.* (1960) for possible toxic effects showed a fall to 1,500 per c.mm. which is at the very bottom of normality even though the counts rose smartly after withdrawal. The efficacy of metronidazole is by no means diminished in pregnancy and in a series from Washington, D.C., of 206 pregnancies[16] the cure rate was even higher than what we normally expect, but over 15 per cent recurred until the husbands were concomitantly treated. Since there is no placental barrier to the passage of metronidazole into the fœtus uneasiness about possible teratogenic effect continues, but still without proof.

In this series the abortion and prematurity rate overall were the same, as was also the incidence of fœtal abnormality, but if analysis is restricted to treatment given in the first trimester of pregnancy then

this series showed that there were no less than 4 fœtal abnormalities, although there was little similarity between any of them. This would be much higher than expected. Our own preference is still, therefore, to withhold all metronidazole during the period of organogenesis within the first 11 weeks of pregnancy. Later the drug can be prescribed with confidence.

A severe discharge may be associated with a very distressing crop of vulval warts (condylomata acuminata) which are due to a specific virus operating in an area first sensitized by a discharge of almost any type. The primary treatment is of the underlying discharge and the warts may be treated by the local application to their surfaces of podophylin (25 per cent) on one or more occasions. They tend to clear up after delivery but if persisting are best removed by the diathermy cutting loop postnatally.

Vaginitis due to *Candida albicans* (*monilia albicans*) is relatively more common in pregnancy than *trichomonas vaginitis* and is favoured by the very acid state of the vagina (Fig. 3). In moniliasis the patient complains predominantly of pruritus vulvæ and secondarily of vaginal discharge, and the vulva may become extensively

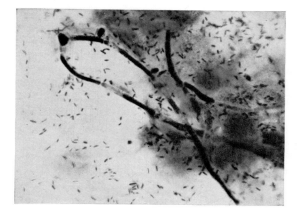

8/Fig. 3.—*Candida albicans.* (× 750.)
(By courtesy of Prof. I. Lominski)

excoriated and eczematised. The diagnosis can be easily clinched by a simple culture at room temperature on Nickerson's medium (Ortho) for five days. No special apparatus is required and a positive culture shows black colonies on naked eye inspection. This condition can be extremely distressing and resistant to treatment, although it usually clears fairly rapidly after pregnancy is over. These patients show a remarkable tendency to become sensitised to a wide variety of local

applications, and 0·5 per cent aqueous gentian violet still remains a safe stand-by in treatment. It is applied daily, if necessary, in the form of a paint. The condition will improve almost immediately with gentian violet, but recurrences up to the time of delivery are by no means uncommon. The most severe cases, accompanied by serious degrees of eczematisation of vulva and thighs, should be admitted to hospital, where the condition will often be found to clear up in half the time taken with ambulant treatment.

Mycostatin (Nystatin-Squibb), a substance isolated from *Streptomyces noursei*, has been found to inhibit mycelial growth and its clinical efficacy in vulvo-vaginal moniliasis has been fully demonstrated by Barr (1957). Fungilin (amphotericin B) is similarly effective.

The relief afforded by properly used nystatin pessaries in these cases is truly dramatic within a few hours and relapses are relatively infrequent. The preparation is colourless and spares the patient the inconvenience of clothing and bed linen indelibly soiled with the depressing colour which gentian violet always spreads.

Gentersal cream which contains gentian violet 0·05 per cent and a similar concentration of alkyldimethylbenzylammonium is almost colourless and can be inserted with an applicator.

Cases which persist after delivery are usually due to reinfection by the husband who may have a monilial balanitis or a scroto-crural dermatitis or the source may be in the patient's intestinal canal and peri-anal region. In the former case the husband should use an ointment containing amphotericin B (Fungizone) and pay close attention to genital and digital hygiene and use a condom at coitus. In the case of intestinal reinfection, which can be very intractable, especially if antibiotics have destroyed the normal bacteriology of the gut, Mycostatin 500,000 units orally t.i.d. can be prescribed.

In the postnatal period the cervix may harbour the infection for a long time. This is best dealt with by diathermy conization of the endocervix.

OVARIAN TUMOURS

Ovarian tumours are common at all stages of reproductive life, and their discovery in pregnancy is not surprising. The commonest varieties are dermoids, pseudomucinous cysts and simple serous cysts. Pregnancy renders the patient particularly susceptible to the risk of complications occurring in the tumour itself. Torsion of the cyst is an ever-present risk, especially in the puerperium, when the rapid change in the anatomical relations of the pelvic viscera, combined with the lax abdominal musculature, particularly favours twisting. Ovarian cysts may also rupture, especially in the course of labour, or they may, from mechanical pressure, undergo necrosis and infection. Likewise, hæmorrhage may occur into the substance of the

tumour. Apart from these complications the tumour may suffer incarceration within the pelvis, possibly causing acute retention of urine as in the case of the incarcerated retroverted gravid uterus. Their presence within the pelvis also favours malpresentation and may obstruct labour. Very large cysts can add enormously to abdominal distension as pregnancy advances, so that the patient is hardly able to get about.

One can never be certain that an ovarian tumour is not malignant until it has been inspected, so that, whether pregnant or not, at any time in life a patient with an ovarian tumour requires laparotomy.

The diagnosis is not difficult, if the tumour can be palpated separately from the uterus. Ultrasonography may reveal a cyst lying alongside the gravid uterus with its fœtal echoes and so clinch the

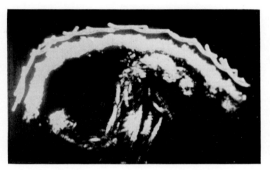

8/Fig. 4.—Ultrasonogram. Transverse section of pregnancy showing large ovarian cyst on left and fœtal echoes on right. (By courtesy of the Editor, *Brit. J. Radiol.*)

diagnosis beyond all doubt (Fig. 4). The following conditions enter into the differential diagnosis:

1. The retroverted gravid uterus may be hard to distinguish from an ovarian cyst in the pelvis, especially when the bladder is distended and painful, but examination after the passage of a catheter should help to resolve the diagnosis. My own record for a "cyst" which vanished on catheterization is 105 fluid ounces.

2. A hæmatocele, either in the pouch of Douglas or peritubal, may simulate ovarian cyst, but its margins are less discrete and definite than in the case of an ovarian tumour.

3. Fibroids in pregnancy when pedunculated may be soft enough to give the impression of being cystic (the distinction is important, because the treatment of fibroids in pregnancy is, if possible, conservative).

4. Other less common sources of confusion are a double uterus; and

5. A uterus distended by hydramnios.

In the early months a perfectly normal pregnancy may yet have

such uterine asymmetry that at first one may be inclined to think that the patient has an ovarian cyst, but again careful examination should distinguish the two. Ultrasonography is invaluable, of course, but in the absence of this modern diagnostic aid, the demands made upon careful palpation are all the greater. Sometimes it is possible to discern a groove between the fundus of the gravid uterus and an ovarian cyst if the patient is placed in the head down Trendelenburg position.[8]

An X-ray of the abdomen is usually worth taking when an ovarian cyst is found in pregnancy, because a tooth may show up and indicate the diagnosis of a dermoid straight away (Fig. 5). Many cases have

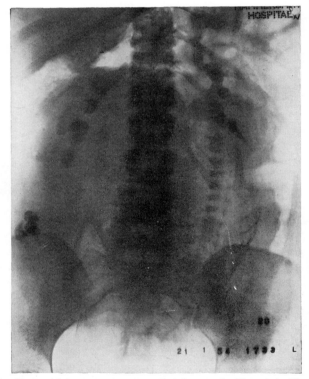

8/FIG. 5.—Dermoid in pregnancy revealed by tooth. Found incidentally in course of I.V.P. Proved at operation to be a parasitic cyst.

(By courtesy of Prof. R. E. Steiner).

no symptoms when first seen, and the tumour is only diagnosed on routine pelvic examination. This constitutes one of the principal indications for examining the patient *per vaginam* in early pregnancy.

Later on the cyst may not be so easily identified once it has escaped from the pelvic cavity.

Treatment of Ovarian Cysts in Pregnancy

Elective operation is better than being forced to perform laparotomy in the face of emergency caused by a complication in the cyst, because there is a strong likelihood that the patient will abort after such emergency surgery. The absolute reasons for operating have already been made clear, and this matter brooks no argument. The only debatable point is the optimum time for doing so. The ideal time is about the 18th week, because the risk of post-operative abortion is thereby much reduced. In the case of a cyst within the pelvis, to delay much after this time would make access to it very difficult because of the size of the uterus. As a matter of practical fact, however, the correct time for operating is "now".

If the cyst is discovered within the last five weeks of pregnancy, one has the choice of removing it there and then (which is preferable, since who can say before laparotomy, except in the case of a radiologically proven dermoid, that an ovarian cyst is benign) and leaving the patient to go spontaneously into labour, or of waiting until term and performing Cæsarean section and removal of the cyst at the same time. If the tumour is discovered right at the end of pregnancy the second of these alternatives is the only sensible choice. It may be argued that at term it is better to remove the cyst and then allow the patient to continue with her labour in order to save a scar in the uterus, but this is sheer inhumanity. Munro Kerr and Chassar Moir stated "one procedure is quite unthinkable, to perform ovariotomy and allow the labour to continue after that operation".

A previously undiagnosed cyst may come in for some very rough handling during the third stage of labour in the belief that it represents the uterine fundus. It is true that the cyst may not be observed until after the patient is delivered, and because of the great liability to torsion, infection and formation of adhesions in the puerperium, it is better to operate fairly soon and before these complications have a chance to develop.

In operating, wherever possible, and especially in the case of dermoids, an attempt should be made to resect the cyst conservatively and preserve the remainder of the ovary. The patient, after all, has demonstrated by her pregnancy the integrity of the rest of her pelvic organs, and they deserve to be conserved as far as possible.

REFERENCES

1. AVERILL, L. C. L. (1955). *J. Obstet. Gynaec. Brit. Emp.*, **62**, 421.
2. BARNES, H. F. (1947). *Brit. med. J.*, **1**, 169.
3. BARR, W. (1957). *Practitioner*, **178**, 616.

4. DONALD, I. (1952). *Brit. med. J.*, **2,** 1223.
5. FAULDS, J. S. (1964). *Lancet*, **1,** 655.
6. GEMMELL, A. A. (1936). *J. Obstet. Gynaec. Brit. Emp.*, **43,** 715.
7. GREEN, G. H. (1966). *J. Obstet. Gynaec. Brit. Cwlth.*, **73,** 897.
8. HINGORANI, VERA (1966). *J. Obstet. Gynaec. Brit. Cwlth.*, **73,** 155.
9. HUNTER, J. W. A. (1955). *J. Obstet. Gynaec. Brit. Emp.*, **62,** 809.
10. HUNTER, W. (1960). *Brit. med. J.*, **2,** 1124.
11. KINCH, R. A. H. (1961). *Amer. J. Obstet. Gynec.*, **82,** 45.
12. MACGREGOR, W. G. (1957). *J. Obstet. Gynaec. Brit. Emp.*, **64,** 888.
13. McLAREN, H. C. (1967). *J. Obstet. Gynaec. Brit. Cwlth.*, **74,** 487.
14. MARTIN, R. T., and KENNY, MEAVE (1950). *J. Obstet. Gynaec. Brit. Emp.*, **74,** 487.
15. MOIR, J. C. (1964). *Munro Kerr's Operative Obstetrics*, 7th edit. London: Baillière, Tindall and Cox.
16. PETERSON, W. F., STAUCH, F. E., and RYDER, CONSTANCE D. (1966). *Amer. J. Obstet. Gynec.*, **94,** 343.
17. RODIN, P., KING, A. J., NICOL, C. S., and BARROW, J. (1960). *Brit. J. vener. Dis.*, **36,** 147.
18. WILSON, D. C., and HARRIS, G. H. (1961). *J. Obstet. Gynaec. Brit. Cwlth.*, **68,** 841.

CHAPTER IX

TOXÆMIAS OF PREGNANCY

by Prof. H. M. CAREY, M.Sc., M.B., B.S., D.G.O. (Syd.), F.R.C.S. (Ed.),
F.R.A.C.S., F.R.C.O.G.

*Head of School of Obstetrics and Gynæcology, University of New South Wales,
Sydney, Australia*

THE concept of a circulating toxin as the cause of raised blood pressure and albuminuria in pregnancy has now been discarded and it is to be hoped that the term "toxæmia" will suffer a similar fate. However, this term is commonly used to encompass a number of syndromes occurring in the second half of pregnancy when hypertension with or without œdema and albuminuria are the main signs.

The main "toxæmia" syndromes are:

1. Pre-eclampsia and eclampsia;
2. Essential hypertension associated with pregnancy;
3. Chronic nephritis complicated by pregnancy.

PRE-ECLAMPSIA

Definition

Pre-eclampsia is characterised by the appearance, during the second half of pregnancy, of two of the following three signs; œdema (or excessive weight gain), hypertension, and albuminuria (proteinuria).

This definition is an arbitrary one and results in the inclusion of more than one pathological entity within the syndrome. As an exception to the above rule, pre-eclampsia may occur in early pregnancy as a complication of hydatidiform mole.

Differential Diagnosis

If the blood pressure was elevated above 85 mm. Hg diastolic before pregnancy or during the first trimester it has been customary to refer to the case as one of essential hypertension. If albuminuria and/or œdema developed in such a case, in the latter half of pregnancy, the case would be classified as pre-eclampsia superimposed on essential hypertension. This definition, however, only segregates the manifest cases of essential hypertension.

Patients classified as suffering from essential hypertension have a raised blood pressure before the start of pregnancy and/or during the

first trimester, but the urine is clear. If raised blood pressure in the first trimester is associated with proteinuria, the case is diagnosed as one of chronic nephritis.

TABLE III

IN THE FIRST TRIMESTER

	Raised diastolic blood pressure	Proteinuria
Pre-eclampsia	—	—
Essential hypertension	+	—
Chronic nephritis	+	+

Clinical Classification

This clinical classification is based on the presence or absence of clinical signs such as hypertension and proteinuria rather than on the pathology of the case. Many cases classified in this way as patients with essential hypertension are ætiologically cases of chronic pyelonephritis.

Some cases of chronic pyelonephritis may start pregnancy with a clear urine and a normal blood pressure, but because of a rise in blood pressure with the development of œdema or proteinuria during the later months of pregnancy, they are diagnosed as cases of pre-eclampsia.

The above classification based on the presence or absence of clinical signs produces considerable confusion because different pathological conditions can produce the same clinical signs. Consequently a pathological classification must be attempted.

Pathological Classification

1. **Placental type.**—In primigravidæ there is sometimes a fairly rapid rise in blood pressure over one or two weeks in the later months of pregnancy. Because of the rapidity with which the blood pressure rises and the level to which it reaches, there is almost invariably an appreciable amount of proteinuria. It is this type of pre-eclampsia which is most commonly associated with eclamptic fits. The fulminating varieties of pre-eclampsia usually belong to this group.

The basic pathology is located in the placenta in the form of infarction or vascular disturbances. For this reason recurrences in subsequent pregnancies are uncommon.

2. **Latent essential hypertension.**—In the early stages of essential hypertension the blood pressure may be normal before pregnancy and during the first trimester. Only in the later weeks of pregnancy does the blood pressure rise. This may occur fairly gradually and

initially may not be associated with either œdema or proteinuria (Adams and MacGillivray, 1961). As the blood pressure reaches higher levels, protein may occur in the urine. There is frequently a family history of hypertension.

This type of pre-eclampsia is common in a first pregnancy, falls in incidence in the second pregnancy and becomes progressively more frequent in later pregnancies due to the increasing age of the patient.

3. **Renal pathology.**—Chronic pyelonephritis may produce a clinical picture very similar to latent essential hypertension; the blood pressure may rise slowly in the later stages of pregnancy. The urine is frequently free of gross proteinuria and œdema is not prominent.

There may be a history of previous pyelitis. Often there is an elevated leucocyte excretion rate or a raised urinary bacterial count.

Occasionally the milder varieties of chronic glomerular nephritis or nephrosis may fall into this group but as a rule proteinuria is more prominent and is frequently encountered in the earlier months of the pregnancy.

Congenital renal abnormalities and fibro-muscular hyperplasia in the arteries can also produce this type of pre-eclampsia.

4. **Venous type.**—Even in a normal pregnancy there is considerable compression of the major abdominal veins, especially the inferior vena cava, with the development of collateral venous drainage (Scott and Kerr, 1963). In some patients this collateral development is not as adequate as in others. Multiple pregnancy, hydramnios and the severe forms of blood group incompatibility cause further embarrassment to the venous return through the abdomen. In some cases the pressure in the renal veins is raised.

As a consequence œdema especially of the lower trunk and lower extremities is marked and proteinuria is present. Hypertension may not be very prominent.

These pressure changes are accentuated in the primigravida because of the better tone of her abdominal wall muscles and the fact that this is the first time this load has been thrown on the collateral circulation.

5. **Diabetes and pre-diabetes.**—Diabetes is associated with vascular lesions which involve the placental circulation. Simultaneously there is often a larger fœtus than normal with some degree of hydramnios. The increased rate of growth makes additional demands on the placental circulation.

6. **Hydatidiform mole.**—The rapidly growing placental tissue in hydatid mole creates excessive demands on the placental circulation and the rate of vascularisation of the uterus which is stimulated to an increased rate of growth in cases associated with the signs of pre-eclampsia.

PATHOLOGY

Placenta

Placental insufficiency is an important basic factor in pre-eclampsia. It may be primary or secondary, but, irrespective of the type, it leads to impairment of the nutritional supply of the fœtus producing babies smaller than normal, some of whom die *in utero* before term.

Dixon and Robertson (1961) studied the vascular supply to the placenta by taking biopsies at the time of Cæsarean section from the wall of the uterus opposite the centre of the placenta. The first stage in the development of the vessel lesion in pre-eclampsia was found to be an acute fibrinoid necrosis. Later the damaged vessel became dilated. There was also an infiltration of lipophages into the damaged wall.

In essential hypertension, hyalinisation of the true arterioles and intimal hyperplasia with medial degeneration and proliferative fibrosis in the small arteries was observed.

When pre-eclampsia was superimposed on essential hypertension the changes associated with both conditions occurred together.

Browne and Veall (1953) observed a reduced placental blood flow in both pre-eclampsia and essential hypertension.

Using improved fixation and staining methods Wigglesworth (1962) demonstrated that the Langhans (cytotrophoblast) layer of the normal placenta persists to term. In pre-eclampsia the Langhans cells proliferate and show a greater degree of variation in size than normally, while at the same time there is degeneration of the syncytium (plasmoditrophoblast).

Hormonal Changes

One aspect of the impaired placental function associated with severe pre-eclampsia is reduced in progesterone production and urinary pregnanediol excretion (Russell *et al.*, 1957).

Progesterone inhibits the action of aldosterone, so with a lowered progesterone level, a given concentration of aldosterone will be more effective in producing sodium conservation by the kidneys (Laidlaw *et al.*, 1962).

Aldosterone secretion rate is elevated throughout a normal pregnancy and is responsive to changes in sodium intake (Watanabe *et al.*, 1963). In mild pre-eclampsia (diastolic pressure of 90 to 105 mm. Hg) the aldosterone secretion is within the range found during normal pregnancy, but in severe pre-eclampsia, the aldosterone secretion rate is depressed to non-pregnant levels. Administration of large doses of progesterone or salt depletion increases the aldosterone secretion rate (Watanabe *et al.*, 1965).

The placenta forms œstriol from dehydroisoepiandosterone sul-

phate (DHA) synthesised in the fœtal adrenal. Absence of the fœtal adrenal or failure of the fœtal circulation causes a fall in maternal urinary œstriol to low levels (Strand, 1963; Diczfalusy, 1964).

Urinary œstriol levels are related to fœtal weight and as the growth of the fœtus is often retarded in severe pre-eclampsia, the maternal urinary œstriol levels are lower than in normal pregnancies of the same period of gestation.

In the experience of Booth et al., (1965) the œstriol levels did not always accurately reflect the condition of the fœtus. This may have been due to the methods used for estimating the œstriol levels. Metabolites from barbiturates and other therapeutic agents can interfere with œstriol readings when some of the shorter chemical techniques are employed in the estimation of œstriol (Greenstreet, 1966). A diuresis produced by thiazide diuretics may produce a temporary rise in the œstriol level while impaired renal function may be associated with low readings. Nesbitt et al. (1965) claimed that in most cases serial œstriol readings showed a drop in level a week or more before fœtal death.

Antidiuretic hormone appears in the plasma and urine in increased amounts only when pre-eclampsia is associated with œdema (Paterson, 1960).

Kidneys

Serial renal biopsies have revealed that the earliest and most consistent pathological change found in pre-eclampsia occurs in the glomerular capillaries. The cytoplasm of the endothelial cells is swollen, probably due to œdema, without any increase in the thickness of the basement membrane. In the early stages these changes affect only occasional cells. Even when severe, however, the endothelial cellular enlargement is not homogeneous throughout the kidney, but varies from glomerulus to glomerulus and even within the same glomerulus there may be variation among the different capillary loops. The capillaries appear bloodless even when the endothelial cellular changes are of only moderate severity. The elevation of the serum uric acid levels is in proportion to the degree of severity of the glomerular lesion (Pollak and Nettles, 1960).

In addition to this specific lesion, amorphous material derived from fibrinogen is deposited below the basement membrane i.e. between the basement membrane and the endothelial cytoplasm. Phagocytosis of this material by adjacent endothelial cells has been observed.

A third component is an increase in the number of intercapillary (mesangial) cells and in their cytoplasmic mass.

The specific lesion has been found only in pregnant patients, and Hopper et al. (1961) have shown that it reverts to normal usually

within ten days following delivery. The lesion has been found in cases of pre-eclampsia without albuminuria and when pre-eclampsia has been superimposed on essential hypertension.

It has persisted in pregnancies complicated by pre-eclampsia in spite of vigorous therapy with diuretics, low salt diet, hypotensive drugs and in spite of clinical improvement expressed in terms of blood pressure, œdema and the amount of proteinuria (Altchek, 1961).

The main afferent arteriole in the stalk of the glomerular tuft shows the same swelling of the endothelial cells which may be sufficient to narrow the lumen of the vessel.

The glomerular filtration rate normally increases during pregnancy but in pre-eclampsia it may be at or below the non-pregnant value. Renal blood flow is also reduced. Following delivery, glomerular filtration returns to normal within two weeks, but normal values for renal blood flow may not be obtained in some cases for several months (Bucht and Werko, 1953).

When effective blood volume falls, the enzyme renin is released from renal juxtaglomerular cells to split angiotensin I from an alpha-2 globulin. A converting enzyme in the plasma then removes two aminoacids to produce angiotensin II, the most potent pressor substance and the stimulator of aldosterone secretion. When angiotensin II is infused into non-pregnant normotensive subjects, oliguria and inhibition of salt excretion occur even at doses too low to affect blood pressure.

In normal pregnant women an increase of plasma renin concentration occurs without hypertension (Brown *et al.* 1966 *b*), and because of the higher level of endogenous angiotensin, a normal woman during pregnancy is two to three times less sensitive to infused angiotensin than in the non-pregnant state (Chesley *et al.*, 1965 *a*).

In mild pre-eclampsia the plasma renin concentration is within the range found in normal pregnant women, but in the severe forms of pre-eclampsia, the renin values are below the mean for normal pregnant women (Brown *et al.*, 1966 *a*). When the endogenous angiotensin level is low, the patient is more sensitive to exogenous angiotensin II (Chesley, 1965 *b*).

Water and Salt Metabolism

MacGillivray and Buchanan (1958) have demonstrated an increase in total body water in pre-eclampsia compared to normal pregnancy but no increase in total exchangeable sodium, so that exchangeable sodium per litre of body water fell from 78·1 to 72·7 mEq.

Davey *et al.* (1961) from a study of five cases of pre-eclampsia followed throughout pregnancy observed an excessive increase in

total exchangeable sodium from 16 to 26 weeks but a return to normal pregnant levels by the time signs of pre-eclampsia appeared.

In contrast to the findings of MacGillivray, Plentl and Gray (1959) claim to have demonstrated increased sodium retention in pre-eclampsia. Chesley (1966) has criticised the results of MacGillivray *et al.* and Davey *et al.* on the grounds that the exchangeable sodium was calculated from the specific activity of urine rather than that of plasma or serum in which both sodium and radio-active counts are usually much higher than in urine. Moreover Chesley contends that the urinary sodium levels in pre-eclampsia are depressed.

The plasma volume is reduced in pre-eclampsia (Friedberg, 1958; MacGillivray and Buchanan, 1958) with a corresponding rise in the hæmatocrit. The plasma proteins and especially plasma albumin are reduced.

The protein in tissue fluid compared to serum levels is very much reduced but the percentage of albumin in tissue fluid is much greater than in the serum.

Arterioles

During the second half of a normal pregnancy there is a progressive increase in peripheral blood flow but in pre-eclampsia the increase at any given stage of pregnancy is less than that normally encountered. This is due to the fact that the decrease in peripheral vascular resistance as pregnancy progresses is less in pre-eclampsia than in a normal pregnancy.

These changes are a consequence of higher tone of the smooth muscle and not the result of a structural change. The capillary filtration rate is unaltered in pre-eclampsia (Spetz, 1965).

In severe cases of pre-eclampsia there is exudation of plasma constituents into the wall of the capillary end of the arterioles producing local œdema. With more advanced lesions there are fibrinoid deposits or necrotic changes in the media of these small vessels and frequently small thrombi form in these areas. Extreme cases are associated with necrotic vessel walls and hæmorrhage into the surrounding tissues.

It is this lesion in the terminal arterioles that produces the pathological changes in the brain.

Brain

In most cases of eclampsia there is a vascular reaction which in its mildest form produces focal œdema of the brain tissue and in its more severe form necrosis, thrombosis and even rupture of the vessel, leading to hæmorrhages of various sizes. These lesions antedate the onset of convulsions and sometimes occur without producing fits.

In about one-third of fatal cases of eclampsia macroscopic hæmorrhages occur in the pons or basal nuclei. Multiple small hæmorrhages mainly in the cortex are found in a few cases.

Sheehan (1958) thinks that puerperal eclampsia is usually associated with thrombosis of one of the cerebral veins. Recovery may be associated with the development of a scar in the cortex which can predispose the patient to epilepsy in a subsequent pregnancy.

Liver

At the time a lesion can be demonstrated in the renal glomerulus, liver biopsies are often normal. The classical changes in liver pathology are as follows:

Macroscopic.—Only a few petechial hæmorrhages appear on the surface, being more prominent in severe cases. On section the lesion resembles that of venous congestion.

Microscopic.—Blood or plasma escapes from the portal vein and displaces the adjacent liver cells. Clotting of the blood occurs and the liver cells adjacent to the clot may be compressed and undergo necrosis. In some cases the blood or plasma, infiltrating towards the centre of the liver lobule, separates the liver cells from the incomplete walls of the sinusoids. During the following 48 hours, these areas of hæmorrhage are first infiltrated by polymorphonuclear leucocytes and later invaded by large phagocytes. By the fourth or fifth day the lesion has disappeared. In fatal cases, the lesions in the liver probably develop within the 48 hours prior to death.

The levels of factor VII, and fibrinogen, are increased in late pregnancy resulting in the more prompt and efficient operation of the coagulation mechanism dependent on tissue thromboplastin. The higher concentrations of fibrinogen and globulins in late pregnancy lead to higher red cell sedimentation rates.

Fåhraeus (1962) has suggested that if, against this background, there is a rapid rise of blood pressure, the hæmoconcentration encountered in pre-eclampsia is accentuated and there may be aggregations of red cells to form hyaline masses, obstructing the circulation in some of the smaller vessels in the liver, kidney, brain and other areas.

Lungs

The lungs show varying degrees of œdema and congestion, with the development of bronchopneumonia in many of those cases of eclampsia dying after the first day (Sheehan, 1958).

Pulmonary complications occur in 40 per cent of deaths due to eclampsia and in 30 per cent of fatal cases pulmonary œdema is present (Menon, 1961).

Cause of Death

Death in eclampsia is usually due to circulatory failure, pulmonary œdema or cerebral hæmorrhage.

Circulatory Changes

During normal pregnancy there is an increase in blood volume and the hæmatocrit reading is lower due to the relative increase in plasma over red cell volume. In pre-eclampsia of rapid onset, the increase in blood volume is not so marked, and sometimes there is an increase in the hæmatocrit reading just before an eclamptic convulsion. The hæmatocrit level sometimes falls when a severe pre-eclamptic patient starts to show improvement. However, the hæmatocrit level also rises with the onset of labour so that the change is not a very specific one. The increase in blood viscosity and the rise in the hæmatocrit reading are manifestations of hæmoconcentration which may be due to the movement of water into the cells.

In normal pregnancy the plasma albumin is diluted as the plasma volume expands, and this change is more marked in cases of slowly developing pre-eclampsia. The œdema fluid has a low protein content, which implies that the permeability of the capillaries to protein is not increased (Page, 1957).

Cerebral vascular resistance is increased in pre-eclampsia (McCall, 1953), but this may be secondary to the rise in blood pressure.

Enzyme Concentrations

The plasma levels of histaminase and oxytocinase (Riad, 1962) are reduced in pre-eclampsia. If these enzymes are derived from the placenta, this reduction in concentration is probably another manifestation of depressed placental function.

Mono-amine activity is also reduced (de Maria and See, 1966), but the administration of drugs that inhibit this enzyme do not produce pre-eclamptic signs in normal pregnancies, so the reduced level of this enzyme cannot be incriminated as one of the factors in the pathogenesis of this syndrome (Sandler and Coveney, 1962).

SYMPTOMS

The symptoms of pre-eclampsia usually are of late onset, and consist of headache, blurred vision and spots before the eyes. Occasionally vomiting and epigastric pain are experienced.

SIGNS

1. Hypertension

Hypertension is the central sign. A diastolic pressure of 90 mm. Hg or above, or a rise of 15 mm. Hg above the first trimester diastolic reading, is traditionally accepted as being abnormal.

A distinction must be drawn between a casual blood pressure reading such as is recorded in the clinic or consulting room and a semi-basal reading which is obtainable only after bed rest and sedation and is based on the average level of a series of four hourly readings. It is this latter reading which should be used to assess the patient and as an index of the need for therapy.

In determining the blood pressure, allowance must be made for differences in arm circumference. Corrections based on measurements made by Ragan and Bordley (1941) have been published by Pickering et al. (1954). However Holland and Humerfelt (1964) found that the correlation between the difference in intra-arterial and cuff blood pressures and arm circumference was barely significant.

2. Proteinuria

The following table based on data from Lorincz et al. (1961) indicates that plasma globulins as well as albumin are passed into the urine. For this reason the term proteinuria is more accurate than albuminuria.

Average Percentage of Total Protein in Urine

	Albumin	Alpha 1 Globulin	Alpha 2 Globulin	Beta Globulin	Gamma Globulin	A/G Ratio
Essential hypertension	62%	9%	8%	16%	7%	1·5
Chronic glomerulonephritis	52%	8%	7%	18%	14%	1·1
Pre-eclampsia	52%	7%	14%	18%	8%	1·1
Eclampsia	36%	3%	12%	15%	34%	0·6

In pre-eclampsia and eclampsia the alpha 2 globulin forms a larger percentage of the proteins in the urine than is the case in other conditions associated with proteinuria. The gamma globulin urinary excretion is increased in eclampsia.

The corresponding figures for serum are as follows:

Average Percentage of Total Protein in Serum

	Albumin	Alpha 1 Globulin	Alpha 2 Globulin	Beta Globulin	Gamma Globulin	A/G Ratio	Total Protein Gm. 100 ml.
Essential hypertension	38%	8%	16%	22%	15%	0·62	6·2
Chronic glomerulonephritis	45%	5%	13%	19%	17%	0·82	5·9
Pre-eclampsia	36%	8%	14%	21%	20%	0·57	5·7
Eclampsia	42%	8%	16%	22%	11%	0·73	5·5
Normal	49%	4%	13%	17%	18%	0·96	5·5

Five per cent of the first pregnancies are complicated by hypertension and proteinuria but only 1 per cent to 1·5 per cent of subsequent pregnancies are associated with these two signs.

3. Weight Gain

Data from Thomson and Billewicz (1957) indicate that the rate of weight gain in primigravidæ between the 20th and 30th weeks of pregnancy has little predictive value in the individual patient.

In the 30th to 36th week period primigravidæ gaining more than 1·4 lbs. a week show an increased incidence of pre-eclampsia but less than one in five women gaining this excessive amount of weight do in fact develop pre-eclampsia.

The lowest incidence of obstetrical complications occurred in the group which gained on the average of 1 lb. a week.

PROGNOSIS

1. Immediate

(a) *Maternal prognosis.*—The maternal mortality from "toxæmia" is 0·2 per 1,000 births and only one in six toxæmic deaths is associated with eclampsia.

(b) *Fœtal prognosis.*—Carey and Liley (1958) studied cases of pre-eclampsia which developed prior to the 36th week and found that the fœtal prognosis was related more to the duration than to the severity of the pre-eclamptic signs. The level of the basal diastolic pressure by itself had a prediction value of only 4 per cent with regard to the occurrence of intra-uterine death.

With hypertension of the order of 100 mm. Hg diastolic uncomplicated by albuminuria, the risk of fœtal loss prior to delivery is probably no more than 1 per cent a week rising to 2 per cent a week near term, especially in the more severe cases of hypertension. However, the risk of intra-uterine death is 50 to 100 per cent greater when hypertension is accompanied by a significant amount of proteinuria.

In determining the overall fœtal prognosis in cases of pre-eclampsia developing prior to the 36th week, the risk of intra-uterine death from carrying on the pregnancy for any given number of weeks must be balanced against the reduction in the risk of neonatal death from the diminished degree of prematurity.

At 34 weeks the neo-natal mortality from prematurity in pre-eclampsia is 15 per cent and this risk is doubled for each additional two weeks of prematurity and halved for each additional fortnight of maturity.

Data from the 1958 British Perinatal Mortality Survey indicate that in the absence of proteinuria a rise in the diastolic blood pressure up to 110 mm. Hg increases the perinatal mortality from 2·5 per cent to 3·6 per cent, while diastolic readings in excess of 110 mm. Hg carry a 5 per cent perinatal mortality rate. When proteinuria is also present the perinatal mortality rate rises to 10 per cent. However, much of this perinatal loss is due to prematurity resulting from the higher

P.O.P.—9*

frequency of induction of labour at an earlier stage of pregnancy in these more severe cases.

2. Remote

Pre-eclampsia does not produce residual renal damage in the mother, and the proteinuria disappears within a few weeks of delivery (Assali, 1958).

Gibson (1956) failed to demonstrate any correlation between the duration of the pre-eclamptic signs and the incidence of residual hypertension in the mother. Browne (1958) and Dieckmann *et al.* (1952) are of the opinion that pre-eclampsia does not produce residual hypertension, but that the 30 per cent of cases who do have an elevated blood pressure in later life represent cases of mild or latent hypertension which have progressed with age to the same extent as they would have done had they not become pregnant. Study of identical twins has confirmed this view by the finding that the nulliparous twin frequently has the same level of blood pressure as her sister who has had "toxæmia" (Platt, 1958).

Light (1948) and Gibson (1956) have presented evidence indicating that the incidence of residual hypertension is related to the age of the patient rather than to the duration of the pre-eclamptic signs.

Chesley (1956) who originally taught that prolonged pre-eclampsia often caused chronic hypertension, now believes that a pre-eclamptic woman who is found to have hypertension at follow-up probably had this predisposition before pregnancy.

TREATMENT

Frequent Antenatal Visits

Very mild cases and cases who have responded satisfactorily to hospital treatment and have been discharged, should be seen at least once or preferably twice a week in the antenatal clinic. They should be weighed, the blood pressure recorded, urine tested for protein and the patient examined for evidence of œdema. Special care should be taken with cases of diabetes, hydramnios, twins, essential hypertension and with primigravidæ.

If protein is detected in an ordinary specimen of urine, the vagina should be swabbed out with a wet and dry swab and the vulva likewise cleaned, and a midstream specimen collected and tested for protein. Catheterisation carries the risk of introducing urinary tract infection and should be employed only when contamination of a midstream collection is unavoidable. Test papers sometimes give false positive results so confirmation by boiling after acidification is required.

Criteria for Admission to Hospital

(*a*) An increase above the non-pregnant or first trimester diastolic blood pressure of 15 mm. Hg, or a persistent blood pressure of 140/90 or above indicates the need for admission.

(*b*) Proteinuria in a midstream specimen of urine.

Co-operative patients who have domestic help may be treated at home if signs of pre-eclampsia are minimal. However, treatment at home is rarely satisfactory and any patients with obvious signs of pre-eclampsia should be admitted to an antenatal bed.

Bed Rest

This is the most effective means of treating pre-eclampsia. Bed rest increases placental blood flow (Morris *et al.* 1956), reduces the venous pressure in the lower extremities and allows reabsorption of a considerable quantity of fluid from these areas. It also reduces the demand on the circulating blood volume, and removes the stimulus to sodium retention.

The position adopted by the patient in bed may be of some relevance. A normal pregnant woman, when given a water loading test, will excrete 100 per cent of the test dose in 3 hours provided she lies on her side; the percentage output falls to about 50 per cent with the patient in the dorsal position and to 30 per cent or less if she stands or moves about.

In a pre-eclamptic subject the output of water is reduced to 20 per cent of the test dose in the supine position, but with the patient lying on her side it may not increase above 50 per cent (Govan, 1962).

Low Salt Diet and Diuretics

On the assumption that depletion of body sodium relieves œdema, it has been traditional to restrict the intake of salt in pre-eclampsia and to prescribe diuretics to increase the elimination of sodium. Such treatment further accentuates the reduction in plasma volume that is part of the disorder of pre-eclampsia. Excessive loss of sodium is limited by the action of the increased amounts of aldosterone secreted in response to the sodium loss.

The intravenous infusion of saline solutions will accentuate the signs of pre-eclampsia, but the amounts of salt in an ordinary diet have no effect on the clinical course of pre-eclamptic patients (Bower, 1964; Mengert and Tacchi, 1961).

Diuretics will accelerate the disappearance of œdema but there is no evidence to indicate that they improve placental function (Mac-Gillivray *et al.* 1962).

The most commonly employed diuretics belong to the thiazide

group. They produce a diuresis which commences about 2 hours after administration, reaches a peak in 6 to 12 hours and lasts for 18 to 24 hours.

Their initial effect is to increase the excretion of sodium and chloride. The chloride loss may exceed the sodium excretion and thus produce a rise in plasma bicarbonate. The increased secretion of aldosterone stimulated by the sodium loss causes the excretion of potassium. A rise in blood urea and uric acid can be produced by the excessive use of thiazide diuretics (Healey *et al.* 1959) and hyperglycæmia and glycosuria in diabetic or prediabetic patients may be aggravated (Shapiro *et al.*, 1961; Hollis, 1961). Thiazides probably produce their effect on glucose tolerance by exerting a direct inhibitory effect on the pancreatic islet cells.

The potency of the other members of the group are indicated by their therapeutic dose in relation to that of chlorothiazide.

Chlorothiazide (Chlotride).	. .	500 mg.
Hydrochlorothiazide (Esidrex)	. .	50 mg.
Hydroflumethiazide (Naclex)	. .	50 mg.
Methyclothiazide (Enduron)	. .	5 mg.
Bendrofluazide (Aprinox)	. .	5 mg.
Cyclothiazide (Doburil)	. . .	5 mg.
Cyclopenthiazide (Navidrex)	. .	0·5 mg.
Polythiazide (Nephril)	. . .	2 mg.

Differences in action between members of the group are of only a minor nature. Polythiazide has a duration of action extending over 24 to 48 hours, while cyclopenthiazide and cyclothiazide exert their actions for only 12 hours.

Chlorthalidone (Hygroton) differs in chemical structure from the thiazides but its mechanism of action is the same except that its effect may last 48 hours. Due to its prolonged action intermittent dosage is possible. Quinethazone although differing in structure from the thiazides has a similar action for about the same period of time, but nausea, vomiting and diarrhœa may be associated with its use.

In clorexolone the 6-membered thiadiazole ring of the thiazides has been replaced by the 5-membered isoindole ring. Its mode of action is similar to the thiazides.

Clopamide (Brinaldix) is a N-amino-heterocycle which acts selectively on the proximal convoluted tubule preventing the reabsorption of sodium and cloride.

Ethacrynic acid (Edecril) acts on the ascending limb of the loop of Henle and the first portion of the distal convoluted tubule where it inhibits active sodium transport. It may work in patients refractory to other diuretics with a duration of action of 6 to 8 hours.

Frusemide (Lasix) is a substituted sulphonamide derivative of anthranilic acid containing the sulphamoyl-benzene group which is also found in the thiazide diuretics. Frusemide is more potent than the thiazides. It has an action which lasts about 4 hours after oral administration and 2 hours after intravenous injection.

Aldosterone antagonists include spironolactone (Aldactone-A) and triamterene (Dytac).

By competitive inhibition spironolactone blocks the activity of aldosterone thus decreasing potassium loss. It has a slow onset of action which may extend over 3 to 7 days.

Triamterene though chemically unrelated to spironolactone is an orally active antagonist of aldosterone but weaker in action than the thiazides. It increases the excretion of bicarbonate and uric acid.

Carbonic anhydrase inhibitors like acetazolamide (Diamox) are less effective than the thiazide diuretics. They produce an acidosis and when this develops they become ineffective. Ethoxyol amide (Cardrase) is twice as active weight for weight as acetazolamide. Dichlorphenamide is another carbonic anhydrase inhibitor. Chlorobenzol disulphonamide (Salco) is a mild carbonic anhydrase inhibitor that acts on the proximal convoluted renal tubule.

The thiazide group of diuretics and chlorthalidone, after several weeks' administration, produce a small drop in blood pressure by reducing peripheral vascular resistance (Villarreal et al., 1962; Pickering et al., 1961). They also potentiate most hypotensive drugs by reducing the plasma volume.

Diazoxide, a thiazide derivative with sodium retaining properties, decreases arterial blood pressure (Rubin et al. 1962; Dollery et al., 1962).

Sedatives

Morphia is frequently given on admission and when there is an exacerbation of the pre-eclamptic signs, but morphia is not a good anticonvulsant, and it suffers from the objection that it stimulates the supra-optic nucleus, and in this way increases the secretion of the posterior pituitary antidiuretic hormone. Its stimulating action produces vomiting in about 20 per cent of patients. It is preferable to restrict its use to patients in labour when its analgesic action reinforces its sedative effect and compensates for its other disadvantages.

Amylobarbitone sodium (Sodium Amytal) helps to reduce the blood pressure, but phenobarbitone is a better anticonvulsant. In a moderately severe case of pre-eclampsia, phenobarbitone 60 mg. b.i.d. and Sodium Amytal 200 mg. six hourly, will usually be found to be a satisfactory method of sedation.

Although paraldehyde is a safe and satisfactory sedative and anti-convulsant, its odour and taste are objections to its routine use.

Magnesium sulphate has been popular in the past as part of the Stroganoff treatment. It has no significant hypotensive action but has a central depressant action (Seller, 1957).

Large doses of magnesium sulphate may produce depression of the vital centres. Small doses can be used to reinforce the action of other sedatives and anticonvulsants. However, intramuscular injections often produce abscesses and the margin of safety of magnesium sulphate is less than that of barbiturates or paraldehyde and hence it has been largely replaced by the barbiturates.

Menon (1961) of Madras has claimed good results from the use of phenothiazine derivatives in the management of eclampsia. On admission he administered 25 mg. of chlorpromazine and 100 mg. pethidine intravenously and 50 mg. of dietazine (Diparcol) intramuscularly. This was followed by chlorpromazine 50 mg. intramuscularly every eight hours and in the interval between the injections of chlorpromazine, 50 mg. of Diparcol was given intramuscularly. In addition, 200 mg. pethidine in 1,000 ml. of 20 per cent glucose was given by slow intravenous drip over a period of 24 hours.

Recurrence of fits occurred in 15 per cent of cases treated in this way, especially if the treatment was started only a few hours before the onset of labour. Maternal mortality due to eclampsia was reduced from 4·8 to 2·2 per cent in a group of 402 cases, mainly by the reduction of pulmonary complications.

Various modifications of the phenothiazine type of sedation have been used in the management of pre-eclampsia.

The guiding principle is to give sufficient sedation to prevent or control fits but not sufficient to encourage the development of hypostatic or other pulmonary complications.

Hypotensive Drugs

(*a*) **Reserpine.**—The hypotensive action of reserpine is partly due to its sedative action. When a hypertensive pregnant patient has been at bed rest for some days under sodium amylobarbitone sedation, the administration of reserpine produces very little further fall in the diastolic blood pressure, a fall of 10 mm. Hg being the best that can be expected.

When given by mouth, the full effect of reserpine may not be evident for up to six weeks, although some effect is usually obvious within three or four days. This latency can be reduced by giving the drug by intramuscular or intravenous injection.

Reserpine reduces the storage of noradrenaline in the peripheral

tissues and of serotonin in the brain; the time taken to produce this effect explains the latency in hypotensive action.

A dose of 0·5 to 0·75 mg. daily will produce better clinical results than larger doses, as the latter only accentuate the side-effects of depression and vagal stimulation without a proportionate increase in hypotension. Reserpine also facilitates sodium retention.

Reserpine by itself is not a sufficiently potent hypotensive agent to be of much value, but is useful as an additive to other drugs. A satisfactory result with the minimum of side-effects can frequently be obtained with small doses of a series of hypotensive agents given together.

(*b*) **Ganglionic and noradrenaline release blockers.**—All members of this group act by inhibiting the normal compensatory vasoconstriction that comes into play on adopting the erect position, so their effect is to pool blood in the peripheral circulation with a consequent decrease in venous return and cardiac output. Glomerular filtration and renal blood flow is reduced as is placental blood flow. With patients lying flat in bed a fairly large dose of any of these drugs is required to lower the blood pressure. If a patient under treatment in this way sits up on a bed pan or gets out of bed and stands up, there may be a marked fall in blood pressure with serious impairment of placental circulation.

Most of the ganglionic agents have been replaced by the noradrenaline release blockers, the former produce the effects of blocking both the sympathetic and parasympathetic innervations, while the latter spares the patient the side-effects resulting from blocking the parasympathetic fibres.

Bretylium tosylate (*Darenthin*) blocks the release, but does not deplete the stores, of noradrenaline from the sympathetic nerve endings. Oral absorption is variable and tolerance develops so that blood pressure control with this agent is erratic. The initial oral test dose is 100 mg. Administration is increased progressively by increments of 100 mg. The blood pressure drops in 3 to 4 hours after administration and the effect of a single dose lasts for 8 to 10 hours.

Guanethidine (*Ismelin*) depletes the noradrenaline content of the peripheral tissues as well as blocking the release of noradrenaline. Unlike reserpine it does not cross the blood brain barrier.

The onset of its hypotensive effect is slow, a week being required to establish satisfactory blood pressure control. Its intravenous administration should be avoided as it may raise the blood pressure by liberating catecholamines if given in this way.

The initial oral dose of guanethidine is 10 to 25 mg. Administration can be increased at weekly intervals to 150 mg. a day. After the drug has been stopped, the hypotensive effect may persist for two or three days.

Side-effects include diarrhoea, especially if the dose is increased too rapidly, weight gain, œdema and mental depression.

The effects of both bretylium tosylate and guanethidine are more marked in hot weather or after a large meal, and diurnal variations in blood pressure when these drugs are being used are also marked. Blood pressure readings are low in the mornings but rise as the day progresses.

Bethanidine sulphate (*Esbatal*) blocks the release of noradrenaline from post-ganglionic nerve terminals without depleting the storage of catecholamines at these sites as do both guanethidine and reserpine. Thus, onset of action is more rapid and the duration of bethanidine is not as prolonged as that of guanethidine.

Duration of Action.—After a single dose by mouth supine blood pressure is not affected but standing blood pressure will commence to fall after $1\frac{1}{2}$ hours, reaching a maximum effect in 4 to 6 hours and returning to control levels within 12 hours.

Dose.—The average dose is 25 mg. in the morning and this is repeated in the early afternoon. The range of the daily dose is 20 to 150 mg. An initial dose of 10 mg. is increased by daily increments of 5 to 10 mg. until control is achieved. The use of diuretics enables a lower dose to be employed. A combination of methyldopa and bethanidine may be useful in resistant cases. Tolerance of the type associated with bretylium has not been a problem. Isolated cases of complete insensitivity occur.

Other Actions.—Bethanidine has local anæsthetic effects and large intravenous doses cause paralysis of voluntary muscles. After administration for some days a hypersensitivity to catecholamines is exhibited.

(*c*) **Methyldopa (Aldomet)** blocks the conversion of DOPA (dihydroxy-phenylalanine) to dopamine (di-hydroxy-phenethylamine), the precursor of adrenaline. This drug also inhibits the decarboxylation of 5-hydroxy-tryptophan (5-HTP), tyrosine, tryptophan and phenylalanine. It reduces the excretion of the amines derived from tyrosine (tyramine), tryptophan (tryptamine) and 5 HTP (serotonin) and lowers the concentration of serotonin in the brain and noradrenaline in the tissues, but does not possess adrenergic neural blocking action.

250 mg. b.i.d. is the initial dose which can be increased by 250 mg. twice weekly to a maximum of 700 mg. daily. The main side-effect is drowsiness. One-third of patients respond to methyldopa with a blood pressure drop in the supine position, while half of the patients given this drug will show a drop of blood pressure in the erect position.

Methyldopa reduces the peripheral resistance, decreases cardiac output and reduces glomerular filtration rate, renal and placental blood flows.

(*d*) **Hydralazine (Apresoline)** has mental binding properties and binds certain organic acids, mercaptans and primary amines. It antagonises some enzymes (e.g. dopa decarboxylase and histaminase) and relaxes smooth muscle, producing its hypotensive effect by acting directly on the wall of the blood vessel. Hence it will produce its hypotensive effect with the patient lying flat in bed.

When given intravenously there is a drop in the diastolic, followed by a reduction in the systolic blood pressure and an increase in the pulse rate. Cerebral, renal and uterine blood flows are increased (Johnson and Clayton, 1957). With intravenous administration, severe headaches are produced in a large percentage of cases. Tolerance develops fairly quickly and this limits the usefulness of the drug.

The initial intravenous dose is 20 mg. given slowly. As tolerance develops this may have to be increased to 60 mg.

Oral administration usually produces disappointing results as the hypotensive effect of the tolerated doses is not very great. However, when combined with reserpine and protoveratrine a useful hypotensive effect may be produced. Prolonged administration may give rise to the hydralazine syndrome consisting of rheumatoid symptoms or lupus erythematosus, but these effects are reversible when therapy is stopped.

(*e*) **Protoveratrine.**—Although not an ideal hypotensive agent, protoveratrine is the most useful of the available hypotensive agents in the control of hypertension during pregnancy.

In cases of eclampsia or severe pre-eclampsia occuring after the 35th week, the object is to control the blood pressure for the short period that it takes to effect delivery.

A reduction of blood pressure can be produced very quickly and satisfactorily by adding 1 mg. of protoveratrine A to a pint of 5 per cent glucose in water and administering it intravenously at the rate of 40 drops a minute until the blood pressure starts to fall. The drop rate is then slowed and adjusted to produce the required level of blood pressure. Alternatively, 0·3 mg. can be given intramuscularly with a further 0·1 or 0·2 mg. every hour until satisfactory control of the blood pressure is obtained. The effect of a single injection lasts about three hours.

For long-term treatment, injections given every three hours are not practicable and protoveratrine A has to be given by mouth. The most satisfactory preparation for oral administration is a retard preparation, each tablet of which contains 0·1 mg. which is liberated following ingestion, a further 0·1 mg. is released in two to four hours, and the third 0·1 mg. is liberated in four to six hours. The emphasis must be on protoveratrine A, as protoveratrine B is poorly absorbed.

Protoveratrine acts by irritating the sensory fibres in the vagus and in particular those which arise from the carotid sinus, the aortic

body and the heart. In this way a reflex fall of blood pressure is produced and the heart is slowed due to reflex stimulation of the motor fibres in the vagus. Protoveratrine may also have some central action.

Unfortunately, there is only a small margin between the hypotensive and the emetic thresholds and unless the blood levels of the drug are kept fairly constant and within this narrow range results are unsatisfactory.

When excessive doses of protoveratrine are given parenterally, acute falls of blood pressure are likely to occur. These can be counteracted by giving atrophine to abolish the vagal effect, raising the foot of the bed, and administering methedrine or ephedrine. Excessive falls in blood pressure are usually transitory and, as a rule, do not jeopardise the fœtus. With oral therapy it is almost impossible to produce serious hypotension, as vomiting occurs when two or more of the 0·3 mg. retard tablets are given every hour. On the other hand, one tablet an hour rarely produces any hypotensive effect, and the average patient requires one and a half to one and three-quarter tablets per hour. With oral treatment, an average reduction of 20 mm. Hg in the basal diastolic blood pressure can be obtained in about one-third of patients, while an equal number will show a drop of 10 mm. Hg in the diastolic pressure.

Value of Hypotensive Therapy

There is no evidence that the employment of hypotensive therapy reduces perinatal wastage from pre-eclampsia or eclampsia. The main justification for its use is to try and protect the mother while conservative treatment is continued or until such time as the pregnancy can be terminated. Reducing the blood pressure without the simultaneous administration of anticonvulsants and other lines of treatment will not prevent the development of fits.

The use of guanethidine is restricted to the ambulatory treatment of severe cases of essential hypertension during early pregnancy. Methyldopa may be of some value in the one-third of patients who will respond to this drug when lying in bed.

For the acute treatment of hypertension in severe pre-eclampsia or eclampsia, protoveratrine given parenterally is the drug of choice. The dose is critical and the duration of effect short, so it requires close supervision and this is its main limitation.

If hypotensive therapy is to be continued for more than 2 or 3 days oral administration is the only practical approach to the problem. A hypotensive effect can frequently be produced with minimal side-effects by the combination of a thiazide diuretic, 0·5 mg. reserpine a day, the maximum oral dose of protoveratrine that will not produce nausea and oral hydralazine.

Intravenous Glucose

The parenteral administration of 1 litre of 20 per cent glucose in water in the space of 20 minutes was once recommended. A more satisfactory alternative was the intravenous injection by means of a syringe of 100 ml. of 50 per cent glucose in water within a period of a few minutes. Advocates of these types of therapy claimed that the osmotic pressure of the plasma was increased and œdema fluid was drawn back into the capillaries and excreted. This is not true as glucose diffuses through the capillary walls and is distributed throughout the extracellular fluid. So long as the plasma concentration is about double the normal level, an osmotic diuresis will be produced and some sodium and potassium excretion will occur. An elevated blood glucose level stimulates insulin secretion so that the excess glucose is rapidly converted into glycogen or fat. Thus the main effect of intravenous glucose is to replenish liver glycogen and relieve the ketosis which may occur in a patient so heavily sedated that she has had little to eat.

Intravenous Dextran, Sucrose or Concentrated Plasma

In an effort to elevate the plasma osmotic pressure, various substances have been given which diffuse through the capillary walls less readily than glucose. Only the larger "dextraven" molecules stay in the circulating plasma for any length of time, as even administered plasma proteins disappear fairly rapidly due to metabolism and the activity of the liver. With the increase in plasma osmotic pressure there is a reduction in glomerular filtration so that what is "gained on the swings is lost on the roundabout".

TERMINATION

As there is no evidence that the duration of the pre-eclamptic signs makes any appreciable contribution to the risk of residual hypertension, only the immediate prognosis has to be considered. With adequate bed rest, hypotensive therapy and sedation, the maternal risk of recurrent eclamptic fits is not great and therefore it is the fœtal prognosis which influences the method of management. The risk of intra-uterine death from placental insufficiency is considerable, and although it is proportional to the duration of the pre-eclamptic signs, this risk has to be balanced against that of neonatal death from prematurity. This latter is of the order of 7·5 per cent at 36 weeks and is doubled for each additional two weeks of prematurity, being 15 per cent at 34 weeks and over 30 per cent at 32 weeks. Consequently, if labour is induced before about the 35th week, it is important to be sure that the degree of placental insufficiency and hence the risk of intra-uterine death is sufficiently great to justify the very high risk of

neonatal death from prematurity that is associated with delivery before this period of gestation. Unfortunately, the severity of the pre-eclamptic signs are an unreliable guide to the risk of intra-uterine death and more reliance must be placed on the duration of the signs when assessing prognosis.

The most useful index of the urgency for the induction of labour to avoid intra-uterine death is the serial estimation of urinary œstriol levels. So long as twice weekly or alternate daily œstriol readings continue to rise or remain level above 6 to 8 mg. per 24 hours there is no immediate risk of intra-uterine death from placental insufficiency.

Once the 38th week has been reached in moderately severe cases of pre-eclampsia, the fœtus should be delivered.

In cases which have been well controlled and are not causing immediate anxiety, labour can be induced by artificial rupture of the membranes followed by an intravenous oxytocin infusion. This should be run during the day and discontinued at night.

Even pure synthetic oxytocin is antidiuretic and if there is the simultaneous intravenous administration of large volumes of fluid, without allowing periods for the uninhibited renal excretion of the excess water, fits may be precipitated by water intoxication.

A reduction in urinary output during oxytocin administration is to be expected and should not be misinterpreted as a deterioration in the clinical condition of the patient.

Intramuscular oxytocin for the induction of labour should not be used as it is ineffective and dangerous. It carries a very high risk of producing short periods of raised uterine tone with impairment of placental circulation.

When shortage of staff renders it difficult to run an intravenous oxytocin infusion with adequate supervision, oxytocin can be given as an intranasal spray following rupture of the membranes. This should not be given more frequently than once every half hour until the patient is conscious of uterine contractions. Once the patient can indicate how often contractions are occurring, the frequency of administration can be increased until a contraction is produced every 3 to 4 minutes. Oxytocin can also be administered as a sub-lingual tablet. A 200 unit tablet placed under the tongue is associated with the continuous absorption of a very small quantity of the oxytocin, about 0·1 per cent of the administered dose reaches the uterus.

A cervix that is long and not taken up (the "unripe" cervix) should not discourage the induction of labour by rupture of the membranes and the use of intravenous or intranasal oxytocin. Under these circumstances, the latent period of the first stage of labour will be prolonged, but the overall incidence of successful vaginal deliveries should not be significantly reduced.

Mild cases of pre-eclampsia should be induced at or shortly before

term and post-maturity complicated by mild degrees of placental insufficiency should be avoided.

ECLAMPSIA

The term eclampsia means "a sudden flash", a graphic description of the epileptiform convulsion, with its tonic and clonic stages, that has been held in so much dread by the obstetrician.

Twenty per cent of eclamptic convulsions occur with very little warning, but the remainder present the signs of pre-eclampsia for a variable period and therefore cases likely to develop eclampsia can be detected by conscientious antenatal care and the development of fits avoided by preventive treatment.

PROGNOSIS

(a) *Maternal.*—Pulmonary œdema has been a common terminal manifestation of eclampsia in the past, but Corkill (1957) in analysing cases which have occurred in New Zealand since 1950, found that the eclamptic state *per se* was not the outstanding feature of the fatal cases. The principal causes of death were massive cerebral hæmorrhage, sudden cardiac failure and anuria following accidental hæmorrhage. Hyperpyrexia is a further cause of death.

Since 1953, only one in six of the toxæmic deaths has been associated with eclampsia. In other words, while the incidence of toxæmic deaths was 0·18 per 1,000 births, the frequency with which eclamptic patients died was 0·03 per 1,000 births

The maternal mortality with antepartum eclampsia was 6·6 per cent, while with intra- and postpartum eclampsia it was 1·5 to 2 per cent.

(b) *Foetal.*—The fœtal loss in New Zealand during 1950 to 1955 was 45 per cent with antepartum eclampsia, 11·6 per cent with intrapartum convulsions, and 5·3 per cent in cases where the mother had the first fit following delivery.

(c) *Remote.*—Chesley *et al.* (1962) carried out a long term follow-up of 270 cases of eclampsia and found a marked difference between the primiparous eclamptic and those who had eclampsia as multiparæ. The latter group had a high incidence of hypertension antedating their eclamptic pregnancies; at follow-up they were found to have suffered a marked increase in remote mortality and the surviving women had a high incidence of hypertension. Primiparous eclamptic women suffered no increase in remote deaths nor was the incidence of residual hypertension higher than in a control group of normal women.

About one-quarter of those who developed eclampsia in their first pregnancy suffered from a mild elevation of blood pressure in a subsequent pregnancy.

Less than 10 per cent experienced moderate to severe toxæmia in a later pregnancy. The higher incidence of hypertension amongst women who had eclampsia as multiparæ was reflected in a recurrence of toxæmia in 50 per cent of subsequent pregnancies.

INCIDENCE

In New Zealand eclampsia is notifiable, and from 1953 to 1955, 206 cases occurred in 164,629 deliveries, a rate of 1·25 per 1,000. There were equal numbers of antepartum, intrapartum and postpartum cases, but whereas two-thirds of the antepartum cases were severe, two-thirds of the intrapartum and postpartum cases were mild.

TREATMENT

The immediate management of an eclamptic fit is a matter of nursing technique, as a member of the nursing staff rather than a doctor is more likely to be present at the time a fit commences.

Nurses are instructed to insert, if possible, a gag or padded peg between the patient's teeth, to turn the patient on her side and give oxygen while awaiting the arrival of the doctor. The principle involved is to maintain a clear airway and reduce anoxia.

The most effective way of aborting a fit is to give a small dose of Pentothal intravenously, just sufficient to stop the convulsion. The patient then requires sedation with tribromethanol (Avertin) rectally.*

Rectal Avertin has the advantage of ease of administration, adequate sedation with reduction of the blood pressure, and once the patient is under its influence she can be moved to an eclamptic room and examination and assessment carried out without fear of precipitating another convulsion. Avertin suffers from the disadvantage that it takes a few minutes to make up the 2½ per cent solution from the concentrated fluid. 0·075 mg. of this concentrated reagent per kilo of body weight are dissolved in water warmed to nearly 40°C. If the temperature goes above this figure, the reagent may break up into toxic products. For this reason, a few millilitres of the 2½ per cent solution must always be tested with congo red. If the colour remains orange red, it can be given to the patient with safety, but if the indicator turns blue the solution must be discarded. Avertin also suffers from the disadvantage of variable rates of absorption when given rectally.

If heavy barbiturate sedation is used in place of Avertin, the blood

---

* The manufacturers of Avertin, namely The Bayer Products Company, have recently drawn attention to the difficulty of maintaining supplies of this useful drug, but have assured us that it will continue to be available for the treatment of eclampsia. (I.D.)

pressure can be lowered by administering protoveratrine by intravenous drip or intramuscularly every three hours.

A close watch is kept on the amount of urine excreted and the patient allowed a fluid intake of one litre a day in addition to a volume equal to her urinary output. She should be nursed in an environment where stimuli are kept to a minimum i.e. the room should be darkened and quiet. Hyperpyrexia is dangerous and must be controlled, and in extreme cases it may be necessary to induce hypothermia by active cooling.

Induction of labour should be delayed for a few hours or a day, until there has been an opportunity of treating the hypertension and adequately sedating the patient. As soon as the maternal condition ceases to show evidence of progressive improvement, the membranes should be ruptured and, if labour does not commence within six hours, an oxytocin drip used to stimulate cervical dilatation.

During labour, a potent analgesic such as diamorphine gr. 1/6 (10 mg.) or morphia gr. $\frac{1}{4}$ (15 mg.) is required to relieve pain which acts as a nociceptive stimulus. As soon as the baby is born it should have 0·1 mg. of levallorphan (Lorfan) injected into the cord before it stops pulsating to counteract the respiratory depressant effect of the opiates.

After the cervix is one-third dilated it is preferable to rely on opiates for sedation for although they are not good anticonvulsants, their increased analgesic efficiency is some compensation, but, most important, if opiates are used as the main sedative for six to eight hours prior to delivery, the depressant effect on the respiratory centres of premature babies can be antagonised with levallorphan.

HYPERTENSION DURING PREGNANCY

Hypertension encountered during pregnancy may be due to:

1. A disorder developing during pregnancy, e.g. the placental type of pre-eclampsia.

2. Pathology antedating the pregnancy but only causing hypertension during pregnancy, e.g. latent essential hypertension.

3. Hypertension preceding the pregnancy may be due to:

(a) Established essential hypertension.

(b) Established renal hypertension including the various types of chronic nephritis.

(c) Endocrine disorders such as phæochromocytoma, Cushing's syndrome, aldosteronism, hyperthyroidism.

(d) Coarctation of the aorta.

Hypertension Developing During Pregnancy

When the blood pressure rises for the first time during pregnancy and there is no associated generalised œdema or proteinuria, the

condition cannot, strictly speaking, be classified as one of pre-eclampsia for, by definition, at least two signs must be present in pre-eclampsia. When hypertension is the only sign, the patient must be classified as suffering from hypertension. If subsequently, proteinuria develops then the criteria of pre-eclampsia are fulfilled. Many obstetricians do not adhere strictly to the academic definition of pre-eclampsia but include in this category patients who develop raised blood pressure as the only abnormality during the latter part of pregnancy.

Pathology developing during pregnancy.—In a small minority of cases of hypertension developing during pregnancy no pathology is present prior to the pregnancy; the ætiological factors are in the placenta or produced by the mechanical effects or hæmodynamic changes of the pregnancy.

Pathology antedating pregnancy.—In the vast majority of cases, some abnormality of the vascular or renal systems is present before the patient becomes pregnant. None the less, the blood pressure may be normal before pregnancy and during the first two trimesters. It may require the hæmodynamic changes of a normal pregnancy to bring to light the reduced vascular reserve. This is often the position with early cases of chronic pyelonephritis and essential hypertension.

Hypertension Antedating Pregnancy

Essential hypertension.—The diagnosis of essential hypertension is usually made by excluding other causes of hypertension such as renal pathology. A family history of hypertension is often accepted as evidence supporting this diagnosis.

As a rule, the more advanced pathological changes of essential hypertension, such as enlargement of the heart, arteriosclerosis and "silver wire" vessels in the retina are not found at the age at which pregnancy is common. Apart from an elevation of blood pressure, these patients appear quite normal.

PROGNOSIS

Harley (1966) has shown that neither the age nor the parity of the hypertensive mother have any influence on fœtal mortality. However those mothers with an initial diastolic blood pressure reading of over 100 mm. Hg lost a quarter of their babies compared to 1 in 10 amongst those with an initial diastolic blood pressure reading below 100 mm. Hg. The presence of proteinuria independent of high blood pressure did not increase perinatal mortality.

It is the height of the initial diastolic pressure rather than proteinuria that is the important factor affecting fœtal mortality.

Reserpine 0·25 mg. twice daily and hydrallazine 25 mg. four times

daily increased if necessary to 400 mg. a day had no effect on fœtal mortality.

Dunlop (1966) found that there is no significant increase in maternal mortality when a woman with essential hypertension becomes pregnant and the perinatal mortality is not increased except in those patients with a systolic pressure of 180 mm. Hg or more on several occasions or who develop proteinuria which appears more commonly with high blood pressure readings or where there has been a marked increase in the blood pressure during the second half of pregnancy.

The development of proteinuria occurs in about 12 per cent of pregnant patients with essential hypertension compared to an incidence of 9 per cent in patients who start pregnancy with a normal blood pressure. Although the overall risk of developing proteinuria is only slightly increased, the possibility of the appearance of a severe degree of pre-eclampsia increases from 0·5 per cent in women normotensive early in pregnancy, to 3·5 per cent in those who start pregnancy with an elevated blood pressure.

Because proteinuria occurs in a higher proportion of cases of pre-eclampsia, this disorder carries a higher perinatal mortality than does essential hypertension. This increase in perinatal mortality is due, not so much to the increase in the number of intra-uterine deaths, as to the increase in neonatal deaths due to the induction of labour at an earlier stage of pregnancy. Many obstetricians are frightened to treat these cases conservatively and, when labour is induced before 34 to 36 weeks gestation, the risk to the fœtus from prematurity usually outweighs the risk it runs from intra-uterine death prior to the 35th week.

The overall picture is one of a hypertensive woman having an 80 per cent chance of producing a child that will live.

Dunlop (1966) observed that the risk of an accidental hæmorrhage lethal to the fœtus was not increased except in the severe forms of essential hypertension.

TREATMENT

The management of cases of essential hypertension follow much the same lines as those outlined for the treatment of pre-eclampsia.

Bed rest, sedation, and the use of hypotensive therapy in the severe cases is the approach usually followed until the stage is reached when the risk of intra-uterine death from continuing conservative management is as great as the reduction in the risk of neo-natal death produced by reducing the degree of prematurity.

If, for example, labour is induced at 34 weeks gestation, 15 per cent of the babies will die from prematurity. For each fortnight induction is postponed, the neonatal death rate will be cut by half. This advantage must be discounted by the number of intra-uterine deaths that

will occur during each two-week period. In mild cases this may be only one per cent while in severe cases it may be as high as 8 or 10 per cent. Serial urinary œstriol readings may be a rough guide to the magnitude of the risk of intra-uterine death. So long as the levels are steady above 6 mg. per 24 hours or are rising, conservative management is justified till after the 36th week. If this method of evaluation is followed, it should be remembered that administration of barbiturates to these patients interferes with the estimation of urinary œstriol unless a saponification step is included in the technique used for the measurement of this steroid.

The above approach is one based on what is best for the fœtus. This philosophy is, however, only acceptable if it can be accomplished without prejudice to the maternal prognosis.

Hypotensive therapy is of no value to the fœtus and under some circumstances it reduces placental circulation. Its use is only indicated when it may play some part in protecting the mother from cerebral hæmorrhage or pulmonary œdema due to the additional load on the left ventricle.

Under most circumstances, conservative treatment aimed at obtaining the best for the fœtus can be followed without affecting the immediate or remote maternal prognosis.

Women with hypertension should be encouraged to plan their pregnancies at as early an age is possible. As they become older the severity of the hypertension often increases.

CHRONIC NEPHRITIS COMPLICATED BY PREGNANCY

Chronic pyelonephritis.—The clinical manifestations of chronic pyelonephritis may closely resemble those of early essential hypertension.

A history of previous urinary tract infections may suggest the possibility of chronic pyelonephritis and be an indication to determine the leucocyte excretion rate and a urinary bacillary count.

A renal biopsy may be the only method of arriving at an accurate diagnosis, but as the methods of management of these varieties of hypertension are all much the same, an accurate diagnosis is not essential and it is doubtful if the performance of this procedure is justified in view of the risks involved. About 4 to 5 per cent of apparently healthy pregnant women have a urinary bacillary count in excess of 100,000 organisms per ml. These individuals are very likely to develop frank urinary tract infections later in the pregnancy or to manifest in later years the features of chronic pyelonephritis.

PROGNOSIS

Fœtal prognosis is similar to that in essential hypertension.

The main risk to the mother is recurrence of urinary tract infection

with further fibrosis of the kidney. The physiological changes which occur in the urinary tract during a normal pregnancy produce a reduced rate of urinary flow with dilatation of the upper urinary tract and these changes predispose to recurrence of infection. For these reasons rotating courses of chemotherapy periodically throughout each subsequent pregnancy are indicated.

TREATMENT

The principles of management additional to those indicated above are similar to those outlined for essential hypertension.

Following delivery patients should be referred for investigation, especially if they have a significant degree of hypertension and are in the younger age group. In about 8 per cent of cases a unilateral renal lesion may be detected and, with correction of the disorder, they may return to a normal blood pressure with a marked improvement in the prognosis for a subsequent pregnancy as well as for their general health and life expectancy.

Chronic glomerular nephritis.—Chronic glomerular nephritis complicates pregnancy far less commonly than does chronic pyelonephritis. A previous history of acute glomerular nephritis or an appreciable amount of proteinuria without an increase in pus cells in the urine during early pregnancy will suggest the possibility of chronic glomerular nephritis.

The glomerular filtration rate can be determined most conveniently by the creatinine clearance. The extent to which the glomerular filtration rate is reduced will give some indication of the reduction in renal reserve. It is only when renal reserve is almost exhausted that the blood urea will rise.

In patients with a semi-basal diastolic pressure of over 100 mm. Hg and a marked reduction in glomerular filtration rate (less than 50 per cent of normal) the perinatal mortality is high.

Serial urinary œstriol readings can be used as a guide to the intra-uterine health and progress of the fœtus. When an ultrasonic echograph is available serial observations can be carried out to assess the rate of growth of the fœtus. All this information can be used as a guide to the optimum time for the induction of labour.

Phæochromocytoma.—Phæochromocytoma is a tumour arising from chromaffin tissue. 90 per cent occur in the adrenal medulla and almost all are benign. They constitute about 0·5 per cent of all cases of hypertensive disease in both sexes. When they complicate pregnancy a high maternal and fœtal mortality result unless the diagnosis is established.

The prompt surgical removal under cortisol cover of a phæochromocytoma in pregnant women is recommended as a matter of urgency in all cases, except those diagnosed in the last few weeks of

pregnancy when the lesion may be removed in conjunction with elective Cæsarean section.

The hypertension produced by phæochromocytomas may be paroxysmal or sustained. The elevated blood pressure may be associated with other manifestations of noradrenaline or adrenaline e.g. perspiration, tachycardia, nausea, severe headaches, visual disturbances, anxiety states, pallor. Two of the neurocutaneous syndromes, multiple neurofibromatosis and von Hippel-Lindau's disease are associated with phæochromocytoma; consequently every diagnostic means should be used to exclude the presence of phæochromocytoma when any of the neurocutaneous diseases are detected clinically.

The most reliable means of diagnosis is the measurement of the concentration of free catechol amines in the urine. The concomitant measurement of their urinary metabolites, nor-metanephrine and metanephrine and 3-methoxy-4-hydroxy-mandelic acid (vanillylmandelic acid—V.M.A.) will established the diagnosis in most cases.

The vasodepressor (blocking) effect of phentolamine can also be determined, but false positive and negative results are not infrequent (Hutchinson *et al.*, 1958). The histamine vasopressor (provocative) test can be dangerous.

Cushing's syndrome.—In Cushing's syndrome pregnancy is exceptional on account of the amenorrhoea and infertility, but where it occurs the prognosis is better than with phæochromocytoma. Adrenalectomy can be performed during pregnancy.

Coarctation of the aorta.—The essential physiological alterations produced by coarctation are:

    (i)   decreased pulse pressure below the coarcted segment;

    (ii) increased arterial blood pressure proximal to the coarctation;

    (iii) increased left ventricular work;

    (iv) extensive collateral arterial circulation.

Pregnancy complicating coarctation may not increase the maternal mortality but the perinatal mortality may exceed 50 per cent, mainly due to cardiovascular and renal complications. Following surgical correction of the coarctation the perinatal mortality usually does not exceed 10 per cent.

REFERENCES

1. ADAMS, E. M., and FINLAYSON, A. (1961). *Lancet*, **2**, 1375.
2. ADAMS, E. M., and MACGILLIVRAY, I. (1961). *Lancet*, **2**, 1373.
3. ALTCHEK, A. (1961). *J. Amer. med. Ass.*, **175**, 791.
4. ASSALI, N. S. (1958). *Clin. Obstet. Gynec.*, **1**, 383.
5. ASSALI, N. S., *et al.* (1958). *J. Lab. clin. Med.*, **52**, 423.
6. BOOTH, R. T., *et al.*, (1965). *J. Obstet. Gynaec. Brit. Cwlth.*, **72**, 229.
7. BOOTH, R. T., STERN, M. I., WOOD, C., and PINKERTON, J. H. M. (1964). *J. Obstet. Gynaec. Brit. Cwlth.*, **71**, 266.

8. Bower, D. (1964). *J. Obstet. Gynaec. Brit. Cwlth.*, **71**, 123.
9. Brown, A. K., and McGarry, J. A. (1961). *Scot. med J.*, **6**, 311.
10. Brown, J. J., *et al.* (1966 *a*). *J. Obstet. Gynaec. Brit. Cwlth.*, **73**, 410.
11. Brown, J. J., *et al.* (1966 *b*). *J. Endocr.*, **34**, 129.
12. Browne, F. J. (1958). *Lancet*, **1**, 115.
13. Browne, J. C. McC., and Veall, N. (1953). *J. Obstet. Gynaec. Brit. Emp.*, **60**, 141.
14. Brownrigg, G. M. (1962). *Canad. med. Ass. J.*, **87**, 408.
15. Bucht, H., and Werko, L. (1953). *J. Obstet. Gynaec. Brit. Emp.*, **60**, 157.
16. Burt, C. C. (1949). *Lancet*, **2**, 787.
17. Carey, H. M., and Liley, A. W. (1958). *N.Z. med. J.*, **58**, 450.
18. Chesley, L. C. (1956). *West. J. Surg.*, **64**, 284.
19. Chesley, L. C., Cosgrove, R. A., and Annitto, J. E. (1962). *Amer. J. Obstet. Gynec.*, **83**, 1360.
20. Chesley, L. C., Talledo, E., Bohler, C. S., and Zuspan, F. P. (1965 *a*). *Amer. J. Obstet. Gynec.*, **91**, 837.
21. Chesley, L. C. (1965 *b*). *Bull N.Y. Acad. Med.*, **41**, 811.
22. Chesley, L. C. (1966). *Amer. J. Obstet. Gynec.*, **95**, 127.
23. Corkill, T. F. (1957). *J. Obstet. Gynaec. Brit. Emp.*, **64**, 67.
24. Coyle, M. G., Greig, M., and Walker, J. (1962). *Lancet*, **2**, 275.
25. Crosley, A. P., *et al.* (1962). *Ann. intern. Med.*, **56**, 241.
26. Davey, O. A., O'Sullivan, W. J., and Browne, J. C. McC. (1961). *Lancet*, **1**, 519.
27. de Maria, F. J., and See, H. Y. C. (1966). *Amer. J. Obstet. Gynec.*, **94**, 471.
28. Diczfalusy, E. (1964). Symposia *Fed. Proc.*, **23**, 791.
29. Dieckmann, W. J., and Pottinger, R. (1957). *Amer. J. Obstet. Gynec.*, **74**, 816.
30. Dieckmann, W. J., Smitter, R. C., and Rynkiewicz, L. (1952). *Amer. J. Obstet. Gynec.*, **64**, 850.
31. Dixon, H. G., and Robertson, W. B. (1961). *Path. et Microbiol. (Basel)*, **24**, 622.
32. Dollery, C. T., *et al.* (1962). *Lancet*, **2**, 735.
33. Douglas, A., *et al.* (1961). *Brit. med. J.*, **2**, 206.
34. Fåhraeus, R. (1962). *Acta obstet. gynec. scand.*, **41**, 101.
35. Finnerty, F. A. (1956). *J. Amer. med. Ass.*, **161**, 210.
36. Ford, R. V. (1961). *Med. Clin. N. Amer.*, **45**, 961.
37. Frantz, A. G., *et al.* (1960). *Proc. Soc. exp. Biol. (N.Y.)*, **105**, 41.
38. Friedberg, V. (1958). *Zbl. Gynäk.*, **80**, 159.
39. Gibson, G. B. (1956). *J. Obstet. Gynaec. Brit. Emp.*, **63**, 833.
40. Govan, A. D. T. (1962). *Postgrad. med. J.*, **38**, 214.
41. Greig, M., Coyle, M. G., Cooper, W., and Walker, J. (1962). *J. Obstet. Gynaec. Brit. Cwlth.*, **69**, 772.
42. Grossman, J. (1960). In *Edema: Mechanisms and Management*, edited by J. H. Moyer and M. Fuchs, p. 223. Philadelphia: W. B. Saunders Co.
43. Healey, L. A., *et al.* (1959). *New Engl. J. Med.*, **261**, 1358.
44. Hellman, L. M. (1961). *Path. et. Microbiol. (Basel)*, **24**, 555.
45. Holland, W. W., and Humerfelt, S. (1964). *Brit. med. J.*, **2**, 1241.

46. HOLLIS, W. C., (1961). *J. Amer. med. Ass.*, **176**, 947.
47. HOOPER, J., *et al.* (1961). *Obstet. and Gynec.*, **17**, 271.
48. HUDSON, C. N. (1961). *J. Obstet. Gynaec. Brit. Cwlth.*, **68**, 68.
49. HUNTER, C. A., and HOWARD, W. F. (1960). *Amer. J. Obstet. Gynec.*, **79**, 838.
50. JOHNSON, G. T., and CLAYTON, C. G. (1957). *Brit. med. J.*, **1**, 312.
51. KUMAR, D., and BARNES, A. C. (1960). *Obstet. gynec. Surv.*, **15**, 625.
52. LAIDLAW, J. C., RUSE, J. L., and GORNALL, A. G. (1962). *J. clin. Endocr.*, **22**, 161.
53. LANDESMAN, R., *et al.* (1961). *Obstet. and Gynec.*, **18**, 645.
54. LIGHT, F. P. (1948). *Amer. J. Obstet. Gynec.*, **55**, 321.
55. LORINCZ, A. B., McCARTNEY, C. P., POTTINGER, R. E., and LI, R. H. (1961). *Amer. J. Obstet. Gynaec.*, **82**, 252.
56. MACGILLIVRAY, I., and BUCHANAN, T. J. (1958). *Lancet*, **2**, 1090.
57. MACGILLIVRAY, I., HYTTEN, F. E., TAGGART, N., and BUCHANAN, T. J., (1962). *J. Obstet. Gynaec. Brit. Cwlth.*, **69**, 458.
58. MAHRAN, M. (1961). *J. Obstet. Gynaec. Brit. Emp.*, **68**, 597.
59. McCALL, M. L. (1953). *Amer. J. Obstet. Gynec.*, **66**, 1015.
60. MENGERT, W. F., and TACCHI, D. A. (1961). *Amer. J. Obstet. Gynec.*, **81**, 601.
61. MENON, M. K. K. (1961). *J. Obstet. Gynaec. Brit. Emp.*, **68**, 417.
62. MORRIS, N., OSBORN, S. B., PAYLING-WRIGHT, H., and HART, A. (1956). *Lancet*, **2**, 481.
63. NESBITT, R. E. L., *et al.* (1965). *Amer. J. Obstet. Gynec.*, **93**, 708.
64. NAIRN, R. C., FRASER, K. B., and CHADWICK, C. S. (1959). *Brit. J. exp. Path.*, **40**, 155.
65. PAGE, E. W. (1957). *West. J. Surg.*, **65**, 166.
66. PATERSON, M. L. (1960). *J. Obstet. Gynaec. Brit. Emp.*, **67**, 883.
67. PICKERING, G. W., CRONSON, W. I., and PEARS, M. A. (1961). *The Treatment of Hypertension*. Springfield, Ill.: Chas. C. Thomas.
68. PICKERING, G. W., ROBERTS, J. A. F., and SOWRY, G. S. C. (1954). *Clin. Sci.*, **13**, 267.
69. PLATT, R. (1958). *J. Obstet. Gynaec. Brit. Emp.*, **65**, 385.
70. PLENTL, A. A., and GRAY, M. J. (1959). *Amer. J. Obstet. Gynec.*, **78**, 472.
71. POLLAK, V. E., and NETTLES, J. B. (1960). *Medicine (Baltimore)*, **39**, 479.
72. RAGAN, C., and BORDLEY, J. (1941). *Bull. Johns Hopk. Hosp.*, **69**, 504.
73. RIAD, A. M. (1962). *J. Obstet. Gynaec. Brit. Cwlth.*, **69**, 409.
74. ROBINSON, M. (1958). *Lancet*, **1**, 178.
75. RUBIN, A. A., *et al.* (1962). *J. Pharmacol. exp. Ther.*, **136**, 344.
76. RUSSELL, C. S., PAINE, C. G., COYLE, M. G., and DEWHURST, C. J. (1957). *J. Obstet. Gynaec. Brit. Emp.*, **64**, 649.
77. SANDLER, M., and COVENEY, J. (1962). *Lancet*, **1**, 1096.
78. SCOTT, D. B., and KERR, M. G. (1963). *J. Obstet. Gynaec. Brit. Cwlth.*, **70**, 1044.
79. SELLERS, A. M. (1957). *Amer. J. med. Sci.*, **233**, 709, 717.
80. SHAPIRO, A. P., BENEDEK, T. G., and SMALL, J. L. (1961). *New Engl. J. Med.*, **265**, 1028.
81. SHEEHAN, H. L. (1958). *Clin. Obstet. Gynec.*, **1**, 397.
82. SPETZ, S. (1965). *Acta obstet. gynec. scand.*, **44**, 227.

83. STEWART, W. K., and CONSTABLE, L. W. (1961). *Lancet*, **1**, 523.
84. STRAND, A. (1963). *Acta obstet. gynec. scand.*, **42**, (Suppl 6), 96.
85. VENNING, E. H. (1958). *Clin. Obstet. Gynec.*, **1**, 359.
86. VILLARREAL, H., *et al.* (1962). *Circulation*, **26**, 405.
87. WATANABE, J., *et al.* (1963). *J. clin. Invest.*, **42**, 1619.
88. WATANABE, M., *et al.* (1965). *J. clin. Endocr.*, **25**, 1665.
89. WRAY, P. M., and RUSSELL, S. C. (1963). *J. Obstet. Gynaec. Brit. Cwlth.*, **70**, 4.
90. WIGGLESWORTH, J. S. (1962). *J. Obstet. Gynaec. Brit. Cwlth.*, **69**, 355.

CHAPTER X

URINARY COMPLICATIONS

THE urinary system derives no benefit from pregnancy and occasionally the reverse. Certain physiological and anatomical changes occur as a result of pregnancy which may bring latent pathology to light or may encourage the development of a fresh urological handicap. In a previously healthy woman, control of micturition may be undermined, and subsequently recurring attacks of urinary infection originate in the urinary stasis which is an inevitable part of normal physiology in pregnancy.

Anatomical and Physiological Changes

Atony and dilatation of the renal pelvis and ureters occurs, and the latter are not only displaced somewhat laterally in the abdominal portion of their course, but are liable to develop kinks. Fortunately, the ureteric dilatation is to some extent compensated for by smooth muscle hypertrophy. This effect is partly due to hormonal influences and partly due to the mechanical pressure exerted by the enlarging uterus, and the changes are, therefore, more marked on the right side than the left because of the usual right obliquity of the uterine axis, the protection which the sigmoid colon and its mesentery afford to the left ureter, and the fact that the right ureter crosses the common iliac vessels at a more abrupt angle than its partner. These differences in pressure effects are, therefore, most noticeable at the level of the pelvic brim (Fig. 1).

Some degree of ureteric kinking is very common in pregnancy, occurring most often just below the renal pelvis and at the lower part of the upper third of each ureter.

Urinary stasis is greatest between the 20th and 24th weeks, and although the mechanical effects of the enlarging uterus continue to operate right up to term, stasis lessens somewhat in the second half of pregnancy, thanks mainly to the muscular hypertrophy of the ureteric walls. Ureteric dilatation is only partly to blame for stasis which often persists for months after delivery, and although dilatation occurs in the multipara, stasis is much less common, possibly because of her more lax abdominal musculature.

Progesterone is mainly responsible for ureteric dilatation and urinary stasis by reducing ureteric tone and peristalsis, so that the capacity of the renal pelvis and ureters is greatly increased from the usual 6–15 ml. to four times that amount. The rising level of œstro-

gen, however, as pregnancy advances is believed to encourage smooth muscle hypertrophy and, consequently, ureteric tone.

Since the ureter in pregnancy is less sensitive than normal to the usual stimuli, only a high fluid intake and consequently a high fluid output will encourage it to exert a healthy peristalsis. The implications, therefore, in the treatment of pyelitis are obvious, since stasis and bad drainage must inevitably aggravate and prolong the illness.

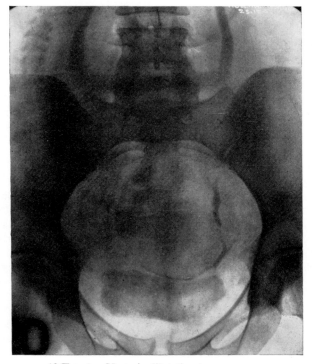

10/Fig. 1.—Ureteric dilatation in pregnancy.
(By courtesy of Prof. R. E. Steiner.)

The bladder is an accommodating organ, and, after an initial protest in the form of frequency due to the local pressure of the enlarging uterus within the pelvis during the first twelve weeks, it settles down to the rest of pregnancy and merely develops an increased volume tolerance which reaches its maximum at the 8th month. It again becomes irritable towards the end of pregnancy with the descent of the presenting part, and occasionally stress incontinence may be a troublesome symptom. It is during labour, however, that the bladder and urethra may suffer their real ordeal. It is not true

that in labour the bladder becomes a wholly abdominal organ with elongation of the urethra and displacement of the bladder neck above the symphysis pubis. Radiological studies[48] in labour indicate that, although the bladder neck is displaced closer behind the symphysis, it is not in fact drawn up. Such displacement as occurs is most marked in mid-cavity dystocia, and depends, not upon the degree of cervical dilatation nor the stretching of the lower uterine segment, but purely on the descent and tight fit of the presenting part. In other words, there is no escape for the bladder neck in hard labour from its potentially dangerous position behind the symphysis pubis, and this accounts for the usual position of obstetrical vesico-vaginal fistulæ.

During pregnancy the ability of the bladder to empty itself is usually complete, in marked contrast to its state during the early days of the puerperium, when the recently acquired tolerance of the bladder to large quantities of urine is liable to be aggravated by traumatic bruising and mucosal congestion, so that retention commonly occurs and encourages puerperal urinary sepsis.

Renal Function

The patient who presents in pregnancy with clearly impaired renal function is not common. Chronic nephritis, as generally understood in medicine, is almost a rarity in obstetrics. It is far more often that renal function tests will be invoked to explain some incidental complication developing later in pregnancy. Unfortunately there is no overall test which will give all the answers.

The **blood urea levels** do not begin to indicate renal pathology until disease is very far advanced. The normal level of blood urea in pregnancy is very much lower than out of it and, in fact, figures over 20 mg. per cent are regarded as significant. At the other end of the scale in full-blown uræmia the levels do not reflect the full extent of renal damage.

The **water excretion test** has a certain limited value, but again is crude and may be highly inconvenient for the patient. After a night's deprivation of water, the specific gravity of the urine should be normally as high as 1,025, although abnormal constituents such as protein may confuse the result. If the patient then drinks a litre of water, 800 ml. should be recovered in the urine within the next four hours if the kidneys are normal. With such a diuresis the specific gravity should go down to as low as 1,002 but, where the kidneys are defective, these wide variations in specific gravity will not be achieved and there will be a tendency for the figure not to deviate from 1010.

The **urea clearance test** has enjoyed a long innings. Here the amount of blood cleared of urea in one minute is expressed as a percentage of normality. For the test to have any semblance of reliability the rate of

urinary excretion should be not less than 2 ml. per minute because of the reabsorption of urea by the tubules if given time to do so. Diuresis is promoted by the patient drinking $\frac{1}{2}$ a litre of water and the bladder is emptied. Exactly one hour later the bladder is emptied again and at the same time a specimen is taken for blood urea estimation (B). After a further exact period such as an hour, the bladder is again emptied and the measure of urine obtained this time divided by the number of intervening minutes gives the volume of urine excreted per minute (V). The concentration of urea in this specimen is then estimated (U). The urea clearance will therefore be $\frac{UV}{B}$. Normally this figure in a healthy individual comes to about 75.

The percentage of normality will therefore now be expressed as $\frac{UV}{B} \times \frac{100}{75}$. If the urinary excretion is less than 2 ml. per minute the formula has to be suitably amended. Urea clearances of less than 70 per cent suggest renal deficiency.

The **creatinine clearance test** is now much more popular as a routine method because creatinine levels in the plasma do not alter as much as plasma urea levels do and because one is not faced with the same problem of reabsorption in the tubules. Furthermore the dietary intake of protein does not alter the level of plasma creatinine as happens in the case of urea. The blood urea level does not start to rise until long after the creatinine clearance rate shows a marked reduction and simultaneous plots of creatinine clearance against plasma urea show the former to be a far more sensitive index.[63] The creatinine clearance test normally lies between 90 and 130 ml./min. and is calculated in the same manner as the urea clearance rate. Great care must be taken in recording the exact amount of urine passed per minute, which depends upon strict technique of collection and on the patient emptying her bladder completely. If specimens are collected over a long period of time, the addition of a few crystals of thymol to the collected urine will act as a suitable chemical preservative.

Intravenous pyelography, although only used with great reluctance in pregnancy gives an incidental indication of renal excretory ability by the concentration of dye achieved in the lower urinary tract. In the course of searching for some structural abnormality by pyelography an impression of renal functional capacity may thus be obtained.

INFECTION OF THE URINARY TRACT

Although the term "pyelitis" is commonly used, the infection is seldom confined to the renal pelvis, but often involves the renal parenchyma as well as ureters and bladder. In fact, the severity of

the patient's constitutional disturbance depends mainly upon the level in the urinary tract at which the infection operates. Nevertheless, in deference to long-established usage, the term pyelitis will be retained.

Chief among the ætiological factors is urinary stasis, which, as already explained, is part of the normal physiology of pregnancy, but this operates more in primigravidæ than in multiparæ, and the incidence of the disease is, therefore, higher in the former. A previous history of urinary infection is significant, and this includes attacks of pyelitis in infancy as well as similar complications in earlier pregnancies. Urinary infection demonstrates the iceberg phenomenon in which the greater body of ice lies below the clinical surface and the ice appears above the surface only in peaks of provocation. Pregnancy is such a provocation. The chances of pyelitis developing during any given pregnancy are doubled in cases who have a history of previous infection.[30] Bacilluria is common in pregnancy, and Gladys Dodds (1931) found an incidence of 11 per cent, quite apart from clinical disease. Kass (1957) defined bacteriuria as the presence of more than 100,000 bacteria per ml., which is grossly in excess of what could be found by contamination provided the urine is examined at once or frozen solid since urine is a surprisingly good culture medium. On this basis he too found a similar incidence of bacteriuria at term. The suggestion is that the urinary tract is likely to be damaged to some extent by previous infection and is, therefore, more susceptible to a recurrence. Structural abnormalities, for example hydronephrosis, urinary calculus, etc., both encourage infection and certainly discourage its elimination.

Intestinal stasis is probably not a very serious factor in itself, but since constipation is more often due to an inadequate fluid intake than anything else, the resultant urinary stasis is more likely to be the direct cause in these cases.

Infection may reach the urinary tract either directly by the regurgitation of infected urine up the ureter from the bladder, which, however, is more common in the puerperium than during pregnancy, or it may be blood borne, or, thirdly, it may reach the renal pelvis by the lymphatic route either from the neighbouring colon, particularly the ascending colon on the right side, or from the bladder via the periureteral lymphatics.

Asymptomatic Bacteriuria.

The significance of bacteriuria as a source of trouble during this particular pregnancy and of later morbidity is worth reviewing at this stage. It is reckoned that in about 5 per cent of all necropsies, pyelonephritis is a major contributory cause of death and that there is

at least some evidence of infection of the kidneys in about 20 per cent of all female post-mortem studies. Although women as a rule live longer than men, their kidneys are nevertheless more vulnerable. The main source of trouble in men lies in the complications of prostatic enlargement.

In the life history of women there is no doubt that symptoms of pyelonephritis become less and less severe with each successive attack. It is possible that a kidney once infected never fully regains its health and that the dangers of latent or persistent sub-clinical infection deserve wider recognition. Radiology may be of limited help by showing enlarged kidneys or calyceal abnormalities, but the fundamental test of latent infection depends upon a demonstration of an abnormal number of bacteria, usually coliforms, in a fresh specimen of urine. Gladys Dodds found bacteriuria present in 11 per cent of all pregnant women very many years ago, and no subsequent series has yet produced a figure much lower than 5 or 6 per cent of all patients examined in the first trimester and it is reckoned that if this symptomless infection is left untreated as many as 35 per cent of such cases are likely to develop pyelitis during pregnancy, whereas less than 5 per cent will develop acute infection if adequately treated by long term sulphonamide therapy. This figure is strikingly different from those without bacteriuria in early pregnancy of whom less than 0·5 per cent will flare up.[42] If the case for routine screening of all women in early pregnancy is accepted, the load upon departments of bacteriology is daunting indeed. It is all very well for teaching hospitals such as my own to preach, backed as they are by large departments of bacteriology, so it is tempting indeed to search for short cuts which achieve adequate screening without causing much extra work. Such an idea, of course, is anathema to many pukka bacteriologists who, not without reason, regard the chemical tests as unreliable and consider that the only genuine method is by colony counting, using the standard wire loop technique from which false negatives are rare and false positives can be eliminated by repeating the test. A large proportion of patients, however, never come within range of a proper bacteriological department and for these the practice of posting off a possibly highly contaminated midstream specimen to the laboratory, either incubating warmly in the husband's pocket, or mislaid in the post, is a poor substitute for sending the patient herself to hospital, there to produce a fresh specimen. Yet even specimens collected in hospital have a trick of lying around for a dangerously long time if they are not discarded without trace, a phenomenon by no means unknown even in the best of departments. What is often forgotten is that urine is a splendid culture medium for most of the bacteria likely to infect it.[1] Pregnant urine is an even more suitable culture medium than the non-pregnant, because the pH is commonly higher than 6 whereas it

is only at lower and more acid levels that the growth of *E.coli* is inhibited—so much for the traditional futility of making the urine more alkaline with potassium citrate as a form of treatment! If one adds to this the fact that clinicians tend to work longer than the office hours of most laboratory staff, it can readily be seen that a specimen not received before about 3 o'clock in the afternoon may well get bacteriologically out of hand waiting for the next morning, or perhaps even a Monday morning or Tuesday following a Bank Holiday, unless it is refrigerated meanwhile at 4°C.

The accuracy and care with which a midstream specimen of urine is collected from a woman is also important and many patients and not a few nurses cannot be trusted to achieve what is called a "clean catch" specimen into a wide-mouthed honeypot jar or some such suitable receptacle. Where there is need to confirm the diagnosis of a significant degree of bacteriuria, there is much to be said for aspirating the urine suprapubically through a fine bore needle, rather than subjecting the patient to the now recognised hazards of wanton catheterisation.

Investigations designed to find the site of urinary tract infection by ureteric catheterisation have indicated that the kidney substance itself is the source in about half the patients and that the affected side or sides usually show some radiological evidence as well.[28]

What is somewhat depressing is that those who are found to have bacteriuria in early pregnancy, if untreated, will persist with the condition throughout pregnancy and into the puerperium. Apart from the risk of an acute flare-up already mentioned, an important series from Melbourne[40] shows that the incidence of prematurity is strikingly increased to 13·3 per cent in the bacteriuric as against only 5 per cent of those with clear urines, i.e. with less than the statutory number of 100,000 bacteria per ml., and furthermore that fœtal loss and pre-eclamptic toxæmia were also commoner. This Australian work also showed that these figures were not affected by the treatment of the bacteriuria in pregnancy; from which the very reasonable deduction was drawn that bacteriuria of itself is not harmful but simply reveals underlying chronic renal disease which itself was responsible for the complications—in other words that the bacteriuria is an effect and not a cause. A series from Hammersmith, although confirming the incidence of asymptomatic bacteriuria, found, however, that only about 32 per cent of cases developing acute pyelonephritis were predictable by bacterial colony counting and that the prematurity and fœtal disaster rates were not so related and that the true value of bacterial counting had been overstated.

For some time I remained in doubt myself about starting a screening programme at the Queen Mother's Hospital and looked forward to the true estimate of the value being furnished by the work of

others, but we have since decided to institute such a screening pro-gramme ourselves, as shall be described later.

Because of the work load already on antenatal clinics such as our own and most major centres, a review of quick, trouble-free screen-ing methods is forgivable, in spite of the withering comments of bacteriologists. Of the chemical tests, the Griess nitrite test is much favoured in some quarters because of the known ability of Gram-negative bacilli, including the *E. coli*, to reduce nitrates in the urine to nitrites.[61] This test may have to be repeated if false negatives are to be eliminated and does not work in the case of streptococcal infections, enterococci, nor pseudomonas. Sometimes the urine, however, does not contain enough nitrate for the test and therefore Sleigh in Edin-burgh has adopted the practice of fortifying the urine with nitrate and incubating to allow sufficient time for the nitrate to be reduced to nitrite before testing with the Griess reagent. Bacterial counts can then be employed to confirm the existence of infection in all urines giving such a positive screening test.

Another quick test is the triphenyl tetrazolium chloride test (TTC) a substance which is colourless and soluble and is reduced to triphenyl formazan by the active respiratory processes of rapidly dividing bacteria in infected urine. The reagents have to be carefully stored at low temperature and 0·5 ml. of the reagent is added to 2 ml. of fresh or refrigerated urine and incubated for 4 hours at 37°C. The pre-cipitate is red and easily recognised. An extensive experience of this test has been gained in Belfast,[53] where the urine of all antenatal patients was routinely examined at the first visit and at the thirtieth and thirty-fourth week, the specimens being collected by the mid-stream technique. This is the test described by Simmons and Williams (1962).

The main purpose of such tests is after all to provide a rapid method of screening and to restrict the labour of a fuller bacteriol-ogical examination to a smaller and more relevant number, but our own bacteriologists will have none of it.

An attractive, purely bacteriological, method has since appeared from the Royal Free Hospital,[8] in which a pre-sterilised disposable and commercially available swab of standard size is dipped into the urine to absorb a standard quantity thereof, with which to inoculate a single dried MacConkey plate. The inoculum consists of four parallel sets of streaks, each made up for strokes, without rotating the swab. This achieves progressive dilution of the urine by the time the final streak is made and from which the test is read, because colony counting at this dilution becomes possible without any bacteriological expertise. These cultures can be made on the spot in the clinic and ensure the use of absolutely fresh urine. The organisms most likely to be responsible for urinary infection are not discouraged even though

the plates are left for some time at room temperature and immediate incubation is not necessary. In fact, plates clearly negative may require no further examination. Although we have no experience of this test it sounds attractive, if only because it must in many cases eliminate the need for confirmatory bacteriological culturing, as the colonies are available for direct identification by the bacteriologist where necessary.

In our own screening programme midstream urine samples are collected at the clinic and immediately refrigerated until the end of the clinic, when they are gathered up and sent to the Department of Bacteriology at the Western Infirmary, to arrive within two hours of collection. A specimen is divided into two, one of which goes to the bacteriology department and the other to the Renal Unit where a modified Addis count is performed, i.e. the count of white cells, casts, and red cells from a spun 10 ml. specimen. In those with counts of over 100,000 organisms per ml., two groups are selected at random for treatment and control, the former receiving sulphadimidine 0·5 g. twice a day throughout pregnancy, provided the treatment can be started before the 20th week. Those in the treated group are re-examined a month later and their urine is checked for sulphonamides to see if they are taking the medication and if, in spite of treatment, the bacilluria is not resolving, the drug is changed to nitrofurantoin 100 mg. twice a day. Needless to say the division between treated and control cases is interrupted in the event of an acute complication such as pyelonephritis developing. This is likely to be a long term project to try and assess for ourselves the importance or need for routine screening and treating of asymptomatic cases, because the cut and dried answers for which we had been hoping seem unlikely yet to materialise.

Estimates of the incidence of pyelitis in pregnancy vary according to the criteria employed, but 2 per cent is a fairly conservative figure.

In over 90 per cent of cases *E. coli* is the responsible organism, though in chronic forms of the disease other organisms are commonly associated. A mixed bag of other organisms also comes into the picture during the puerperium, for example *B. proteus*, *B. ærogenes*, *Str. fæcalis*, *Staph. pyogenes* and *Ps. pyocyaneus*, the last, together with typhoid and paratyphoid bacilli, being uncommon. Rarely the gonococcus may be responsible.

Clinically the disease has an acute onset, often with rigors, abdominal pain, vomiting, and pain in the back, particularly in the costo-vertebral angle. A temperature of 103° F. is common, while it may occasionally be as high as 105° F. and the patient looks ill, with flushed cheeks and dirty tongue. Deep breathing is often painful, and a dry cough may be troublesome. The pain, in its distribution, tends to be referred in accordance with the situation of the naturally occurring ureteric kinks. Bladder symptoms, in the form of frequency and dysuria, may co-exist or may precede the attack, but are

commonly absent. On examining the abdomen, the most characteristic feature is tenderness in the loin and particularly in the costo-
vertebral angle. Abdominal rigidity is usually not marked but is very
variable. Urinary output is reduced, at first due to inflammatory
congestion and œdema of the ureters in addition to dehydration, and
the urine is strongly acid. The finding of large numbers of pus cells
and organisms settles the diagnosis. It must be remembered, however, that pus may not be found in the urine for the first forty-eight
hours due to temporary ureteric blockage.

Signs and symptoms occur more often on the right than on the
left, even though the infection may be bilateral. Bowel sounds are
usually audible, and the uterus, apart from referred and apparent
tenderness, does not reveal clinical abnormality.

The differential diagnosis is chiefly concerned with acute appendicitis, which fortunately is not a common complication of pregnancy.
In the case of appendicitis, vomiting is more usual, the initial temperature is lower, rigors are absent, and tenderness is more marked
laterally at the level of the umbilicus rather than in the costo-
vertebral angle. Rigidity, in so far as it can be assessed, is more
marked, the pulse is relatively faster and urine examination is
negative.

Retro-placental hæmorrhage also comes into the differential diagnosis. In this instance, the patient is not febrile, the tenderness is
restricted to the uterus or some part of it, the uterus is often tense,
and although albumen may be present in the urine, pus cells are unlikely. Some cases of pyelitis of pregnancy present with hyperemesis,
and the urinary source of the trouble may be overlooked unless
the patient is properly examined. A urinary calculus may produce acute symptoms, but is also often associated with a urinary
infection.

Pneumonia and pleurisy can easily be mistaken for pyelitis and
vice versa, hence the importance of examining the urine under the
microscope.

Less acute cases of pyelitis may present with only mild pain and
pyrexia and are more difficult to diagnose; in fact, one may first
become aware of the condition by the presence of albumen in the
urine due to pyuria. Chronic pyelonephritis may present as refractory iron deficient anæmia.

The role of pyelography in assessing these cases is reserved for
those in whom the infection persists in spite of treatment or in whom
it recurs. By its use, an underlying ætiological factor may be un-
earthed. Its employment during the acute phase of the disease is
contra-indicated, as it is undesirable to deprive the patient of fluid
in order to secure clear-cut radiographs. If there is nitrogen retention, the dye is unlikely to be satisfactorily excreted, but otherwise

pyelitis does not contra-indicate intravenous pyelography, when this is considered necessary.

Prophylaxis

To the patient with a history of previous recurrent attacks of urinary infection, prophylactic measures are often worth while. In these cases bacteriuria, as defined above, should be sought in a freshly collected midstream specimen of urine. It is clear from the observations of Kass that about 40 per cent of patients with bacteriuria will subsequently get a pyelonephritis and conversely if bacteriuria can be eliminated this complication is unlikely to arise. Similar observations have been made in Aberdeen[66] which also indicate that the high risk cases should be screened in this way and a powerful attempt made to eliminate the bacilluria by treatment with long-acting sulphonamides or nitrofurantoin, or, if necessary, by both. It would appear that by securing a sterile urine while the infection is still latent and not clinically manifest the renal parenchyma is likely to be spared yet another inflammatory insult and that this may make an appreciable difference to the patient's renal prognosis in middle age and later life.

There are three main long-acting sulphonamides, namely, sulphamethoxypyridazine (Lederkin) or Midicel, sulphaphenazole (Orisulf) and sulphadimethoxine (Madribon). Their action is bacteriostatic and interferes with the utilisation of para-aminobenzoic acid. They are very slowly excreted hence their prolonged action, but they are less useful for acute infections since they are readily inactivated in plasma by becoming protein bound. However, sulphadimethoxine is excreted as a very soluble glycuronide and is therefore probably the most useful in the long term prophylaxis of E. coli urinary infections. The dose is 0·5 to 1 g. daily in a single dose. Not only will such ambulant treatment reduce the chances of an acute infection developing but may succeed in sterilising the urine at least for many months to come. Resistant cases may respond equally well to nitrofurantoin therapy.

The dangers of catheterisation in women are now becoming increasingly recognised. Kass reckoned that the likelihood of subsequent bacteriuria was somewhere between 2 and 4 per cent after a single catheterisation. In this country the team in Bristol have amply demonstrated the dangers of catheterisation and there is no such thing as a totally sterile catheterisation and a bladder that has already been once infected is readily infected again.[32, 59] To us in Glasgow it also became apparent that the infection rate is likely to be related to the number of catheterisations and that indwelling catheters in particular are the worst offenders of the lot. We also incriminated the soft rubber catheter wielded by a nurse with naked, wet hands.[25, 50]

The only excuse now for using a catheter is as a therapeutic measure, for example, before the application of forceps or at some other obstetrical operation. This need cannot be eliminated because of the known interference with uterine activity which a full bladder causes, but the danger of cross-infection in a properly isolated maternity hospital is very much less than in the case of a gynæcological unit where the patients are subjected to a much greater risk of hospital strains of resistant organisms.

The Glasgow method described by Paterson *et al.* of catheterising with clean, dry, but not necessarily sterile hands, using a solid catheter held only by the hilt and instilling 60 ml. of aqueous chlorhexidine (1: 5,000), but without the wetting agents in commercial hibitane (which may provoke hæmaturia) has been found to reduce the infection very materially in obstetric patients. An alternative method of preventing infection from catheterisation has also been tried by the Bristol team, by disinfecting the urethra a few minutes before passing a catheter by injecting up the urethra a lubricant containing chlorhexidine jelly.

Of all the prophylactic measures which may be adopted during pregnancy, a satisfactory daily intake of fluid is the most important.

Latent Urinary Infection

Once a urinary infection, always a urinary infection. It is very doubtful if the kidney ever wholly recovers from a previous infection and a lifelong subclinical, chronic interstitial pyelonephritis is the likely result. Such a kidney under times of stress, for example, in pregnancy or the puerperium and after genito-urinary operations such as repairs for prolapse is then very liable openly to declare its chronic infection. What is much more serious is that hypertension in later life may be due to this factor and the condition may ultimately shorten life. By the time renal excretion tests are positive, already about 80 per cent of the renal parenchyma has been damaged beyond repair. As a practical measure, therefore, it would be much more rewarding to detect latent interstitial pyelonephritis at a time when active treatment could help towards preventing further damaging infections. It is therefore more sensible to investigate an apparently "essential" hypertension in early pregnancy with this in mind than for biochemical evidences of renal failure. Fortunately the work of Pears and Houghton (1958 and 1959) has provided us with a means of unearthing chronic pyelonephritis which as Rosenheim (1960) and de Wardener have pointed out smoulders on as a continuing infection but commonly with a sterile urine. This is the pyrogen test in which, following an intravenous injection of "Pyrexal" (which is a purified lipopolysaccharide prepared from *Salmonella abortus equi* in a dose of 0·007 micrograms per kilogram of body

weight), produces within the next few hours an outpouring of leucocytes, epithelial cells and protein in the urine. Bacteria follow later, often the next day. The white cell excretion rate is likely to rise to a total of over 200,000 per hour when the test is positive and the test serves to distinguish chronic pyelonephritis from glomerulo-nephritis in which it is usually negative. Leather *et al.* (1963) in Bristol have questioned its specifity in this latter respect, although they admit that the test is of great diagnostic value in those cases in which the urine is apparently normal.

Because "Pyrexal" can sometimes produce quite a reaction, especially in pregnancy, alternative provocative techniques have been developed, for example, the injection over a period of up to five minutes of 40 mg. of prednisolone phosphate dissolved in 10 ml. of saline and the test has been found superior in all respects.[20, 38, 46] It is worth counting the renal epithelial cells excreted separately from the leucocytes because any type of chronic urinary infection, includ-ing one of the lower urinary tract, might give a positive result, but that if there is a large excretion of renal epithelial cells it would strongly suggest that the damage is situated within the kidney itself.[54] The importance of this work lies in the opportunity which it affords to prevent deterioration in a patient's renal well-being by adequate prophylaxis and later stringent follow up of cases who have suffered a clinically overt attack.

Treatment

Once an acute attack of pyelitis has developed, the patient should be put to bed, and fluid intake should be sufficient to ensure the passage of not less than 1500 ml. a day because dehydration, which is otherwise likely to occur, encourages urinary stasis. In the early stages of the disease the diet should consist only of milk, fruit juices and carbohydrates. Often the patient can be made more comfortable and drainage of the infected renal pelvis assisted by making her lie on the unaffected side. An aperient is given, and, if the temperature is very high, tepid sponging may be necessary, especially since hyperpyrexia may cause intra-uterine foetal death. Potassium citrate and sodium bicarbonate are said to increase the efficiency of sulphonamides. Since Meave Kenny in 1937 introduced sulphona-mides in the treatment of pyelitis in pregnancy and the puerperium, they have become our main therapeutic standby. In standard dosage they produce an improvement in the patient's condition within 48 hours. The more soluble preparations, such as sulphadimidine are efficiently excreted and concentrated in the urine.

The usual dosage is 2 g. initially, followed by 1 g. four-hourly usually for a minimum of five days. If improvement is not obtained with this treatment by the time 30 g. of such sulphonamides have

been given, it is dangerous to persist blindly without a fuller urological investigation to identify the underlying cause or insensitive organisms. The early hazards of such treatment are anuria from crystallisation, skin rashes and other sensitisation phenomena, to say nothing of nausea and vomiting which are common indeed.

After more than ten days' treatment on full dosage of sulphonamides there is the further danger of granuloleucopenia, aplastic anæmia and thrombocytopenia.

The search for safer, more soluble and more potent sulphonamides continues and sulphafurazole, for example, has been shown by Svec *et al.* (1954) to be about twenty times more soluble in urine of pH 6-7 than sulphadiazine. Furthermore, about 70 per cent of it is excreted in the urine in active, i.e. non-acetylated form. In the body, this drug is mainly confined to extracellular fluids and does not readily penetrate cells. This may account for its very low toxicity in addition to its efficacy in urinary infections. The dose is as given above.

A sustained temperature for more than a week often indicates ureteric blockage, which is preventing drainage of the infected renal pelvis. It is in these rare cases that ureteric catheterisation is called for, and nowadays the need for this must be very rare indeed.

Organisms which prove to be insensitive to sulphonamides should be identified by culture, and their sensitivity to different antibiotics should be assessed in order to determine appropriate antibiotic treatment. The sulphonamides are so effective, however, in the majority of cases of pregnancy pyelitis that the field for antibiotic treatment is relatively restricted. This state of affairs, however, may not long continue since resistance both to sulphonamides and antibiotics is rapidly increasing in many organisms which until recently could be trusted to succumb to such treatment. Even the *E. coli* now shows, from time to time, an unexpected resistance.[32] This is particularly likely to occur if the urine is not rapidly made sterile by the first chemotherapeutic or antibiotic attack. Empirical treatment with the antibiotics is therefore not only likely to be ineffective but may breed resistant strains of organisms, prolong the illness, prejudice later cure and at the same time distract attention from the need to eliminate underlying genito-urinary pathology, for example hydronephrosis, calculus or tuberculosis. Furthermore, the prolonged and indiscriminate use of broad spectrum antibiotics may make the patient more sick than the original illness with nausea, vomiting, diarrhœa and occasionally intestinal moniliasis or staphylococcal enterocolitis.

Before embarking therefore upon anything more drastic in the treatment of urinary infection than a five-day course of sulphonamide, full sensitivity reports should be obtained from the bacteriologist. Where such reports indicate them, streptomycin 0·5 g. injected twice daily may be very effective. One of the troubles with

streptomycin is that resistance very readily develops and therefore the dose must be adequate, and the urine, in order to achieve the best effect immediately, should be rendered alkaline. Because of the danger of toxic accumulation streptomycin should never be used in any case in which renal output is impaired.

The tetracyclines are now taboo in pregnancy because of their adverse effects on the baby's teeth. Liver damage in the mother is another possible complication following high dosage. Nitrofurantoin (Furadantin) produces a very rapid and effective antibacterial concentration in the urine and because of its safety and absence of toxicity, enjoys wide popularity. It is given by mouth 100 mg. q.d.s. in five-day courses. Ampicillin where bacteriologically appropriate has a notable advantage in parenchymatous lesions because of the high levels of concentration achieved in tissue as well as in urine.[9]

Certain organisms infecting the urinary tract are notoriously difficult to eradicate. The B. proteus for example is capable of developing resistance within a day or two and treatment with streptomycin should aim at sterilising the urine within the first twenty-four hours if possible by a high loading dose of 3 g. within that period, followed by 1 g. daily thereafter. Even so resistance may develop. Nalidixic acid (Negram) may prove useful against B. proteus as well as other common urinary pathogens and would appear to be reasonably free of toxic side-effects. The usual dosage is 1 g., four times daily, for a five day course. Ps. pyocyanea which is a very refractory organism, fortunately uncommon in obstetrics, responds well to colistin methane sulphonate (Colomycin) given by intramuscular injection 120 mg. 8-hourly.[26] Another line of attack on these very difficult infections is Polymyxin B sulphate (Aerosporin 250,000 units by intramuscular injection four-hourly for four days).

The emergence of resistant strains in chronic urinary infections treated with antibiotics can be considerably postponed by the combined use of two antibiotics, to both of which the organisms have previously been shown to be sensitive. This is because of the much smaller statistical chance of a doubly resistant variant emerging.

Termination of pregnancy on account of urinary infection is now very rare and is restricted to cases in which only one kidney is present or functionally active and in which a severe degree of infection threatens to undermine what is left of renal function. The tuberculous kidney comes into a separate class and will be discussed presently.

One should not be satisfied with merely obtaining symptomatic relief for the patient, but a genuine attempt should be made to sterilise the urine by thorough treatment before term and certainly before the patient starts another pregnancy. In spite of modern treatment, however, the recurrence rate in the same pregnancy is high, and it is

likely to complicate the puerperium in about 10 per cent of cases. In other respects the maternal prognosis is good, although even after apparently adequate chemotherapy the urine is likely to yield a positive culture several months later in a significant number.[31] Patients suffering from cardiac diseases are at greater risk because the acute infection may precipitate cardiac failure, and diabetics very easily get out of control, as with any acute infection, and are liable to go into diabetic coma. The fœtal prognosis is, to some extent, adversely affected by the risk of abortion, premature labour or intra-uterine death as the result of hyperpyrexia.

Puerperal Pyelitis

Urinary stasis in the upper tract is less of a factor after delivery, but the bladder is likely to be insensitive and guilty of retention, so that puerperal cystitis, together with residual urine, encourages an ascending urinary infection. Stagnant urine in the first days of the puerperium is liable to be regurgitated past a temporarily incompetent uretero-vesical meatus. There is therefore great danger in using parasympathomimetic drugs.

Pyelitis in the puerperium is much more common than in pregnancy, and represents one of the chief causes of puerperal pyrexia. There is now a more varied bacteriology, although E. coli is still the chief offender. Characteristically, fever does not appear before the end of the first week unless the urine was already infected at the time of delivery. Localising symptoms are often absent, and although cystitis is present in the majority of cases, the patient complains of no urinary symptoms at all. Loin tenderness or pain are hardly ever to be found in such cases at this time. The treatment follows the same lines as in pregnancy pyelitis, except that there is no need to deal with ureteric blockage by catheterisation of the ureters.

It is not usually too difficult to sterilise the urine, at least temporarily, in cases of acute urinary infection, provided the appropriate antibiotic is given in a course lasting from 5 to 10 days, but the chances of recrudescent infection are very high and there is much truth in the statement "once a urinary infection, always a urinary infection." Apart from the risk of recurrence in pregnancy the reality of a chronic infection may only come to light postnatally. This raises the question of how long chemotherapy should be maintained, as even 6 months low-dose treatment with a suitable antibiotic may fail to produce a permanent effect. In such cases a very full search must be made for some persisting cause, such as vesico-ureteric reflux or structural abnormality of the urinary tract. Even so the best efforts may be rewarded with no more than a 10 per cent permanent cure in the well-established chronic case.

RETENTION

This is occasionally hysterical, but in early pregnancy the commonest cause is incarceration of the retroverted gravid uterus or an impacted pelvic tumour. The subject has been dealt with fully in the chapter on local abnormalities, under "retroversion". Retention may be masked by apparent incontinence which is due to overflow. The characteristic time of onset is about the 13th or 14th week of pregnancy, and the physical signs, as described, should make the diagnosis obvious enough.

Retention does not again complicate the obstetrical picture until labour is well advanced. It can now be very troublesome and interfere with progress and uterine activity, and repeated catheterisation may be necessary. Neglect in labour of the bladder which is incapable of emptying itself, quite apart from the other penalties, is simply asking for cystitis in the puerperium.

After delivery, bladder tone is always diminished, and there is great tolerance of large quantities of retained urine, so that the puerperal patient can hold up to a pint and a half of urine without feeling any urgent desire to micturate. Labial lacerations and perineal sutures reflexly discourage micturition, and bruising and œdema of the bladder neck interfere with it in the first few days. The patient should, therefore, be firmly encouraged to perform, and if she fails to pass her water within the first 20 hours after delivery she should be catheterised. Catheterisation is both safer and more certain than the use of drugs, such as carbachol and doryl, which are often ineffective or may encourage the regurgitation of stagnant urine up the dilated ureters. One of the great arguments in favour of early rising in the puerperium is the more thorough spontaneous emptying of the bladder thereby encouraged.

Finally, the height of the fundus must only be recorded after one is satisfied that the bladder is empty, because a full bladder raises the level of the fundus and consequently gives the impression that involution is not proceeding normally.

HÆMATURIA

The vesical causes of hæmaturia include trauma, especially after difficult delivery or Cæsarean section, hæmorrhagic cystitis, varicosities within the bladder, papilloma and stone. Cystoscopy will clear up doubtful cases.

The source of blood in the urine when it originates in the upper urinary tract is not always so clearly defined. There is a not uncommon type of hæmaturia which results from no recognisable pathology, appears to be peculiar to pregnancy and clears up after

delivery. This condition is sometimes due to the pregnancy engorgement of superficial veins in the region of the renal pyramids. Crabtree suggested that this may be due to œstrogens, and mentioned the case of hæmorrhagic cystitis resulting from massive stilbœstrol dosage.

Renal tuberculosis is one of the most important causes of hæmaturia and should be thought of first (see later). Other causes include renal infarction, papilloma, hydronephrosis, polycystic kidney and calculus. Hæmaturia also occurs in acute and chronic nephritis, and blood cells in the urine are often found in cases of severe hyperemesis and renal cortical necrosis.

TUBERCULOSIS OF THE URINARY TRACT

This is a very serious complication of pregnancy, far more so, in fact, than pulmonary tuberculosis. Childbearing favours a miliary spread of the disease, either in pregnancy or in the puerperium; a chronic infection may become active and a unilateral case may be converted into one that is bilateral. Tuberculous cystitis develops readily, and tuberculous pyonephrosis may occur. Fortunately, it is not a common complication of pregnancy. One is more often confronted with the problem of a patient who has already had one kidney removed because of tuberculosis and who has now become pregnant. Although she may be regarded as apparently cured, it is vital to assess the health of the remaining kidney, and pregnancy is absolutely contra-indicated unless one is reasonably certain that the other kidney is free from the infection (Fig. 2). Even then, the advent of the common or garden type of pyelitis in the remaining kidney affects the outlook sufficiently to warrant considering termination of the pregnancy. Fortunately, the advent of streptomycin and chemotherapy has brightened the outlook. Any woman who has had a kidney removed for tuberculosis should avoid pregnancy for a minimum of three years, in order to enable follow-up examination to be conclusively reassuring. With these provisos, the prognosis of pregnancy following successful nephrectomy would appear to be good.[29]

The symptoms are often indefinite, but hæmaturia or a pyelitis which is resistant to the usual sulphonamide and potassium citrate treatment should raise one's suspicions. Red blood cells are nearly always present on microscopic examination of the urine, and albuminuria may be of greater degree than one normally encounters in E. coli pyelitis. A sterile pyuria is very significant. The presence of the tubercle bacillus is often overshadowed by secondary invasion by other organisms, and guinea-pig inoculation may be necessary to identify it. Cystoscopy will clarify the diagnosis where there are bladder involvement or characteristic signs at the ureteric orifice.

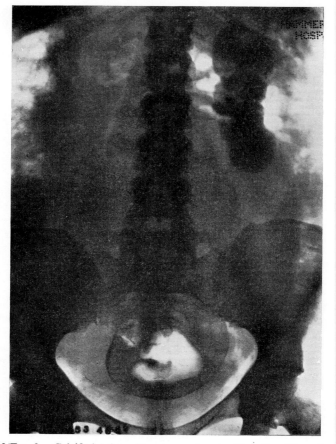

10/Fig. 2.—Calcified tuberculous pyonephrosis. Gestation 37 weeks.
(By courtesy of Prof. R. E. Steiner.)

Intravenous pyelograms, though very necessary, are often difficult to interpret, but provided there is an adequate secretion of dye there may be noted abnormalities of the calyces, ureteric rigidity and less lateral displacement of the ureter than is usual in pregnancy (Figs. 3 and 4).

Once the diagnosis of active renal tuberculosis is made, termination of pregnancy may be considered in order to save the lesion from becoming bilateral. Nephrectomy is then performed later. This is far safer than performing nephrectomy and allowing the pregnancy to continue, because then one cannot adequately prevent the infection from spreading to the other side. Whether pregnancy is terminated

or not, treatment with streptomycin combined with INAH and PAS should be conscientously maintained. Calcium benzamido-salicylate

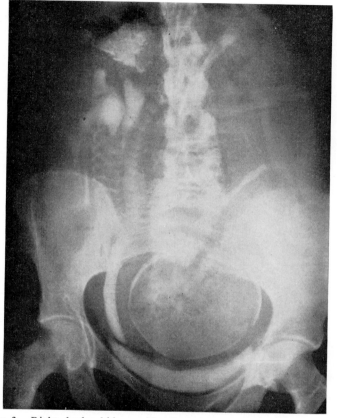

10/Fig. 3.—Right duplex kidney with tuberculous pyonephrosis of the upper component. Both components are still functioning.
(By courtesy of Dr. Ellis Barnett.)

is recommended by Hanley (1957) in place of PAS since it is better tolerated. This drug, after oral administration, is hydrolysed to PAS.

Structural Abnormalities of the Urinary Tract

There may be congenital absence or hypoplasia of one kidney, the kidney may be congenitally cystic, ectopic or horse-shoe. Other abnormalities include cases of double ureter and bifid renal pelvis and aberrant renal vessels. The majority of these cases pass through

pregnancy and delivery without trouble, and many are only diagnosed because of a full urological investigation necessitated by the persistence of an infection. The case of single kidney following nephrectomy has to be considered in the light of the indications for

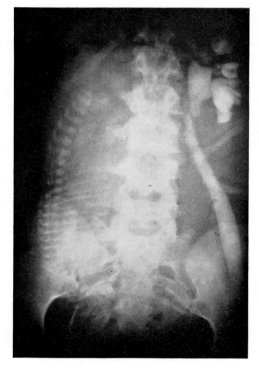

10/FIG. 4 (a).—INTRAVENOUS PYELOGRAM.

Non-functioning right kidney due to chronic infection.

which the original nephrectomy was done, for example, renal tuberculosis.

Hydronephrosis is bound to be aggravated by pregnancy, but one should be chary of diagnosing hydronephrosis for the first time in pregnancy because of the physiological dilatation of the renal pelvis which normally occurs. These remarks, of course, do not apply to gross cases. Whatever the reason for which previous nephrectomy was performed, the functional capacity of the remaining kidney should be carefully assessed, and serious notice should be taken of any complicating pyelitis during pregnancy, however mild.

Polycystic disease of the kidneys is an uncommon complication of pregnancy, partly because such cases are not very fertile, but in recent years we have had two such cases in our unit, one of which is

illustrated in Figs. 5a and 5b. Pregnancy only indirectly worsens what is in any case a bad ultimate prognosis and there is seldom any advantage to be gained by terminating it, since deterioration is inevitably a matter of time. The immediate risks, however, are a super-

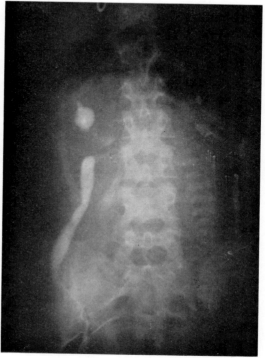

10/Fig. 4 (b).—Retro-grade Pyelogram.

Same case as Fig 4 (a). Ureter is dilated up to the renal pelvis which does not, however, show the usual dilatation of pregnancy. In the kidney there is only a blob of dye representing the dilated calyces. Suggests a chronically infected right kidney shrivelling in size.

(Figs. 4 a and b by courtesy of Mr. W. S. Mack.)

imposed urinary infection to which these patients are liable and which must be watched for and treated early and energetically. Hypertension is also a likely complication and must be taken very seriously. Prolonged periods of hospitalisation during pregnancy are likely to be needed for either or both of these reasons and the chances of a successful pregnancy are largely determined by the degree of renal failure present.

Calculi

These are not common in pregnancy mainly because of age incidence. Stones in the bladder are very rare. In the upper urinary tract calculi not only encourage infection, but may be responsible for its persistence.

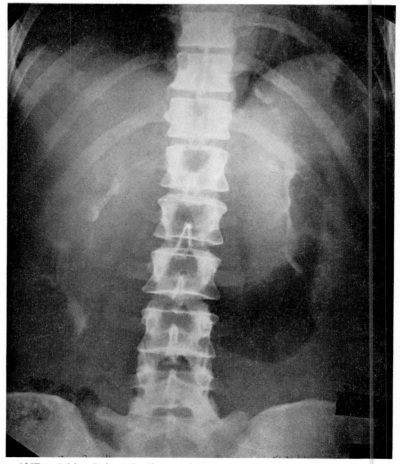

10/Fig. 5 (*a*).—Polycystic disease of kidneys—non-pregnant. I.V.P. at 20′.
(By courtesy of Dr. J. Innes.)

Pain is complained of more frequently during the first half of pregnancy than the latter half, mainly because the physiological dilatation of the upper tract in pregnancy accommodates the stone more comfortably. Hæmaturia is variable and often absent. The diagnosis usually comes to light in the course of full urinary investigation because of persistent infection. The best time to remove a calculus is between pregnancies, especially in the patient who manages to go through her pregnancy without trouble. Nevertheless, there is much to be said for removing at once a calculus which first comes to

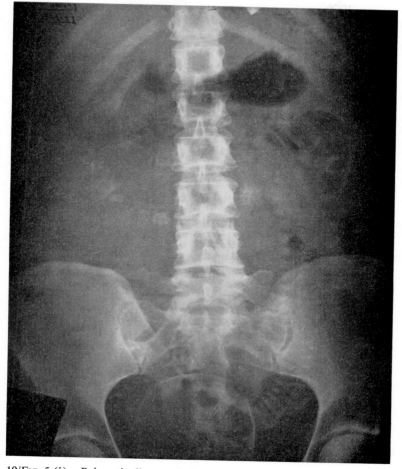

10/Fig. 5 (b).—Polycystic disease of kidneys in pregnancy. I.V.P. at 40'. Same case. Both kidneys markedly enlarged. Calyces spidery and elongated with calcified glands on right. Some calyces show smooth concavities due to cyst distortion.

(By courtesy of Dr. Ellis Barnett.)

notice during the early months, before ureteric dilatation allows it to slip down the ureter, where it is likely to lodge at the level of the pelvic brim and be difficult to reach surgically because of the bulk of the gravid uterus. If the stone is first discovered in the latter half of pregnancy, it is best to temporise if possible and remove it in the postnatal period; but when active steps are called for in late preg-

nancy on account of severity of symptoms, there is much to be said for draining the renal pelvis by nephrostomy until after delivery.

OLIGURIA AND ANURIA

Urinary suppression is an extremely grave sign, and it is necessary, if possible, to deduce into which of the two main pathological classes the case falls. These classes are, on the one hand, cases of acute cortical necrosis and, on the other, those of acute tubular nephrosis. Suffice it to remark here that, clinically, cortical necrosis greatly resembles anuria due to other causes, but there is a world of difference in the prognosis, inasmuch as it is almost invariably fatal.

The great difference between cortical necrosis and acute tubular nephrosis lies in the irreparable damage which occurs in the former, while in the latter recovery will occur in time provided that the patient can be prevented meanwhile from dying of uræmia or from the effects of injudicious treatment. Even in these days when hæmodialysis is almost commonplace the gravity of acute renal failure of obstetric origin should not be underestimated, and the mortality would appear to differ according to whether the renal failure occurs in the first half of pregnancy (mainly due to induced abortion) or those in the last trimester often complicated by pre-eclamptic toxæmia. These findings were brought to light by a study of a series of 70 patients with renal failure, all of whom had required some form of dialysis, and excluding all those that recovered or died without being dialysed.[62] Of the former group, i.e. in early pregnancy, 27 per cent died and 8 out of the 11 deaths were directly attributable to infection which had occurred either after recovery from renal failure or at a time when the fluid and electrolyte disturbances were under control. The infections were mainly clostridial or staphylococcal. What is particularly interesting is that no patient in this abortion group died with evidence of irreversible renal damage. Surgical intervention was eschewed because of the danger of converting a local infection to a general one in conformity with more or less universal practice today, but because of the deadly significance of infection, particularly some gas-forming organisms, a policy of full doses of penicillin and ampicillin together was advocated as soon as swabs had been taken for culture and sensitivity testing. Of the cases of renal failure in late pregnancy the mortality was much worse at 45 per cent and at autopsy more than half were found to have renal cortical necrosis. The main causes were pre-eclamptic toxæmia, eclampsia, abruptio placentæ and postpartum hæmorrhage. Infection in these cases played a very much smaller part and there was also the factor of hepatic necrosis and one disaster from the complications of hæmodialysis. In other words, one is dealing with a different pathology. Of those that were

dialysed, not all by any means received the treatment on an artificial kidney machine, but peritoneal dialysis found increasing favour among the later cases in the group. This method was recommended for daily use and it was claimed that it permitted very efficient removal of excess sodium and water, allowing a smooth control of blood chemistry. It also allowed unrestricted fluid intake and Hammersmith workers have come to regard this as the method of choice, hæmodialysis being reserved only for cases in which technical failure prevents the peritoneal route.

ACUTE CORTICAL NECROSIS

Although this condition has been described in connection with specific fevers and dioxan poisoning, for all practical considerations it will be found that its association with pregnancy is almost invariable, and its relationship with eclampsia, the pre-eclamptic state and retroplacental hæmorrhage is well known.

Pathology

A narrow band of cortex immediately beneath the capsule and portions in the region of the junction of cortex and medulla are the only parts of the cortex to survive, being able to derive their blood supply from sources other than the usual glomerular afferent vessels which undergo hyaline necrosis. These latter are the intralobular arterioles and their branches, and they are to be found widely dilated with small points of rupture and perivascular hæmorrhages (Fig. 6). Small thrombi may occur within the lumina. The necrosis is primarily the result of ischæmia whether it be due, as Trueta (1947) asserted, to a shunt mechanism whereby renal blood flow is diverted from the cortical nephrons to the juxtamedullary nephrons by a reflex spasm of the interlobular arteries supplying the former, followed by their later vasoparalysis and dilatation; or whether, as de Navasquez (1935) stated, vasoparalysis occurs in the first place due to some operative toxin which so retards circulation as to produce necrosis. Young (1942) considered that autolysis in the separated and ischæmic placenta may supply such an agent.

The glomerular afferent vessels are end arteries, and damage is irrevocable, hence the ultimate issue.

ACUTE TUBULAR NEPHROSIS

Bull (1950) pointed out the striking clinical uniformity in this condition despite the wide variety of causes, ranging from shock to acute poisoning, and the pathological picture of acute necrosis is common to all.

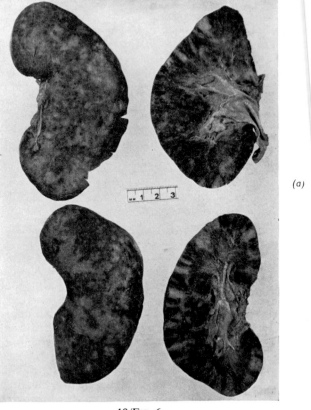

(a)

10/Fig. 6

(*a*) Acute cortical necrosis of kidneys.

(*b*) Bilateral cortical necrosis of kidneys. Infarcted cortex showing an enormously distended thrombosed interlobular artery giving off two afferent glomerular arterioles. (× 40.)

(*c*) Bilateral cortical necrosis of kidneys. Œdematous congested renal capsule separated by a thin hyperæmic zone infiltrated with polymorphs from underlying infarcted cortex. (× 60.)

(By courtesy of Prof. I. Doniach and Dr. H. Walker, and the Editor, *J. Obstet. Gynaec. Brit. Cwlth.*)

The cases can be divided (Dible, 1950) into those with pigment deposition and those without. Instances of the former include mismatched blood transfusion, transfusion of hæmolysed, stale or overheated blood, intravascular hæmolysis from any cause, blackwater fever, circulating myohæmoglobin as in the crush syndrome, cases of hæmolysis resulting from criminal abortion using intra-uterine soap

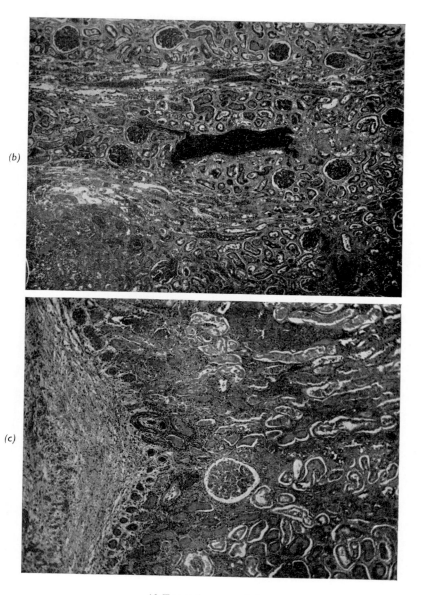

(b)

(c)

10/Fɪɢ. 6 (*see opposite*)

solution injections, which is a common practice today, quinine poisoning and *Cl. welchii* septicæmia, in which the exotoxin is hæmolysing. Those cases without pigment include protracted shock from any cause, producing severe hypotension, as may occur, for example, in induced abortion or very traumatic delivery. Acute septicæmia may also be a cause. In a series of twenty-six obstetrical cases quoted by Chambers (1961), thirteen followed abortion, eight were due to accidental hæmorrhage, three were associated with severe pre-eclampsia or eclampsia and two were transfusion accidents. The average duration of the oliguric phase (to 1 litre of urine) was nine days.

It is to be noted here that a systolic blood pressure which remains for long below 75 mm. of mercury is insufficient to produce secretion of urine in the absence of diuretic substances.

In all the above, recovery is to be sought, and is possible provided the case is correctly understood and treated.

Cases of oliguria resulting from acute nephritis, malignant hypertension and sulphonamide crystal obstruction have different mechanisms and do not belong to this class.

Pathology

In the first 30 hours the kidney is congested and the cortex appears full of blood. The lesion begins in Henle's tubules, especially in the intermediate zone, involving particularly the ascending limb and second convoluted tubule, and is fully developed after 48 hours. It is essentially degenerative in type.

Thereafter pigment, either myohæmoglobin or a hæmolytic blood derivative, appears in the tubular casts, especially in the second convoluted tubule, though the whole nephron is to some extent affected with collections of necrotic cellular debris (Fig. 7).

After five or six days local inflammatory changes supervene, chiefly in the boundary zone, and finally some degree of fibrosis remains.

Pigment deposition is held to be a secondary phenomenon rather than the cause (Dible, 1950) as, in all cases, the tubular casts are not at first pigmented, though the later presence of pigment worsens the outlook because of its own toxic action. According to Darmady (1950) renal failure is not due to tubular blockage with pigment casts, as can be proved by micro-dissection of the nephron.

Death commonly occurs in about a week, but the full pathological picture would probably be seen more often if many candidates for the condition did not first die from additional causes such as sepsis, hæmorrhage, shock and cardiac failure.

Toxic damage or primary ischæmia are the likely initial causes,

and regarding the latter Bull (1950) does not consider, as some do, that the Trueta or Oxford "shunt" mechanism is responsible. His investigations have shown that the renal blood flow, at any rate in the human species, is markedly reduced and the blood removed by catheterisation of the renal vein is very low in oxygen content, thus differing from experimentally produced shunts in animals. Bull, in fact, considers that there occurs a passive fluid diffusion through damaged tubular walls, which leads to increased intrarenal tension, thereby compressing the capillary vessels and retarding circulation still further. This low renal blood flow persists in spite of a normal cardiac outflow which may be restored to the rest of the body, and remains peculiar to the kidneys, and cannot, therefore, be relieved by extrarenal agencies. If the Trueta shunt were still operative, splanchnic block or spinal analgesia would abolish it, but none of Bull's eight cases so treated did in fact respond. This does not disprove the existence of the shunt earlier. The tension within the kidney is "splinted" by the relatively rigid vascular stroma rather than by the renal capsule, and for this reason decapsulation of the kidney is unlikely to be effective.

Any apparently successful results to such treatment (which are, therefore, without rational foundation) must be viewed in the light of possibilities of spontaneous recovery.

Clinical Picture

Bull distinguished four definite phases. Firstly, there is the phase of abrupt onset sometimes preceded by a short-lived diuresis. Secondly, there follows the oliguric or anuric phase which may last from a few hours up to three weeks. Thirdly comes the early diuretic phase in which errors of treatment can ruin what is now a good prognosis. In this phase tubular reabsorptive function is delayed for a period proportional to the duration of the oliguric phase, and an important loss of sodium, potassium and chloride ions is likely to occur if this danger is not met. In the fourth or late diuretic phase tubular function returns and catches up with the already established glomerular activity. It is to be noted that in the second phase both glomerular and tubular function are absent as a result of reduced renal circulation, and the above-mentioned ions tend to accumulate, and in the case of potassium this may be highly dangerous. Treatment has to be modified, therefore, as the different phases of the process are recognised.

Treatment

It goes without saying that any case in whom oliguria does not resolve spontaneously within 48 hours should be transferred to a renal unit; in fact the sooner the better.

It is now believed that there is initially a stage of functional renal failure before organic blockage of the renal tubules becomes established and it is during this very early stage when emergency treatment with mannitol may nip the process in the bud. Mannitol is a polyhydric alcohol, is inert, is rapidly excreted and is relatively nontoxic. Nevertheless if given over a long period it can produce necrosis. Its effect is thought not to be due to osmosis but to lowering of blood viscosity and renal vascular resistance. It is also believed to dilate the afferent arterioles to the glomeruli.

Oliguria after a surgical or obstetrical insult may be due either to

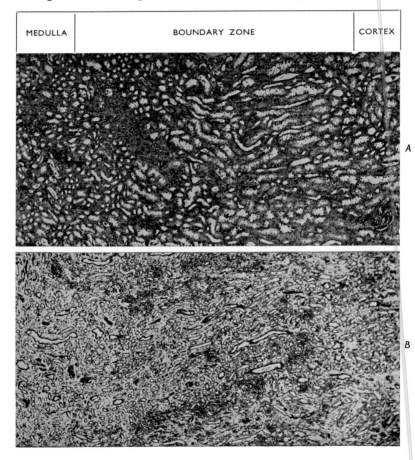

10/FIG. 7 (a).—Boundary zones of (A) normal and (B) anuric kidneys, showing degenerate and atrophic tubules, œdema and fibrosis of the intercellular tissue and widespread cellular infiltration. (× 36.)

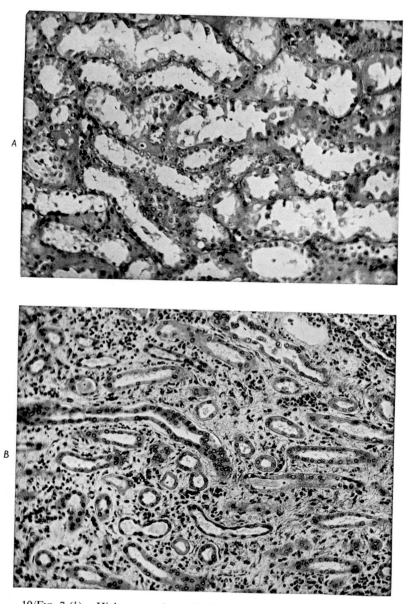

A

B

10/Fig. 7 (b).—High-power view of fields seen in preceding figure. (× 160.)

(Fig. 7 a and b from *Hadfield's Recent Advances in Pathology* by courtesy of Prof. J. H. Dible and J. & A. Churchill.)

post-operative dehydration or to renal shut-down and the stimulation of antidiuretic hormone from the posterior lobe of the pituitary may also play a part. It is important to be able to distinguish the two clinically, as dehydration simply requires intravenous fluid whereas renal shut-down requires the reverse. The distinction is simply made by estimating the ratio of the urinary urea over blood urea. If this is high it suggests occult dehydration but if it is low, i.e. below 14, it suggests renal functional failure for which the treatment is immediate infusion intravenously of 100 ml. of 20 per cent mannitol, i.e. 20 g. This should be given very slowly,[47, 44] taking about 10 minutes over the injection. If the treatment is going to be successful there will be a diuresis within the hour, but if the hourly urine excretion does not increase by at least 50 per cent within two hours, the treatment may be repeated once. Further failure now indicates major organic renal damage. The strength of solution should not exceed 20 per cent because of the danger of crystallisation and repeated or overdosage may precipitate congestive cardiac failure because of the rapid increase in extracellular volume which results.

The main use of mannitol is simply as an emergency prophylaxis, which must be applied within the first 48 hours of oliguria if it is going to be effective. It will achieve nothing once organic pathological changes within the kidneys have set in.

On no account should mannitol be mixed with a blood transfusion drip because it will cause crenation of the red cells which may be irreversible and hence cause agglutination. [55] This is another reason for giving the injection very slowly in case it achieves the same unpleasant effect within the lumen of the vein.

On the biochemical side three facets have to be considered, namely those of water, mineral and nitrogen imbalance, of which the last is the least important, although we still use the term "uræmia" in describing the patient's deterioration.

Many cases are actually killed with water. Lattimer (1945) pointed out that the body was not a tank into which water could be forced until it finally burst out through the kidneys, yet, until recently, over-hydration was common in incorrectly treated patients who were driven into an œdematous condition, with bulging neck veins, cardiac dilatation, gallop rhythm, liver enlargement and crepitations at the lung bases, in fact, a state of cardiac failure. In addition, drowsiness, twitchings and coma can be provoked by water retention. Lattimer found that of his 33 anuric cases none died where the fluid intake was less than 2 litres a day, whereas 75 per cent of those to whom over $3\frac{1}{2}$ litres were given succumbed.

Mineral loss occurs only to a minor extent during the anuric stage and then only through fæces, vomit and sweat; that due to vomiting can be simply replaced. Any diet at this stage should be free, or

nearly so, of electrolytes. The danger of building up a high potassium level is enormously increased by administering such apparently harmless drugs as potassium citrate, while it must be remembered that many bottled fruit drinks and coffee contain enough potassium to jeopardise recovery. When early diuresis starts in the third phase, however, electrolyte loss must be quantitatively replaced.

The level of blood urea naturally rises during oliguria, but urea itself is not toxic, although other end products of protein breakdown may well be, and an accumulation of potassium ions occurs in the body from both exogenous and endogenous protein metabolism. Borst (1948) advised that endogenous protein catabolism can be reduced to a minimum in cases on a non-protein diet by ensuring an adequate number of calories by giving a high carbohydrate diet. However, a limited protein intake can be overdone and in the end will produce the undesirable effects of hypoalbuminæmic œdema, anæmia and asthenia; but these late effects are confined to chronic cases of uræmia rather than the condition under discussion.

Infection has a disastrous effect in stimulating protein catabolism, and must be controlled by antibiotics, bearing in mind that those that are excreted in the urine may accumulate excessively during anuria and after the first few days the dose should be drastically cut.

The scheme of treatment originally advocated by Bull and his colleagues was firstly, during the anuric phase, to limit water intake to 1,000 ml. in 24 hours, which approximately replaces the daily loss through the lungs, skin and fæces. All vomited material was collected, filtered and returned through a nasal stomach tube. This replaced lost electrolytes. More recently a daily water intake of 1,000 ml. plus the previous day's measure of urinary output has come to be regarded as excessive, and the basic figure has been reduced from a litre to 500 ml. Barr and Chambers (1958), in a very full and detailed scheme of treatment, recommend the immediate stopping of all oral feeding and fluids and the administration by intragastric tube of 500–700 ml. of 50 per cent glucose per 24 hours, plus 500 mg. ascorbic acid and vitamin B complex preparation. Alternatively lactose 150 g. per day is better tolerated orally (Chambers, 1961). Vomiting can be reduced by the anti-emetic cyclizine hydrochloride 50 mg. by mouth. The original peanut oil mixture devised by Bull has now been superseded by carbohydrate feeding only. When vomiting is present, as is often the case, it is better to proceed forthwith to intravenous or intracaval therapy.

To meet the double difficulty of restricting the fluid intake and yet maintaining the high carbohydrate provision without producing thrombosis in a vein, Evans et al. (1953) recommended a drip of 1 litre a day of 40 per cent glucose directly into the superior vena cava using a cardiac catheter, a method based on that of de Kayser

in Holland. This provided a daily intake of 1,600 calories. Additional water could be given by mouth or in the drip in amounts equal to the previous day's urinary output, if any. The fact of placing the end of the catheter within a very large blood channel like the vena cava enables the irritant effect of the concentrated glucose solution to be sufficiently diluted by the large volume of blood flowing past. Heparin (10,000 units per 500 ml.) had to be added, even so, to the caval drip. We then came to use more commonly the inferior vena cava for this type of administration as recommended by Scott Russell *et al.* (1954), the cannula being introduced through the upper end of the internal saphenous vein under rigid aseptic conditions. The drip had never to be allowed to stop, even momentarily, for fear of clotting and a reserve supply had to be available through a Y-piece connection to maintain the flow, however slowly, while the bottles were being changed. One such polythene catheter usually managed to serve for about a week or more. The treatment certainly had the advantage of leaving one in no doubt about what was going into the patient, whereas absorption through an intragastric drip was more problematical.

Today the method of controlling calorie and fluid intake has been simplified even further by replacing glucose with 20 per cent fructose, of which 600 millilitres are now given intravenously daily without the need for catheterising the inferior vena cava. The fluid volume is increased by the amount of urine passed or fluid vomited in the course of the previous day. When all danger of vomiting, however, has ceased the patient may take concentrated solutions of sugar in control quantities and in palatable form such as Glucozade.

Parsons and McCracken (1959) recommend the synthetic anabolic steroid norethandrolone (Nilevar) in dosage of 30 mg. a day because of its ability to reduce protein catabolism and thereby to reduce or postpone the need for artificial kidney dialysis.

Under this scheme the blood urea will only rise about 17 mg. per cent a day in the first week and 10 mg. per cent in the second and thereafter, whereas in patients treated otherwise the daily rise in blood urea may exceed 50 mg. per cent. In other words this treatment is one of playing for time—time for kidney function to recover before uræmia carries off the patient.

When diuresis starts, in addition to replacing electrolytes quantitatively the procedure is to add water to the basic ration in the same quantity as the previous day's urinary output, and when the diuresis exceeds 1 litre per diem, the drip feed may be discontinued and a low protein diet commenced. The blood urea does not start to fall until a diuresis of at least 1 litre is achieved, as the urine filtrate during the third phase is, as yet, too dilute to rid the body of sufficient quantities.

If the hæmoglobin level is at any time below 70 per cent, transfusion of packed red cells is given, as anæmia of itself reduces renal function.

In severe cases it may be anything up to four weeks before the kidneys begin to excrete urine, which shows what this treatment can achieve. Bull frequently found himself initially handicapped by receiving cases that had been ill-advisedly waterlogged with glucose-saline intravenous therapy (personal communication).

As a rule the rise in serum potassium is not marked under the above regime and, if present, can to some extent be offset by giving 50 units insulin. This encourages the transfer of potassium, together with the glycogen thus formed, within the cell, where it is harmless. Nevertheless, cardiac arrest due to hyperkalæmia is still a potent cause of death and, where the potassium levels cannot adequately be controlled as above, an ion exchange resin such as Resonium-A may be used as a temporary expedient pending artificial kidney dialysis.

Resonium-A is a polystyrene sulphonate cation-exchange resin in sodium form[5] and liberates 3·0 mEq. of sodium per gram of resin. It is not without its dangers in renal failure because it acts as a powerful sodium donor and may precipitate heart failure, œdema and severe hypertension. For this reason the use of a calcium form of cation-exchange resin is recommended (calcium-zeokarb 225) in a daily dose of 60 g. which is superior in renal failure to the sodium resin. It can be made more palatable if finely powdered and suspended in honey. Instead of replacing the potassium of hyperkalæmia with sodium, the ion exchanged is calcium, which, in any case, is less readily absorbed, and hypercalcæmia has not been encountered.[6] These resins do not affect the rise in blood urea but help to control the serum potassium levels. They act within the lumen of the intestine and are by no means rapid. Unfortunately in obstetrical anuria, hyperkalæmia may quickly assume emergency proportions requiring even more urgent treatment short of dialysis. In fact in the seriously ill case one may have little enough time even to wait for electrolyte balance studies. The quickest method of deciding treatment is to undertake electrocardiography, because the signs are if anything more important than high biochemical levels, to which the degree of cardiac danger is not directly related.

The signs of dangerous hyperkalæmia are as follows:

Gross peaking of the T-waves.
Absent P-waves.
Widening of QRS complex to 0·2 seconds.

Under these circumstances treatment is urgent with either 10 per cent calcium chloride intravenously, up to 60 ml. given slowly over 5 minutes, or 10 per cent calcium gluconate (60 ml.). The effect on the

E.C.G. is almost immediate. Calcium chloride is possibly more potent than calcium gluconate because the calcium is completely ionised, but the gluconate solution which is also adequate is less dangerous from the point of view of tissue necrosis due to perivenous extravasation. In either case the intravenous injection should be given very slowly with continuous electro-cardiographic monitoring and should be stopped as soon as the E.C.G. appearances indicate improvement.[14]

During the diuretic phase the rapid loss of potassium may be serious. To some extent this can be made good by giving fruit juices, but if the loss is urgent potassium chloride 5 g. in a day can be given by mouth.

Electrolyte levels must be estimated twice daily and corrected quantitatively where possible. Barr and Chambers give warning of the additional danger of calcium depletion in prolonged treatment and recommend calcium gluconate if the serum calcium falls seriously.

It goes without saying that all cases of anuria should be transferred, as soon as possible, to centres where the necessary biochemical investigations can be undertaken daily and where facilities for dialysis exist. Dialysis is no longer the dangerous and formidable procedure of only a few years ago. In fact, it is no longer a last and desperate resort but the treatment of choice in cases of anuria lasting more than a week.

The following are nowadays accepted as the indications for artificial kidney dialysis:

1. Serum potassium higher than 6·5 mEq/l.
2. Electrocardiogram showing widening of the Q.R.S. complex.
3. Acidosis with bicarbonate reserve below 15 mEq/l.
4. Blood urea more than 350 mg. per cent.
5. Mental changes and confusion.
6. Vomiting in spite of drip treatment (see above).

By the time twitching, fits and a falling blood pressure are observed it can be said that dialysis has been too long delayed. About six hours' treatment with the artificial kidney will restore an almost normal blood urea and electrolyte state which will tide the patient over for many more days and thus allow more time for the recovery of renal function.

REFERENCES

1. ASSCHER, A. W., SUSSMAN, M., WATERS, W. E., DENIS, R. H., and CHICK, SUSAN (1966). *Lancet*, **2**, 1037.
2. BAIRD, D. (1935). *J. Obstet. Gynaec. Brit. Emp.*, **42**, 577, 774.
3. BAIRD, D. (1936). *J. Obstet. Gynaec. Brit. Emp.*, **43**, 1, 435.
4. BARR, J. S., and CHAMBERS, J. W. (1958). *Scot. med. J.*, **3**, 123.

5. BERLYNE, G. M., JANABI, K., and SHAW, A. B. (1966). *Lancet*, **1**, 167.
6. BERLYNE, G. M., JANABI, K., SHAW, A. B., and HOCKIN, A. G. (1966). *Lancet*, **1**, 169.
7. BORST, J. G. C. (1948). *Lancet*, **1**, 824.
8. BRADLEY, J. M., CROWLEY, N., and DARRELL, J. H. (1967). *Brit. med. J.*, **2**, 649.
9. BRUMFITT, W., PERCIVAL, A., and CARTER, M. J. (1962). *Lancet*, **1**, 130
10. BULL, G. M. (1950). *Brit. med. J.*, **1**, 1263.
11. BULL, G. M. (1954). *Proc. roy. Soc. Med.*, **45**, 848.
12. BULL, G. M., BYWATERS, E. G. L., and JOEKES, A. M. (1950). *In Modern Trends in Obstetrics and Gynaecology*. London: Butterworth & Co.
13. BULL, G. M., JOEKES, A. M., and LOWE, K. G. (1949). *Lancet*, **2**, 229.
14. CHAMBERLAIN, M. J. (1964). *Lancet*, **1**, 464.
15. CHAMBERS, J. W. (1961). *J. Obstet. Gynaec. Brit. Cwlth.*, **68**, 1059.
16. CRABTREE, E. G. (1942). *Urological Diseases of Pregnancy*. Boston: Little, Brown & Co.
17. CRABTREE, E. G. (1944). *J. Amer. med. Ass.*, **126**, 810.
18. DARMADY, E. M. (1950). *Brit. med. J.*, **1**, 1263.
19. DE NAVASQUEZ, S. (1935). *J. Path. Bact.*, **41**, 385.
20. DE WARDENER, H. E. (1960). In *Recent Advances in Renal Disease*, p. 157, edit. by M. D. Milne. London: Pitman Med. Pub. Co.
21. DIBLE, J. (1950). *Brit. med. J.*, **1**, 1262.
22. DODDS, GLADYS (1931). *J. Obstet. Gynaec. Brit. Emp.*, **38**, 773.
23. DODDS, GLADYS (1932). *J. Obstet. Gynaec. Brit. Emp.*, **39**, 46.
24. DODDS, GLADYS (1945). *Proc. roy. Soc. Med.*, **38**, 655.
25. DONALD, I., BARR, W., and McGARRY, J. A. (1962). *J. Obstet. Gynaec. Brit. Cwlth.*, **69**, 837.
26. EDGAR, W. M., and DICKINSON, K. M. (1962). *Lancet*, **2**, 739.
27. EVANS, B. M., HUGHES JONES, N. C., MILNE, M. D., and YELLOWLEES, H. (1953). *Lancet*, **2**, 791.
28. FAIRLEY, K. F., BOND, A. G., and ADEY, F. D. (1966). *Lancet*, **1**, 939.
29. FELDING, C. (1964). *Acta Obstet. gynec. scand.*, **43**, 152.
30. GABE, J. (1945). *Proc. roy. Soc. Med.*, **38**, 653.
31. GARROD, L. P., SHOOTER, R. A., and CURWEN, M. P. (1954). *Brit. med. J.*, **2**, 1003.
32. GILLESPIE, W. A. (1956). *Proc. roy. Soc. Med.*, **49**, 1045.
33. GILLESPIE, W. A., LENNON, G. G., LINTON, K. B., and SLADE, N. (1962). *Brit. med. J.*, **2**, 13.
34. GILLESPIE, W. A., LINTON, K. B., MILLER, A., and SLADE, N. (1961). *J. clin. Path.*, **13**, 187.
35. HANLEY, H. G. (1945). *Proc. roy. Soc. Med.*, **38**, 660.
36. HANLEY, H. G. (1957). *Recent Advances in Urology*, pp. 39–48. London: J. & A. Churchill.
37. KASS, E. H. (1957). *Arch. intern. Med.*, **100**, 709.
38. KATZ, J. J., VELASQUEZ, A., and BOURDO, S. R. (1962). *Lancet*, **1**, 1144.
39. KENNY, MEAVE, JOHNSTON, F. D., HAEBLER, T. VAN, and MILES, A. A. (1937). *Lancet*, **2**, 119.
40. KINCAID-SMITH, PRISCILLA, and BULLEN, MARGARET (1956). *Lancet*, **1**, 1144.

41. LATTIMER, J. K. (1945). *J. Urol.* (*Baltimore*), **54**, 312.
42. LAWSON, D. H. (1967). Personal communication.
43. LEATHER, H. M., WILLS, M. R., and GAULT, H. M. (1963). *Brit. med. J.*, **1**, 92.
44. LINDSAY, R. M., LINTON, A. L., and LONGLAND, C. J. (1965). *Lancet*, **1**, 978.
45. LINTON, K. B., and GILLESPIE, W. A. (1962). *J. Obstet. Gynaec. Brit. Cwlth.*, **69**, 845.
46. LITTLE, P. J., and DE WARDENER, H. E. (1962). *Lancet*, **1**, 1145.
47. LUKE, R. G., LINTON, A. L., BRIGGS, J. D., and KENNEDY, A. C. (1963). *Lancet*, **1**, 980.
48. MALPAS, P., JEFFCOATE, T. N. A., and LISTER, URSULA M. (1949). *J. Obstet. Gynaec. Brit. Emp.*, **56**, 949.
49. PARSONS, F. M., and MCCRACKEN, B. H. (1959). *Brit. med. J.*, **1**, 740.
50. PATERSON, M. L., BARR, W., and MACDONALD, S. (1960). *J. Obstet. Gynaec. Brit. Emp.*, **67**, 394.
51. PEARS, R. A., and HOUGHTON, B. J. (1958). *Lancet*, **2**, 128.
52. PEARS, R. A., and HOUGHTON, B. J. (1959). *Lancet*, **2**, 1167.
53. PINKERTON, J. H. M., HOUSTON, J. K., and GIBSON, G. L. (1965). *Proc. roy. Soc. Med.*, **58**, 1041.
54. PINKERTON, J. H. M., WOOD, C., WILLIAMS, E. T., and CALMAN, R. M. (1961). *Brit. med. J.*, **2**, 539.
55. ROBERTS, B. E., and SMITH, P. H. (1966). *Lancet*, **2**, 421.
56. ROSENHEIM, M. L. (1960). In *Recent Advances in Renal Disease*, p. 137, edit. by M. D. Milne. London: Pitman Med. Pub. Co.
57. RUSSELL, C. S., DEWHURST, C. J., and BRACE, J. C. (1954). *Lancet*, **1**, 902.
58. SIMMONS, N. A., and WILLIAMS, J. D. (1962). *Lancet*, **1**, 1377.
59. SLADE, N., and LINTON, K. B. (1960). *Brit. J. Urol.*, **32**, 416.
60. SLEIGH, J. D. (1965). *Brit. med. J.*, **1**, 765.
61. SLOWINSKI, E. J., and SMITH, L. G. (1966). *Amer. J. Obstet. Gynec.*, **94**, 906.
62. SMITH, K., BROWNE, J. C. M., SHACKMAN, R., and WRONG, O. M. (1965). *Lancet*, **2**, 351.
63. STILL, B. M. (1966). *Proc. roy. Soc. Med.*, **59**, 157.
64. SVEC, F. A. RHOADS, P. S., and ROHR, J. H. (1954). *Arch. intern. Med.*, **85**, 83.
65. TRUETA, J., BARCLAY, A. E., DANIEL, P. M., FRANKLIN, K. J., and PRICHARD, M. M. L. (1947). *Studies of the Renal Circulation*. Oxford: Blackwell Scientific Publications.
66. TURNER, G. C. (1961). *Lancet*, **2**, 1062.
67. YOUNG, J. (1942). *Brit. med. J.*, **2**, 715.

CHAPTER XI

TWINS AND HYDRAMNIOS

TWINS

TWIN pregnancy is due either to the fertilisation of two separate ova, in which case the twins are called binovular, or from the division of one fertilised ovum into two separate embryos, which are thus uniovular. The former are five or six times as common as the latter. As might be expected, uniovular twins are like two beans out of the same pod and are always of the same sex, whereas binovular twins bear only fraternal resemblance to each other.

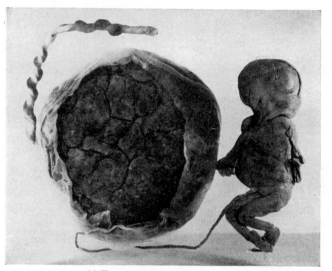

11/FIG. 1.—Fœtus papyraceus.
(By courtesy of Dr. E. W. L. Thompson and R.C.O.G. Museum.)

Where two ova are thus fertilised it is usual for them to be produced simultaneously from one Graafian follicle, so that only one corpus luteum is present. Such twins have completely distinct sets of membranes of their own, so that the membranous septum between the two amniotic sacs consists of the amnion and chorion of one fœtus, then the chorion and amnion of the other, and the two placentæ, although contiguous in 9 out of 10 cases, are nevertheless structurally separate and their circulations are practically always

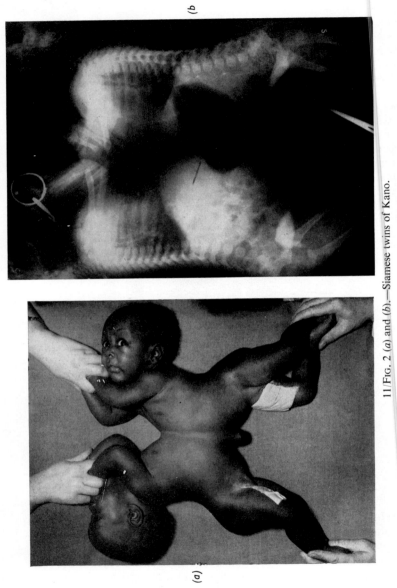

11/FIG. 2 (a) and (b).—Siamese twins of Kano.

(By courtesy of the late Prof. Ian Aird and the Editor, *Brit. med. J.*)

distinct from each other. In uniovular twins the double placenta, though not entirely common to both, has a varying degree of anastomotic circulation, and the membranous septum between the two fœtal sacs, provided it has not been broken down, consists only of the two layers of amnion, one from each fœtus.

Instead of the terms uniovular and binovular, therefore, it is also common to use the terms monochorionic and dichorionic. Careful

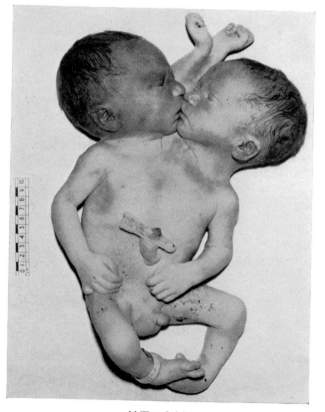

11/Fig. 3 (a)

inspection of the septum between two amniotic sacs often leads to mistakes however, which histological section would place beyond all doubt, because the chorion shows up well. This sort of information may be valuable one day as uniovular twins can in later life share a certain amount of transplantation surgery between them without fear of rejection.

P.O.P.—11*

All the above would be of little more than academic interest were it not for the fact that certain well-known disadvantages operate in the case of uniovular twins. For instance, intra-uterine death of one fœtus is not uncommon, and if it takes place relatively early in

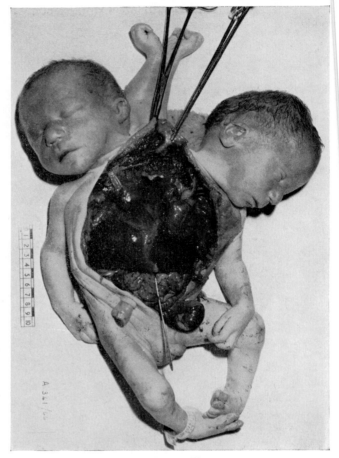

11/Fig. 3 (b)

pregnancy, the dead fœtus is usually retained *in utero* as a shrivelled and compressed object; hence its name, fœtus papyraceus or compressus (Fig. 1). It is finally expelled with its surviving brother at delivery. It is thought that this phenomenon may be due to the overpowering of the circulation of the unsuccessful fœtus by the more powerful cardiac output of the survivor through the placental ana-

stomosis. On a lesser scale it is possible for one uniovular twin to exsanguinate itself into the circulation of the other, producing polycythæmia. Kerr (1959) reported four such cases occurring

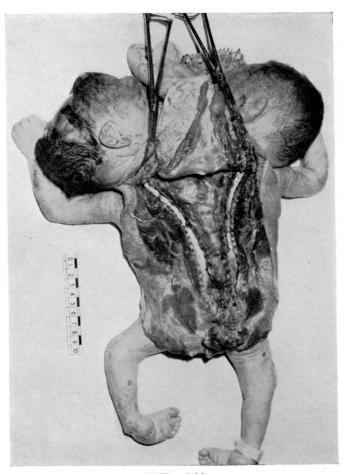

11/Fig. 3 (c)

within three years at the Glasgow Royal Maternity Hospital. In two of them transfusion was required for the anæmic twin.

One can only speculate about the origin of uniovular twins, but this phenomenon may be due to some minor arrest in the very early development of the fertilised ovum, so that the embryonic streak divides by a sort of binary fission. In rare instances this division may

not be complete, and all manner of double monsters, for example thoracopagus and Siamese twins, may result (Figs 2 and 3). The incidence of fœtal abnormality is higher in uniovular twins, and may be due to something in the nature of this mechanism or to a blood circulation overpowered by the stronger fœtus.

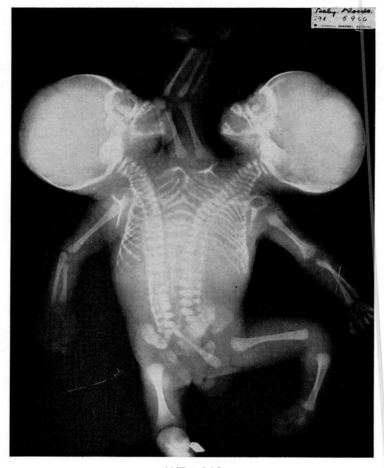

11/Fɪɢ. 3 (d)

11/Fɪɢs. 3 (a), (b), (c) and (d).—Siamese twins delivered at 36½ weeks gestation. Their existence was unsuspected until after the spontaneous delivery of the first head when difficulty with delivery of the shoulders was encountered. At this point the second head was found on examination. Delivery was completed with an intact perineum! The monster survived only a few minutes.

(By courtesy of Dr. R. M. Still and Mr. Waldie, Stobhill Hospital, Glasgow.)

Hydramnios, although associated with twins of both varieties, is relatively more often found in the uniovular variety, and tends to occur with the larger twin, whose greater cardiac output results in increased renal excretory activity.

Superfecundation and superfœtation are freak occurrences, more often than not of doubtful authenticity. In the first, fertilisation of

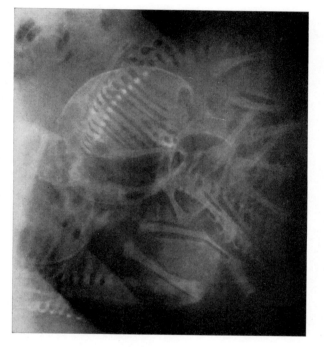

11/Fig. 4.—Triplets.
(By courtesy of Dr. J. W. McLaren.)

two separate ova occurs during the same intermenstrual period by separate acts of coitus. In superfœtation credulity is stretched a great deal farther, because the twins are derived from separate ovulations as well as separate acts of coitus during different intermenstrual periods, as a result of which a woman may simultaneously carry two fœtuses of markedly different gestational ages. In theory such a phenomenon is mechanically feasible up to about the 12th week, after which the fusion of the decidua vera and decidua reflexa should make it impossible, except in the case of a double uterus.

Twins tend to run in families, and heredity plays a very important

part. Oddly enough, paternal as well as maternal influences may be responsible.

The incidence of twinning varies with race, with population fertility and with age, and is more often encountered in fertile negro populations than among the white races. Moreover, as women get older they become less likely to have twins, in spite of the fact that multiple pregnancy is commoner in multiparæ. The average incidence

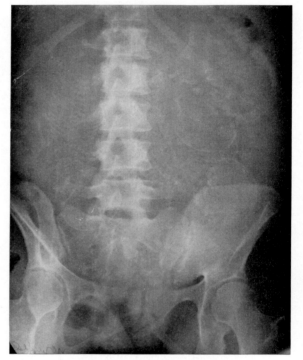

11/Fig. 5.—Quadruplets.
(By courtesy of Dr. Ellis Barnett.)

of twins, therefore, works out at about 1 in 80 pregnancies. The variations in different parts of the world are mainly composed of differences in the binovular incidence.

Triplets occur no more than about once in every 8,000 pregnancies, and quadruplets about once in every three-quarters of a million (Figs. 4 and 5). Quintuplets are a very extreme rarity, of which the Dionne sisters were by no means the only cases, although they were remarkable for their survival. The highest score yet recorded for human litter is six!

The remaining possible combinations are too uncommon to be worth listing, the least common of all being the double transverse position.

LABOUR

An anæsthetist should always be present throughout the second and third stages of all viable twin deliveries, prepared to induce an anæsthetic at a minute's notice.

Labour is usually normal, but it is as well to be on the look-out for trouble. Because of the overdistension of the uterus there is some tendency towards uterine inertia, but this is to a certain extent offset by the smallness of the babies as a result of prematurity. Post-maturity with twins, incidentally, is very uncommon. If it appears that overdistension is handicapping uterine function, especially in association with hydramnios, it is sometimes worth relieving it by puncture of the forewaters, provided the lie of the first child is longitudinal. Hindwater rupture is inadvisable because the second sac may be thereby drained instead of the first. This may not only interfere with longitudinal alignment of the second twin in the second stage of labour but may also precipitate fœtal distress in it as well. The membranes tend to rupture early, and it is a good rule to perform vaginal examination as soon as this occurs to ensure that the cord has not been washed down, and to satisfy oneself as to the identity and engagement of the presenting part; provided this is either breech or vertex, no further action is required for the time being, but otherwise treatment appropriate to the particular malpresentation will be necessary. If the first child presents by anything other than the vertex, it is as well to conduct the first stage in bed and to withhold an enema in order to preserve the membranes as long as possible.

When labour is premature an episiotomy should be performed in good time during the second stage in order to save the head from damage, particularly if the first child presents by the breech. In this last instance the aftercoming head cannot be assisted in delivery by suprapubic pressure because the second twin, of course, is in the way, and the forceps should be ready for immediate use if necessary. The complication of locked twins preventing delivery of the first child captures the imagination of every student but is exceedingly rare. Here, the aftercoming head of the first child is prevented from entering the pelvis by the presentation of the head of the second child. Anæsthesia must be immediately induced and the treatment has to be both very prompt and lucky if the first child is to be saved, and consists in pushing the second head out of the way so that the first head can enter the brim, by no means an easy manœuvre if the babies are of any reasonable size. More often the attempt fails or can only be made too late, and the first child dies of asphyxia, in

which case the treatment is to decapitate the first child, deliver the body and retrieve the head after delivery of the second twin. Rather more common, but still rare, is collision of heads at the brim, in which neither head will make way for the other. For this the treatment is simply to push one of the heads up and out of the way.

After the first child has been born the cord is divided between two ligatures. Every textbook makes much of this because of the risk of a second uniovular twin bleeding to death through the placental anastomotic circulation and cord of the first, but the practice of dividing the cord between clamps or ligatures is so universal in every delivery that it hardly needs stressing.

The Second Twin

After the delivery of the first child the first step is to palpate the abdomen and to ensure that the lie of the second child is longitudinal, if necessary performing external version. It is important that, on the return of contractions, the second bag of membranes should not rupture with the child in an uncorrected transverse position, for in that case the cord or an arm, or both, might prolapse.

There now follows a brief period of waiting for the contractions to return. Provided there is no maternal hæmorrhage meanwhile, all that has to be done is to observe the fœtal heart of the second twin in order to detect signs of fœtal distress, which, of course, demands immediate intervention.

The placentæ nearly always come together after the delivery of the second twin. Occasionally, however, the first placenta is extruded, often to the accompaniment of bleeding, with the second twin still unborn. Under these circumstances the second bag of waters should be ruptured and the remaining child delivered in order to empty the uterus and arrest hæmorrhage by uterine retraction.

All of us have long recognised that the second twin is at far greater risk than the first; in fact a review of the literature shows that the increase to the hazard is of the order of about 50 per cent.[1] Failure to correct malpresentation by external cephalic version is one cause, but prolonged hypoxia jeopardises the second baby's chances the longer the interval between delivery of the first and second. Any general anæsthesia given for the delivery of the first twin has longer in which to affect the second, and wherever possible anæsthesia should be restricted to regional methods for the first and instantly available by a general technique for the second.

The use of epidural anæsthesia in twin deliveries has its own peculiar hazards. Firstly, it is commonly held that the uterus may clamp down too tightly on the second twin and endanger it, but more important is the sharp reduction in blood pressure which may be

associated with epidural and spinal anæsthesia. Tipping the patient's head downwards may be all very well to maintain maternal cerebral circulation, but does not help placental circulation which normally carries a double requirement load. Epidural and spinal anæsthesia therefore require a very close watch upon maternal blood pressure, bearing in mind the needs of two fœtuses rather than one.

The second twin, for as long as it remains *in utero* after the first has been expelled, continues at risk due to reduction in utero-placental circulation, and fœtal distress must be watched for vigilantly and anticipated by early delivery rather than late.

A waiting period of half an hour used to be recommended, provided there was no bleeding and no fœtal distress unless contractions returned earlier. Most of us are now agreed that this delay is not only unwise but excessive. After all, the cervix is fully dilated, and if one were conducting a normal single delivery one would rupture the membranes forthwith. The same argument applies to the second twin and it is now our practice to push the presenting part of the second twin into the pelvis about five minutes after the separation of the first and to rupture the membranes there and then. If delivery does not occur within a further ten minutes we proceed to operative delivery forthwith while the undelivered child is still well. Macdonald (1962) in a review of 500 consecutive cases in Glasgow showed that this practice not only lowers the complication rate but does not even encounter uterine inertia, as was once thought. If the presenting part is not well in the pelvis, or in any case if there is hydramnios, the cord may easily prolapse with membrane rupture and a look-out for this should be kept. Should this happen the child should be extracted forthwith, otherwise natural delivery is allowed to proceed.

If a general anæsthetic has been necessary in the course of delivery of the first child, one has a choice of action. The older teaching was to discontinue it while awaiting the arrival of the second. The modern practice, however, is to rupture the second amniotic sac at once, to insert the hand and perform internal podalic version and breech extraction.

This type of version is both safe and easy because of the newly-found room available. The latter type of treatment is also to be preferred to rupturing the second sac and failing to push the head well into the pelvis, usually because of a deflexion attitude of the fœtus. The temptation to press on with the delivery by high forceps extraction must be resisted. Having manœuvred oneself into this ugly dilemma with the second head high and the membranes newly ruptured, it is still better to perform internal version before it is too late, rather than awaiting spontaneous descent of the presenting part or embarking upon what may prove to be a hazardous and difficult high forceps delivery, in spite of the small size of the baby. The

Ventouse, or vacuum extractor, has, however, proved a useful alternative in our unit and is infinitely to be preferred to high forceps application, especially if the cervix is attempting to shut down. Its use leads to an easy and gentle delivery without general anæsthesia and with full co-operation from the patient and her stimulated uterus.

In such cases the traditional method of internal version and breech extraction may prove hazardous if the cervix is not fully dilated or if the second twin is unexpectedly larger than the first.[11]

The *third stage* of labour is undoubtedly the most dangerous in twin delivery. For several reasons the risks of postpartum hæmorrhage are enhanced, firstly, because the very size of the double placenta may delay its spontaneous expulsion; secondly, the placental site is larger in area and therefore capable of more profuse bleeding; thirdly, the placental site may partially occupy the lower uterine segment where retraction is inefficient; and fourthly, the uterus may demonstrate a marked degree of inertia following its recent over-distension. A syringe already loaded with ergometrine should therefore be at hand, and the intravenous injection of 0·25 mg. after the birth of the second twin is increasingly used as a prophylactic measure against postpartum hæmorrhage.

It occasionally happens that ergometrine is given at the end of the second stage to a woman in whom the presence of twins has been hitherto unsuspected, and this risk constitutes one of the few serious objections to this excellent routine practice in normal labour. If such a mistake is made, the risks to the undiagnosed twin are very great as a result of uterine spasm, and the child should be extracted at once.

The treatment of any postpartum hæmorrhage should be prompt and energetic, and whether or not ergometrine is used before the delivery of the placenta, half a milligramme of ergometrine should certainly be injected intramuscularly at the completion of the third stage in all cases of twins in order to maintain uterine retraction. The uterus is very liable to soften after a twin delivery and to fill with blood, and it is not really safe to relax vigilance for 4 hours after delivery. The patient should certainly not be left without first expressing any clots of blood which may have accumulated within the uterine cavity.

Triplets

The problems are similar to those of twins but considerably magnified, particularly the risks of premature labour. Admission from the 28th week of pregnancy is therefore desirable if reasonable maturity is to be achieved.

It is particularly inadvisable to waste much time between the

births of each child and as soon as breech or vertex of the next appears in the pelvis the membranes should be ruptured artificially. If neither pole presents, then internal version and breech extraction should be carried out forthwith.

The use of a slow running oxytocin drip is an admirable precaution throughout the second and third stages of such cases in order to discourage any inertia or undue hold-ups. I watched the Glasgow quadruplets being delivered in splendid succession, placentæ and all, in 28 minutes with a well-regulated drip, and postpartum bleeding was minimal.

Prognosis and Aftercare

The maternal prognosis is somewhat adversely influenced by the complications of pregnancy already enumerated, for example pre-eclamptic toxæmia and antepartum hæmorrhage, but even more so by the dangers of postpartum hæmorrhage and collapse. As a result, puerperal morbidity is to some extent increased.

The fœtal prognosis is worse than in single delivery mainly because of prematurity. To a lesser extent the influence of malpresentation and the treatment thereof is also a factor to which cord prolapse, too, may contribute adversely. Intra-uterine death, especially in the case of one of uniovular twins, also occurs from time to time. Fœtal distress in the second child during the second stage of labour often results in the aspiration of liquor and meconium because of asphyxia due to retraction at the placental site, and possible placental separation, so that the second child is frequently more in need of clearance of the upper air passages than the first.

Lastly, twins may be more difficult to rear than single infants, because the maternal milk supply is often inadequate for both, and rickets and anæmia are commoner, because during pregnancy the increased demands for iron and calcium may not have been fully met.

HYDRAMNIOS

The official name for this condition is "polyhydramnios" but the word hydramnios is universally used.

The degree to which an excessive amount of liquor should be regarded as pathological is not mathematically fixed, and in normal cases the amount varies, increasing a little in the third trimester as compared with the second.[3] The usual range is from 300 to 800 ml. and is determined by a dilution technique, injecting sodium amino-hippurate at amniocentesis and analysing liquor samples by spectro-photometry.[4] Liquor volumes exceeding 1500 ml. are abnormal.

Sonar examination provides a characteristic picture with large "blob" echo patterns within copious clear areas representing liquor

(Fig. 11c). In the second and third trimesters of pregnancy the head can always be found by sonar examination; in fact so confident are we, that in a case of hydramnios in which the head cannot be found by this technique we are prepared to diagnose anencephaly.

To most of us there is little doubt that congenital malformations of the central nervous system, including anencephaly and spina bifida, are more likely to appear again in subsequent pregnancy than in the normal case. I have had one patient with three anencephalic fœtuses and no living children. A second patient, by a variety of male partners, produced three babies with spina bifida, all of whom had ultimately died, and another surviving baby with ectopia vesicæ and incontinence of urine, and who, at the age of 42, became pregnant by yet another man to whom she was not married. The substantial risk that this further pregnancy would end in an abnormal fœtus drove me reluctantly to terminate the pregnancy and with somewhat less reluctance to sterilise her. Another high spinal deformity was found in the fœtus.

For purposes of genetic counselling it has been suggested by Carter and Roberts[67] that the risk after two children with central nervous system malformations in England runs at about one in ten.

Although the term is often loosely used to account for a uterus larger than would correspond to the period of gestation, because of the amount of liquor present, it should really be restricted to those cases in which undue pressure symptoms or malpresentations occur as a result.

The causes of hydramnios are still to some extent obscure, although many complicating conditions are associated with excess liquor. Even the source of normal amounts of liquor is open to some question, but it would appear that hydramnios may owe its origin to maternal or fœtal causes or both.

Whatever the source of excessive liquor, it does not, as a rule, noticeably differ in composition from normal cases. Hydramnios is commoner in multiparæ than in primigravidæ.

Of the maternal conditions more likely to be associated with hydramnios are pre-eclamptic toxæmia, congestive cardiac failure and diabetes. In the case of the last mentioned, it is thought that the presence of sugar in the liquor may irritate the amnion to produce excessive quantities.

Of the fœtal causes of hydramnios the association of twins, especially uniovular, is noteworthy. Gross fœtal abnormality is a prominent ætiological factor, with anencephaly predominating (Fig. 9). The reputed inability of the anencephalic fœtus to swallow and therefore to absorb liquor into its circulation is said to be the cause here, and for the same reason hydramnios may be associated with œsophageal atresia. To a lesser extent other types of gross fœtal abnormality, for

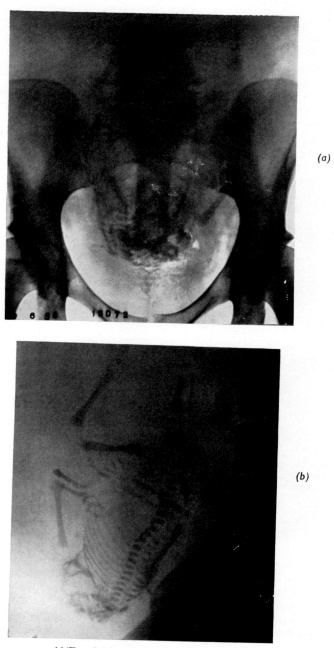

(a)

(b)

11/Fig. 9 (a) and (b).—Anencephaly.

example spina bifida and hydrocephalus, are associated with hydramnios (Fig. 10).

Other associated fœtal conditions are hydrops fœtalis and the very rare condition of chorioangioma, a small tumour growing from a single villus and consisting of hyperplasia of blood vessels and connective tissue. Syphilis is not nowadays regarded as an ætiological factor.

The clinical picture will depend upon the degree of hydramnios and the rapidity of its onset. Acute hydramnios is so rare that

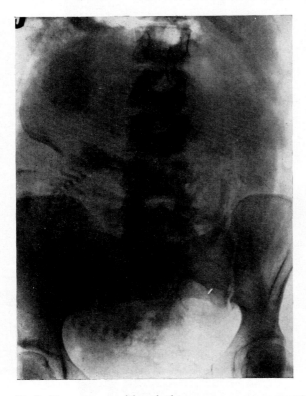

11/FIG. 10.—Hydrocephalus and spina bifida.

(Figs. 9 and 10 by courtesy of Prof. R. E. Steiner.)

F. J. Browne considered that every case encountered was worth reporting in the literature, but subacute varieties are by no means uncommon. Hydramnios occurring in mid-pregnancy should always arouse a suspicion of uniovular twins. The slower the development of the condition the less is the patient likely to complain. The acute variety may present many of the features of an acute abdominal catastrophe, the uterus being hard and tender and causing the patient great distress, so that the picture may resemble abruptio placentæ.

In the usual cases of gradual onset the patient may complain of an unmanageable girth, shortness of breath, considerable digestive discomfort, œdema of the lower extremities, and increasingly troublesome varicose veins. Occasionally hydramnios can cause hyperemesis in late pregnancy, and I have seen a highly parous patient prostrated with vomiting due to this cause, with ketone bodies in her urine, and finally suffering repeated hæmatemesis. Hiatus hernia may well have been a complicating factor but was not proven. Following the surgical induction of labour and delivery, her condition dramatically improved. In mild cases the fœtus can be freely ballotted and a fluid thrill is present. In more severe cases, however, palpation of the fœtus may be very unsatisfactory, and it is most difficult to hear the fœtal heart. Malpresentations are common, the lie may be unstable, and if the vertex presents the head is likely to be high.

The differential diagnosis is concerned firstly with multiple pregnancy. As has been repeatedly stated, all cases of hydramnios should have an X-ray as a matter of course, not only to determine the presence of twins but in order to detect the possible presence of gross fœtal abnormality. If no fœtal abnormality is demonstrated radiologically a further X-ray should be taken after rupture of the membranes, because abnormality is now more readily demonstrated and its recognition might discourage Cæsarean section if fœtal interests should subsequently appear to indicate it. The usefulness of sonar in examining the patient who is "larger than dates" is now beyond all doubt and is routinely employed by us. Not only will such an examination determine that the patient's dates may be wrong, because the fœtal head size gives a very good estimate of maturity, but the question of twins, hydramnios, associated ovarian cysts or fibroids, or even the very full bladder are readily distinguished from each other (Fig. 11).

Using sonar the diagnosis of hydatidiform mole in the abnormally enlarged uterus is easiest of all (see Chapter II).

An ovarian cyst may resemble pregnancy with hydramnios, but careful examination should distinguish the two conditions. There is a well-known story about a London gynæcologist who tried hard and unsuccessfully to induce labour with bougies in a case of ovarian cyst! An ovarian cyst displaces the uterus and pushes the cervix downwards, whereas in hydramnios the lower segment has to ride above the pelvic brim so that the cervix is consequently drawn up. Obesity may confuse the diagnosis of an ovarian cyst in association with pregnancy by making it difficult to palpate the sulcus between cyst and uterus. Examples of two-dimensional ultrasonograms differentiating causes of undue abdominal enlargement in pregnancy are shown in Fig. 11.

A full bladder may be mistaken for hydramnios, but this mistake

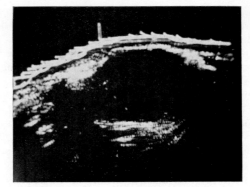

11/FIG. 11 (*a*).—Longitudinal section of abdomen. Umbilicus marked on the surface with a notch. Shows a large ovarian cyst cranialwards (to right) and fœtal echoes to the left.

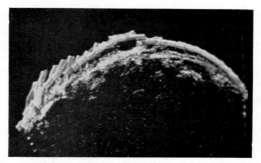

1/FIG. 11 (*b*).—Transverse section of normal though protuberant abdomen. Bowel echoes prevent deeper penetration. Not pregnant.
(By courtesy of the Editor, *Brit. J. Radiol.*)

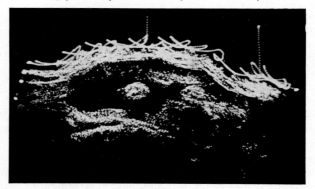

11/FIG. 11 (*c*).—Transverse section of hydramnios. In the centre is a sectional view of the body of an anencephalic fœtus. The enormous distension of the amniotic sac is well shown.

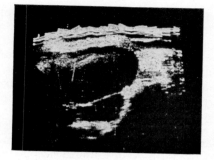

11/Fig. 11 (d).—Longitudinal section (cranialwards to the right). Shows very distended bladder with empty non-gravid, anteverted uterus lying behind it.

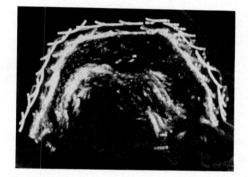

11/Fig. 11 (e).—Transverse section of pregnant diabetic uterus at 32 weeks gestation. Shows hydramnios and huge baby. (Cæsarean section two weeks later: baby weighed 12 lb.)

is not likely to be made provided the possibility is thought of. Lastly, hydatidiform mole, by causing undue uterine enlargement, may suggest hydramnios, but in this case there is usually some bleeding, the patient is ill, no fœtal parts can be ballotted, there is no fluid thrill, and pre-eclamptic toxæmia is more often present.

If the condition is bad enough to warrant treatment, putting the patient to bed is undoubtedly the most important measure. In many cases the excess quantity of liquor appears to diminish as pregnancy advances. Binders have been recommended, but as usual are almost worse than useless and merely increase the patient's misery. It is only when fœtal abnormality is present, or in the unusual instances of great severity, that the question of removal of some of the excess liquor arises. As an alternative, labour may be deliberately induced. The trouble about removing liquor is that the amount removed is liable to be quickly replaced, and the onset of labour is more often than not precipitated. One has the alternative choice of tapping

through the abdominal wall (after catheterisation) or of performing high puncture of the membranes with a Drew-Smythe catheter. Abdominal paracentesis of the amniotic sac is always fraught with the danger of rupturing a large placental blood vessel, although this risk is very much less in the case of hydramnios. Nowadays we seldom employ amniocentesis without first localizing the placenta by ultrasonic placentography.[8] If bloodstained liquor appears, it should be tested for fœtal hæmoglobin at once (see Chapter XV) to identify its source. I recall a case of hæmo-amnion due to fœtal hæmorrhage in which the source was identified by this test and immediate Cæsarean section secured a live birth. At operation a lacerated artery was found on the fœtal surface of the placenta. It follows, therefore, that radiologically demonstrable fœtal abnormality should be ascertained before interfering, Cæsarean section in such a case being ruled out.

When draining liquor gradually in a case of hydramnios through a fine needle inserted through the abdominal wall and connected by a length of narrow tubing to a suitably enclosed receptacle to prevent infection, it is often a helpful plan to thread over the tubing and apply to the abdominal wall the tin core of a wide roll of adhesive strapping. This simple device helps to keep the needle in place and at right angles to the abdominal wall. A very safe and gradual decompression can thus be achieved.

If it is decided in any case to induce labour deliberately, high membrane puncture should be performed first in order to give the presenting part an opportunity to settle into the pelvis before rupturing the forewaters. This simple precaution reduces the chances of the cord prolapsing. Often the forewaters are accidentally ruptured in the process, but an attempt should be made if possible to control the rate of loss since abruptio placentæ with severe accidental hæmorrhage may follow the sudden release of large quantities of liquor amnii. A late colleague of mine was once reckless enough to rupture the membranes in the patient's own house in a case of gross hydramnios and complained that he put the fire out. When anencephaly is associated with hydramnios there should be no hesitation in inducing labour by artificial rupture of the membranes. These cases do not fail to go into labour provided that the period of gestation is not less than thirty-four weeks.

Labour is usually normal, but may be complicated by uterine inertia, in which case hindwater rupture may enable the uterus to operate to better mechanical advantage. The patient should be nursed in bed during the first stage, until it is certain that the presenting part has settled well into the pelvic cavity, and a vaginal examination is indicated as soon as the membranes rupture to exclude the presence of a prolapsed cord. Labour may be complicated by malpresentation in this sort of case, and external version

during labour may deal with the situation. Treatment appropriate to the nature of the malpresentation (if any) may be called for. Lastly, the risk of postpartum hæmorrhage, though not as great as in the case of twins, is a very distinct possibility, and ergometrine should be immediately available, if needed, for intravenous injection.

After birth the baby should be tested for œsophageal atresia by the passage of a soft rubber catheter into the stomach. Failure indicates immediate further investigation since the surgical prognosis depends upon prompt recognition.

REFERENCES

1. CAMILLERI, A. P. (1963). *J. Obstet. Gynaec. Brit. Cwlth.*, **70**, 258.
2. CARTER, C. O., and ROBERTS, J. A. F. (1967). *Lancet*, **1**, 306.
3. CHARLES D., JACOBY, HANNAH, E., and BURGESS, FLORENCE (1965). *Amer. J. Obstet. Gynec.*, **93**, 1042.
4. CHARLES, D., and JACOBY, HANNAH E. (1966). *Amer. J. Obstet. Gynec.*, **95**, 266.
5. DONALD, I., and BROWN, T. G. (1961). *Brit. J. Radiol.*, **34**, 539.
6. DONALD, I. (1965). *Amer. J. Obstet. Gynec.*, **93**, 935.
7. DONALD, I. (1965). *J. Obstet. Gynaec. Brit. Cwlth.*, **72**, 907.
8. DONALD, I., and ABDULLA, U. (1967). *Brit. J. Radiol.*, **40**, 604.
9. KERR, M. M. (1959). *Brit. med. J.*, **1**, 902.
10. LIGGINS, G. C., and IBBERTSON, H. K. (1966). *Lancet*, **1**, 114.
11. LILLIE, E. W. (1962). *Brit. med. J.*, **1**, 940.
12. MACDONALD, R. R. (1962). *Brit. med. J.*, **1**, 518.
13. SUNDEN, B. (1964). *Acta obstet. gynec. scand.*, **43**, Suppl. 6.

CHAPTER XII

BREECH PRESENTATION

by the late G. W. GARLAND, M.D., F.R.C.O.G., *Obstetric Physician, St. Thomas's Hospital*

"and don't forget, if you find a head which is deeply engaged it may not be there at all" Irish midwifery tutor

THERE are three types of breech presentation, namely the complete breech with both legs flexed, the frank breech with both legs extended, and the footling in which one of the thighs is extended. The frank breech is more frequently seen in practice, and is much commoner in primigravidæ. The complete breech is the more usual in multigravidæ.

The breech presents in some 2–3 per cent of all women at the onset of labour. It is remarkable that this figure remains much the same even though prophylactic external version is being used less and less.

Cause

This is often a matter for speculation; nevertheless, certain facts are significant. Vartan (1945) has pointed out that at 30 weeks' gestation the breech presents in 1 of every 4 women examined. It is, therefore, true that prematurity is associated with a higher incidence of breeches. At about 34 weeks the fœtus, in the majority of cases, turns a somersault, and the cause of persistent breech presentation must, therefore, be that which prevents spontaneous version. It is obvious that the cause so often given in the past, something which prevents engagement of the head in the pelvis, can have no connection, seeing that the head does not normally engage until some time after spontaneous version should have taken place. Moreover, it has been shown that these time-honoured conditions, contracted pelvis, placenta prævia and so on, are altogether only found in about 7 per cent of breech presentations.

Vartan noted that failure of spontaneous version occurred most frequently in association with extended legs. Multiple pregnancy accounted for many others, but no factor whatever could be found in about a quarter of the cases. It is easy to see that the presence of another fœtus in the uterus would prevent version, while extended legs, by acting as a splint to the fœtal trunk, will prevent the flexion of the latter that must occur before the baby can pass the transverse axis of the uterus. Why the legs become extended is still unknown, although a plausible explanation is possible. The fœtus, while lying

as a breech, is always kicking out with its legs. There may come a time, especially with scanty liquor (and this is often notable in breech presentations), when it is unable, because of the resistance of the uterine wall in what is the less roomy part of the uterus, to draw back one or both of its legs, which will then remain extended. This would fit in with the frequent occurrence of this abnormality in primigravidæ, where the tone of the uterus is likely to be greater. Certainly, extended legs are not often, if ever, seen in X-rays when the vertex presents.

Summarising, then, a breech presentation is found either when the onset of labour is premature or, at term, when some factor has prevented spontaneous version. While this factor may often be extended legs or multiple pregnancy, a proportion cannot be so explained. Stevenson has suggested that a cornual fundal insertion of the placenta is responsible in these remaining cases, and he has shown by radiology that this type of placental insertion is common in breech presentations.

THE DANGERS OF BREECH DELIVERY

Labour in breech presentations is usually of normal length, for the frank breech forms a very satisfactory presenting part. The complete breech would be more likely to cause the long labour so common in malpresentations, but since it occurs in the multigravida, the tendency is often cancelled out by the increased efficiency of the uterus. Thus there is little, if any, increased risk to the mother. It is the baby who suffers most. Fœtal mortalities between 10 and 25 per cent have been quoted in the past, but in recent years there has been a marked fall. Now the average of many series of cases is about 3 per cent, with some reports (Todd, 1963; Hall, 1965; Dalrymple, 1965) as low as 1 per cent or less. It must be admitted, however, that these figures are only reached after correction for premature, abnormal or macerated fœtuses. Moreover the Cæsarean section rate is much higher as a result of careful selection of cases. Compared with a precisely similar series of vertex deliveries, it is still more dangerous for a baby to be born breech first.

The baby may die of asphyxia because the head is delivered too slowly; directly the head enters the pelvis the cord is obstructed, and until the mouth and nose are delivered the baby is unable to fend for itself. But by far the most common cause of fœtal death is intracranial damage due to the head being delivered too quickly. It must be remembered that in normal vertex delivery the head takes many hours to pass through the pelvis and has plenty of time to accommodate itself to the rigid bony canal. In breech delivery it must pass through the pelvis in not more than 10 minutes, and such a speedy passage of the head, even in a vertex delivery, can cause death.

Moreover, passing through the pelvic floor and vulva, the pressures acting on the head tend all the time to draw the cranial vault away from the base of the skull. The falx cerebri is attached firmly to the sagittal suture of the vault, and the tentorium cerebelli is attached just as firmly laterally. The falx meets the tentorium in the midline. The effect of the tensions previously described will be to pull the falx upwards, and this causes a bilateral tear in the tentorium, always about a quarter of an inch from the insertion of the falx. It is a very constant injury, and the resultant intracranial hæmorrhage nearly always leads to death of the fœtus.

Intracranial damage and asphyxia, brought about in these ways, are the main reasons for the greater danger of this type of delivery. Moreover, minor degrees of disproportion, difficult to recognise with the fœtal head at the wrong end of the abdomen, will increase the danger. In addition prolapse of the cord, with its great dangers to the fœtus, is commonly seen in complete, though not in frank breech presentations.

As a result of difficult breech deliveries, other fœtal injuries are occasionally seen. Grasping the abdomen in order to rotate the baby may cause rupture of abdominal viscera. Fractures of the humerus and femur or Erb's palsy may also follow difficult extractions.

Antenatal Management

External cephalic version has been used for many years to correct a breech presentation during the latter weeks of pregnancy. Because of the high fœtal mortality of breech delivery in the past every effort was made to avoid it, although version itself carried a small risk. This is negligible when performed without anæsthesia, but the danger to the fœtus when anæsthetic is used is of the order of 1–2 per cent. It is therefore obvious that, however much the use of extra force under anæsthesia is deprecated, it must be very difficult to avoid! The chief cause of fœtal death is separation of the placenta with consequent antepartum hæmorrhage. Often the patient goes into premature labour and, depending on the stage at which the version is being done, this may result in a few fœtal deaths. Rarely a true knot may be tied in the cord.

It has been said that the fœtus tends to undergo spontaneous version at or before the 34th week. This may vary by one or two weeks in either direction, and shrewd judgement is necessary to decide when to perform version. As a general rule a breech presentation found in a primigravida at 32 weeks may be turned if possible in the clinic. She should then be seen weekly in case the malpresentation should recur. In any event failure to correct the breech presentation should not indicate the use of anæsthesia until the 35th week or even later in a multigravida. This will make reversion

to a breech afterwards less likely and make the consequences of premature labour less serious to the fœtus.

Failure of an external version may be due, firstly, to an error of judgement in that the baby has been allowed to grow too big relative to the amount of liquor present. Secondly, version may be unsuccessful because of the extended legs of the fœtus. Other failures may be due to obesity, fibroids, congenital abnormalities of the uterus (e.g. septate uterus) or an unduly short cord. It is my experience, however, that even as early as 28–30 weeks one can recognise the breech that will never be turned.

Version is contra-indicated in pre-eclamptic toxæmia and hypertensive states because of the risk of abruptio placentæ; also following antepartum hæmorrhage, when twins are present, in cases of hydrocephaly and in the presence of a Cæsarean section scar.

Before an external version is performed search should be made for associated abnormalities. The most important investigation is an X-ray photograph. Not only can an accurate diagnosis of fœtal position be made in this way, but also it prevents such an undignified procedure as attempted version on one of twins. I myself saw a houseman trying for some time to do an external version on a fundal fibroid. The X-ray photograph should be taken as late as possible before the attempted version.

In the antenatal clinic it is a good plan to put the patient on a couch tipped to about 15° of Trendelenburg's position. In this way the breech tends to come out of the pelvis, making subsequent version easier. The frank breech, having the shape of a bung, easily settles down in the pelvis, and may cause difficulty in that it will not disengage. This should seldom be a cause of failure of a version, because as a last resort it can be disimpacted by a finger in the vagina, but this is rarely necessary.

With the woman in this position and as relaxed as sensible explanation and reassurance will allow, the breech is pushed with the right hand into the iliac fossa, which has been occupied by the back. In other words, the fœtus should turn head first. With the left hand the head is sought and gently pressed towards the other hand. All movements should be gentle and unhurried. It is essential to realise that rotatory movement of the fœtus is not enough, because the transverse axis of the uterus is usually shorter than the crown-rump length of the fœtus. Therefore, the first movement must be to flex the fœtal trunk, and it is because this is prevented by the splinting action of extended legs that the latter may cause failure.

Once the child is flexed it is surprising how often a sudden kick by it will cause version to take place. If this does not happen the head may be gently displaced downwards, making sure that the breech does not re-engage in the pelvis. Once past the transverse the child

will take up a cephalic presentation without further manipulation. It is useless to follow this manœuvre by attempting to push the head into the pelvis, although this might be thought to discourage reversion. The head is always extended and usually cannot be pushed down. The fœtal heart should be counted after completion of the version, and should it be absent or grossly slow the best thing is to turn the fœtus back to a breech. This complication suggests a short cord. The heart will always be a little slow after version, but its rate should not drop below 100 beats per minute and should return to normal within a minute or two. Lastly, search should be made between the patient's legs for any sign of vaginal hæmorrhage.

If the above technique fails, an attempt to rotate the baby in the opposite direction may succeed. At all events, if pain is caused or the uterine wall becomes tender, all manipulations should cease, and it is prudent to observe the patient in hospital for a day or two. The placenta may well have been disturbed.

If an anæsthetic is to be used the woman is usually admitted for one night. The anæsthetic is a matter of personal preference. A deep ether anæsthetic is unpleasant subsequently for the patient but very good for the job on hand. Cyclopropane is useless, as it tends to increase uterine tone. Pentothal alone may be too short in its action, but is often used nowadays in association with the shorter-acting muscle relaxants, such as "Scoline". It is a good practice always to examine the patient under premedication and before the anæsthetic is started, because version may succeed now when it failed before.

There has been considerable rethinking in recent years about the management of breech presentations and the above policy is tending to be modified. The reason for the change is primarily the dramatic fall in the fœtal mortality of breech delivery, when undertaken on selected cases by experienced obstetricians. It then becomes obvious that external version, especially under anæsthesia, is unjustifiable unless there is a special risk, such as mild disproportion, in the breech delivery. This attitude is strengthened because in practice version under anæsthesia has a considerable failure rate, with the result that often the woman runs the risk of the anæsthetic, the fœtus the risk of the version and both still have the trials of a breech delivery.

Hay (1959) questions whether version is ever justifiable as he considers that the incidence of breech deliveries is unaffected by its routine performance. In other words he thinks that successful versions are only performed on cases in which spontaneous version would eventually have taken place anyway.

Most authorities, however, would still agree to the gentle manipulation of a breech presentation in the clinic at 32–34 weeks. If this fails an X-ray pelvimetry should be done in order to get exact

information about the patient's pelvis. The brim and lateral views are sufficient, the outlet view being unnecessary since the outlet is easily measured on clinical examination. Only in multigravidæ, where there is a history of the normal delivery of a good-sized baby, may this examination be left out. If there is any abnormality in the pelvis then a breech delivery becomes more hazardous to the fœtus and in such a case it is reasonable to try a version under anæsthesia, for the alternative, if the breech persists, is a Cæsarean section. If the pelvimetry shows a normal pelvis then further version is not attempted and preparations are made for a breech delivery.

MANAGEMENT OF BREECH DELIVERY

As has been said the fœtal risk of breech delivery has fallen dramatically in recent years. This has only been brought about by careful selection of cases and supervision of the delivery, always in hospital if possible, by an experienced obstetrician. In the careful selection of cases, all those in which the delivery is likely to be unusually difficult, due to such abnormalities as pelvic contraction or a large baby, are best delivered abdominally. If there is any other complicating factor, such as elderly primigravidity, Cæsarean section may well be preferred and therefore the Cæsarean rate in breech presentations is high.

As X-ray pelvimetry has already been done, the next thing to consider is the size of the baby. Babies of more than 7 lb. birth weight tolerate breech delivery badly, even if the pelvis is normal, and as the birth weight rises, so the mortality goes up by leaps and bounds. In order to obviate this possibility many workers advocate induction of labour before term, should the baby appear to be of reasonable size, and this seems to be a very good plan.

The best method of induction is by rupture of the forewaters and, as most cases will be extended breeches, there will be no danger of prolapse of the cord. Those obstetricians averse to such interference point out that judgement of fœtal size per abdomen is very difficult, and also that even forewater rupture may fail to start labour within a reasonable time. This is admittedly a drawback and routine early induction in breech deliveries may well increase the number of Cæsarean sections. But this is a small price to pay and so much is gained in the majority of cases that induction of labour to prevent the nightmare of a really large breech delivery should be routine, certainly in any case who has not gone into spontaneous labour by term.

The first stage of labour is managed normally. There will be a few cases in which the first stage of labour is prolonged and it has come to be realised that this causes a sharp rise in the fœtal mortality,

almost certainly because it is often due to mild disproportion. Therefore most authorities agree that inefficient uterine action should be an indication for Cæsarean section and very much sooner than in a vertex presentation. Beware of first stages in breech presentation which last longer than 20 hours! It should be stated here that trial of labour in breech presentations, which is often mentioned in the literature, is a reasonable procedure provided it is realised that it is a trial of uterine action and not a trial of the passage of the head through the pelvis.

It may be very difficult to tell when the woman enters the second stage. The pointed breech may protrude some distance through a cervix insufficiently dilated to allow the head to pass. It is prudent, therefore, never to consider the second stage started until the anterior buttock is visible. Again, in a male fœtus the scrotum may be so œdematous that it presents at the vulva some time before full dilatation. Premature diagnosis of full dilatation and therefore delivery of the baby through an incompletely dilated cervix, will lead to extended arms and difficulty in delivery of the head. It is the commonest fault in breech deliveries.

It should be stressed here that if possible an anæsthetist should always be present during the second stage.

When the second stage is considered to have been reached, the woman is encouraged to make voluntary expulsive efforts in any position most comfortable to herself. When the posterior buttock is seen to be distending the perineum, she should be placed in the lithotomy position. Now, during a contraction, the breech will be seen to be making its characteristic climb up the perineum.

Now is the time to do an episiotomy. It should be done in all primigravid and most multigravid breech deliveries, firstly because it eliminates the obstruction of the perineum and thus straightens the curve through which the fœtal trunk has to bend before it can be delivered. Secondly, during delivery of the head much of the pressures acting on it are dissipated. It should be done now and not later, because it is now that the birth of the trunk is being held up. Furthermore, manual manipulations may sometimes be necessary during a breech delivery, and they are usually needed quickly; there is then no time to do an episiotomy, and putting the hand through the vulva when the fœtal trunk is already there will usually result in an ugly tear.

The episiotomy is best done after infiltration with the local anæsthetic of choice. Some practitioners prefer at this stage to do a formal pudendal block, especially if other help is not to hand. Such a block will allow of manipulations to the level of the upper half of the vagina, and it can be strongly recommended.

Immediately the episiotomy is performed (and remember that it

may bleed enough to justify tying bleeding points) the breech will begin to pass through the outlet, usually "climbing up" to a lesser extent in front of the obstetrician. Nothing should be done to help it, neither should any attempt be made to disentangle the legs until at least the umbilicus is seen. Nothing needs self-control so much as delivering a breech. Rarely will unnecessary interference be punished so tragically.

As the umbilicus is born, it is permissible, for the first time, to touch the child, disengage the extended legs and pull down a loop of cord. The latter is traditional. The body will now tend to flop downwards, and the back, up to now facing obliquely, will tend to look directly upwards. Never allow the ventral surface of the child's body to turn upwards at this stage.

During this part of the delivery the midwife should have a hand on the fundus of the uterus. She will not only be able to note the presence of a contraction, but can also follow the descent of the child, and by keeping a slight pressure on the uterine fundus she may prevent extension of the arms.

The shoulder blades of the infant will now be visible, and this is the time to look for the presence of the arms across the chest. Normally they will be there and can easily be flipped out. With a slight bearing down effort from the mother, the child is now born to its neck.

The head has still not entered the pelvis, but from now on it will do so and compress the umbilical cord. From this point, not more than 10 minutes should elapse before the child is in a position to breathe. Conversely at least 5 minutes should be allowed for descent of the head. Older obstetricians used the jaw and shoulder traction variously described by Mauriceau, Smellie and Veit to draw the head into flexion and thus through the brim of the pelvis. The modern method, described by Burns (1934), is to allow the baby to hang by its own weight from the vulva, the woman being in the lithotomy position. In most cases this causes flexion of the head, and the body is seen to drop slowly, signifying descent of the head. Occasionally suprapubic pressure may be necessary to aid descent, but if the head still does not engage it may be made to do so by turning the fœtus so that the head can enter the pelvis in the transverse diameter, which is rather more roomy.

As the hairs on the nape of the child's neck become visible, the obstetrician, standing with his back to the patient's left leg, takes the child's legs in his right hand. Then, exerting a firm outward force, he draws the child over the maternal pubis. The fœtal head is now delivered by a movement of flexion, and the left hand of the obstetrician can be used to guard the perineum and at the same time prevent the head emerging too quickly. Directly the mouth and nose of the fœtus are free, it can breathe, and a suction apparatus should be

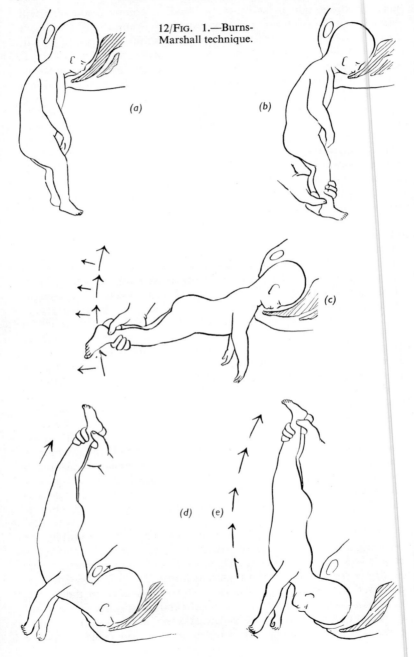

12/Fig. 1.—Burns-
Marshall technique.

(a)

(b)

(c)

(d) (e)

introduced into its airway to remove debris. The head, from now on, should be delivered slowly and carefully (Fig. 1).

This position of the obstetrician prevents the use of undue force while swinging the baby up over the mother's abdomen. Nevertheless, it is necessary to pull the child outwards a little, otherwise instead of the head pivoting on the underside of the pubis, the neck will impinge there and subsequent delivery of the head is difficult. In fact, the head is actively retained (Fig. 1d) and the steps will have to be gone through again, this time in a hurry, and damage is likely to be done. The importance of these manipulations can readily be seen with a model fœtus and pelvis, and the significance of the several details realised.

During delivery of the head, it is a good practice to ask for a quick induction of anæsthesia. Pentothal is very good, as it can no longer reach the fœtus. It is much easier to deliver the head slowly and gently with the patient unconscious, as otherwise a slight involuntary "push" will cause the head to pop out, and the mother's desire to do this must be very great! It is also a good plan to apply Wrigley's short forceps to the head at this stage, as subsequent slow extraction is much easier, and also the forceps may relieve some of the pressure from the fœtal head. However, this necessitates another pair of hands, unless the midwife, guarding the fundus, can hold the baby's legs (Fig. 2). She should be discouraged, however, from lifting the body too high as this encourages extension of the head in the birth canal.

The third stage in a breech delivery is usually very quick, as the slow emptying of the uterus allows the placenta to separate and be expelled before the cervix can shut down.

COMPLICATIONS DURING BREECH DELIVERY

These are considered separately in order to avoid breaking the continuity of the description of uncomplicated breech delivery.

Delay in descent of the breech.—In the past much was made of the inability of the extended breech to undergo the lateral flexion of the trunk necessary to negotiate the birth canal. If such flexion does not take place, descent of the breech ceases. With an episiotomy and in the absence of disproportion this is very rare. If it occurs, then the best thing to do is to insinuate a forefinger into the anterior groin (or preferably both groins) of the fœtus and exert gentle traction. This traction should be such that pressure is not exerted on the fœtal thighs, otherwise a fracture of the femur may result. A breech hook should never be necessary and should never be used on a live child.

In the very rare cases when descent still does not occur, an anæsthetic should immediately be given. The breech is then pushed upwards far enough for the anterior leg to be brought down. The

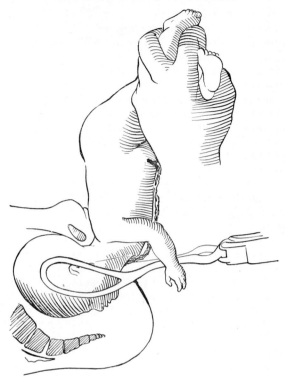

12/Fig. 2.—Forceps applied to the aftercoming head.

fingers of the operator must reach to the popliteal fossa of the particular leg before it can be flexed, and the anterior buttock must be above the symphysis pubis before the thigh can be brought down through the pelvis. Only one leg need be brought down, and the delivery now proceeds as a breech extraction. It is stressed how rarely it is necessary to bring down a leg.

Extended arms.—When the umbilicus is born the arms are looked for across the chest. If they are not there they must be extended, and no time should be lost in bringing them down. An anæsthetic should be given; and it can now be seen why the presence of an anæsthetist at these deliveries is desirable. The body of the fœtus is pulled to the side opposite to its posterior arm and slightly upwards. The operator's hand (the episiotomy has long since been made) can now pass up the child's body to the shoulder and thence along the arm to the elbow. Pressure on the elbow will bring the arm down in front of the face of the baby. A similar procedure can now be carried out on the other side. Nuchal displacement of an arm is very rare, but should it occur

the fœtus is turned towards that arm, when friction will bring the arm beside the baby's face, whence it can be brought down. Failure to bring down arms, which is an easy procedure in the absence of disproportion, is due to timidity. One must get up to the elbow of the fœtus before trying to pull the arm down, and consequently anæsthesia is essential.

Løvset (1937) described a method of dealing with extended arms which does not entail so much manipulation, nor an anæsthetic. He pointed out that the posterior shoulder will be below the promontory of the sacrum when the anterior shoulder is above the symphysis pubis. If, therefore, when the inferior angle of the anterior scapula is seen the baby is pulled gently downwards and at the same time rotated so that the back looks upwards, then the posterior shoulder turns and, being in the pelvis already, is seen under the symphysis pubis. Turning the child in the opposite direction will now bring the erstwhile anterior shoulder under the symphysis. The technique is seen in the accompanying sketches. It is easy to learn and works whether the arm is extended or nuchally displaced. Similarly, it can be used if disproportion is such that manual manipulations are difficult. Løvset claimed that he had no failures (Fig. 3).

Difficulty in descent of the head.—This can only be due to disproportion, if flexion is encouraged as already suggested. Having got into this uncomfortable position, the obstetrician can now only resort to force. Either the head can be drawn into the pelvis by strong jaw and shoulder traction, or the forceps can be applied to the head above the pelvic brim. The latter is very bad practice. If the head cannot be made to enter the pelvic brim, then almost certainly the baby will now be dead, and the best treatment is perforation. In fact, the impossibility of adequate treatment at this stage, if the head is too big for the pelvis, makes us even more likely to ensure that disproportion is not present before embarking on a breech delivery.

At the other extreme, however, a breech is much the most favourable presentation in cases of hydrocephaly, for the aftercoming head is more easily deflated than the forecoming head. It is, unfortunately, rather uncommon, should the head be presenting, for the diagnosis to be certain at a stage when external podalic version is feasible, but, if possible, it should be done.

In these cases the delivery proceeds normally until the body and arms are delivered. The body is then pulled down and a transverse incision made over the highest available cervical spine of the fœtus. A straight metal catheter can then be introduced into the spinal canal and thrust through the foramen magnum to drain the excess cerebrospinal fluid. This operation is made much easier if a spina bifida is present, which is often the case. After deflation of the head, the delivery is quickly completed.

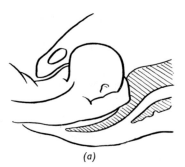

(a)

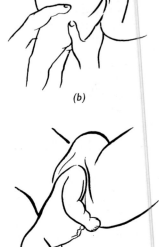

(b)

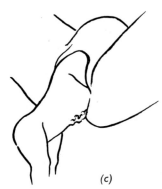

(c)

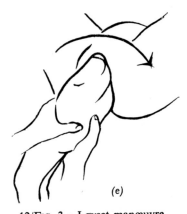

(d)

(e)

12/Fɪɢ. 3.—Løvset manœuvre.

(Figs. 1–3 drawn by Miss Pat Burrows, and by courtesy of the Editor, *J. Obstet. Gynaec. Brit. Emp.*)

It is true that some authorities now favour a little more action in the delivery of a breech, as against the policy of non-intervention preached above. Their results are so good that they cannot be ignored and obviously the important factor is the experience of the operator. This is, however, a different thing from breech extraction, which Macafee (1956) still insists is dangerous and only to be done if absolutely necessary.

Lastly, in nearly every published series of breech deliveries, the fœtal mortality is higher in multigravidæ than in primigravidæ. This should be pondered.

REFERENCES

1. BURNS, J. W. (1934). *J. Obstet. Gynaec. Brit. Emp.*, **41**, 923.
2. DALRYMPLE, IAN J. (1965). Clinical Report, Rotunda Hospital, Dublin, **20**.
3. HALL, J. E., *et al.* (1965). *Amer. J. Obstet. Gynec.*, **91**, 665.
4. HAY, D. (1959). *J. Obstet. Gynaec. Brit. Emp.*, **66**, 529.
5. LØVSET, J. (1937). *Ibid.*, **44**, 696.
6. MACAFEE, C. H. G. (1956). *Med. Press*, **236**, 268.
7. MARSHALL, C. McI. (1934). *J. Obstet. Gynaec. Brit. Emp.*, **41**, 930.
8. STEVENSON, C. S. (1951). *Amer. J. Obstet. Gynec.*, **62**, 488.
9. TODD, W. D., *et al.* (1963). *Obstet. and Gynec.*, **22**, 583.
10. VARTAN, C. K. (1940). *Lancet*, **1**, 595.
11. VARTAN, C. K. (1945). *J. Obstet. Gynaec. Brit. Emp.*, **52**, 417.

CHAPTER XIII

FACE AND BROW PRESENTATION
SHOULDER PRESENTATION
PROLAPSE OF THE CORD

by the late G. W. GARLAND, M.D., F.R.C.O.G., *Obstetric Physician, St. Thomas's Hospital*

THESE, the rarer malpresentations, are now seen infrequently enough for few obstetricians to be adept at their diagnosis and treatment. One tends to talk from a personal experience which is too limited to embrace all contingencies. Information about them is only to be obtained from series of cases extending over many years; and these are conspicuously lacking in agreement on many points—even on the incidence of the abnormalities—and the number of cases is still comparatively small.

MALPRESENTATIONS IN GENERAL

Causes

Most authors agree that disproportion under one guise or another is the most important factor (Dede and Friedman, 1963). Face and brow presentations occur frequently as an end result of a posterior position of the occiput in a borderline pelvis, consequently mento-anterior positions are seen at least as often as mento-posterior positions. The mechanism would appear to be that the deflexion already present is increased as the uterus pushes from above while the occiput is prevented from descending into the pelvis. The same thing occurs in a flat pelvis, especially if the foetal back is to the right, and the uterus, as is usual, inclines to the right; in such a case the head swivels on its parietal eminences and extension of the head results.

Even with an anterior position of the occiput, the presentation may, by extension, become a brow or face when the pelvis is contracted or the baby unduly large.

Shoulder presentations may result from disproportion of a more extreme kind, and are due to the inability of the head to engage in the pelvis. In this connection it must be stressed that, in a multigravida who has delivered herself previously of an 8 lb. baby, a 10 lb. baby may cause disproportion.

Coupled with disproportion as a cause of malpresentation is multiparity, and the two are complementary in shoulder presentations because a lack of uterine and abdominal wall tone allows the

350

head, which cannot engage, to swing to one or other side of the mid-line. Over half of all face and brow presentations occur in multi-gravid women.

Similar causes of malpresentations are hydramnios and pre-maturity, as both allow undue mobility of the fœtus.

Fœtal abnormalities are associated frequently with face and brow presentations (Fig. 1). Of course, an anencephalic fœtus must present by the face if the head is the lower pole. But, much more rarely, tumours of the anterior aspect of the neck (Fig. 2), and coils of cord round the neck may cause extension of the head to a brow or face. A dead fœtus may be so flaccid that any presentation can occur.

Stevenson stressed the effect of the site of insertion of the placenta on the presentation of the fœtus. He showed by soft-tissue radio-graphy that when the placenta occupies either the upper or the lower pole of the uterus, especially in multigravidæ, the shape of the amniotic cavity is such that an oblique or transverse lie may easily occur (Fig. 3). But placental insertion can have no effect on the production of a face presentation. Congenital abnormalities of the uterus, for instance septate uterus, can also cause a persistent trans-verse lie, and should be considered in the primigravida.

All the foregoing can be said to cause the malpresentation second-arily. Nearly half of most series of face and brow presentations cannot be explained in this way. It is probable that many of these are primary, being present before the onset of labour with no exciting cause. Gibberd pointed out that the uterus cannot, by its constraining walls, have much effect on fœtal position, as well-flexed babies are frequently seen in cases of hydramnios. Therefore, the tone of the fœtal muscles must be responsible for the position of the baby *in utero*, and more particularly the balance between flexor and extensor tone. He considered that a primary face or brow presentation can result from excessive extensor tone, and that such excess of tone could come on and pass off at odd times during pregnancy. In many cases it is unrecognised. In others an X-ray photograph shows a typical face presentation before labour, yet the child is delivered normally as a vertex presentation; in other words, the excess tone has passed off. In a few cases the tone persists even after delivery, and may take as long as a fortnight to pass off.

LABOUR

As a general rule, the labour with a malpresentation tends to be prolonged. This is obviously true in persistent mento-posterior posi-tions and brow presentations, for with a normal baby such cases can-not be delivered *per vaginam*, nor usually can a shoulder presentation.

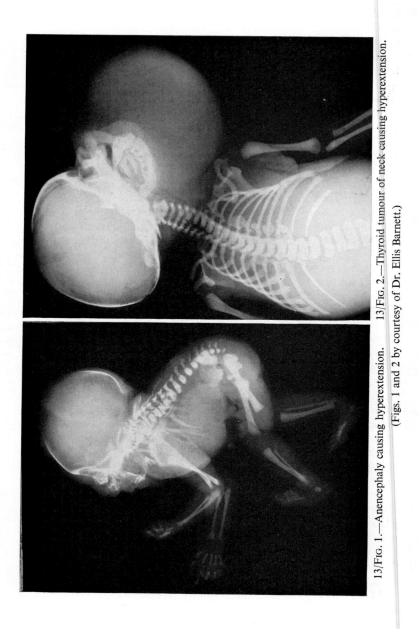

13/Fig. 1.—Anencephaly causing hyperextension.   13/Fig. 2.—Thyroid tumour of neck causing hyperextension.

(Figs. 1 and 2 by courtesy of Dr. Ellis Barnett.)

But even with a mento-anterior position, which is much more favourable, the second stage of labour especially is prolonged. Of course, the exciting cause, if any, of the malpresentation may well increase the length of labour in its own right. The membranes often rupture early in labour, and it is a cardinal rule that a vaginal examination be made immediately this happens to exclude prolapse of the cord.

One of the first concepts, therefore, in the management of these cases is that everything possible should be done to preserve intact membranes. The first stage of labour will be conducted with the patient in bed. In view of the possibility of a protracted labour, the mother's physical strength and morale are supported at all times.

As will be seen later, however, it is not often given to us to be able to carry out these laudable ideas. All too frequently the malpresentation is

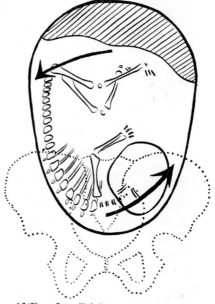

13/Fig. 3.—Ætiology of oblique lie.
(By courtesy of Dr. C. S. Stevenson and the Editor, *Amer. J. Obstet. Gynec.*)

found during labour, may indeed have occurred during labour, and irreparable damage may already have been done to the patient's mind, body and membranes.

FACE PRESENTATION

The incidence of this presentation is probably about 1 in every 600 deliveries. Hospital statistics are not very reliable here because their cases are to a certain extent selected. Mento-posterior and mento-anterior positions occur about equally. In the past a face presentation in labour carried with it heavy risks for both mother and child, but of recent years these have lessened. The fœtal mortality, excluding anencephalics, is still in the region of 10 per cent, largely due to the high incidence of premature babies and because intervention is necessary more often than in vertex deliveries, but the mother is little more at risk than in normal presentations.

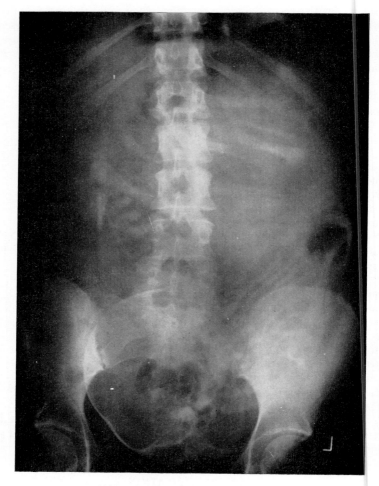

13/Fig. 4.—Primary face presentation.
(By courtesy of Dr. D. McKay Hart.)

Diagnosis

The recognition of a face presentation by abdominal palpation is difficult. It is said that the marked protuberance of the occiput on the same side as the fœtal back is very suggestive, but often the fœtal chest is mistaken for the back. What usually happens is that the doctor is suspicious because the fœtus does not feel quite right and therefore asks for an X-ray examination (Fig. 4).

Much more often the diagnosis is made during labour by vaginal

examination (Cucco, 1966). Even this has its snags, because if the presenting part is high and the cervix only slightly dilated, a face may easily be mistaken for a breech. But when advance has taken place and the cervix has become more dilated, the alveolar margins in the mouth, the nose and the supra-orbital ridges determine the diagnosis.

Management

A mento-anterior face presentation is consistent with a natural and spontaneous delivery, although the second stage is usually prolonged. The diameter of engagement in such cases is the submento-bregmatic, which is no greater than the suboccipito-bregmatic; but delivery is not quite so easy as in a vertex presentation, because moulding of the facial bones does not occur. In most series of cases, however, more than half are delivered spontaneously.

Mento-posterior positions are not nearly so favourable, but anterior rotation, followed by spontaneous or easy forceps delivery, occurs often enough for undue pessimism to be out of place. Failure to rotate leaves a persistent mento-posterior position and labour becomes obstructed.

When the diagnosis is made before the onset of labour it is necessary to exclude all possible causes of the malpresentation, especially contracted pelvis. Such causes, if found, merit treatment in their own right. If one can satisfy oneself that the pelvis is adequate, it is best to allow labour to proceed under strict supervision. In many of these cases the baby will be delivered normally by the vertex, the excessive muscular tone responsible for extension of the head having passed off. If labour starts with the face still presenting, however, spontaneous rectification is unlikely, but normal progress still occurs in the majority of cases. Should delay occur, however, intervention is called for at once.

Methods have been described of flexing the head by abdominal manipulation, but these are uniformly unsuccessful (and mechanically not very sound either) and they will not be described here.

If delay occurs during the first stage in the presence of good pains, it is probably due to a mento-posterior position. It is not recommended that attempts be made to rectify this position with the cervix not fully dilated; the proper treatment is Cæsarean section. Since the membranes have nearly always already ruptured, internal or bipolar version should never be done because of the risk of rupture of the uterus.

Associated factors, such as in the elderly primigravida, may cause one to terminate the labour much sooner, especially if the chin is known to be posterior.

In the absence of disproportion, however, the majority of cases will ultimately reach the second stage. Many will then proceed to spon-

taneous delivery or an easy forceps operation with the chin anterior. Between 30 and 40 per cent of all mento-posterior positions do not rotate spontaneously and so will need operative intervention. The treatment then is either rotation to mento-anterior or rectification to occipito-anterior and forceps delivery. The former is often quite easy, and is performed in the same way as for an occipito-posterior position. When using Kielland's forceps it may be found that rotation occurs more easily at a lower level in the pelvis than in occipito-posterior positions, and it may even be necessary to pull the uncorrected face down before rotation is successful. Sometimes rotation may be impossible, and then it is permissible to attempt rectification. This manœuvre entails pushing the presenting part above the pelvic brim, and deep anæsthesia is therefore essential. The whole hand is passed into the vagina and the face disimpacted. Above the brim of the pelvis the head can be flexed with the external hand assisting by pushing on the fœtal chest. It is a good plan for an assistant to pull the breech in the opposite direction to the force on the chest, thereby assisting flexion. This manipulation is obviously difficult and the average obstetrician sees far too few cases to get any experience in it. It is stressed, therefore, that rather than persist when failure has first occurred, and when manual rotation has already failed, it is better to swallow one's pride and proceed to Cæsarean section, if the baby is still alive. Internal version is an alternative, but is dreadfully dangerous when the membranes have been ruptured for any length of time, as is likely, and Cæsarean section, even in this potentially infected case, is the better procedure.

It may be one's fate to see a neglected case of persistent mento-posterior position with the head deeply impacted, the uterus near to rupture and the baby dead. Perforation through the orbital fossa and, if necessary, crushing of the head is then the only possible procedure.

BROW PRESENTATION

Brow presentation in labour is rare, and estimates of its frequency vary enormously. The average incidence would appear to be about once in 3,000 deliveries.

In this presentation the largest of all the diameters of the fœtal head attempts to engage and descent is impossible with an average baby and pelvis. Occasionally one sees even a normal-sized baby spontaneously delivered *per vaginam* as a brow presentation, but this is only in the presence of a cavernous pelvic cavity; very premature babies may be so delivered through normal pelves.

In the vast majority of cases, however, the brow remains above the brim in labour. The maternal and fœtal risk is obviously high and reflects the high interference rate that is necessary.

Diagnosis

Abdominal palpation is of little help and only serves to verify the non-engagement of the head. As in face presentations the diagnosis is most often made before labour by a radiograph taken because of doubt; frequently the question of fœtal abnormality has arisen because the head feels so big.

After the onset of labour a vaginal examination, performed because of lack of advance with reasonable pains, should reveal the true state of affairs, but as the presenting part is always high, it may be difficult until an anæsthetic is given. The points to note are the root of the nose, the supra-orbital ridges and the anterior fontanelle. If labour has been in progress any length of time, caput formation will obscure these points and make diagnosis difficult. The value of intra-natal radiography here is considerable.

A brow presentation should always be thought of in the grand multipara, if there is delay in labour with the head above the brim. Only too often, lulled into a sense of security by the size of her previous babies, one waits too long for the head to descend. Such patients go downhill surprisingly quickly and Cæsarean section becomes an urgent necessity.

Treatment

If the diagnosis has been made by X-ray before labour commences, it is best to await events, for the head frequently flexes or extends when contractions start, and labour progresses normally with the vertex or face presenting. When the diagnosis is made after the onset of labour, and after the membranes have ruptured, treatment should be instituted at once, there being no reasonable chance of a natural outcome. Occasionally the case may not be seen until she is in frankly obstructed labour and treatment is urgently necessary to prevent rupture of the uterus.

As many of these women have had more than one previous confinement, and thus the capacity of the pelvis is known, it might be thought that internal or bipolar version, according to the dilatation of the cervix, had a place in treatment. But the membranes have nearly always been ruptured some time, and in such cases intra-uterine manipulations are dangerous, because of the risk of uterine rupture, and nowadays quite unjustifiable. If the baby is alive, Cæsarean section is the obvious and sensible treatment.

If full or nearly full dilatation has been achieved, there is a case for manual rectification of the presentation to a face (if the chin is anterior) or a vertex, whichever is the easier, pushing down the head, followed by the application of the forceps, but again this should not be done if the woman has been in long and fruitless labour, the risk of uterine rupture being then too great. If the baby

is already dead, perforation might be considered, but such an operation on a head above the brim is full of pitfalls. Opportunities for the relatively safe delivery of these patients by means other than Cæsarean section are very rare, and the doctor has seldom much experience of the manipulations necessary. I have seen a brow presentation above the brim in a multigravida at full dilatation and the membranes still intact. An internal version and breech extraction was perfectly reasonable here and was performed, but I doubt if I shall ever see another case.

SHOULDER PRESENTATION

This is synonymous with "transverse" and oblique lie, the latter being really the correct term, as the fœtus almost never lies exactly across the uterus. It is difficult to assess the frequency of this complication. It is often found at some time in the antenatal period, but in labour the position is rare. It is very much more commonly seen in multiparæ. In view of the frequency of interference the risk of this presentation to the mother is more than in normal presentations, but the outlook for the child is far worse.

Diagnosis

The very shape of the abdomen on inspection may raise the suspicion of an oblique lie, as the fundus is low and the uterus spread across the whole abdomen. On palpation it will be noted that there is nothing in or over the brim of the pelvis, and the head is found laterally on one or other side of the uterus.

When the case is seen for the first time late in labour there will be all the signs of obstructed labour and almost certainly the cord or an arm or both will have prolapsed. Vaginal examination then is almost academic, but the scapula and ribs will be noted.

THE UNSTABLE LIE

Before considering the treatment of shoulder presentation in labour, a most important and relatively common problem will be discussed, that of the unstable lie late in pregnancy. It goes without saying that the patient is a multigravida of high parity. The fœtus may be found on examination to be in a different position each time. In such a patient the question of disproportion is unlikely to arise although it should be remembered; in fact, the very size of previous children successfully delivered may be an important predisposing factor.

Obviously at each antenatal visit the presentation is corrected by external version, which is performed easily, but the fœtus will not stay put. Near term, however, the question arises as to what will

happen if she goes into labour at home, when the fœtus is in one of its unfavourable positions. To guard against this it is common practice to admit the woman to hospital and to rupture the forewaters after external cephalic version, the head then being pushed into the brim and held there by pads and binder.

This method is not recommended, for the following reasons:

1. Labour does not always immediately ensue.

2. If labour does not start, the pads and binder are useless to prevent the head escaping into one or other iliac fossa, and, as the membranes are ruptured, prolapse of the cord is extremely common.

3. The interference is very often unnecessary.

The method of choice is to admit the woman to hospital and to watch her until she goes into labour spontaneously; during her wait in hospital the fœtal position may be corrected repeatedly. Soft tissue radiography should be carried out to exclude placenta prævia which may not yet have declared itself by antepartum hæmorrhage. When she goes into labour, the increase in tone of the uterine muscle frequently straightens out the lie of the fœtus, especially if the breech occupies the lower half of the uterus.

She should be examined immediately she goes into labour, and if the lie remains oblique the fœtus can now be turned by external version and the membranes ruptured with confidence, because labour is under way.

Occasionally the membranes rupture first while the fœtus is lying obliquely and the cord may prolapse, but as the patient is in hospital immediate treatment is available.

The disadvantage of this method of management is the frequency with which these women go past their expected date of delivery, presumably because they are resting in bed. This has been considered an inconvenience of no great importance. More recently, however, MacGregor has suggested that when postmaturity does occur the fœtal mortality is far higher and he recommends resort to Cæsarean section in such cases. This certainly is safer for the fœtus.

Treatment

The exact method of treatment of a shoulder presentation in labour depends on the dilatation of the cervix, the tone of the uterus, how long the membranes have been ruptured, and the condition of the baby. There are four possible methods:

(a) External version followed by rupture of the forewaters.

(b) Internal or bipolar version.

(c) Cæsarean section.

(d) Decapitation.

Obviously the first will be used if applicable, and it matters little

if the head or the breech is brought over the brim, the easier manœuvre usually being performed. It is the common method of dealing with the second of twins lying obliquely. Internal or bipolar version must never be used if the membranes have been ruptured for more than a very short time or if the uterus does not relax well between contractions. Cæsarean section will, therefore, nearly always be the method of choice if the baby is still alive some hours after the rupture of the membranes and gives by far the best results to mother and child. Internal version, while safe to the mother provided the rules are obeyed, has a high fœtal mortality, because of the breech extraction.

Decapitation is the treatment usually recommended for the neglected case of impacted shoulder presentation when the baby is dead. The important point in this operation is the strong pull on the prolapsed arm which will bring the neck down to the most accessible position. The best instrument to use is Ramsbotham's hook, which has a rounded end and a sharp, instead of a serrated, edge. The position of the back and head having been ascertained, the hook is passed along the palm of the hand until its end is above the neck. It is then turned backwards through a right angle so as to bring the cutting edge across the neck. The tissues are severed by a sawing movement, the end of the hook always being guarded by the finger, so that damage to maternal soft tissues is avoided. Pulling strongly on the hook will, of course, drag the neck even farther down and much of the cutting can more safely be done with strong scissors.

After decapitation the body is delivered by traction on the arm and the head is hooked down with a finger in the mouth. It must be realised that these manipulations may cause rupture or other damage to the uterus especially if, after a long labour, the lower segment is very thin. For this reason alone Cæsarean section is usually preferred, even more so if the obstetrician has no experience of destructive operations.

PROLAPSE OF THE CORD

This complication is seen in association with anything which prevents the presenting part from fitting closely into the lower segment and thus shutting off the forewaters from the hindwaters. It occurs, therefore, in multiparæ, cases of hydramnios, twins, prematurity, disproportion, and, by far the most important, in malpresentations. It will be noted from the above, however, that it is rare in the extended breech, which fits into the lower segment very snugly.

Prolapse of the cord is also encouraged by an unduly long cord or, more often, a first-degree placenta prævia of battledore or velamentous type with the cord entering at the lower pole. This may, of course, be itself the cause of the high head or malpresentation. Prolapsed cord occurs about once in every 400 deliveries.

It is, practically speaking, of little use to differentiate between presentation and prolapse of the cord, the former occurring when the membranes are unruptured. The treatment will nearly always be the same, and it is unusual for presentation even to be discovered. Much more often the prolapsed cord is found by vaginal examination, which has usually been done as a routine at the beginning of labour or after rupture of the membranes in any case where the presenting part is high.

In most cases, except sometimes in flexed breech presentations, the cord, having prolapsed, will be pinched between the presenting part and the pelvic brim, and the blood vessels in it become obstructed. It is, however, the experience of most obstetricians, that fœtal death can occur even if the cord is not so pinched; in fact, the presenting part may be prevented by vaginal manipulation from descending and still the cord ceases to pulsate. Rhodes (1956) suggests that spasm of the cord vessels may be as important a cause of fœtal death as actual mechanical blockage. If this is so, and there is experimental evidence to support it, then the likelihood of its occurrence may be much greater, and the fœtal prognosis therefore much graver, if the cord is actually outside the vagina, because its temperature will then fall. Moreover handling of the cord may also cause spasm, in which case efforts to replace it can do little good.

In any event the outlook for the fœtus is very poor unless delivery is prompt. The maternal risk is nil, except as a result of intervention designed to save the baby.

Treatment

In a large number of cases the cord has already ceased pulsating when the condition is found and no treatment is of any avail. If, however, the cord is still pulsating, the patient should at once be placed in such a position that gravity will tend to prevent the presenting part from obstructing the cord. The knee-elbow position is usually mentioned, but this is most irksome for the patient. It is more practical, therefore, to put her into an exaggerated Sims' position and at the same time to raise the foot of the bed. This first-aid treatment is only to allow time for more radical measures to be planned. If the prolapsed cord has not yet emerged from the vagina it is important to prevent it from doing so by applying a firm vulval pad since exposure to the cold, if it prolapses outside, may quickly extinguish pulsations.

It must be stated at once that there may be some associated abnormality which demands treatment in its own right, but we will consider here only the problem of the prolapsed cord.

The cases are best divided into those with the cervix fully or nearly fully dilated and those where the cervix has only just started to

dilate. In the former cases immediate delivery is the obvious treatment, and it can be done either by application of the forceps, taking care to exclude the cord from inside the blades, or by breech extraction, whichever pole of the fœtus presents. If the head is high, internal version may be the treatment of choice, but only if the membranes have very recently ruptured.

In cases where the cervix is not fully dilated, however, the choice lies between replacement of the cord and Cæsarean section. Replacement of the cord is only feasible if the cervix is at least three fingers dilated, and it is anything but universally successful. Many methods have been advocated in the past and some have leaked through to the present, but only one is of any use at all. This is to wrap the cord in a large piece of sterile roll gauze and then, under an anæsthetic, manually to replace the bundle above the presenting part. After this the presenting part is pushed into the pelvis and a binder put round the patient in the hope that it will stay there. This is sometimes successful and delivery in due course may be awaited.

Cæsarean section is the method of choice. It has been frowned upon in the past as being too radical, especially as the baby's life hangs by its cord if not by a thread. The fear of performing section for a dead baby can be minimised by auscultating the fœtal heart immediately before operating. Obviously, if, at that time, the heart sounds are already absent or very irregular, it is unjustifiable to expose the mother to the operative risk for so little likelihood of a return.

REFERENCES

1. COPE, E. (1951). *J. Obstet. Gynaec. Brit. Emp.*, **58**, 259.
2. COX, L. W. (1951). *Lancet*, **1**, 561.
3. CUCCO, U. P. (1966). *Amer. J. Obstet. Gynec.*, **94**, 1085.
4. DEDE, J. A., and FRIEDMAN, (1963). *Ibid.*, **87**, 515.
5. GIBBERD, G. F. (1939). *Proc. roy. Soc. Med.*, **32**, 1223.
6. HELLMAN, I. M., EPPERSON, J. W. W., and CONALLY, F. (1950). *Amer. J. Obstet. Gynec.*, **59**, 831.
7. MACGREGOR, W. G. (1964). *J. Obstet. Gynaec. Brit. Cwlth.*, **71**, 237.
8. MORRIS, N. (1953). *J. Obstet. Gynaec. Brit. Emp.*, **60**, 44.
9. POSNER, A. C., and BUCH, I. M. (1943). *Surg. Gynec. Obstet.*, **77**, 618.
10. RHODES, P. (1956). *Proc. roy. Soc. Med.*, **49**, 937.
11. STEVENSON, C. S. (1949). *Amer. J. Obstet. Gynec.*, **58**, 432.
12. STEVENSON, C. S. (1951). *Ibid.*, **62**, 488.

CHAPTER XIV

ANTEPARTUM HÆMORRHAGE

MANAGEMENT AND DIAGNOSIS

THIS is one of the complications of pregnancy which very often has to be managed before it can be diagnosed, and an attempt will be made in this chapter to present the subject and its difficulties roughly in the chronological order in which they will greet the practitioner. Most books give an account of the signs and symptoms, diagnosis and treatment of placenta prævia on the one hand and accidental hæmorrhage on the other, but this is of little help or guidance to the doctor who, for the moment, does not know which variety he is dealing with. This chapter, therefore, will start with the patient who presents with a story of bleeding only. After all, this is the commonest way in which these cases are encountered, and, for the moment, we will leave aside all those cases who present with the additional symptoms of pain, tenderness, or shock, which cannot be accounted for by the amount of blood lost; in order to keep the issues clear, we will defer consideration of abruptio placentæ, other intra-abdominal lesions associated with the onset of premature labour and "show".

It is often difficult to distinguish between a show and an antepartum hæmorrhage, and, indeed, many so-called large shows at the beginning of labour are in fact due to placental separation and may furnish the only evidence of, for example, a low-lying placenta. The distinction between show and antepartum hæmorrhage can only be made somewhat arbitrarily on the amount of blood lost.

For bleeding to qualify for the term antepartum hæmorrhage, its origin should be restricted to a portion of the placental site, but since this fact cannot be known when the case first presents it is more practical to refer to all cases of bleeding from any part of the genital tract as cases of antepartum hæmorrhage, provided pregnancy has reached the 28th week. Bleeding earlier than this is called abortion, of one variety or another, threatened or inevitable. The arbitrary dividing line at 28 weeks between antepartum hæmorrhage and abortion represents the earliest accepted chances of fœtal viability.

It was Rigby in the 18th century who first distinguished between cases of antepartum hæmorrhage where the placenta was normally situated and those in which the placenta was situated, in whole or in part, in the lower uterine segment, and the importance of his ob-

servation lies in the fact that the latter type of hæmorrhage is inevitable and is therefore liable to recur until the woman is safely delivered. From Rigby's day until our own this classification has continued, but it is no longer regarded as wholly satisfactory, because far too many cases of antepartum hæmorrhage cannot be explained. In fact, in many cases it can never be proven whether or not the bleeding came from the placental site. It will, therefore, be realised that bleeding appearing at the vulva may be due to:

1. Placenta prævia.
2. Accidental hæmorrhage; abruptio placentæ.
3. Extraplacental incidental sources.
4. Vasa prævia.
5. Origin cannot be determined.
6. Small recurrent antepartum hæmorrhages may be associated with a circumvallate placenta. In such cases the uterus is "small for dates" with a small baby, a well engaged presenting part and a normally placed placental site (Macafee, 1960).

A case can only really be diagnosed as having placenta prævia by feeling or seeing the placenta or by one of the newer methods demonstrating its presence wholly or partly over the lower uterine segment. Even the term "lower uterine segment", however, is not universally agreed. There are, for example, a few who say that the lower uterine segment is not properly developed until labour actually starts. There are three definitions, as follows:

Lower Uterine Segment

1. The physiological definition: "It is that part of the uterus which passively stretches in labour and takes hardly any active, contractile part in the expulsion of the fœtus." The importance of this definition lies in the word "stretches". In stretching, the placenta comes adrift from its attachment much as a postage stamp would come off a piece of elastic if the latter were stretched. This type of hæmorrhage is inevitable, because the lower uterine segment must sooner or later start to stretch.

2. The anatomical definition: "It is that part of the uterus which lies below the level at which the peritoneum on the anterior surface of the uterus ceases to be intimately applied to the uterus, and is reflected via the utero-vesical fold on to the dome of the bladder." This definition only serves at laparotomy, as, for example, in performing Cæsarean section.

3. Metric definition: "It is that portion of the uterus which towards term lies within three inches of the internal os." This is a rough-and-ready definition, but it is the one of most practical value in diagnosis, because it represents the distance over which the

uterine cavity can be explored by the examining finger passed through the cervix. Therefore, if no placenta can be felt, one can be reasonably certain that the case is not one of placenta prævia.

The diagnosis of accidental antepartum hæmorrhage, on the other hand, is often made only by exclusion of placenta prævia, and is open to a good deal of error. In recording such a diagnosis, evidences of placental changes following separation and hæmorrhage should be sought after delivery, though it will often be found that, following quite severe hæmorrhages, no trace can be found by examining the placenta.

The accidental group should be subdivided into cases of bleeding associated with pre-eclamptic toxæmia, hypertension or renal disease, as against those cases of accidental hæmorrhage in which no such toxic association is present.

Premature separation of a normally situated placenta occurs no more than once in 133 non-toxæmic pregnancies, while with toxæmia the incidence rises to 1 in 18, and in eclampsia to 1 in 3. The ætiological significance of pre-eclamptic toxæmia in accidental hæmorrhage becomes obvious. Often there is no more than a record of a systolic blood pressure of 150 mm. Hg or more occurring some time before the antepartum hæmorrhage. Murdoch (1952) observed this in 29 out of 339 cases.

Macafee (1945) tabulated 341 cases of antepartum hæmorrhage as follows:

1. Placenta prævia, 108.
2. Toxic cases, 83.
3. Extraplacental local causes, 18.
4. Unclassified, 132.

In a further series of 395 cases he was unable to trace the origin of the hæmorrhage in 163. It will be appreciated, therefore, that the so-called unclassified group forms one of the largest classes. Murdoch's findings were similar, although many of the hæmorrhages, though small, were repeated, yet confirmatory evidence of placenta prævia was lacking. One of the important things about this indeterminate class is that it accounts for almost half of the fœtal wastage. The risks to the fœtus in placenta prævia are obvious, but it is only now becoming recognised that the baby is at even greater risk when the source of antepartum bleeding is not determinable. In Murdoch's series of 339 cases, placenta prævia was found in 85, either at examination under anæsthesia or at Cæsarean section. Of these, 23 cases suffered from associated pre-eclampsia.

There is, of course, no particular reason why pre-eclamptic toxæmia should not be associated with placenta prævia any more than with other pregnancies, and its incidental presence should not put one off the scent. Even though the case proves to be one of

placenta prævia, there is no doubt that the addition of pre-eclamptic toxæmia greatly increases the fœtal risks. Rigby's classification, although it was an important step, has rather helped to cloud the issue, and it is important to recognise that any true case of ante-partum hæmorrhage, of whichever variety, involves greater risk of stillbirth or neonatal death.

PLACENTA PRÆVIA

The incidence of this condition is approximately 1 in 200, but since the majority of these cases find their way into hospital, the published figures of maternity units exaggerate the incidence in pregnancies throughout the country. It is much more common in multiparæ, although 20 per cent occur in primigravidæ; but multi-parous pregnancy is very much more common than first pregnancies and the factor of multiparity has probably been overstressed. More cases occur in the first pregnancy, however, than in any other sub-sequent pregnancy, for example the fourth or the fifth, and this fact encourages one to question the generally accepted factors said to predispose to placenta prævia. This incidence definitely increases over the age of 35 years.

"Chronic endometritis", for example, has been blamed, although it is doubtful if, in actual pathology, this condition is authentic. Likewise sub-involution has been claimed to favour a later and therefore a lower site of implantation. Neither of these conditions is likely to operate in the case of the primigravida. It is more probable that, as a result of some local aberration in uterine blood supply, the distinction between the areas of chorion frondosum and chorion læve does not occur in the normal situation and the developing ovum comes to derive its nourishment from a lower region of the uterus than is customary. The decidual reaction in the lower uterine segment is often inadequate, and this false secondary type of implantation may be defective, so that abortion occurs. Many of these cases, in fact, never reach the degree of maturity which would qualify them for the title of placenta prævia. Moreover, because of the local inadequacy of the decidua, patchy areas of morbid adhesion may occur and complicate the third stage of labour.

The incidence of placenta prævia is, of course, increased in mul-tiple pregnancy, since the placental site, because of its size, has a greater chance of encroaching on to the lower uterine segment. Whatever the factors responsible for the development of placenta prævia, there is no doubt that the grand multipara runs a greater risk of this complication. Placenta prævia can hardly be regarded as a truly recurrent condition, but the chances of having a subsequent pregnancy thus complicated are about 12 times as high as in the normal child-bearing population with no such history.

Degrees of Placenta Prævia

There are four degrees (also called "types"):

1. The placenta encroaches on the lower uterine segment, but does not reach as far as the os.

In these minor degrees there is often a disproportionate amount of blood loss from what is known as marginal sinus bleeding following separation of the lower edge of the placenta, thus exposing a small localised area of the placental site. The amount of blood lost is not necessarily related to the area of placental separation.

2. The placenta reaches to the os, but does not cover it.

3. The placenta covers the os by reaching across to the farther margin, but ceases to do so as the cervix dilates.

4. The placenta covers the os to such a degree that even dilatation of the cervix does not bring its margin over the cervix.

In the majority of cases the placenta mainly lies on either the anterior or the posterior wall. The latter is slightly more common and is also more dangerous because it discourages engagement of the head more readily, and is likely to be compressed in labour.

STEPS TO BE TAKEN WHEN FIRST SEEN

If word is received that a patient, still in her own home, has had an antepartum hæmorrhage, she should be instructed on no account to come to the hospital, or to the doctor's surgery, until visited and until proper arrangements for her transport can be made. She should be told to remain in bed and instructed not to clear up sheets, etc., soiled by blood. This will, at least, give the doctor or midwife a chance of estimating how much blood has been lost. She should be visited as soon as possible and her general condition noted.

There is a curious but natural tendency on the part of those in attendance on the patient to clean her up before the doctor's arrival, so that traces of blood from thighs and legs have already been removed. When a patient finds herself bleeding in bed, her first reaction is to jump out of it and stand on the floor, so that blood runs down her legs and collects on the soles of her feet and between her toes.[34] Professor Parks of Washington, D.C., who, as far as I know first made this observation, happened to be visiting the Queen Mother's Hospital one day and saw a woman recently admitted by the Flying Squad with antepartum hæmorrhage. He immediately asked whether the nursing staff thought she had lost more or less than 150 ml. of blood. He thereupon pulled back the bedclothes from her feet and legs which looked impeccably clean and demonstrated the clotted blood still on the soles of her feet and between her toes, signifying a very sizeable hæmorrhage. His triumph was almost as great as the consternation of my nurses.

If she arrives at the antenatal clinic either bleeding or with a history of having bled recently, she should be persuaded to remain in hospital and not to go home to pack her things. Patients are often reluctant to take this advice because, from their own point of view, they usually feel perfectly well; they are in no pain and the hæmorrhage has often been no more than slight, and not a few will, in their own minds, rightly attribute it to the effects of coitus. The significance of antepartum bleeding, however, cannot be dismissed on the grounds of recent coitus, because placenta prævia bleeding is particularly easily provoked thereby.

If the patient is still bleeding when first seen she should, in the first instance, be given a quarter of a grain of morphia (15 mg.) by injection and put to bed. Only the briefest examination is called for at this stage, but it will include the recording of blood pressure and pulse and any general signs of exsanguination. The abdominal wall is only lightly palpated, mainly to exclude the presence of any areas of uterine tenderness or to observe the presence of rhythmical contractions signifying the onset of labour or a hard consistency indicating abruptio placentæ. The fœtal heart is auscultated, and the urine, if necessary a catheter specimen, is examined for the presence of albumen. By now the injection of morphia already given will have begun to take effect. The same procedure is to be followed if the patient is first seen in her own home, and neither in clinic nor in private dwelling is any form of pelvic examination permissible.

If the patient is bleeding seriously at home it is far safer to send for "flying squad" assistance from a neighbouring hospital than to send the patient in before the necessary restorative treatment. One such case "posted in" to us by her doctor, continued bleeding on the journey and became so shocked that she could not be got over the doorstep alive but died as she was being lifted out of the ambulance. She should, of course, have been properly sedated and liberally transfused first until fit to make the journey.

Many general practitioners feel that, on being summoned by a midwife to a case of antepartum bleeding, they are not making much of a contribution to treatment by restricting their activities to arranging admission to hospital on a telephone. But the more experienced will realise the great value of such forbearance.

This is one of the emergencies in which the administration of morphia before admission is not only permissible but positively indicated, and a note to the effect that this drug has been given should accompany the patient. A clean vulval pad should be applied, abdominal binders should be eschewed and the patient's clothing should be disturbed as little as possible before transfer.

While awaiting admission, a history can now be taken, particular note being made of the presence or absence of any associated pain,

when movements were last felt and what the patient was doing at the time when the bleeding first occurred. In many cases of placenta prævia bleeding the patient will state that the first thing she noticed was that the sheets were damp with blood or that the bleeding started during a visit to the toilet.

All cases of bleeding *per vaginam* should be admitted for observation and, in the vast majority, expectant treatment is employed in the first instance unless the bleeding is very severe or labour is actually in progress.

REASON FOR ADMISSION OF ALL CASES OF ANTEPARTUM HÆMORRHAGE

Since many patients are unwilling to go to hospital, it is as well to be conversant with the reasons for insisting. Firstly, every case of antepartum hæmorrhage is to be regarded as due to placenta prævia until the contrary has been proven, because, in this event, further bleeding is bound to occur sooner or later and none can predict its severity. Even the smallest initial warning hæmorrhage may be the herald of a loss so catastrophic as to cause not only the baby's death but that of the mother as well, and only a properly equipped institution is in a position to deal adequately with such an emergency.

Let us discuss the likely fate of the untreated case. Admittedly, she will most probably deliver herself ultimately in a variable state of exsanguination, although a small number would die from hæmorrhage before delivery. Labour, moreover, would probably be premature, and in all but the lesser degrees of placenta prævia the child would be stillborn. In delivering herself, the placenta would be likely to come adrift completely before the delivery of the child and to present first at the vulva. Malpresentation too is common in placenta prævia, and the complications of this have to be added to the process of labour. If she failed to deliver herself of the placenta at the same time as the baby, it is more than likely that the placenta would remain partially detached within the uterus and cause still further bleeding. Even though she survived the second stage of labour, postpartum hæmorrhage, not necessarily excessive, might prove more than her exsanguinated condition could stand. Lastly, having negotiated all these hazards, she would now find herself a ready prey to puerperal sepsis because of her anæmia. This sequence of events is not uncommon in outlying parts of the world where medical aid is not readily available.

MATERNAL AND FŒTAL MORTALITY

Until recently, antepartum hæmorrhage came fourth in the list of causes of maternal death. Much of this is preventable with proper

antenatal supervision and institutional care. The incorrectly treated case of placenta prævia is in far more peril than that of accidental hæmorrhage, but modern treatment has reversed the order of importance of these two as causes of maternal death. The majority of deaths from placenta prævia are due to mismanagement. Macafee, more than anyone else in this country, demonstrated what can be done in this respect by achieving a maternal mortality of 0·57 per cent in contrast to the previously accepted figures of 6 or 7 per cent. The fœtal mortality was also impressively reduced from over 50 per cent to 23·5 per cent (1945). In his later series of 200 cases there has been no maternal death and nowadays the fœtal mortality should not exceed about 10 per cent.

One of the commonest causes of death in cases of antepartum hæmorrhage, whether placenta prævia or accidental, is postpartum hæmorrhage, for even a small loss of blood after delivery may tip the scales against an exhausted, shocked and exsanguinated patient. Areas of morbid adhesion of the placenta (placenta accreta) in the lower uterine segment are not uncommon in placenta prævia and can cause very dangerous postpartum bleeding[27] and even without difficulties of separation, bleeding can be very free. Another common cause of death is puerperal sepsis, to which the patient is particularly prone as a result of the interference which may have been occasioned in the course of delivering her and as a result of her diminished resistance to infection from anæmia. These patients often succumb to shock, operative or otherwise, the effects of which again are magnified by blood loss and, finally, both shock and hæmorrhage invite the possibility of tubular nephrosis of the kidneys, so that the patient may die of anuria. The case of toxic accidental hæmorrhage runs the additional risks of acute cortical necrosis of the kidneys and the possibility of eclampsia.

Murdoch reported a maternal mortality in the toxic group, including cases of hypertension, of 6 per cent, and the improvement in outlook in this group in no way matches yet the results in cases of placenta prævia. The reduced maternal mortality in recent years is mainly attributable, firstly, to the increased use of blood transfusion, secondly, to effective chemotherapy, thirdly, to a better understanding of the management of shock, fourthly, to the more rational management of anuria, and lastly, to the abandonment of many of the older practices which, in the past, made midwifery such a blood-and-thunder subject.

Until recently attention was mainly concentrated upon the mother's chances of survival, but now increasing note is being taken of the means of improving fœtal prospects.

All types of antepartum hæmorrhage jeopardise the fœtus, and until the 1939–45 war the fœtal mortality was over 50 per cent. Since

then, in the case of placenta prævia, the increased use of Cæsarean section, preceded by expectant treatment as advocated by Macafee, has been universally adopted and Stallworthy as long ago as 1951 declared that it should be our aim to reduce maternal mortality to nil and the fœtal mortality to less than 10 per cent. Unfortunately, although in accidental hæmorrhage there has been some improvement, it is nowhere near so impressive, and in the toxic variety fœtal loss remains between 40 and 50 per cent, while in non-toxic cases the fœtal loss is very much lower, about 14 per cent. Where the cause of the bleeding cannot be determined the baby is at greater risk than in placenta prævia and if the bleeding is recurrent the risks are greater still. We have, in the past, been so blinded by the hazards of placenta prævia that it is only now that the importance of this very unsatisfactory, unexplained group has fully come to light.

Causes of Fœtal Death

1. *Intra-uterine asphyxia*, due to placental separation, howsoever caused. This is the commonest mechanism, but hypotension in the mother, as a result either of hæmorrhage or shock, may also starve the fœtus of oxygen. In toxic antepartum hæmorrhage the reduced maternal placental circulation, as a result of pre-eclampsia, also plays a part.

2. *The hazards of delivery*. Malpresentation, if present, confers its own penalties, particularly in the case of the premature infant who is very prone to intracranial hæmorrhage, especially in breech delivery.

3. *Prematurity*. This, too, often takes its toll, and the modern expectant treatment of placenta prævia has gone a long way towards minimising this hazard.

4. *Fœtal abnormality*. This is more common in placenta prævia, and Macafee quoted a 3·4 per cent incidence. The most likely forms are spina bifida, hydrocephalus and anencephaly.

5. *Atelectasis neonatorum*. This is very commonly associated with prematurity, particularly with a history of antepartum hæmorrhage.

6. *Hyaline membrane*. This condition is really a sub-variety of atelectasis neonatorum, and is dealt with more fully in the chapter on prematurity.

7. *Fœtal exsanguination*. Usually ruptured vasa prævia are responsible for the fœtal blood loss which does not have to be large to kill the baby or to make it seriously anæmic. The foolish use of hindwater rupture as a method of surgical induction of labour in cases of placenta prævia producing a "bloody tap", is another potent source of this trouble.

The possibility that the bleeding may be of fœtal origin must be determined or eliminated at once. Fortunately this can be carried out

within about 20 minutes by the alkali denaturation test for fœtal hæmoglobin, as described in the chapter on "Induction."[28]

Normally the fœtal abnormality rate is not more than 0·94 per cent, so that it will be seen that the incidence is more than trebled in placenta prævia. Most of the neonatal deaths are due to prematurity with its associated risks, particularly atelectasis and intracranial hæmorrhage, and lastly fœtal abnormality.

There are certain special dangers, apart from injudicious treatment, which confront the fœtus in placenta prævia in the course of vaginal delivery, and these are associated with battledore insertion of the cord, which is by no means uncommon and may even take the form of a velamentous insertion (Fig. 1). When, as is very often the

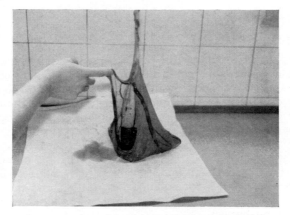

14/Fig. 1.—Velamentous insertion of the cord. This baby had the good fortune to escape through a rent between the large foetal vessels running in the membranes. Otherwise rapid foetal exsanguination would have occurred.

case, the insertion is at the lower pole of the placenta, the fœtal mortality is greatly increased, even with placenta prævia of only first degree. This combination of circumstances is even more dangerous if the placenta is situated posteriorly and encourages the acceptance of Stallworthy's term, the "dangerous low-lying placenta". In these instances, the fœtal mortality is very much greater than in more frank degrees of placenta prævia, which are treated by Cæsarean section.

MANAGEMENT ON ADMISSION

Macafee's great contribution lay in his advocacy of expectant treatment, thereby reducing prematurity. As a rule, the first hæmorrhage is not lethal either to the mother or the child, particularly in

the case of the primigravida, and with morphia and rest in bed it presently ceases in practically every case. The separated area of placenta becomes infarcted and the maternal vessels supplying the exposed portion of the placental site thrombose. Provided too great an area of placenta is not detached, that is to say more than about a third, the fœtus readjusts itself and probably some compensatory mechanism, if given time, meets its oxygen requirements. For this reason, small repeated hæmorrhages are far less dangerous than single large ones. The words "if given time" are important, and hence unwarranted interference may defeat the process. The first warning hæmorrhage is not an indication necessarily for active investigation, which is almost bound to provoke the need for immediate treatment. Diagnosis must, therefore, be deferred.

The first step to be taken in hospital is to ensure that the patient's blood group and Rh grouping is known and that a supply of compatible blood is available for transfusion at any moment. It is safer to keep the patient strictly in bed, not to allow her to have a bath and to forbid visits to the toilet, at least for five days after the cessation of bleeding. The colour of the blood appearing at the vulva is noted, and its increasing darkness will reassure one that no fresh bleeding is occurring.

If on examination of the abdomen it is found that a malpresentation is present, no steps must be taken to correct it by external version.

The hæmoglobin is estimated on admission and again repeated two or three days later to assess, firstly, the patient's general blood state, and secondly, the anæmia which will be manifested at the second reading by hæmodilution. No vaginal examination nor even a rectal examination may yet be made. The fœtal heart is auscultated, the blood pressure is recorded twice daily, and the urine is examined every day for albumin, unless the specimen is contaminated with blood, in which case a clean swab specimen is tested.

It is important that the admitting officer or house surgeon on the ward should inform the consultant in charge of the patient's admission, rather than act upon his own initiative. Provided fresh bleeding does not occur, the patient is left alone for five days at least before proceeding farther, during which period no purgative should be given.

It is commonly taught that a speculum should be passed on admission and the cervix inspected, but with this practice we strongly disagree except in the very mildest cases of bleeding. For one thing, if there is any appreciable amount of blood in the vagina, it will not be possible to see the cervix without resort to mopping, which in itself may be almost as bad as a full vaginal examination. Secondly, further bleeding may be provoked. Where the bleeding amounts to no more than a slight stain, however, a cautious speculum examina-

tion is often worth while, because it may not be possible later to ascertain whether the blood was issuing from the cervical canal or otherwise. In most cases, therefore, speculum examination is deferred until five days after the cessation of bleeding. This is done in order to exclude lesions of the cervix and vaginal vault which might have been the source. A large Fergusson speculum is admirable for the purpose.

After the first few days, the patient may be allowed to go outside to the lavatory, but she must be forbidden to lock the door. It occasionally happens that a patient thus closeted has a severe hæmorrhage and may lose consciousness; therefore a prolonged absence from the ward calls for inquiry. I recall one such case in which the patient collapsed on the lavatory floor in a pool of blood and the door had to be broken in. She lost both her twins as a result of the severe hæmorrhage. It is this fear of severe, inevitable and recurrent hæmorrhage which necessitates this cautious attitude as long as the existence of placenta prævia remains a possibility.

Soft tissue X-ray placentography may be undertaken at any time from the 34th week onwards (see later). This may not only determine the site of the placenta but may help to exclude fœtal abnormality, or twins with which placenta prævia is more frequently associated. An assessment of fœtal maturity may also be made at the same time. Ultrasonic localization of the placenta can be undertaken several weeks earlier and with us has become standard practice. The discovery of a fœtal abnormality will render further expectant treatment somewhat pointless, and will make one loath to deliver the patient by Cæsarean section, although in fourth-degree placenta prævia this is the only safe method of delivery.

Any anæmia should be appropriately corrected during the patient's wait in hospital, so that intervention, if and when it has to be undertaken, is performed under optimum conditions.

After the first few days the patient is allowed up and about in the ward, and there now follows a very irksome period of waiting. Not a few, for domestic reasons, will refuse to remain any longer in hospital and will take their discharge on their own responsibility. This is very understandable, and one cannot do more than advise them at least of some of the risks and the steps to be taken if they materialise, but on no account should a patient's desire to leave hospital precipitate one into trying to exclude the presence of placenta prævia at this stage by vaginal examination. For one thing, it is impossible to be certain without passing a finger through the cervix, which at this stage is unthinkable, and, for another, one's curiosity in those very cases where it was most warranted will provoke the very disaster against which one is trying to insure the patient.

As it is, the patient may have to spend many weeks of apparently fruitless imprisonment in hospital, only to find at the end that there was no placenta prævia after all. This is a serious matter, but in the present state of our knowledge the rule can only be broken in face of the risk of an occasional disaster. The end results of this expectant treatment speak for themselves, but they are achieved at a great price in inconvenience to the patient, and not infrequently we are prepared to take a chance on the patient who has a deeply engaged vertex and a history of very slight bleeding on one occasion only. Deep engagement of the head does not, of course, completely exclude placenta prævia, but makes it very much less likely.

In the absence of modern diagnostic facilities (see later) this period of waiting and observation is maintained until the 38th week, that is to say until the question of prematurity no longer applies, and the patient is then examined under an anæsthetic as described below.

Should bleeding not cease within a few hours of admission, or should it at any time become profuse, expectant treatment is out of place. If the patient is already in labour she should be examined under an anæsthetic, in an operating theatre prepared to undertake immediate Cæsarean section should the findings indicate it. It may be found, for example, that the patient is farther on in labour than expected and that the cervix is already appreciably dilated, in which case artificial rupture of the membranes or pulling down a leg may meet the case, especially in a multiparous patient. But this carries a prohibitive fœtal mortality rate and may cause deep lacerations of the cervix and more hæmorrhage and shock ultimately than the procedure is designed to prevent. It is only worth considering if the fœtus is already dead or if the patient is parous with a cervix at least 3 fingersbreadth dilated and where the child is either grossly premature or deformed. Even after pulling down the leg through the vulval outlet it is better to await spontaneous delivery with just sufficient light traction to stop further bleeding rather than to hurry it by unnecessary and dangerous manipulation. If, however, the patient is not in labour and bleeding continues or is profuse at any time and shows no signs of abating, it is safer, provided that the fœtal heart is still present, to omit the diagnostic examination and to proceed forthwith to Cæsarean section in the interests chiefly of the child. The importance, therefore, of having previously excluded fœtal abnormality by X-ray is now obvious. Lastly, if bleeding continues as described above and there is strong presumptive evidence that the baby is already dead, morphia and a blood transfusion should be given in a determined attempt to encourage its arrest. If, in fact, the baby is dead, the bleeding almost certainly will stop in due course, but if not, more active measures, however unwelcome,

may have to be undertaken. Personally, I have not yet been confronted with this last situation.

So far we have only considered the patients who have actually bled, but it must be remembered that a certain number of cases of placenta prævia do not bleed until the cervix starts to dilate or vaginal interference is undertaken. The possible existence of the condition, therefore, should not be forgotten in the course of obstetrical examination, particularly in cases of otherwise unexplained variable lie.

INCIDENTAL AND EXTRAPLACENTAL CAUSES OF BLEEDING

It is to be assumed that bleeding is coming from a portion of exposed placental site unless or until some lesion of the cervix or vagina can be found on speculum examination to account for it. It has already been noted that this examination is usually deferred until five days after bleeding has stopped, but this rule is broken if bleeding persists, or in cases in which it is very slight, and it is hoped to avail oneself of the opportunity of identifying its site of origin before all traces have disappeared.

Most important of the incidental causes is carcinoma of the cervix, which is by no means rare and has a very serious prognosis, since it grows with great rapidity. By observing the above rules, diagnosis will not be delayed more than a few days at the most. The appearance of the cervix is fairly characteristic, and certainly not by any stretch of imagination will it ever look normal. Friable and vascular growth will be seen which bleeds very readily on touching, and a small portion should be removed for biopsy. Microscopy of sections of the cervix in pregnancy can play notorious tricks on an inexperienced pathologist, who can be misled into wrongly diagnosing malignant disease.

Cervical erosions are a fairly common cause of blood-staining in pregnancy, but the hæmorrhage is never more than slight. Although the erosion bleeds on gentle swabbing, it is not friable and, in any doubtful case a small portion should be removed for microscopy. Radical treatment of an erosion is not possible during pregnancy for obvious reasons, and there is no danger in the condition. Nevertheless, some employ superficial cautery as a temporary measure. It does no good.

Cervical polyps, both mucous and fibroadenomatous, are occasional causes of slight bleeding, while fibroid polyps, rarely, may be found. The last-mentioned are very uncommon, because their very existence tends to discourage conception. One is tempted to avulse such polyps by twisting, but this should never be done in the out-patient department, firstly because, as already stated, the examina-

tion should only take place in hospital, and secondly because bleeding may continue from the base after removal. This will always stop in time, but the possibility is enough to discourage one from dealing with polyps in an out-patient clinic.

Varicosities may bleed quite profusely on occasion, especially if traumatised. They are usually situated at the introitus or at the lower end of the vagina, although occasionally they may be found in the vaginal vault. Local gentle pressure will quickly arrest the bleeding.

Occasionally a well-marked vaginitis, particularly trichomonas infection, is found to account for slight bleeding, but usually there is an associated discharge as well. In 16 out of Murdoch's 339 cases a lesion on the cervix or marked vaginitis was responsible for the blood loss.

Many so-called shows of blood are due to rupture of the small vessels in the lower segment decidua, which bleed when the overlying chorion is disturbed in the course of stretching of the segment. This mechanism also accounts for the slight amount of bleeding which often occurs when one passes a finger through the cervix and sweeps the membranes from the uterine wall, as, for example, in surgical induction of labour. Lastly, in a few cases there is a marked decidual reaction in the upper portion of the endo-cervix from which a small blood loss can be provoked by minor trauma.

The history of recent coitus is of very little help in clarifying the diagnosis, since all varieties of antepartum bleeding can be provoked thereby.

ATTEMPTS AT PROVISIONAL DIAGNOSIS

Without the aid of special methods and of examination under anæsthesia, it is only possible to guess in deciding whether the case is one of accidental hæmorrhage or placenta prævia. The history is of only partial assistance. Characteristically, bleeding from placenta prævia is unrelated to activity on the part of the patient and often takes place at night. It is absolutely painless. The only symptoms which can be attributed to placenta prævia are those resulting directly from hæmorrhage and no others. The fact that a patient associates the bleeding with activity or coitus, or that hæmorrhage may have followed external version, does nothing to exclude placenta prævia. Further presumptive evidences of this condition are afforded by the fact that bleeding is often recurrent, although recurrence is not by any means restricted to placenta prævia.

With placenta prævia, the patient's general condition is directly related to the amount of blood actually lost. The uterus is normally relaxed and soft, so that fœtal parts are readily palpable and no areas of tenderness can be found. In about a third of the cases, malpresentation will be observed, and in the remainder the head is usually

not engaged. Often, however, a placenta prævia is very thin; under these circumstances the head may be able to settle in the pelvis, but it is very rare for it to do so deeply. A useful measure is to listen to the fœtal heart at the same time as endeavouring to force the head into the pelvis. If, in doing so, it is found that the fœtal heart becomes slow or irregular, it strongly suggests that the baby's oxygen supply is being pressed upon. This sign is very often found, according to Stallworthy, in cases of posterior placenta prævia, especially with a low insertion of the cord. It bodes ill for the baby in the course of a vaginal delivery, even though the placenta prævia may be only of the first or second degree, and, of itself, is a sound indication for deciding upon elective Cæsarean section. I have often observed this sign, however, in women in whom there was no such abnormality and in whom perfectly safe and normal delivery, without fœtal distress, took place later and I agree with Percival (1959) who reckons that any fœtal heart rate will slow if the head is pushed hard enough regardless of placental situation. The sign, nevertheless, encourages one to carry out placental localization by one specialized technique or another. Lastly, signs of pre-eclamptic toxæmia should be looked for. The association of this complication is no commoner than usual in placenta prævia, but in cases of accidental hæmorrhage it will be found in approximately one-third of the cases. Not only is the presence of toxæmia a pointer in the diagnosis, but because of its own inherent risks, both to mother and child, its discovery may determine treatment.

Bleeding from torn vasa prævia is impossible to diagnose before delivery without special alkali denaturation tests to determine the presence of fœtal hæmoglobin, and is necessarily of small amount. In this instance it is the fœtus and not the mother that is losing blood. The condition occurs as a result of velamentous insertion of the cord in association with placenta prævia. The baby may bleed to death before delivery, and there is no doubt that if, in the course of examination under an anæsthetic, pulsating vessels synchronous with the fœtal heart are palpated through the cervix, the child should be delivered by Cæsarean section, so great is its peril. It is, unfortunately, rare for one to have the luck to make this diagnosis in time to prevent the death of the child.

LOCALISATION OF THE PLACENTA

Considering how often a patient has to be kept in hospital for no other reason than that she might have placenta prævia, it is natural that great efforts are being spent on methods to identify the position of the placental site, short of adopting the obvious measure of passing the finger through the cervix and feeling it, a procedure which,

as already stated, must be deferred until the last two or three weeks of pregnancy.

Radio-isotope Localisation of the Placenta

This method was first used by Browne and Veall (1953) at Hammersmith. Radiosodium in a dosage, which would not now be acceptable, of 50 microcuries was injected intravenously and, with the help of a Geiger Muller counter, revealed the large collections of blood which would normally be found in the placental site as well as the liver and heart. Since that time a number of others have used this as a localising method, e.g. Hibbard (1962) using [132]I, but in nearly all units soft tissue placentography has proved itself more popular. The isotope technique is not without its pitfalls especially when the placenta is situated wholly posteriorly and therefore less accessible to gamma ray counting and because the lower dosages which are to-day acceptable are often insufficient to compete with natural background interference.

Ultrasonic localisation of the placenta can be undertaken several weeks earlier and, with us, this method has become standard practice.[8, 9] Certainly [132]I is a more suitable isotope of iodine than the more traditional ^{131}I with its much longer half-life of a matter of days instead of a few hours; consequently there is no need to block the thyroid of mother or baby with Lugol's iodine and the radiation dose is acceptably low. One nuisance, however, is that the [132]I has to be prepared fresh from tellurium, thus calling for facilities which are by no means universally available.

Technetium 99 is a more recently used isotope for the same purpose and is said to involve the fœtal gonads in no more than one to two weeks natural background radiation dose and about one hundredth that of a single X-ray exposure. It has the advantage of being rapidly excreted in the bladder urine, but this in itself may, by producing a high count at the lower pole of the uterus, tend towards a false diagnosis of placenta prævia. Radiochromium (^{51}Cr) labelled red cells, from donor or patient, can also be used and the isotope does not cross the placenta.

Automatic scanning methods and print-outs are much in vogue, but they are more cumbersome and slower than ultrasonic scanning (see later).

All isotope methods have one thing in common, namely, reliance upon the identification of a pool of maternal blood from which to infer the placental site. They also require the available services of hospital physicists at weekends too. The isotopes have to be ordered and dispensed, and permission to use them has to be obtained through the Medical Research Council; nor can the method be used on an occasional or casual basis and therefore its use is restricted to units

with a reasonably large and stable turnover; in other words the occasional case cannot be undertaken without planning and it is for reasons such as these that the radioisotope methods of locating the placenta have only a limited acceptance, mainly confined to large services with other interests in nuclear medicine as well. I must admit to some prejudice myself, but, to our practised eyes, a well taken ultrasonic placentogram with its clean edges and positive identifiability in the majority of cases, seems greatly preferable to the fluffy mess which sometimes passes for an isotope localisation.[7]

Soft-tissue Radiography

This is a more generally available method which has been employed with increasing success during the last 20 years, although it is not yet universally reliable. As Chassar Moir has pointed out, the radio-opacity of the placenta differs very little, if at all, from that of uterine wall and liquor amnii, so that it requires skilful exposure to reveal it (Fig. 2).[5, 6, 15, 39, 40, 42] Occasionally there is a sufficient degree of calcification in the placenta to make its localisation an obvious matter, but this is unusual. The accuracy of soft tissue radiography is adversely affected by gross obesity, hydramnios and twins, for obvious technical reasons.

This method is best employed after the beginning of the 34th week before which it may be unreliable.

Arteriography

Of all radiological methods this is probably by far the most accurate and, carried out in highly specialised units, gives excellent results with minimum hazard. The necessary expertise, however, is not by any means widely distributed and the procedure has the status of a minor surgical operation at least, since it involves retrograde cannulation of the aorta usually by the Seldinger technique via the femoral artery.[12]

These radiological techniques are described in more detail later in the chapter by Dr. Ellis Barnett.

Infra-Red Thermography

This is a wholly nonsensical method of locating the placenta. It is based on the old idea of localising maternal blood pools to signify the placental site, but differs from the common sense of gamma ray emitting isotopes in relying upon the theory that the overlying skin of the abdominal wall would emanate more heat from an area overlying the placenta and incidentally fat abdominal wall, peritoneum and uterine musculature. The method seems to have crept into the textbook literature without verification. We at least undertook a large trial[26] in a series of 150 patients, and found it useless.

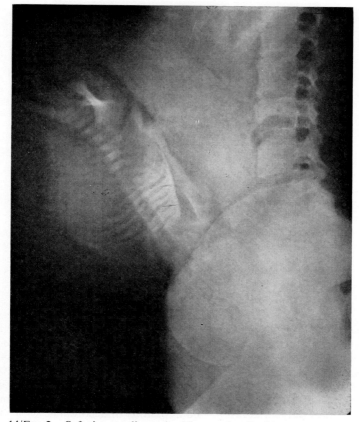

14/Fig. 2.—Soft-tissue radiography. Placenta localised in upper segment
posteriorly.

Ultrasonic Placentography

If one is possessed of a two-dimensional B-scan apparatus (and I
predict that the day will come when all diagnostic units are so
equipped) localisation of the placenta by sonar has enormous
advantages. For one thing the patient is in no way disturbed and can
be examined even in her bed. All that is necessary is to switch on the
machine and smear the abdominal wall with olive oil, and the results
can be obtained within a few minutes. A small quantity of urine in
the bladder is a help in delineating the lower pole of the uterus and its
relationship to the presenting part (Fig. 3). The apparatus must be
very expertly adjusted but the placenta shows up first of all as a
space occupying structure which gradually fills with speckles from

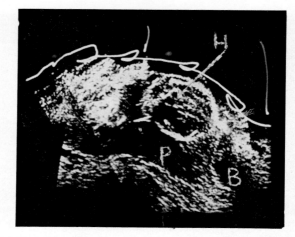

14/Fig. 3.—Posterior placenta prævia, type II, at 37 weeks gestation. Ultra-sonogram in longitudinal section, cranialwards to left, confirmed at Cæsarean section.

B = Bladder
H = Fœtal head
P = placenta.

in front backwards as the time-varied gain-setting of the machine is increased. Furthermore with correct positioning of the scanning direction the fœtal surface can be revealed as a characteristic white line. Our experience at the time of writing now extends to over 400 cases and we only resort to other methods of placentography if clinical evidences throw doubt upon the ultrasonic diagnosis. Some care is necessary in adjusting the apparatus in accordance with the obesity or otherwise of the patient's abdominal wall and it is a wise precaution to take 2-dimensional ultrasonograms in both longitudi-nal, transverse and, if necessary, oblique section before jumping to conclusions.[8, 9, 14]

There could be no more convincing testimony to the average obstetrician's dissatisfaction with fancy and expensive methods of localising the placenta than the sheer number and variety of techniques at present being exploited and to the practical physician no diagnostic method is as reliable as the use of the God-given digit which, un-fortunately, must await the maturity of the 38th week. Nevertheless there is great value in knowing rather than suspecting that a placenta is in fact prævia, or conversely that it is safely situated in the upper segment.[7]

Where placenta prævia can be confidently excluded and where bleeding has been slight and has not recurred, it is permissible to

allow the patient home from hospital, at least until the 38th week. So far we have not had cause to regret this procedure and from the patient's point of view it saves much unnecessary and tedious hospitalisation. In the large series quoted by Crawford and Sutherland (1961) there was a very material difference in antenatal hospitalisation before delivery or vaginal examination without increasing perinatal mortality, which is the acid test. It is, therefore, our practice to confirm or eliminate the diagnosis of placenta prævia as soon as possible and to review the advisability of allowing the patient home at least until the 38th week. If there is any doubt about the position of the placenta or the bleeding has recurred or is more than slight, then we consider it reckless to allow the patient out of our sight. In quite a significant number of patients, nothing further happens and the cause of bleeding is never finally explained. It might be argued that it was unnecessary to readmit them at the 38th week for examination, but we feel that this is a wise plan because any bleeding from, or damage to the placental site must to some extent have, damaged the baby's chances and we are more than ever inclined to take the opportunity not only of checking the accuracy of the placentography, which is usually well over 90 per cent, but we usually rupture the membranes and induce labour at the same time for fear that the baby may outstrip the reserve of an already damaged placenta, whether it be prævia or normally situated.

Notwithstanding the increasing reliance which so many units, including our own, are placing upon this method Macafee (1960) stated that in his hospital placentography had not been carried out for years. He evidently regarded it as both unnecessary and dangerously misleading. If one is going to take this attitude one must do as he did and keep the patients in hospital until safely delivered. It rather depends upon how much store one places on the woman's liberty to be out and about during pregnancy and whether one is prepared to accept with equanimity and in retrospect an unnecessary period of incarceration within an antenatal ward. Safety may be purchased at too high a price. I am indebted to Dr. Ellis Barnett for the following account of radiological localisation of the placenta, as these techniques are likely to be the most commonly used, at least for a few more years.

RADIOLOGICAL METHODS OF PLACENTAL LOCALISATION

by ELLIS BARNETT, F.F.R., D.M.R.D.
Radiologist, Glasgow Royal Maternity Hospital.

The degree of accuracy of placental localisation by radiographic methods, and the resultant saving of valuable bed space, fully justifies the radiologist's contribution to this problem.

The radiological methods of placental localisation are:
1. Amniography.
2. Soft tissue localisation, using plain films.
3. Outlining of the bladder and rectum with contrast medium.
4. Pelvic arteriography.

AMNIOGRAPHY

This procedure involves the injection of a water soluble contrast medium into the amniotic sac, to opacify the amniotic fluid. The patient empties her bladder, and an antero-posterior film of the abdomen is taken to show the position of the fœtal parts. A fine lumbar puncture type of needle is inserted through the anterior abdominal wall in the para-umbilical region under local anæsthesia, in such a position as to avoid the fœtal parts. 40 ml. of liquor amnii is aspirated and replaced by an equal amount of contrast medium (Diodone 70 per cent or Hypaque 60 per cent). The patient is rotated to facilitate mixture of the contrast medium with the liquor. Antero-posterior, postero-anterior, lateral and oblique films are taken as indicated. The placental site is recognised by the finding of a localised area of flattening of the contour of the amniotic sac, and a corresponding thickening of the "uterine wall" (Fig. 4). But this method has fallen into disrepute, largely because the ideal contrast medium has not yet been found which will mix freely with the liquor, will have a high degree of opacity, and yet be completely non-irritant. Even with modern water soluble media there is a likelihood of inducing labour. There is also a danger of damage to fœtal parts. Also, the method rather defeats its own purpose in so far as one would prefer to exclude an anterior situation of the placenta before inserting the needle through the anterior abdominal wall.

SOFT TISSUE LOCALISATION

This is the method of choice in routine practice. One great advantage of this method is that the procedure can be incorporated into the routine examination of patients, and does not necessitate highly specialised apparatus or conditions, or a high radiation dose to the patients.

Before describing this method certain basic facts must be considered, namely:

1. As indicated by Chassar Moir (1944) the radiopacity of the placenta is exactly the same as the liquor amnii, and therefore we cannot actually see the placenta separate from the liquor on a plain radiograph, but can only infer its presence.

2. The placenta in the average case is a large organ covering about one-third of the inner wall of the uterus and radiologically the placental shadow may be as much as seven centimetres thick at its centre.

3. The majority of placentas are implanted on the anterior or antero-lateral, or posterior or postero-lateral uterine wall. Only about 2 per cent are situated mainly on the lateral wall. It follows that in most cases the placenta can be localised on a lateral film only, and therefore this view is by far the most important.

4. Calcification of the placenta in varying degree is not uncommon, appearing as a fine filigree pattern (Fig. 5). Blair Harltey (1954) claims that about 30 per cent of placentas after 32 weeks are calcified to some extent, and this can be demonstrated on a plain film. This statement is undoubtedly true, but with the present accepted trend towards faster films and faster X-ray screens to reduce radiographic exposure to a minimum, placental calcification is less likely to be demonstrated on a radiograph.

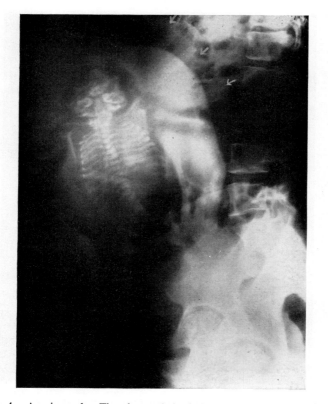

14/Fig. 4.—Amniography. The placental site is indicated by localised flattening of the contour of the amniotic sac posteriorly, with a corresponding thickening of the uterine wall.

From a practical point of view reduction of X-ray exposure is more important than the demonstration of placental calcification. Although the detection of placental calcification will indicate the general placental site, it may not permit the observer to exclude placenta prævia, unless the calcification is extensive, and obviously involving the whole of the placenta.

5. During the last two or three months of pregnancy, and before the onset of labour, the junction of the upper and lower uterine segments

probably lies in the pelvic cavity and within a few centimetres of the brim. For radiological purposes it can be accepted that this junction lies at the level of the pelvic brim. Therefore, any placenta which extends below this level is a placenta prævia, and the extent of encroachment determines the degree.

6. As we cannot actually visualise the placenta as a separate organ but determine its presence by inference, it seems logical that we should delay

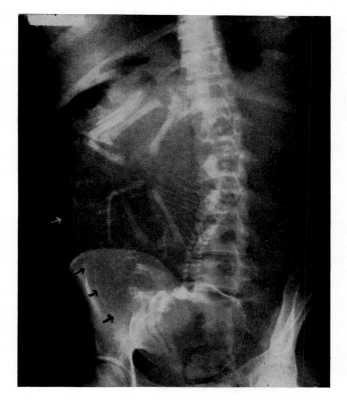

14/Fig. 5.—Placental calcification. Fine filigree calcification in the placenta which is implanted on the right lateral uterine wall.

localisation by the soft tissue method until the pregnancy is well advanced. In other words, until the fœtus is large enough to occupy most of the available space. It is particularly important to delay the examination until the subcutaneous fat line of the fœtus has become visible, thus enabling the observer to differentiate between the fœtal soft tissues and the surrounding liquor. The fat line usually appears at about 32 weeks, therefore, if possible, we prefer to delay placental localisation by this method until the maturity is 34 weeks or more.

7. In a vertex presentation, the occiput tends to be directed towards the uterine wall opposite the placenta. But this occurs only in about one-third of cases, and therefore is not sufficiently consistent to be of value in determining the placental site.

Technique

The following films may be taken:

(a) Postero-anterior film with the patient prone.
(b) An antero-posterior film with the patient supine.
(c) An erect lateral film.
(d) Oblique views. Prone or supine.
(e) Semi-inclined view.

However, the routine use of all these views is neither necessary nor desirable. In practice it is rarely necessary to take more than three views, and, in fact, often only one film, namely, the erect lateral view, will permit adequate localisation of the placenta. At the Royal Maternity Hospital, Glasgow, the initial examination involves the taking of a postero-anterior view and an erect lateral view. These two films will permit not only adequate placental localisation in most cases, but will also give routine information as regards the fœtal lie presentation and position, fœtal anomalies, fœtal maturity and cephalo-pelvic relationships. These two films are examined before any other views are considered and the vast majority of placentas can be localised from them. Sometimes a posterior situation of the placenta may indicate the necessity for a semi-inclined view. This view can be taken with the patient sitting, and leaning backwards, or may be taken with the patient lying supine on the X-ray table, which is then tilted to an angle of thirty degrees from the horizontal. The film is placed at the side of the patient and an exposure made using a horizontal beam (Fig. 6).

From a practical point of view localisation of the placenta may be considered in two stages:

1. Determination of the general placental site.
2. Diagnosis of placenta prævia.

Determination of the general placenta site.—As already indicated, we cannot actually visualise the placenta as a structure distinct from the liquor amnii. Therefore, we can only infer its presence by finding of a part of the uterine cavity which could possibly accommodate such a large organ as the placenta. We do this by noting the outline of the uterine wall on the postero-anterior and lateral views, and consider the relationship of the subcutaneous fat line of the fœtus to the uterine wall on both films. It is usually found that in one part of the uterine cavity there is a fairly substantial gap between the fœtus and the uterine wall. This gap is noted to be thickest at one point, and tapers off above and below. It is inferred that this corresponds with the placental site (Figs. 7 and 8).

Diagnosis of placenta prævia.—Having decided upon the general situation of the placenta, the next step is to determine whether the placenta is encroaching upon the lower segment. i.e. extending below the level of the

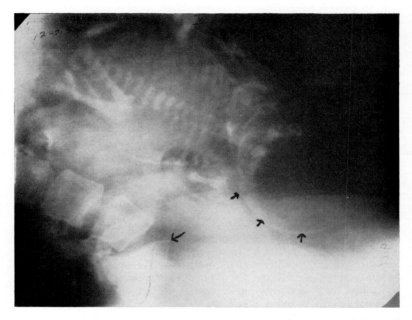

14/Fig. 6.—Semi-inclined view. Posterior placenta prævia. Note the failure of the presenting part to descend into close relationship to the sacral promontory.

pelvic brim. We evaluate this point by invoking gravity as much as possible.

The specific gravity of the fœtus is greater than the liquor amnii, therefore the fœtus will tend to descend to the most dependent part of the uterine cavity in all positions. Thus, in the erect position the fœtus tends to descend into close relationship to the symphysis pubis and sacral promontory. The only structures intervening are:

(a) The thickness of the amniotic lining.
(b) The thickness of the lower uterine segment.
(c) The bladder anteriorly and the rectum posteriorly.

Therefore, if the bladder and rectum are known to be empty, the presenting part of the fœtus should descend to within about $1\frac{1}{2}$ cm. of these bony landmarks. We usually allow 2 cm. as the normal limit for this gap.

Displacement of the presenting part away from these bony landmarks implies the presence of a low lying placenta, and, as a rule, the greater the degree of displacement the greater is the extent of encroachment upon the lower segment (Fig. 9). One can usually deduce the degree of placenta prævia by noting the extent of the shadow on the upper segment in conjunction with the size of the gap between the presenting part and the bony landmarks. The normal presence of air in the rectum can be of value

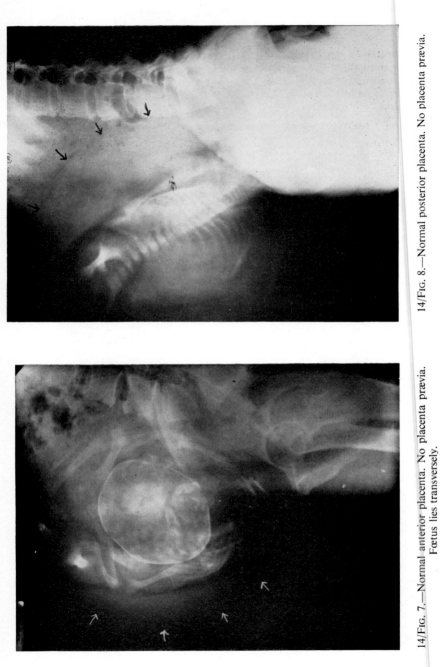

14/Fig. 7.—Normal anterior placenta. No placenta prævia.
Fœtus lies transversely.

14/Fig. 8.—Normal posterior placenta. No placenta prævia.

in the exclusion of posterior placenta prævia, but in doubtful cases the insufflation of air into bladder and rectum, depending upon whether the general placental site is anterior or posterior, can greatly assist an assessment of the degree of low implantation. Insufflation of air permits the lower uterine segment to be outlined clearly in the erect lateral view, and the exact distance between the air shadow and the presenting part is

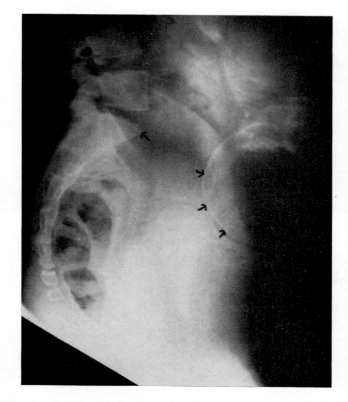

14/Fig. 9.—Erect lateral view. Posterior placenta prævia, grade three. (Fig. 6 shows the semi-inclined view of the same patient.)

shown. This gap should be very small (average measurement is 1·2 cm.), (Fig. 10). As a general rule engagement of the presenting part in the pelvic brim would tend to rule out placenta prævia, but occasionally extension of placenta on to the lower segment may be suspected under these conditions. In these circumstances air insufflation is again useful. Displacement of the presenting part away from the mid line is confirmatory evidence of a low lying placenta (Figs. 11a and b), although absence of this sign does not exclude the diagnosis.

Failure to find a placenta on the upper segment in the presence of displacement of the presenting part from the symphysis pubis and sacral promontory should lead one to suspect a major degree of placenta prævia with almost the whole placenta implanted on the lower segment.

Placenta membranacea is, fortunately, rare, and is likely to be missed using the soft tissue method of localisation. In this anomaly no adequate "placental bed" is evident above the brim and the relationship of the

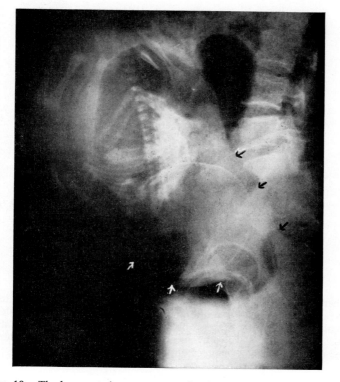

14/FIG. 10.—The lower uterine segment outlined with air in the bladder and rectum. No placenta prævia.

presenting part to the bony landmarks may be normal. A succenturiate lobe of placenta may also cause confusion, but this possibility may be suspected if the shadow above the brim suggests that the whole placenta is situated on the upper segment and yet there is a significant displacement of the presenting part; provided, of course, that the possibility of a pelvic mass such as a fibroid or ovarian cyst can be excluded. Again insufflation of bladder and rectum may be of value, but pelvic arteriography to outline the placental sinuses may be necessary.

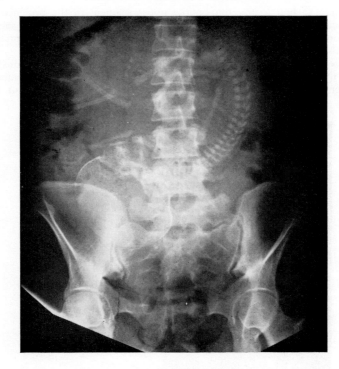

14/Fig. 11 (a).—*See opposite.*

There is no doubt that exclusion of placenta prævia is easiest in the presence of a vertex presentation. A breech presentation introduces difficulties unless the subcutaneous fat around the buttocks is well developed. A transverse lie creates even more difficulty. But no matter the presentation the basic principles outlined still apply.

OUTLINING OF BLADDER AND RECTUM WITH CONTRAST MEDIUM

The use of cystography in placental localisation was first described many years ago (Ude and Weum Urner, 1934). In the original technique the bladder was filled with sodium iodide and the distance between the bladder and the presenting part measured. In placenta prævia the distance is increased by the intervention of the thickness of the placenta and there may be loss of parallelism between the bladder outline and the presenting part, but this procedure is only of use where the placenta is situated on the anterior or antero-lateral uterine wall.

As already mentioned, we have found the simple insufflation of air into

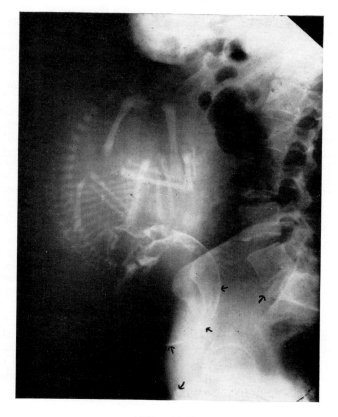

14/Fɪɢ. 11 (*b*).

14/Fɪɢ. 11.—Left lateral placenta prævia. (*a*) The postero-anterior view shows displacement of the presenting part upwards and to the right. (*b*) The erect lateral view shows displacement of the presenting part away from both the symphysis pubis and the sacral promontory.

bladder and rectum to be of value in doubtful cases. The procedure is simple and if performed carefully is considered to be devoid of risk.

Pᴇʟᴠɪᴄ Aʀᴛᴇʀɪᴏɢʀᴀᴘʜʏ

This method involves the percutaneous catheterisation of the femoral artery after the method of Seldinger (1953). A catheter is introduced into the femoral artery through a special cannula, and is advanced into the abdominal aorta until the tip lies approximately at the level of the second lumbar vertebra. This positioning of the catheter will ensure filling of the ovarian arteries, in addition to the uterine arteries, as they may take part in

the blood supply to the uterus during pregnancy (Borell *et al.*, 1963). The femoral arteries are then compressed by means of sphygmomanometer cuffs, to dam back the contrast medium and 25 ml. of 60 per cent Hypaque is injected rapidly, filling the pelvic arteries and eventually outlining the placental sinuses. A single film taken at 3 seconds after the end of the injection, with the patient lying in the true lateral or 5 degree off-lateral position, permits low implantation of the placenta to be accurately diagnosed.

A similar picture can be obtained by the intravenous injection of a large bolus of contrast medium into an antecubital vein. The success of this method depends upon an accurate preliminary calculation of the circulation time.

These methods are not extensively used in this country, largely because such a high degree of accuracy has been achieved using the soft tissue method. Nevertheless, in doubtful cases, particularly with an abnormal lie of the fœtus or where placental localisation is essential in the earlier stages of pregnancy, visualisation of the placental sinuses by injection of contrast medium should be considered.

With some experience a high degree of accuracy of placental localisation can be achieved, using the soft tissue method. For example, in my own Department the analysis of all the cases referred for placental localisation during the year 1961 shows that a correct diagnosis was recorded in 97·6 per cent of 283 cases, errors being confined to seven cases only.

From Dr. Barnett's account it will be seen that there are many pitfalls with which to reckon. Firstly, the placenta may be too thinned out to contribute much of a significant shadow between the fœtal outline and the uterine wall. Secondly, the coexistence of hydramnios spoils definition and confuses the diagnosis. Thirdly, the lax abdominal wall, as in the case of a multipara, may allow the unengaged head too much mobility to permit of a reliable assessment, and, lastly, the presence of any pelvic tumour will, of course, vitiate the results. In the next place it may not be possible to obtain a true profile view of the placenta, especially if there is uterine obliquity or rotation, and, finally, in any but vertex presentations the X-rays are very much less reliable.

It has been suggested[36, 52] that the hazards attendant upon encountering a major degree of placenta prævia when exploring the lower uterine segment with the finger can be eliminated altogether if the radiological diagnosis is accepted.

That such a diagnosis can now be more readily accepted is revealed in the succession of reports which have appeared in the last few years from a number of centres as the technique is more widely adopted, but as far back as 1949 Stevenson, in a large series of cases, demonstrated an accuracy in placental localisation of 95·3 per cent, the mistakes being confined to the lesser degrees of placenta prævia.

Examination under Anæsthesia at the 38th Week

Let us assume that a patient has now reached the 38th week of pregnancy without further serious blood loss. One has the choice of continuing the supervision in hospital until she goes spontaneously into labour at term, with the question of placenta prævia still in doubt, or of making the diagnosis by vaginal examination. The latter course is usually to be preferred, because if, in fact, placenta prævia is present in severe degree, there is little to be gained by sitting any longer on a volcano. On the other hand, fœtal interests may be best served in cases of earlier accidental hæmorrhage by artificial rupture of the membranes at the 38th week because of the higher incidence of stillbirth already discussed.

The examination is conducted in an operating theatre, where the instruments are all laid out in readiness for Cæsarean section should it be necessary. A slow saline drip should be set up in advance. Compatible blood should be available for immediate use if required, and the anæsthetic should be such as will permit proceeding to operation without further delay. It is better not to put the patient in the lithotomy position. I have been badly caught out with a massive hæmorrhage which was provoked in this position and valuable seconds were lost in replacing the patient's legs on the operating table. For the same reason an assistant should be standing by ready gloved to open the abdomen while the surgeon changes his own gown and gloves, in order to save precious time, and blood. If hæmorrhage is really profuse it is tempting to dispense with the examination under anæsthesia altogether and proceed forthwith to Cæsarean section. Occasionally I have been in that much of a hurry, but I can recall a case in which the hæmorrhage was, in fact, coming from some large, torn varicose veins just inside the introitus which was fortunately observed before proceeding to a section which would have been wholly inappropriate.

Our own rules about working only in operating theatres for all surgical procedures, however minor, including, of course, all cases of antepartum bleeding whatsoever the diagnosis, was on one occasion disastrously ignored by a junior colleague who had excellent clinical reasons for diagnosing abruptio placentæ and set out to rupture the membranes in one of our small normal delivery rooms, in which surgical procedures are forbidden. He was greeted with such torrential hæmorrhage from placenta prævia that the patient had a cardiac arrest within a minute or two and before any kind of effective action could be undertaken. The usual three-hour programme of resuscitative techniques was gone through before life was finally pronounced to be extinct.

Another precaution to bear in mind when one's hand is forced into

carrying out an examination under anæsthesia or some vaginal procedure in the acute case with a full stomach, is the danger of passing
a stomach tube in a laudable attempt to reduce the hazards of inhaled
vomit. The placenta prævia case already bleeding may in fact bleed
very much more heavily as a result of gagging with the passage of the
tube and it is far safer to induce the anæsthetic with the patient lying

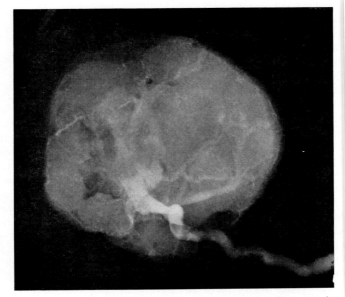

14/FIG. 12.—X-ray of placenta after delivery showing fine granular
calcification.

on her side and to intubate as soon as she is unconscious. Rapid head
down tilt facilities are, of course, mandatory, as in all modern anæsthesia.

While the most important part of the procedure is the presence of
established anæsthesia before starting, the instrument packs for
immediate Cæsarean section should be at hand. The bladder is
drained and the usual aseptic and antiseptic ritual carried out. The
vaginal examination is now made.

The head is pressed into the brim, and first of all the fornices are
thoroughly explored to see if there is any intervening thickness
in the lower uterine segment between finger and the fœtal head or
presenting part. If the head can be felt clearly through all fornices,
one may then proceed to pass a finger through the cervix with increasing confidence. If, on the other hand, a suggestive mass of tissue

is felt through the fornices in the lower segment, one should proceed to the rest of the examination with great deliberateness and care. If there is any difficulty in making a thorough examination, the whole hand should be inserted into the vagina. If the placenta is lying over the internal os, in other words it is of the third or the fourth degree, quite severe bleeding may be provoked at this stage unless one proceeds with great gentleness. The presence of the placenta in this position is not always as easy to diagnose as one would think, and blood clot may easily be mistaken for it. However, on careful palpation the stringiness of the placenta will be observed, which is lacking in the case of blood clot, which feels more friable.

If no placenta is felt over the os, the finger is now passed inside the lower segment and proceeds to explore by sweeping gently in a concentric fashion of ever-widening radius until as much as possible of the region within 3 inches of the os has been carefully investigated.

Furious bleeding may occur as a result of detaching the placenta, in which case the examining finger should be kept within the cervix to act as a temporary plug. This hæmorrhage has plenty of volume but very little pressure, and it is not difficult to hold it in check with the finger *in situ*, unless the cervix is already more than one finger dilated. Cæsarean section must in this case be undertaken at once, and since we have waited patiently until the 38th week the question of prematurity need not further concern us. While waiting for the final preparations for Cæsarean section, the finger should be kept *in situ* as long as the bleeding threatens to continue. The gloves are then changed and the operation is begun. Occasionally it is not possible to control the hæmorrhage by keeping the finger in the cervix, and in this case roll gauze, 6 inches wide, can be quickly packed into the vagina. If this is not immediately available, one should proceed with the utmost expedition to operate. If the placenta is found over the internal os, but bleeding is not provoked, the occasion still demands Cæsarean section forthwith.

Sometimes bleeding is only slight, usually with the lesser degrees of placenta prævia, and, provided that there are no other obstetrical contra-indications, the forewaters should be ruptured. This will bring the head or the presenting part on to the detached placenta, and should very quickly control further bleeding. The patient should now be watched for about ten minutes, to make sure that bleeding is not going to start again, before she is allowed to come round from her anæsthetic and proceed to vaginal delivery. If, on the other hand, artificial rupture of the forewaters does not control the bleeding and the patient is not already in labour, Cæsarean section is undoubtedly the safest course in preference to version, pulling down a leg, or applying Willett's forceps.

If no placenta prævia is felt and no bleeding is provoked, and the

cervix is unfavourable, i.e. like the spout of a teapot, one may decide against rupturing the membranes at this time and return the patient to her bed to await the spontaneous onset of labour.

TREATMENT OF PLACENTA PRÆVIA

It will have been noted that thus far nothing has been done in the actual treatment of placenta prævia, only a conservative policy of "watch and wait" in the hope of getting past the hazards of prematurity. However, there is an account from Scandinavia[13] of an idea first suggested by Løvset, that an encircling suture of the cervix using thick, braided nylon might be used, as in the Shirodkar operation, to prevent the lower segment of the uterus and the internal os from dilating and allowing further separation of the placenta. The patients so treated were thereafter allowed home. I have no experience of such a technique and am not likely to acquire it, because if the patient did not have a placenta prævia, and it is quite likely I might not yet know, the operation would have been unnecessary; if I knew she had a placenta prævia I would be afraid of triggering off a massive hæmorrhage, if one was not already in force demanding evacuation of the uterus in its own right, and even if I succeeded in inserting the suture as suggested I would be terrified to let her home with an established diagnosis of placenta prævia. In fact the dividend of a few weeks extra shopping in the world outside would hardly seem worth the anxiety entailed.

The outlook in antepartum hæmorrhage, in general, has been transformed for the better in recent years, firstly by the ready availability of blood, secondly by the advent of chemotherapy, thirdly by the improved methods of anæsthesia, and, fourthly, by the increased use of lower segment Cæsarean section. Unfortunately Cæsarean section is no guarantee of neonatal survival as babies so delivered in these cases have an increased susceptibility to the respiratory distress syndrome due to hyaline membrane atelectasis.

Most undergraduates have been trained to invoke Cæsarean section in their answers as the last resort in treatment, but in this condition it should be the first. This is not to suggest that Cæsarean section is always the treatment of choice, and we will presently review the indications for the alternative methods. The advantages of Cæsarean section in placenta prævia are that the fœtal prospects are good, that maternal mortality is reduced, the cervix is not torn (a danger to which it is exposed by the increased vascularity as a result of placenta prævia), and, in the end, the patient is delivered as a rule with far less loss of blood. In the five-year period 1955–59 we had 288 cases of placenta prævia with one maternal death and a perinatal mortality of 11·5 per cent. Cæsarean section was carried out in 164 of

them (57·7 per cent). In the first two years after opening the Queen Mother's Hospital we lost only one baby in 32 cases of placenta prævia and the section rate was 84 per cent.

Although the lower segment operation is now almost universally preferred it is as well to beware of two hazards in placenta prævia. Firstly, the placenta, if encountered, should be spared from damage as far as possible because the baby may lose a dangerous amount of blood before the cord is clamped. It is far better to find an edge to the placenta and push it aside in order to extract the baby rather than to cut through it, if this is at all feasible, and in either case because of the danger of fœtal hæmorrhage the cord should be clamped as soon as possible. Secondly, maternal hæmorrhage may be very brisk. The best way of coping with this is to get on with the operation and finish it! Louw recommends packing or ligation of the uterine vessels to control severe bleeding, but fast, determined and accurate suturing of the uterine incision should be adequate in most cases.

Unfortunately the placenta may be morbidly adherent to the lower segment in patches and in the course of trying to separate it hæmorrhage may be very profuse. This is not uncommon and the surgeon is torn between the desire to get the uterus sewn up as quickly as possible and at the same time to satisfy himself that the source of the bleeding from within the uterus has been dealt with before it is shut from view. Having closed the abdomen it may now be seen that a patient is bleeding fairly freely *per vaginam*. Three alternatives have now to be faced; hopeful expectancy, hysterectomy or packing.

Usually the blood transfusion rate is accelerated and the patient is allowed to surface from her anæsthetic, in the hope that with further ergometrine and squeezing the blood out of the uterus all will yet be well and this is often the case, but sometimes bleeding continues or recurs and in my own experience I have met two such cases of the utmost severity. In the first of these, I saw the patient several hours after her original Cæsarean section for placenta prævia and she was now pulseless with a blood pressure of 40/0 mm. Hg and receiving her 14th pint of blood. I was put under great pressure to undertake hysterectomy forthwith, but it was fairly obvious that her condition could not stand such a procedure. She was still bleeding, and under a very brisk and light cyclopropane anæsthetic I packed the uterus firmly from top to bottom with a further reinforcement of ergometrine, trusting to my colleague's suturing. The effect was dramatic and with further blood transfusions she rapidly improved and left hospital fourteen days later none the worse for her experience. The pack was removed after twenty-four hours under morphine and this would appear to be the treatment of choice, as in this case she was a young primigravida aged 27.

A more recent case was a grand multipara in her late thirties who continued to bleed furiously after lower segment Cæsarean section for placenta prævia at the hands of a junior but experienced colleague. He called one of his seniors, who, two hours later, removed the uterus. Her condition, nevertheless, continued to deteriorate although there wasn't much visible bleeding from the vagina. Six hours later her condition was truly desperate and intraperitoneal bleeding was strongly suspected. She was curarised, intubated and put onto intermittent positive pressure inflation, while hypothermia was induced with ice packed round the axillæ and neck. In this condition she hovered between life and death for several hours more and I was invited to see her. I might say here that although there were strong grounds for suspecting continued intraperitoneal bleeding in spite of the perfectly routine hysterectomy, with complete confidence about the integrity of the pedicles, the diagnosis was extraordinarily difficult to make in a frozen patient, totally relaxed under curare. The fearful decision had to be made whether to open the abdomen for the third time in eighteen hours in her present very parlous condition. To be mistaken might well prove disastrous. Her circulating blood volume was rapidly estimated by a physicist using a standard dilution technique with radioiodine and he announced what was, to him, the highly improbable result of 1 litre. Considering the patient's condition I was only too ready to believe this and with the help of one of my ultrasonic machines there could be no doubt that the abdomen was full of fluid, presumably blood. On opening the abdomen there was an enormous quantity of blood everywhere, both retroperitoneal and intraperitoneal, and on examining the pedicles all were perfectly secure, but the raw surface of the bladder and every possible blood vessel in the region of the vaginal vault was streaming blood and it was impossible to overtake the situation by suturing. The condition seemed to be particularly bad on the left side. I therefore ligated the anterior division of the left internal iliac artery, passing an aneurysm needle under it, blind, loaded with strong silk and taking great care not to rupture the underlying internal iliac vein. This did the trick and we had no further trouble. She left hospital seventeen days later with full recovery of her renal function and again apparently none the worse for her terrible experience.

In retrospect I feel that hysterectomy in this case should not have been undertaken and it would have been far better to have packed the uterus firmly and deliberately from top to bottom, but my friend who called me in said that he had had the most tragic experiences from this procedure but, of course, he was referring to the desperate 1930s, when this measure was often undertaken as a last resort in the absence of blood transfusion. This case just described had, in all, 26 pints of blood, which, to date, is my record.

All cases of third- and fourth-degree placenta prævia should be delivered by Cæsarean section, not only in the interests of the mother but chiefly in the interests of the child. In deciding the delivery route, the relationship of the presenting part to the brim is of more importance than the nearness of the placenta to the internal os, and an anterior placenta prævia case can be more safely delivered by the vaginal route than cases where the placenta is posterior. If the head can be made to engage in the brim without upsetting the fœtal heart, it is an additional indication that the membranes can be ruptured safely. As a general rule, therefore, vaginal delivery is nowadays more and more restricted to those cases of the first and second degree, in which the placenta is anteriorly situated.

Local anæsthesia has been recommended by many for carrying out Cæsarean section, but there are several reasons against its use. It is, of course, not applicable for vaginal examination, and it takes too long to induce. Also, it is less easy to operate at speed should this presently become necessary. Moreover, if bleeding continues unabated after extracting the child, it is impossible to resort to more drastic measures, such as packing of the lower segment or proceeding to hysterectomy without waiting for general anæsthesia to be induced.

Occasionally, a patient's condition may be so moribund from hæmorrhage that one may be tempted to defer operation until her condition has been restored by blood transfusion. This procrastination, however, is only permissible if bleeding has already stopped, otherwise matters can only be made worse by every minute's delay. No case is ever so moribund from placenta prævia bleeding as to contra-indicate Cæsarean section. In this desperate emergency, rapid classical Cæsarean section is indicated. I much regret not having done so in a very acute case who died on the table just after the uterus had been emptied and tragedy might, in fact, have been averted by saving even a few precious seconds involved in carrying out the more formal lower segment operation. Clearly I had underestimated the gravity of the patient's acute blood loss and encountered the immediate period of primary shock, the signs of which are described in a later chapter as usually appearing about ten minutes too late.

If the patient when first seen is bleeding and already in labour, a vaginal examination should be made, preferably under an anæsthetic, so as to permit the pulling down of a leg if a foot presents and the placenta is not covering the internal os. If the vertex presents, rupture of the forewaters may suffice. This is particularly useful in the case of the multipara. If this simple measure arrests the hæmorrhage, nothing further should be done to expedite delivery; in fact, any hurry will be positively dangerous because of the risk of tearing the lower segment and cervix and also of increasing shock. Having

ruptured the membranes and brought the presenting part down on to the dilating cervix, there are many who favour increasing the local pressure by the use of a binder. But if a binder is going to be efficient it must be put on so tightly that it embarrasses the patient and may aggravate shock, and is, on the whole, better dispensed with. If this does not arrest the hæmorrhage it is better to apply gentle traction to the leg brought down or, as the case may be, to the vertex by means of a Ventouse cup (vacuum extractor), than to resort to the now discredited Willett's forceps. Slow and very gentle delivery may thus be achieved. This is less traumatic to the maternal tissues in a cervix not yet fully dilated than the ordinary obstetrical forceps. Willett's forceps do far more damage to the baby's scalp and personally I have not used them or seen them used on such a case since before the last war. All the more picturesque and bloody methods of coping with placenta prævia during labour have now gone by the board and one is left fundamentally with the alternatives of Cæsarean section and artificial rupture of the membranes with spontaneous labour possibly assisted by vacuum extraction. Any unit without facilities for undertaking Cæsarean section is not really fit to undertake obstetrics.

General Remarks concerning Vaginal Delivery

Labour must not be hurried. By contrast, the advocates of *accouchement forcé* of a century ago reaped a terrible harvest of disaster, both from increased hæmorrhage and shock. All possible steps should be taken to restore the patient's blood volume in order to improve her chances of surmounting the risks of the third stage. Antepartum anæmia, moreover, predisposes the patient to uterine atony. The third stage is full of possible treachery, and a relatively small blood loss now may tip the scales against an already shocked and exsanguinated patient, so that all possible prophylactic steps should be taken, including the use of ergometrine at the completion of the second stage. Not only are the effects of bleeding more marked in placenta prævia delivery, but postpartum hæmorrhage is particularly likely to occur for the following reasons. Firstly, part of the placental site is in the lower segment of the uterus and, therefore, in a non-retractile portion. Secondly, the placenta which is prævia is usually larger and thinner than usual and, as a result, the shearing mechanism, whereby the mass of the placenta is detached from the uterine wall in the normal physiology of the third stage, fails to operate effectively, and one is then faced with all the evils of a partially separated yet retained placenta. Morbid adherence, too, is not uncommon. Lastly, because the placental site is generally larger, there is a greater area from which bleeding can occur. The patient

cannot be regarded as safely delivered until at least a couple of hours after the placenta has arrived.

Because cervical tears are particularly common, preparations should always be at hand for the proper examination and suturing of the cervix if necessary. The incidence of manual removal of the placenta is somewhat increased, because of morbid adhesion.

Attention to asepsis and antisepsis must be punctilious, because puerperal sepsis is very liable to follow, not from local interference but because the placental site, being both lower in the genital tract and larger than usual, provides a portal of entry which is more quickly reached by ascending infection. Often a certain amount of old blood clot will have been retained in the uterus for a considerable period of time, so that intra-uterine infection may be already established before the completion of labour. The patient, because of her exsanguination, will succumb far more readily to infection in the puerperium than the patient who finds herself after delivery still in possession of nearly all her original blood. All the antibiotics in the world are no substitute for a healthy blood state, and 1 pint of blood is worth several million units of penicillin.

ABRUPTIO PLACENTÆ

There is a dying tendency in the reports from obstetrical departments to classify all cases of antepartum hæmorrhage in which evidence of placenta prævia is not established as cases of accidental hæmorrhage. Such a classification is too wide, because in at least a quarter of the cases of antepartum hæmorrhage an accurate diagnosis of its source cannot be made, and when this is the case such patients should be put in the unclassifiable group.

We are concerned in this section with bleeding from the placental site when it is normally situated wholly within the upper uterine segment. Bleeding can only occur if there is some degree of placental detachment, and for this reason the term "abruptio placentæ" is preferred. The process is bound to leave its effect or scar upon the placenta itself, and, unless the clinical evidences before delivery are overwhelming, these placental signs should be looked for and noted after delivery before regarding the case finally as one of abruptio.

The placenta after delivery shows, in a recent case, a depression, usually with a clot firmly attached to it, or, if some time has elapsed between the abruptio and delivery, evidences of a sizeable area of infarction in varying degrees of organisation. Not all cases of abruptio bleed per vaginam, and there are minor degrees which end in no more than a retroplacental hæmatoma, a condition in which the so-called variety of concealed accidental hæmorrhage occurs in miniature.

Placenta prævia and accidental antepartum hæmorrhage have only one thing in common, namely both types bleed as a result of placental separation, but in all other respects they differ totally. In abruptio, the external bleeding is probably the least important feature of the case, and what matters far more is the degree of associated toxæmia, shock, the amount of blood retained *in utero*, and the area of abrupted placenta. In fact, the greater the amount of external, revealed bleeding, the less wide as a rule is the area of placental separation *in utero*, and, conversely, the most severe cases of concealed hæmorrhage result in practically total placental separation.

Abruptio placentæ, therefore, declares itself as concealed intra-uterine hæmorrhage, in which no blood whatsoever appears at the vulva for the time being, or as revealed external hæmorrhage, in which practically no blood is retained within the uterine cavity. Most commonly, a mixture of the two varieties obtains. The gravity of the case is directly proportional to the amount of blood retained within the uterus, because herein lies the source of severe degrees of shock. The extent to which bleeding is concealed or revealed is determined far more by the tone of the uterine muscle and its ability to expel the blood to the outside world than by the actual quantity of blood lost. If all the bleeding were revealed, the patient's general condition would vary directly with the amount of blood lost, but in the concealed variety the patient's general condition is grave out of all proportion to the blood lost, even including the quantity apparently retained *in utero*, which seldom exceeds 2 pints. It is important, therefore, not to be misled into relating the gravity of the condition to the amount of visible hæmorrhage. In placenta prævia, on the other hand, hæmorrhage is often very much more profuse, and its degree directly accounts for the patient's general condition.

The above categorical statements are almost wholly true but alas not totally so, and the clinical differentiation between unavoidable and accidental hæmorrhage, between placenta prævia and abruptio placentæ, is not always absolute and there may be an overlap. We have all seen cases due to placenta prævia bleeding who have had a hard, tender uterus with retained blood within it and conversely cases of accidental hæmorrhage with surprisingly little pain or uterine hardness that have been due to major degrees of placental abruption.

It is difficult to arrive at a reliable estimate of the incidence of abruptio placentæ, and figures should only be accepted from centres in which definite evidences of abruptio are sought and noted, including examination of the placenta after delivery, and to accept the exclusion of placenta prævia as grounds for classifying the case as one of accidental hæmorrhage is to rate the incidence too high. True,

abruptio is very much less common than placenta prævia—certainly less than half. O'Donel Browne, for example, confining himself to toxæmic antepartum hæmorrhage, gave the incidence as 0·6 per cent. In multiparæ the incidence is 4 times as high as in primi-gravidæ. To some extent, this is offset by the fact that there are more multiparæ and they tend to fall into a slightly older age group, with a consequent general rise in the level of blood pressure, but the inci-dence increases markedly after the fifth pregnancy, and rapidly re-peated childbearing is also a factor. Social factors are undoubtedly important and the frequency of abruptio increases the further down the social scale one searches. Abruptio can occur at any time in late pregnancy, but most commonly does so about the 34th week.

The majority of the genuine cases are of the mixed variety, and the wholly concealed hæmorrhage is fortunately an uncommon, though desperate, emergency.

ÆTIOLOGY OF *ABRUPTIO*

In many instances it is impossible to trace the cause; nevertheless the coincidence of pre-eclamptic toxæmia is by far the most import-ant factor. This, however, is only half the truth, for the majority of cases of toxæmia do not suffer abruptio and, in a certain number, the evidences of pre-eclampsia are first seen after the onset of abruptio and not before it. Proteinuria, for example, is frequently found for the first time after shock has supervened. Patients who are already in hospital under observation for pre-eclamptic toxæmia only un-commonly develop abruptio, and there is some doubt in relating pre-eclampsia to abruptio in deciding which is cause and which effect.[19] The number of cases of known pre-eclamptic toxæmia who abrupt is only moderately raised to 1·6 per cent, as against a normal control rate of 1·07 per cent and in the case of hypertension 2·3 per cent.[17] The issue is further fogged by the fact that antecedent hypertension may be masked, when the patient is first seen, by the development of shock, which lowers the blood pressure. Notwithstanding all this, it is generally accepted as one of the entities of the pre-eclamptic state, and it is probable that many more of these cases would actually develop eclampsia were it not for the fact that the blood pressure is reduced first by the shock of concealed hæmorrhage.

The theory underlying the association of pre-eclampsia is that there is hypertensive spasm of the vessels supplying the placental site which results in capillary anoxia. When the hypertensive spasm wears off, the damaged capillaries are unable to cope with the vas-cular engorgement which follows, and bleeding therefore takes place. Both chronic nephritis and hypertension are associated with abruptio and the mechanism here is probably somewhat

similar. In many cases of abruptio there is no evidence of toxæmia. In this type of case the antepartum hæmorrhage may not only recur during pregnancy but may complicate later pregnancies as well. We are largely in agreement with the view emanating from Liverpool that folic acid deficiency may be a major ætiological factor without overt megaloblastic anæmia being present. Seventy-two out of seventy-three cases of abruptio were found by Hibberd to have this deficiency and we too have found a remarkable reduction in the frequency of abruptio placentæ since concentrating upon the early detection of anæmia of all varieties, including folic acid deficiency. As mentioned in Chapter VI the blood of our patients is examined at every antenatal clinic visit and a small but adequate supplementary dose of folic acid is given along with iron therapy, which is reckoned to be about adequate for the Glasgow diet. In fact most of the cases we now see are among the unbooked, and not only those who have had no antenatal care, but perhaps the even more unfortunate who have had inadequate care outside.

There is probably more to the problem than simply folic acid deficiency as an isolated cause and there may indeed be multiple dietetic factors; for example, in Malaysia no increased evidence of megaloblastic erythropoiesis could be found in association with cases of abruptio placentæ.[49]

The "supine hypotensive syndrome", a condition in which the inferior vena cava is obstructed by the pressure of the gravid uterus in late pregnancy when the patient lies on her back, is thought to be associated with occasional abruptio, as has been experimentally produced in animals. Certainly recumbency in the dorsal position aggravates shock and hypotension after abruptio has occurred and before the uterus is emptied. These cases should always be nursed in the left lateral position.[25, 57]

In a few cases, the cause can be related to trauma and, in these instances, the bleeding is mainly revealed. The commonest type of trauma likely to cause bleeding is that of external cephalic version, particularly under anæsthesia where the anæsthetic has been used as a misguided excuse for the employment of more than customary force. In hypertensive and pre-eclamptic patients, therefore, because of their increased tendency to abruptio, external version is contra-indicated.

Direct blows to the abdomen may also cause abruptio, although it is remarkable how much violence the average pregnant uterus can withstand without suffering this complication. Coitus is occasionally incriminated, and in a few cases the bleeding appears to follow some great psychological shock, though the mechanism of the latter is obscure.

Occasionally the existence of a short cord has been blamed, but

this is only likely to operate as a cause if the patient is in labour with the presenting part advancing. In a few cases, fibroids are held responsible in the same way as they may be regarded as causes of abortion.

Because of the generally accepted influence of multiparity, it has been postulated that sub-involution of the uterus may be a cause. But this, on the whole, is unlikely, because conception in the first place is thereby discouraged. Social factors combined with poor life-long dietary habits are often linked with uncontrolled parity. Lastly, separation of the placenta may follow the sudden release of hydramnios.

PATHOLOGY

The changes in the placenta, as observed after delivery, have already been mentioned, and the freshness of the infarcted area will depend upon the time interval existing since separation.

In the full-blown case of concealed hæmorrhage the uterus is distended to an appreciably greater size than would apply to the period of gestation, and contains a large retroplacental clot which may have tracked beyond the confines of the placental margin and may even have burst into the amniotic sac. The characteristic Couvelaire uterus shows ecchymoses on its serous surface which may be heavily fissured and from which blood may be oozing. Bleeding may likewise occur between the layers of the broad ligament, and the muscle bundles of the uterine wall are heavily infiltrated with extravasated blood and œdema fluid. It is not certain whether the hæmorrhages are entirely due to capillary endothelial damage resulting from hypertension, spasm and anoxia or to the direct effects of some toxin, but it can be easily seen how the uterus itself comes to be atonic, which is one of the features of this condition. In the worst cases of Couvelaire uterus there is usually a blood-clotting defect due to hypofibrinogenæmia. The peritoneal cavity usually contains an appreciable quantity of blood-stained fluid, and occasionally the uterus may actually rupture with profuse intraperitoneal hæmorrhage, although this, considering the damage to the uterine wall, is surprisingly rare. The uterine muscle fibres themselves may necrose in patchy areas, yet the case who recovers appears to suffer no residual uterine structural weakness.

The pathological changes of eclampsia may be found in both the liver and the kidneys, even though the onset of eclamptic seizures has been aborted by the shock of the abruptio. Distant organs often show numerous small hæmorrhages, for example the ovaries, tubes, liver, suprarenals, heart and meninges, while hæmatemesis may result from hæmorrhages in the gastric mucosa and hæmaturia may likewise arise from the damaged kidneys. The disturbance, therefore,

is by no means confined to the uterus, but is more general (Fig. 13). The kidneys are liable to suffer further disaster, either in the form of bilateral cortical necrosis, which is a characteristic sequel of concealed accidental hæmorrhage, and is practically always fatal, or a tubular

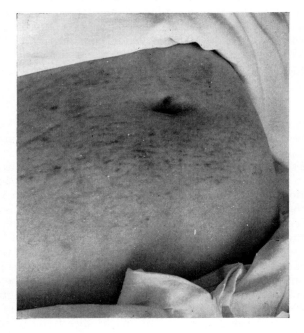

14/FIG. 13.—Purpuric type of rash in a case of abruptio placentæ at 34 weeks, with hypofibrinogenæmia, megaloblastic anæmia, thrombocytopenia and twins. She required 7 pints of plasma and 13 pints of blood. Recovered.

nephrosis may occur as a result of shock. These two causes of suppression of urine and death from uræmia are dealt with more fully in the section on oliguria (Chapter X).

Sheehan's Syndrome

Some cases manage to survive a severe and prolonged period of shock due to abruptio placentæ only to demonstrate later on the signs of anterior pituitary necrosis, namely amenorrhœa, genital atrophy, intolerance to cold, listlessness and premature senility. Murdoch (1962) followed up 94 patients who had severe postpartum hæmorrhage and shock in Glasgow. The follow-up extended up to nine years after the incident and already 11 of them (11·6 per cent) complained of poor health and intolerance to cold although, except

for one patient, amenorrhœa (apart from hysterectomy) was not a feature. The severity of the shock would appear to be less important than its duration and the full-blown picture of hypopituitarism may be delayed until the time of the natural menopause. Conversely Murdoch observed that in 54 cases of Sheehan's syndrome the onset of symptoms had first appeared in almost a half of them between the ages of 41 and 50 years (24 cases) and he reckons that the menopause or an earlier pyrexial illness may act as triggers in the case of latent hypopituitarism from obstetrical causes.

BLOOD COAGULATION DEFECTS

It might not be out of place to consider here briefly the subject of deficient coagulation as it is particularly one of the complications of abruptio placentæ. There are indeed other complications of pregnancy and labour such as amniotic fluid embolism, retained intra-uterine dead fœtus (especially due to Rh-hæmolytic disease) and septic abortion, as will be discussed later, and different mechanisms may operate in producing the ultimate clotting defect according to the causative condition.

The whole subject of blood coagulation has been bedevilled by an inconstant and bewildering terminology, which acts as a "student swamper" and makes the average clinician turn away in frustration and disbelief.

The International Committee for the Nomenclature of Blood Clotting Factors has tied up the terminology in accordance with the table below (*Brit. med. J.*, 1962, **1**, 465), since when two modifications have been made and are herewith included.

These factors have a proven separate identity. So far, in obstetrics, we have only to consider a few, but who knows the degree of complexity with which we may yet have to grapple? There are four major stages in coagulation in some of which groups of the above factors may trigger each other off. The process has, in fact, been likened to a cascade or waterfall phenomenon.

Four Stages of Coagulation

(1) Thromboplastin generation.

(2) Conversion of prothrombin to thrombin.

(3) Conversion of fibrinogen to fibrin.

(4) Later resolution involving the destruction of fibrin by a process of fibrinolysis in order to restore patency to the clotted vessel.

There is thus a balance between clotting and unclotting and since these are both mechanisms which are controlled by powerful enzyme systems, it can be seen how equilibrium can be lost and the whole situation get out of control.

TABLE IV

BLOOD CLOTTING FACTORS

Factor I . . .	Fibrinogen.
Factor II . . .	Thrombin.
Factor III . . .	Thromboplastin.
Factor IV . . .	Calcium.
Factor V . . .	Accelerator globulin, pro-accelerin, labile factor.
Factor VI . . .	Now discarded.
Factor VII . . .	Proconvertin, serum prothrombin conversion accelerator (SPCA), auto-prothrombin I, stable factor.
Factor VIII . . .	Antihæmophilic factor.
Factor IX . . .	Christmas factor, plasma-thromboplastin component (PTC), auto-prothrombin II, anti-hæmophilic factor B.
Factor X . . .	Stuart-Prower factor.
Factor XI . . .	Plasma thromboplastin antecedent (PTA).
Factor XII . . .	Hagemann factor.
Factor XIII . . .	Fibrin stabilising factor.

In obstetrics we are mainly concerned with fibrinogen depletion which may be brought about in one of three ways. Firstly, loss of fibrinogen within a retroplacental clot due to abruptio placentæ. Secondly, intravascular microcoagulation and thirdly, fibrinolysis including fibrinogenolysis.

Hypofibrinogenæmia.—The normal circulating level of fibrinogen in late pregnancy is raised to about 0·45 g. per cent and uncontrolled hæmorrhage occurs if this level falls below 0·1 g. per cent. Many cases of persistent postpartum bleeding in the past were wrongly attributed to the alleged atony of the Couvelaire uterus, when, in fact, they were suffering from hypofibrinogenæmia.

The association between abruptio placentæ and coagulation failure had long been recognised but it was not until Schneider's observations in 1952 that clinicians began to understand the pathology with which they were faced.

At first the generally accepted explanation was that thromboplastins liberated from the retained blood clot or damaged placenta within the uterus, and absorbed into the blood stream, caused widespread microcoagulation throughout the entire vascular tree, too evenly and thinly spread to be clinically noticeable but effectively

using up the available supplies of circulating fibrinogen which the liver cannot replace fast enough. It is known that the uterus and the decidua, as well as the lungs, are important sources of tissue thromboplastins when damaged, and this mechanism of microcoagulation may well, in fact, apply in cases of amniotic fluid embolism and retained intra-uterine dead fœtus.

In abruptio placentæ, however, the observations of Willoughby in this country, Nilsen in Norway and, before these, of Pritchard and Wright in America, have abundantly shown that the loss of fibrinogen from the circulation can, in fact, largely be accounted for by measuring the amount of fibrin within the retroplacental clot. The clot very rapidly retracts, so that its volume at delivery is deceptive simply to naked eye examination. The fluid components from the clot appear to be absorbed and further to dilute the circulating fibrinogen, hæmoglobin and all its other necessary constituents, thereby adding to the patient's anæmia which may become suddenly severe. Coagulation failure is further aggravated. The situation can now be made even worse by the administration of dextran.[44]

It is suggested that quite apart from the factor of fibrinogen dilution by intravenous dextran, the fibrinogen may be precipitated as fibrin or inactivated by forming a fibrinogen-dextran compound. We too have had trouble following dextran infusion in cases of abruptio placentæ and have now ceased to use it altogether. After dextran solutions have been used it is more difficult to cross-match the patient's blood for subsequent transfusion—another though less urgent reason for not using them.

Apart from persistent bleeding, often severe, it will be noticed that the blood is slow to clot, sometimes taking over ten minutes to do so and that a clot once formed often liquefies thereafter on incubation. This, the clot observation test described by Weiner, can be done most cleanly at the patient's bedside simply by withdrawing blood from a vein into a dry test tube.

The diagnosis can be confirmed by the thrombin test (Fibrindex or Thrombin (Maw) on the spot by mixing in a test tube 0·2 ml. each of citrated blood and thrombin solution. Clotting should start within 10 seconds in the case of normal blood and the clot should already be formed within a minute. If clotting takes longer than 20 seconds or the clot liquefies after a minute, severe hypofibrinogenæmia is indicated. The Fi-Test (Baxter) claims specificity by using rabbit antibodies to human fibrinogen combined with polystyrene latex. It is only necessary to add one drop of the patient's whole blood diluted in a glycine-saline buffer (provided) to the antibody reagent and clumping should occur within 20 seconds if normal, but low levels of fibrinogen below 0·1 g. per cent do not clump. No obstetric unit should be without the means of performing this test which, by

indicating the true nature of the patient's peril, may be life saving. It gives only a qualitative rather than a quantitative answer. As soon as possible blood should be sent to the laboratory. Our own practice is to have a stock of labelled tubes containing 1 ml. of fresh 3·8 per cent citrate in the freezing compartment of the matched blood refrigerator. Whole blood from the patient is added to this tube up to the 10 ml. mark and mixed. It is a good plan to take blood from a normal individual at the same time and in the same way. The fibrinogen level can now be very quickly assayed within about 20 minutes by the Schneider test, in which serial dilutions of the patient's plasma are made up in saline and thrombin is added to each tube. The result is read as the highest dilution at which the fibrin clot becomes visible.[56]

In normal plasma clotting should be observed in all tubes up to a dilution of 1 in 128 and certainly 1 in 64, which corresponds to a concentration of about 200 mg. per cent and indicates a safe level of fibrinogen. The clotted tubes are now incubated in order to detect subsequent digestion of fibrin clots. This is one of the main tests which, carried out repeatedly, will indicate whether or not fibrinogen replacement is adequate. A moderate fibrinogen deficiency is revealed at a titre of 1 in 8 to 1 in 32 and severe deficiency may have a titre of 1 in 2, 1 in 4 or no sign of a clot in any of the tubes. A rough and ready guide, however, is immediately furnished as to how much fibrinogen to give the patient in order to correct the defect, and it is recommended that titres below 1 in 8 to 1 in 32 require at least 4 g. of fibrinogen and titres even lower of 1 in 8 require 8 g. initially. The test should be repeated every hour or two to ensure that a safe level of circulating fibrinogen is being maintained. The actual estimation of fibrinogen level requires a complicated laboratory technique, and takes several hours to complete.

Some years ago I saw a case who was admitted with a severe degree of abruptio and delivered herself shortly thereafter of a stillborn fœtus. In spite of a reasonably firm uterus and intravenous ergometrine she continued to bleed after the delivery of the placenta. She required in all one pint of dextrose (at the beginning of the drip), seventeen pints of blood, two of plasma and a further pint of quadruple strength plasma when the diagnosis of hypofibrinogenæmia became known. Her fibrinogen level was estimated as quickly as possible and found to be at the danger level of 0·1 g. per cent. It was the quadruple strength plasma which saved the day and she left hospital well some days later with a satisfactory urinary output, a hæmoglobin level of 10·8 g. per cent and a fibrinogen level of 0·35 g. per cent, thanks to prompt and massive transfusion (through three drips) which kept just ahead of severe and irreversible shock. Today we would have been a little quicker off the mark in recognising the existence of hypofibrinogenæmia.

In the cases who get over this dire emergency the liver quickly restores the fibrinogen level, often within 48 hours.

The treatment, as soon as the diagnosis is made, is to inject pure fibrinogen 4–8 g. intravenously, or, if that is not immediately available, double, triple or even quadruple strength plasma. One bottle of plasma contains 1·1 g. of fibrinogen so that two bottles of double strength plasma will supply 4·4 g. and should suffice to counter hypofibrinogenæmia in most cases. Whole blood should of course be transfused as well to make good the blood lost. Where massive transfusion is necessary, as it often is, the amount of citrate acquired by the patient may be excessive and it is advisable to give calcium gluconate up to 2 g. intravenously to counter the citrate effect. Fibrinogen is nowadays more readily available and is certainly preferable to plasma because it is possible to correct a deficiency rapidly and by infusion of a smaller volume of fluid.

Some have referred to this as the defibrination syndrome and certainly the loss of fibrinogen is the most important cause of coagulation failure in obstetrics, but other deficiences must also be looked for as soon as time allows, for example low platelet counts, low levels of factor VIII (antihæmophilic factor), factor IX (Christmas factor), and factor V (proaccelerin). The platelet count is particularly important in cases where hypofibrinogenæmia is due to abnormal fibrinolysis, which is discussed presently. The latter does not lower the platelet count of itself and the loss of platelets is probably due to a severe degree of intravascular clotting, for example, in the pulmonary bed and, in fact, one may be dealing with a case of amniotic fluid embolism whose mechanism differs from that of abruptio placentæ.

At one time we held the view that the defibrination syndrome could not be reversed until after the uterus had been evacuated, because it erroneously seemed to us that as long as thromboplastins were being absorbed, any circulating fibrinogen was likely to be deposited further as fibrin; but any persistence of hæmorrhage in cases of abruptio in those days was in fact due to inadequate treatment, rather than to the above mechanism.[55] Such a state of affairs may in fact be true with intravascular microcoagulation as may occur after amniotic embolism, but is certainly not true of abruptio placentæ where the urgent need is to replace fibrinogen lost within the retroplacental clot, and adequately treated hypofibrinogenæmia can be permanently corrected by an adequate infusion of fibrinogen. In fact, as Willoughby has pointed out, the very reason that such an improvement can be achieved and maintained in circulating fibrinogen levels supports the conclusion that the condition was due to a straight subtraction effect of lost fibrinogen. In the cases he describes, clotting abnormalities were not in fact accentuated by the administration of fibrinogen and furthermore there was no postpartum hæm-

orrhage. The term "consumptive phase" of fibrinogen has been used to signify that the process of fibrinogen depletion is continuing, usually from a different pathology from what is found in abruptio placentæ, and it is therefore as well to know when, as Scott (1968) has remarked, giving fibrinogen during this phase is like attempting to rebuild a house on fire instead of summoning the Fire Brigade.

It is important to recognise the cause of the hypofibrinogenæmia with which one is faced, because if there is a continuing "consumptive phase" it is likely to be due to the digestion or fibrinolysis of intravascular microcoagulated deposits of fibrin, and stoking up with more fibrinogen will only prolong and aggravate the process. As this hardly happens at all in abruptio placentæ, the question of fibrinolysis and antifibrinolytic agents should not therefore feature in the treatment. The situation is altogether different with amniotic embolism and retained dead fœtus, and in differentiating the various mechanisms the clinical recognition of the likely cause will be of far more benefit than a whole battery of laboratory tests.

Fibrinolysis can include fibrinogenolysis and split products of fibrinogen in themselves may accentuate a clotting defect. Further fibrinogen supplying yet more plasminogen, where activator is still circulating, may magnify and prolong the lytic effect. But more important still perhaps is to recognise that fibrinolysis is a physiological phenomenon designed to restore the patency of the affected blood vessels and as long as the process does not get out of control the effects are entirely beneficial. To reverse them therefore with antifibrinolytic agents may turn a case of incipient recovery into disaster.

I bitterly recall the tragic fate of a patient who represents one of my Cæsarean fatalities. She had a bad obstetric history, hydramnios, a high head and an irregular fœtal heart without demonstrable radiological abnormality. She was well into her thirties and, for better or for worse—worse as it happened—I sectioned her and delivered a healthy baby without incident except for the massive escape of her excess liquor amnii. She must have got an amniotic fluid embolism, because shortly after an apparently normal recovery from her anæsthetic she collapsed with obvious signs of hæmorrhagic shock. On reopening the wound there was total failure of hæmostasis at all levels from the skin downwards and complete absence of clotting. The fibrinogen level was apparently nil and huge quantities of triple strength plasma and fibrinogen were given urgently; in fact, the equivalent of thirteen pints of blood, although hæmorrhage itself had not been excessive. The fibrinogen levels were restored to normal within a few hours and there was no further clinical evidence of bleeding, but her condition progressively deteriorated in spite of the treatment and with steadily deepening cyanosis and clinically solid lungs she died in an oxygen tent, within a few hours. At that time

E.A.C.A. was new to us and we tried it although she was not now bleeding, but she died an hour or two later. Looking back, I think the fibrinogen deficiency must have been due to pulmonary intravascular microcoagulation and that the E.A.C.A. simply prevented the fibrinolysis which might have given her at least a chance. The amniotic embolism was obviously the trigger that set off the whole train of biochemical events, but was not of itself the cause of her deepening cyanosis since the pulmonary signs only developed hours later and after the fibrinogen levels had been restored.

Excessive Fibrinolysis as a Cause of Hæmorrhagic State

Normally, if fibrinogen is present in sufficient quantity it is converted under the influence of thrombin to fibrin monomer which then polymerises to fibrin polymer and this in turn gelates to a firm and visible clot. This is the final stage in the complex business of blood clotting. There might, of course, be no end to this process if it once started inside vessels and theoretically the whole vascular tree could become blocked up by continued propagation of clot were it not for the natural anticlotting mechanisms which exist and are due to fibrinolysin, now better known as plasmin, whose function is to prevent excessive clotting and to maintain the patency of the vascular tree throughout the body. Plasmin does not normally exist in a free and active state, but is derived from a normal plasma globulin called plasminogen. This plasminogen has to be activated by an enzyme known as an "activator" in order to be converted to plasmin. These activator enzymes are present in very small quantities in plasma but in large quantities in damaged tissues, particularly lung, uterus, prostate, thyroid and brain. Major trauma to such tissues or any event which causes their liberation into the blood stream in large quantities will therefore cause plasminogen to be converted into this fibrinolytic substance plasmin. This is fairly unlikely to happen in abruptio placentæ which is promptly treated by rupture of the membranes, but occurs more readily in amniotic fluid embolism as already stated and in the gradual absorption of thromboplastins which can occur with a retained intra-uterine dead fœtus. These activators can also be produced by bacteria, for example, streptokinase and staphylokinase. Such activators, which could theoretically be extremely dangerous in undermining any clotting process, are excreted in the urine as urokinase. It can be seen that plasmin, once liberated, could undermine all clot repair of damaged blood vessels and get completely out of hand were it not for the fact that normal circulating plasma contains antiplasmins which neutralise the fibrinolytic plasmin. The plasmin gets into the clot all right and helps to digest it by becoming absorbed on to the fibrin molecules, but the antiplasmins do not reach them so easily. In this way the fibrinolytic effect is to

some extent restricted to the site of actual clotting. Now the action of plasmin is to digest fibrin into soluble polypeptides and therefore ultimately to destroy clot and restore the patency of the affected blood vessel. This action is to be seen *in vitro* when a patient suffering from a hæmorrhagic state due to this cause has blood which, at first, clots in a test tube and then presently the clot dissolves again, a clinical observation of considerable importance. This would make the diagnosis of an abnormal fibrinolytic state of the blood fairly easy were it not for the fact that plasmin also digests fibrinogen and factors V and VIII (antihæmophylic factor) so that an abnormal fibrinolytic state may in certain instances be associated with hypofibrinogenæmia, but not always. This distinction may be important in treatment.

Fibrinolysis may thus be primary or secondary following intravascular clotting. A platelet count and plasminogen assay may help to differentiate between the two because thrombocytopenia indicates intravascular coagulation with secondary fibrinolysis, but marked plasminogen depletion, being due to conversion to plasmin and utilisation as such, is common to both. Unfortunately this assay is a lengthy business and not likely to be of much immediate help to the obstetrician. Theoretically at least if the trouble was primarily one of intravascular coagulation the treatment, paradoxically, would be heparin rather than an antifibrolytic agent. Heparin acts by direct antagonism of thrombin.

As long as the mechanism of a patient's defibrination remains in doubt antifibrolytic agents should be given with great caution.[11] In deciding the appropriate treatment for such cases, other than abruptio placentæ where the issue is direct and clear, it may be of some help to consider which feature of the case is the more worrying, either the hæmorrhage or the cardiopulmonary embarrassment. Of the two, the latter is probably the more dangerous in amniotic fluid embolism.

Fibrinolytic Inhibitors.—This reaction of converting plasminogen to plasmin under the influence of the liberated activators from damaged tissue can, however, be inhibited by competition from certain natural amino-acids, such as lysine and even more effectively by the less toxic synthetic amino-acid known as epsilon amino caproic acid (E.A.C.A.). Not only does this substance inhibit the activators of the plasminogen to plasmin reaction, but in high concentrations it also directly inhibits plasmin itself in its action upon fibrinogen and fibrin. E.A.C.A. is excreted in the urine rapidly and is also absorbed to a full extent within two hours of administration by mouth, but in many of the hæmorrhagic emergencies in which its use is indicated it is better administered intravenously. A loading dose of 4 to 6 g. is first given and then this is followed on the basis of 1 g. per hour to replace excretion. It can be given with normal saline, 5·5 per

cent glucose, or Ringer's solution, but not with fructose. As a general rule it should not be given in the existing presence of hypofibrino-genæmia until that has been permanently corrected, in which case it may not now be necessary and its use really is confined to cases who demonstrate a continuing clotting defect despite a level of 200 mg. per cent of fibrinogen.

If fibrinogen levels are not reduced and one is confronted with a hæmorrhagic state in obstetrics due to some clotting defect, it will be obvious that to go on pumping fibrinogen into the patient either in the form of triple strength plasma or as pure fibrinogen is only adding fuel to the fire and that what is wanted is something that will inhibit the activators released from the damaged tissues and which are con-verting plasminogen to plasmin. Emptying of the uterus, of course, removes these activators from further absorption into the circulation. For intravenous use a sterile solution containing 5 g./100 ml. is dripped in over 15 to 30 minutes, and the rate of administration there-after reduced to about 1 g. per hour. Oral doses should be dissolved in fairly large quantities of water, but are not likely to be used in the kind of emergency we are considering.

Trasylol is another inhibitor of protein splitting enzymes and thus an antifibrinolytic agent. It is relatively non-toxic apart from occasional urticaria and is rapidly excreted, having a biological half-life of only 150 minutes. It must be given intravenously. Each 5 ml. ampoule contains 25,000 units and 2 ampoules may be given straight away and the infusion thereafter maintained. It acts as a competitive inhibitor of plasminogen activator and also of plasmin itself. It has the advantage also of interfering with thromboplastic degeneration thus producing an anticoagulant effect early on in the coagulation process, so it has the advantages of being both anticoagulant and antifibrinolytic. However, as with E.A.C.A., it is unwise to use it unless the true nature of the coagulation defect is thoroughly under-stood.

These are powerful and interesting drugs, but the clinician who is not backed by a very competent and advanced hæmatological service would do well initially to concentrate on the fibrinogen needs of his patient.

Mortality in *Abruptio*

There is no doubt that under modern conditions the maternal prognosis is appreciably worse than in the case of placenta prævia correctly treated. In 100 toxæmic cases of antepartum hæmorrhage quoted by O'Donel Browne, 7 patients died, and, in spite of im-proved resuscitative facilities, more enlightened obstetrical care and antibiotics, the usual maternal mortality in the more genuine and

serious cases of abruptio is probably not far short of about 7 or 8 per cent. The principal cause of death is shock, and any delay in the treatment of this grave emergency will magnify its influence. In some instances it is very difficult to correct shock, so that active measures have then to be undertaken too late and ill-advisedly when the patient is in even worse condition to withstand them.

It is commonly said that the incidence of postpartum hæmorrhage is no greater than normal after abruptio, but this is misleading, and even a small loss of blood following delivery may be enough to pre-cipitate collapse in a patient whose state was previously parlous. The most torrential postpartum hæmorrhage I ever encountered was in a case of severe abruptio placentæ, and the story is worth telling as a warning of what may happen if delivery is effected in the presence of complete uterine atony. The patient had a minor degree of pelvic contraction and a large baby weighing approximately 10 lb. After a normal and fairly rapid first stage, she failed to deliver herself in the second, and the head became arrested in the high mid-cavity of the pelvis. I decided to deliver her with forceps, and the anæsthetist ran into a lot of trouble during the induction. I happened to notice that the patient's finger-nails looked very blanched and asked one of my students to take her pulse. After what seemed a long time he stated that he could not be sure, but that it was cer-tainly over 200. The midwife in attendance felt the uterus and assured me that she was having a "terrific pain" and, fearing the onset of uterine rupture, I made haste to deliver the patient with forceps. At this stage there had been no external bleeding. It proved a difficult delivery and, considering the very powerful contraction of which I was assured, I was surprised that so much traction was necessary to deliver the head. The baby was stillborn on arrival and almost immediately afterwards a large bulge appeared at the vulva, so that I thankfully prepared to receive the placenta. Instead, an enormous clot came out of the vagina, and there followed a hæmor-rhage the like of which I had read about but had never previously encountered. Nowadays, whenever I see petrol being poured in-correctly from a 2-gallon can, I am reminded of this particular post-partum hæmorrhage, which exactly resembled it. Manual removal of the placenta was a matter of seconds, but the hæmorrhage continued unabated. Bi-manual compression of the uterus was unsatisfactory, because it was so soft that I could not feel what I was compressing, nor was the fundus anywhere to be found. Intravenous ergometrine and pitocin were likewise disappointing, and only a hot intra-uterine douche, coupled no doubt with the patient's extreme hypotension, saved the day. She recovered, and I am thankful that we subsequently had an opportunity to deliver her of a living child by Cæsarean section. In retrospect, it is clear that this patient suffered a massive

concealed hæmorrhage from abruptio, hence the hardness of the uterus mistaken for a uterine contraction, and that I had delivered her in the presence of complete uterine atony.

Another cause of death is suppression of urine, and a very careful watch for diminished urinary output must be maintained both before, during and after delivery. Lastly, these cases may easily succumb from puerperal sepsis, not only because of the need which may arise to intervene, but chiefly because the patient's resistance to infection, as a result of blood loss and shock, is greatly diminished.

The fœtal mortality is also seriously affected by abruptio, and even in revealed cases of bleeding it is hardly better, and often a good deal worse, than the mortality in cases of placenta prævia, and is certainly not as a rule less than 20 per cent. The mortality is very largely influenced, in addition, by the co-existence of pre-eclamptic toxæmia, and prematurity takes its toll during the neonatal period. In concealed hæmorrhage the stillbirth rate is very high, being about 75 per cent even in the milder cases, but in severe cases it is not far short of 100 per cent, and only immediate Cæsarean section carries any prospect of securing a live child, whose hold on life for the first few days may continue precarious from atelectasis, prematurity or both.

THE CLINICAL STATE

Occasionally there are premonitory symptoms, such as cramp-like pains in the abdomen and a small amount of vaginal bleeding, so that the onset of labour may be inferred, but the majority of cases present acutely. The primary symptom is that of abdominal pain to to which bleeding is mainly secondary. By contrast, bleeding due to placenta prævia is always painless. In the most severe cases abdominal pain is agonising and shock is profound, but all gradations of severity may be met, depending upon the amount of blood retained and concealed within the uterus. In the less serious cases pain may not be complained of, but palpation of the uterus will always elicit an area of tenderness.

If revealed bleeding is copious and yet the patient has neither pain nor tenderness, it is very unlikely that the case is one of abruptio, and a presumptive diagnosis of placenta prævia will be made.

As already stated, the level of blood pressure may be misleading because the immediately antecedent level may not be known, and a blood pressure which drops precipitately from 190 to 110 mm. Hg systolic can be just as much associated with shock as one which has dropped from 110 to 70 mm. Apart from this source of error, however, the usual signs of shock are present in varying degree.

The abdomen is tense and the abdominal wall appears to be very

rigid, while the uterus itself has the well-known hard "wooden" consistency, together with great tenderness, so that in severe cases it is quite impossible to identify any fœtal parts or to determine the presentation. If the case is seen early enough this wooden hardness may be seen to develop within about half an hour. This hardness of the uterus is a remarkable phenomenon when one considers that it is in a state of acute atony which is by no means due to the mechanical distension of its cavity with blood clot, because the membranes on vaginal examination are not found to be bulging under pressure. In most instances the fœtus is already dead, and in any case in which more than one-third of the placenta is abrupted fœtal death is inevitable. If the patient is seen almost immediately after the onset of concealed hæmorrhage, the fœtus may yet be alive, and every now and then can be saved by prompt Cæsarean section, but such good fortune is unusual.

Other evidences of pre-eclamptic toxæmia may be present; for example, there may be œdema, but this is variable and is only noteworthy in about half the cases. The bladder should be catheterised and the urine examined, not only for albumin, but its quantity, specific gravity, and the presence of casts or blood should be noted. In the majority of cases albumin is present, but if associated with a concentrated scanty amount of urine, it may be a shock phenomenon and is not necessarily indicative of pre-eclampsia. Shock albuminuria is probably due to renal anoxia, and can be distinguished from pre-eclampsia by the fact that it usually disappears within 2 days after delivery, whereas pre-eclamptic albuminuria tends to persist for longer.

So great and continuous may be the patient's pain that it is impossible to tell whether or not labour has actually started without resorting to a vaginal examination, and there should be no hesitation in performing this, after adequate sedation with morphia has been achieved, in order to identify the fœtal lie and to confirm the prospects of expeditious vaginal delivery.

If signs of cervical dilatation are already present, so much the better, since the patient who is in a state to initiate spontaneous labour has a far more favourable prognosis. The worst cases are those in which pain is severe and hæmorrhage slight or absent.

DIAGNOSIS

The diagnosis of abruptio is not usually difficult, and the history of pain associated with bleeding should make one think of it first. The fact that bleeding may be recurrent does not exclude the possibility of abruptio, since the full-blown attack may be preceded by warning hæmorrhages. Co-existing signs of pre-eclamptic toxæmia

make the diagnosis more likely, although cases of placenta prævia may be incidentally associated with toxæmia. The essential part of the diagnosis depends upon examination of the abdomen for uterine hardness and tenderness, which may be either localised or generalised. The size of the uterus, the height of the fundus and the abdominal girth should all be recorded at the first examination, because an increase in uterine size will accompany and indicate a deterioration in the patient's condition due to the accumulation of still further concealed bleeding.

It is less likely that the diagnosis will be missed than that other abdominal catastrophes will be wrongly attributed to concealed hæmorrhage, and I have myself made the classic mistake of diagnosing a ruptured appendix in late pregnancy as a case of abruptio. By the time I had changed my mind and decided to operate it was already too late, and the patient died before active measures could be undertaken. The patient in question was a young primipara at about the 30th week in pregnancy, who had been admitted a few days previously with signs of pre-eclamptic toxæmia. She collapsed with acute abdominal pain, had a rigid board-like exquisitely tender abdomen, while the fœtal heart could not be heard, and it is depressing to reflect that one could easily repeat the same mistake. She was treated with morphia and blood transfusion which availed her nothing, and at necropsy there was generalised peritonitis.

A ruptured uterus may simulate concealed hæmorrhage, since both produce severe continuous pain and shock, and in both there is likely to be at least some revealed bleeding *per vaginam*. A history of previous classical Cæsarean section complicated by a septic puerperium would, of course, bring this possibility to mind, but uterine rupture can occasionally occur spontaneously in the previously intact organ, especially in grand multiparity. If the patient is fairly obese, it may be very hard to distinguish between the two, but the presence of albuminuria may be of some help in indicating concealed hæmorrhage, and a blood pressure higher than the state of shock would suggest may also be a help.

A retroperitoneal hæmatoma in the broad ligament may simulate a concealed hæmorrhage, but, in this instance, the uterus is pushed to one side and is not itself tender nor necessarily hard in consistency, although the area over the hæmatoma is acutely painful.

A hæmatoma of the rectus abdominis muscle is by no means rare and may produce the pain, shock and abdominal signs of abruptio, but there is no vaginal bleeding, the fœtal heart is not affected, evidences of pre-eclampsia are absent, and the uterus itself is of normal consistency.

Acute hydramnios may have to be considered, but there is no vaginal bleeding and no shock. The fœtal heart can usually be

heard though sometimes with difficulty and sonar puts the matter beyond all doubt.

Volvulus of bowel and the rupture of any of the hollow viscera must also be taken into account in the differential diagnosis. These matters are more fully dealt with in the chapter on acute abdominal pain in pregnancy. Rarities, such as a ruptured splenic aneurism, may enter the diagnostic field about once in a practitioner's lifetime.

Acute pyelitis should not be mistaken for this condition, because it is associated with fever, usually with pyuria, and the pain is situated more to one side than the other. In spite of all that has been said so far in this chapter, placenta prævia may be diagnosed when in fact the case is one of abruptio, even after vaginal examination. The common mistake here is to palpate a boggy mass of clot within the lower uterine segment and, because of the hæmorrhage which is likely to accompany the examination, further identification of the mass is forgone, and it is assumed that one is feeling the placenta itself. But even fairly well organised clot should not be mistaken for placenta, because the latter is definitely stringy and is not broken up by the examining finger. What makes the differential diagnosis of concealed hæmorrhage so serious a matter is the fact that most of the conditions with which it may be confused call for very definite lines of active treatment, as witness the disastrous case above described, whereas in the majority of cases of concealed hæmorrhage conservatism applies.

MANAGEMENT OF *ABRUPTIO PLACENTÆ*

In the case of revealed hæmorrhage, in which there is very little abdominal pain or tenderness, it is impossible at this stage to diagnose abruptio, and, in fact, a presumptive diagnosis of placenta prævia bleeding will be made and the treatment will follow the lines outlined earlier. In other words, if morphia, complete rest in bed and blood transfusion, where necessary, result in a cessation of bleeding and an improvement in the patient's general condition, she will be kept in hospital until such time as proper examination can be carried out, including, if necessary, examination under anæsthesia later, as in the routine treatment and observation of placenta prævia. If, on the other hand, bleeding continues, it is almost certain that labour will supervene, and on the indication of hæmorrhage alone it will be necessary to examine the patient under an anæsthetic in the operating theatre. If this examination reveals that the cervix is already dilating, all that is necessary is to rupture the membranes, after which delivery will proceed even more expeditiously and the use of oxytocin is seldom necessary.

If, on the other hand, the cervix has not started to dilate and the

fœtal heart is still present, it is safer to perform Cæsarean section forthwith, regardless of the variety of continuing antepartum hæmorrhage. In the rare cases in which artificial rupture of the membranes fails to control bleeding in the already labouring patient, Cæsarean section is preferable to vaginal manipulations designed to extract the child before full dilatation, but this is a rare combination of circumstances.

When signs of concealed hæmorrhage predominate over those of revealed external bleeding, the first requisite is to restore the patient's general condition as soon as possible and before labour supervenes. To this end, morphia 15 mg. (gr. $\frac{1}{4}$) is given to relieve pain and reduce restlessness, the patient is nursed on her left side to prevent aggravating the hypotension by the weight of the gravid uterus on the inferior vena cava, and blood is transfused. The amount of blood is varied according to the case, but it is reasonable to give up to a litre at once, followed by slower transfusion, being guided by the patient's pulse rate which falls as adequate replacement is achieved. Most cases are seriously undertransfused. These patients are severely hypovolæmic at first and respond with vasoconstriction. Therefore vasoconstrictor drugs are neither necessary nor indicated and the first attack should be on the reduced circulating blood volume. This results in a low venous return and consequently a low cardiac output. The only way to get rid of the vasoconstriction which, of course, is protective only to the brain and heart, is not to aggravate it by giving vasoconstrictor drugs but to get rid of the stimulus by restoring the blood volume. I have toyed with the idea of buying expensive apparatus for measuring circulating blood volumes by isotope dilution or dye dilution detectors, but these emergencies don't tolerate much waste of time and the best gauge of adequate restoration of blood volume by transfusion is the measuring of the central venous pressure. As O'Driscoll and McCarthy describe it the method is simple, costs no time and can be combined with massive transfusion using the same apparatus. The aim is to go on transfusing until the central venous pressure is elevated to 10 cm. of water. This is more important even than early delivery. Furthermore blood volumes below 60 ml. per kg. body weight indicate a critical state and below 40 ml. give warning of likely renal failure unless hypovolæmia is urgently corrected within the next two or three hours.[50]

The size of the uterus is noted and repeatedly checked, for it may be increasing, and the blood pressure and pulse are recorded every half-hour. No full-blown case of abruptio placentæ should receive less than a 2 litre blood transfusion. Many will require much more. In this condition blood accountancy never makes sense and the patients always require very much more than can ever be accounted for by hæmorrhage, revealed and concealed.

By far the majority of cases will respond dramatically to this treatment, and, in most cases, labour supervenes within the next 12 hours.

Because of the patient's extreme pain, which is continuous, it is
often difficult to know with certainty when labour has started, but
increasing restlessness is an indication. The appearance of blood at
the vulva in renewed amount signifies, at least, that the uterus has
some contractile power, otherwise the blood would have remained
concealed, and at this point it is worth making a vaginal examination, because the unremitting hardness of the uterus makes it impossible to observe rhythmical labour contractions.

At this stage, if not before, the membranes should be ruptured
artificially, after which labour usually proceeds apace. We used to
advise against too early rupture of the membranes while the uterus
was still allegedly atonic because of the fear that the escape of liquor
would be replaced by more blood lost into the uterine cavity, ren-
dering the last state of the woman worse than the first.

It is now realised, however, that the longer the delay between
abruptio and delivery the greater the liability of afibrinogenæmia and
deepening shock. Douglas et al. (1955) pointed out at the 14th
British Congress in Oxford that almost three-quarters of their cases of
Couvelaire uterus identified at Cæsarean section occurred in patients
whose delivery was delayed more than 3 hours after placental
separation, and they recommended delivery, by one means or another
(Cæsarean sections were performed in 40 per cent), if possible within
6 hours of the emergency, to improve fœtal salvage and decrease the
chances of anuria and hypofibrinogenæmia. The truth of this was
brought home to me vividly and tragically shortly after my arrival
in Glasgow when I hung on to conservative treatment too long.
The patient became anuric 24 hours after admission although
copious blood transfusion appeared to have restored her general
condition. She failed to go into labour and with a rapidly rising
blood urea I undertook Cæsarean section, in spite of an absent fœtal
heart, on the third day. She died on the table and necropsy showed
complete renal cortical necrosis. At that time we consoled ourselves
with the reflection that death would have been inevitable in any case,
but I now consider that had I secured delivery earlier on her kidneys
would not have failed.

The use of oxytocin has frequently been advocated, but there is only
a limited place for it in the treatment of concealed hæmorrhage, since,
if the uterus is already contracting, there is no need for it, and if the
uterus is atonic it will be incapable of reacting favourably to the drug;
it is futile to flog a sick horse and may encourage the absorption of
thromboplastins. Theoretically this risk may be higher while the
uterus is still in the earliest phases of abruptio than when it has recovered its ability to contract and expel its contents, which it now

Prematurity

Another common risk is that of prematurity due to a mistaken impression of the child's size and an inaccurate history of the menstrual cycle and last period, and induction for "postmaturity" may actually result in premature labour. I once asked all female candidates at an examination how many women were absolutely sure of their dates and the usual answer was "about half". This did not surprise me. When a patient presents herself at a clinic she is often intimidated and anxious not to appear stupid. She therefore produces a date for her last period and after that she "sticks" to her story.

Unforeseen Disproportion

More serious are the clinical mistakes so easily made in assessing relative disproportion. Often, following induction of labour for this reason the fœtal head at delivery shows so little evidence of moulding that one may wonder whether it had ever been necessary to interfere with the course of pregnancy. However, it should be remembered that the premature head, because of its bony pliability, very quickly loses its moulded shape, so that the observation is not quite fair, nor, for that matter, is moulding a desirable occurrence in the premature, even as a vindication of the obstetrician's diagnosis of disproportion. There is no doubt, however, that such cases are often induced unnecessarily early, and babies are just as likely to be lost because of prematurity as saved by preventing a difficult labour at term. In the other direction, a mistaken assessment of disproportion may reveal itself after induction in the course of labour when it becomes clear that the head will not mould through the pelvis. Such disproportion is itself a cause of inert uterine action, so that the trial of labour is no true test at all, and the Cæsarean section, now necessary, would have been better left deliberately until term. It is for this reason that many obstetricians hold that trial of labour should be reserved for spontaneous labour only.

Inertia

Inertia following induction is a very real risk which statistics do not fully reveal. Averages can be misleading, and even though the majority of cases do not become inert, the effects of inertia are so much worse, particularly when labour has been surgically induced.

The following risks are peculiar to surgical as distinct from medical methods of induction.

Sepsis

With modern methods this risk is negligible, provided that the time interval between induction and delivery does not exceed 48

hours, after which time the morbidity rate rises steeply whatever method has been employed. The older practices of leaving foreign bodies, such as bougies, stomach tubes and rubber bags, in the uterus have left too long a trail of misfortunes due to sepsis to make their use any longer desirable. Drew Smythe, long ago, placed methylene blue in the vagina after introducing Kraus' bougies, and at the end of the third stage noted that the membranes from the upper portions of the uterus were stained blue, and he argued that if the dye could track up alongside the bougies, so could infection.

So long as the amniotic sac is intact the risks of intra-uterine infection are very much less, but when the forewaters have been ruptured, the chances of infection mount steadily with the passage of time and prejudice the safety of Cæsarean section should it become necessary. For this reason induction-delivery intervals of more than 48 hours are a cause for concern, and to await signs of established infection may be hazardous procrastination. The baby is at much greater risk than the mother and may acquire either an active infection before birth or a latent infection which declares itself weeks later but whose bacteriology incriminates the maternity hospital as its source. All cases having an induction/delivery interval of 48 hours or more have histological evidence according to Govan of placentitis and amnionitis. There can be no such thing as an aseptic surgical induction, whatever the precautions, and in nearly 38 per cent of the series of surgical inductions reported by McCallum and Govan (1963), pathogenic organisms were present in the vagina before surgical interference.

Where the fœtus is dead *in utero*, surgical methods of induction are so dangerous as to be absolutely contra-indicated. Quite apart from being strictly unnecessary, nothing could be more inviting to gas-forming organisms than the presence of a dead fœtus and placenta, and many disasters in the past have occurred with dramatic rapidity.

Placental Site Retraction and Fœtal Asphyxia

Nowadays, surgical induction is chiefly limited to methods of tapping the amniotic sac and removing varying amounts of liquor, which reduces the volume of the uterine contents as a whole. The uterus must, therefore, shrink to some extent to compensate for the loss of liquor, and this shrinkage and retraction are mainly confined to the upper uterine segment in which the placenta is normally situated. Some reduction, therefore, of the area of the placental site will occur, but what is more important is that the volume of maternal blood flow through the placenta will be reduced. This may not matter very much for a number of hours, but if, as is occasionally the case, the fœtus is already on the verge of asphyxia (and some

degree of hypoxia is physiologically present at the end of all pregnancies), then a delayed or protracted labour may tip the scales and
result in a stillbirth which is the consequence of prolonged though
mild asphyxia.

Partial Placental Detachment and "bloody tap"

Where the placenta is sited low in the uterus, surgical induction
commonly provokes antepartum hæmorrhage if placental attachment to the uterine wall is disturbed. Fortunately the bleeding usually
stops spontaneously on removal of the catheter, but if prolonged may
call for forewater rupture, and if uncontrollable may require delivery
at once by Cæsarean section.

The other cause of a "bloody tap" is the rupture of vasa prævia
or fœtal blood vessels encountered in a low-lying placenta. It is
clearly a matter of the most urgent importance to decide whose
blood is being lost, mother's or baby's. Fœtal exsanguination, as an
uncommon but serious possibility, has been pointed out by Russell
et al. (1956) who reported two fœtal deaths from this cause following
surgical induction by hindwater rupture.

Fortunately it is now possible to identify the blood within little
more than ten minutes by the use of the Singer test for fœtal hæmoglobin as modified by Anderson. The test depends upon the fact that
fœtal hæmoglobin is more resistant to denaturation by alkali than is
adult hæmoglobin. The following description of the test is given by
Mitchell, Anderson and Russell (1957):

ANDERSON'S MODIFICATION OF SINGER TEST FOR FŒTAL HÆMOGLOBIN

Principle.—A sample of blood is allowed to react with an alkali for
a set period of time. The reaction is then stopped by an acid solution
which also precipitates non-hæmoglobin chromogens. The mixture is
filtered immediately and the filtrate examined by the naked eye and in a
colorimeter.

Reagents.—Alkali: N/12 NaOH or N/12 KOH. Acid-precipitating
solution: 800 ml. of 50% saturated $(NH_4)_2SO_4$ plus 2 ml. of 10 N HCl.
Blood: The sample is either pure blood or a mixture of blood and other
contaminants issuing from the vagina. It should be collected in a clean
heparinised bottle. If collected in an oxalated tube or by means of a
siliconed syringe, there is a danger of "fœtal results" being obtained from
adult blood.

Technique.—The hæmoglobin level of the blood sample is first determined. To 2 ml. of alkali, 0·1 ml. of blood is added and the mixture is
shaken. The reaction is allowed to proceed for one minute at room temperature, when 4 ml. of acid-precipitating solution is added and the mixture again thoroughly shaken. It is then filtered through a No. 1 What-
man filter paper and the filtrate collected.

The results are usually obvious by naked-eye examination. With adult-type hæmoglobin the filtrate is either clear and colourless or a faint brown amber colour. With fœtal-type hæmoglobin it varies from a faint pink to a distinct cherry red, depending on the amount of hæmoglobin in the sample.

A colorimeter may be used for greater accuracy, especially when both types of blood are mixed and for the elimination of false positive results for fœtal hæmoglobin which might be obtained by naked-eye inspection.

The timely discovery that the bleeding is of fœtal origin may be life saving if Cæsarean section is promptly undertaken within the next hour or two. A longer period of grace before the fœtal heart stops cannot be counted upon.

Accidental Hæmorrhage (Abruptio placentæ)

Full-blown abruptio placentæ may occur following the sudden release of enormous quantities of liquor in cases of hydramnios. For this reason, severe cases should, if possible, be decompressed by "controlled rupture". This is usually attempted with a Drew Smythe catheter before finally rupturing the forewaters. Unfortunately the forewaters in such cases are often ruptured accidentally, thus defeating one's purpose. An alternative is to decompress the uterus by abdominal paracentesis first, with a lumbar puncture type of needle.

Dry Labour

The risks of a dry labour are potentially very great. Quite apart from fœtal asphyxia, already discussed, labour may be prolonged for a variety of reasons. The uterus may come to mould itself round the irregular fœtal outline and lose much of its expulsive efficiency thereby; it will discourage rotation, particularly in occipito-posterior positions; it will become more irritable, presumably because of the uneven stimulation of the fœtal foreign body, and constriction ring may develop. During all this unfortunate sequence, infection increases, and eventually operative intervention is likely to be called for in ugly circumstances.

Fœtal Pneumonia

This is a common penalty of prolonged retention of the fœtus *in utero* with ruptured membranes, particularly in association with prolonged labour. The combination of fœtal anoxia and the inevitable presence of infected meconium invites deep inspiratory efforts on the baby's part, so that it may be born with an established aspiration bronchopneumonia, which can be fatal. It is customary to give prophylactic chemotherapy before delivery in such cases, but although this may protect the mother from the most vicious forms of sepsis, it

is less likely to save her child. For one thing the antibiotic must be capable of traversing the placental barrier and reaching the liquor in high concentration and for another the organisms, whose nature is not yet known, should be sensitive to it. So great are the risks, however, that we feel some guesswork is indicated here and for a time it was our practice to give ampicillin prophylactically after 24 hours with artificially ruptured membranes, but we have since switched to cephaloridine.[3]

Cord Prolapse

This should not occur unless either the head fails to engage or there is malpresentation, particularly with oblique or transverse lie, in which case surgical induction is plainly contra-indicated until the lie has been converted to the longitudinal and the presenting part has been made to engage firmly in the pelvis. With a high head the forewaters should not be ruptured unless the head is first made to engage, but even hindwater rupture with a high head is not devoid of this complicating risk, and a careful examination should always be made at the end of the operation to exclude the presence of a prolapsed cord. If indeed the cord does prolapse at amniotomy, immediate Cæsarean section is the only really rational treatment (another reason for carrying out surgical induction of labour only in surgical conditions). We make a rule of carrying out this simple operation in one of our operating theatres and have had reason to be grateful for such strict caution.

Amniotic Embolism

Lastly, amniotic fluid embolism may occur, either at the time of amniotomy or some hours later. It occurs more readily if the uterine contractions are very strong, usually in a multipara, and amniotic fluid is squeezed into a maternal sinus through a hole in the membranes. I know of such an accident which befell a colleague's patient who collapsed immediately following this simple operation and died within a few minutes. In another case on my own unit the patient's doctor had ruptured the membranes on the previous day. She suddenly became very ill, was admitted deeply cyanosed with pyrexia 105° F. and gross tachycardia. She died within 45 minutes of delivery by forceps from amniotic fluid embolism, presumably a sequel to her previous amniotomy. Admittedly these hideous complications are uncommon but their incidence should not exceed nil if the operation is done for inadequate reasons.

Fœtal Mortality

This is, in most centres, higher than in spontaneous delivery, but considering the very large number of reasons for which labour may

be induced it is not really fair to blame the induction without taking into account the indication, which has its own fœtal mortality.

HISTORY OF INDUCTION OF LABOUR

Since antiquity various methods, many bizarre and some frankly dangerous, have been used in an attempt to bring on labour.

Massage of the breasts and uterus are very old but inefficient methods. Something approaching the use of tents dates back to the sixth century, and stretching of the cervix digitally has been long employed. The last century brought with it more ingenuity and at one time electricity was thought of. As far back as 1838 rubber tubing was pushed into the uterus, only to be revived in the form of a stomach tube about ninety years later by Fitzgibbon.

Scanzoni used a hot carbolic acid douche in 1856, and at this time Kraus introduced his bougies, which only in recent years have fallen into disuse because of their relative inefficiency, their sepsis rate and the oft-encountered risk of harpooning or detaching placenta.

Kraus' bougies had, however, one virtue over the other foreign-body methods in that they did not displace the presenting part. The writer used them frequently before the last war, and had little serious trouble with them apart from occasionally encountering the placenta, which called for reintroduction of the bougies in another direction and the delay sometimes of many days before labour started; it is not safe to leave them in the uterus for more than two days. It is now generally recognised, however, that their use is not justified.

Barnes in 1861 used rubber bags filled with water, but this was only an extension of the more traditional method of using pigs' bladders. It must be remembered that none of these weapons was sterilised in their heyday, and some of the results must have been frightful.

Artificial rupture of the forewaters stands in a class by itself, for it has stood a prolonged test of time, being first used by Denman in 1756 for cases of contracted pelvis, and being known since then as the "English method". It remains to this day the most efficient and most widely used method in spite of the sacrifice of an intact amniotic sac which it entails.

Hindwater rupture with the Drew Smythe catheter was introduced in 1931, but what it gains in safety, in forewater preservation, in reduced amniotic fluid infection and in discouragement of cord prolapse, it loses in efficiency when compared with forewater rupture.

Paracentesis of the amniotic cavity via the abdominal wall remains to be mentioned. It is seldom indicated, and when used labour is usually induced only incidentally, as the method is most often em-

ployed simply to relieve the pressure symptoms of a severe hydramnios without the intention of inducing labour, which is very likely to supervene, nevertheless. The same may be said, by the way, of attempts to date at amniography.

PRESENT-DAY METHODS OF INDUCTION

There are four main classes:
(1) Use of drugs.
(2) Use of hormones.
(3) Mechanical stimulation.
(4) Reduction of uterine volume by withdrawal of liquor.

What is surprising is that the psychiatrists do not yet appear to have tilted at this problem. After all, when one thinks of the effects of air-raids, thunder-storms and emotional stimuli in provoking labour, it would seem that there is scope here, and it is certainly no more ambitious than trying to make labour both brisk and painless.

Drugs.—Castor oil is the traditional aperient, and is supposed to stimulate the uterus to act by reflex overflow from the activity of the large bowel. Castor oil, however, exerts its direct effects only on the small intestine and the large bowel is only secondarily affected. No aperient will induce labour in a woman who is not already on the brink of it.

A so-called simple induction consists of giving castor oil in doses of 1 to 2 ounces, followed by a soap and water enema and, after the mess has died down, a hot bath to restore the patient's morale and in the interests of sound æsthetics. It has for long been known as giving the patient an O.B.E. It would be more exact to call it an O.E.B. because of the order of procedure. Such a time-honoured practice is now somewhat under a cloud for a variety of reasons which do not in every instance make sense. The castor oil is regarded as an assault upon the dignity of the patient reminiscent of the punitive practices associated with Fascism before and during the last war; even the soap traditionally put in the enema is thought by some to be useless and, in fact, the French commonly manage to their own satisfaction on water alone, and the hot bath is regarded as the most useless of the lot. So the patient is offered, as a more scientific alternative, an oxytocin drip. Now this iconoclastic attitude is not entirely fair. For one thing a so-called O.B.E. commonly works when a pregnancy is ripe for labour and the omission of castor oil undoubtedly reduces its efficacy. This has been demonstrated by tocographic study by Mathie and Dawson (1959) and certainly fits in with my own clinical impression. If one is talking in terms of kindness to patients I regard an oxytocin drip as anything but a soft-

hearted procedure, since the contractions so produced can be just as painful as those of labour and the patient lies apprehensively at the mercy of something over which she has no control. All such treatments are tolerable provided they work and the patient forgets about them in the success of her labour. It is in the failed cases that their unpleasant effects should be compared and on this basis it is nonsense to condemn castor oil as an inhumane procedure without similar reservations about the oxytocin drip. There is still a case, therefore, for retaining the O.B.E. in obstetric practice.

Quinine undoubtedly increases uterine irritability, and its use was often routine in medical induction some years before the war, when, as far as can be remembered, the success rate was nearly 80 per cent after the 38th week of gestation, which is far better than we obtain nowadays since abandoning it. The prewar practice was to prescribe quinine hydrobromide in 10-grain doses three-hourly following the usual oil, bath and enema, up to a maximum of three doses or until the ears buzzed or labour started, whichever was the sooner, and if labour did not start, half-hourly injections of oxytocin were given.

An alternative method of giving quinine was to prescribe it in 3-grain doses with Mist. Acidæ Strychninæ thrice daily for three days before the rest of the medical induction was given. The baby, nevertheless, frequently suffered and occasionally died as a result of its use; in any case, fœtal distress was often marked and meconium was copiously passed, so that it has now been abandoned. It is still well worth administering, however, in cases of intra-uterine fœtal death when the above disadvantage does not apply.

Hormones.—We believe, in a vague sort of way, that the onset of labour results from a combination of mechanical and endocrine factors with some degree of over-riding emotional control. It is surprising that modern biochemistry has not brought us nearer to the brink of success in finding a method of infallibly inducing labour, accurately controlling uterine activity and ushering in the dawn of elective delivery. Acetylcholine is of course useless because of its immediate destruction by choline esterase. Anticholinesterases, the basis of the most deadly war gases which, fortunately, were never put to the test in the last war, are much too dangerous and have far too many other side-effects on the autonomic nervous system to be considered for the purpose. Oestrogens are on the whole ineffective because any therapeutic dose, however massive, is trivial compared with the patient's own endogenous production, but they may help to sensitise the uterus to subsequent quinine and oxytocin in cases of intra-uterine fœtal death. In this case, where it is most desirable to avoid surgical induction, several days initial priming with œstrogen can be attempted by administering doses of 5 to 10 mg. of stilbœstrol or its equivalent every four hours up to a total of about 300 mg., or

œstradiol benzoate in 2 mg. doses can be injected eight-hourly for eight days, followed, if necessary by quinine and oxytocin.

The oxytocic factor from the posterior lobe of the pituitary is nowadays prepared in great purity, free of vasopressor substances and synthetic ocytocin has an established popularity and usefulness.

Oxytocin is destroyed very rapidly, it is believed, by the enzyme oxytocinase, so that intra-muscular or subcutaneous injections are highly unpredictable. It should never be used as long as there is a living fœtus *in utero*, because the rapidity of absorption and how much of the drug will reach the uterus cannot be foreseen and the response may be disappointing or frankly alarming. Absorption of oxytocin is more rapid and predictable through the nasal and buccal mucous membranes, as will presently be described, but for downright reliability and control the intravenous dilute drip method must be employed. This is an every-day ceremonial in most maternity hospitals and its usefulness is almost matched by the degree to which it is abused.

Oxytocin Intravenous Drip

Given intravenously it is essential to dilute oxytocin at least to 1:1,000 (1 ml. containing 10 units in 1,000 ml. of 5 per cent glucose). Dilutions of 1:2,500 or 1:5,000 are even safer and the drip rate should not exceed 40 drops per minute at first until the patient's response and sensitivity to the drug can be assessed by observation. The drip rate cannot be safely stabilised in less than half an hour, during which time the doctor must not leave the patient.

It is a good plan to connect two bottles of glucose solution to the delivery tube by means of a Y-piece, the one with oxytocin and the other without. The drip is started with the dummy solution and then switched to the other. It is often combined with other induction techniques, e.g. sweeping or artificial rupture of the membranes or both or it may be reserved for those cases who fail to go into labour within 24 hours.

Even with the above precautions the accurate control of oxytocin infusion is anything but precise and furthermore involves the infusion of large amounts of fluid which may, especially in pre-eclampsia, be undesirable. Even switching off the oxytocin bottle, and by means of the Y-piece transferring to the dummy solution, does not immediately cut off an exaggerated response as the remaining tubing may still contain a good deal of oxytocin before it is finally flushed out, even though the Y-piece is kept as near the vein as possible.

We are making increasing use of an "escalation technique" which would horrify Theobald with his long-established doctrine of very dilute physiological dosage, but there are occasions when the uterus continues refractory to even high doses and a relatively concentrated

or fast running drip, particularly in cases of intra-uterine death. We have found the small, variable speed syringe pump of Sage Instruments a very elegant and useful way of achieving accurate control, instantaneous cut-off, if necessary, and relatively high dosage.[14] Initially two units of Syntocinon (synthetic oxytocin)[1, 17] are drawn into a 10 ml. syringe which is made up with water, and 5 ml. of this dilution is drawn into a disposable syringe and connected to the pump and a manometer. The speed of the pump is set at the lowest point and gradually increased every five minutes, initially aiming to increase from 0·16 to 0·40 units per hour rate of infusion, which approximates to a fluid drip containing 4 units of Syntocinon per litre being increased from 12 to 30 drops per minutes over half an hour.[14] The dose is thereafter stepped up progressively according to the uterine response and if by the time the first 5 ml. syringe is exhausted and uterine activity has still not been provoked, the concentration in the next syringe is doubled with the dials again being set at the lowest point and gradually increased. Apart from its elegance and control the main advantage seems to be that the dose can be stepped up without intimidating the patient or her attendants.

The somewhat bolder approach has certainly reduced the number of failed inductions in our unit, but the pump must be stopped instantly if the uterus gets a tetanic spasm, and slowed down if contractions come more frequently than once every two minutes. If intravenous oxytocin is being used in the course of the second stage, it must be maintained until the completion of the third stage and after, as otherwise an atonic third stage hæmorrhage may result.

The oxytocin drip now enjoys enormous popularity, and since it was popularised by Theobald and his colleagues it has won enthusiastic and vociferous support which some of us feel is not wholly deserved. Obviously the more widely it is used the better will be the results since any number of cases that would have laboured satisfactorily anyway swell the number of successes and dilute the hard core of refractory cases. If, as is our practice, its use is restricted to the latter, disappointment is common. We have found that it always succeeds in stimulating uterine contractions but that labour may not supervene nevertheless, and after several hours of fruitless suffering on the part of the patient the cervix is found to be no more dilated than before and the drip has to be taken down for the sake of the patient's morale. In such cases we recommend calling a halt and returning to the attack next day or even later, meanwhile giving back the patient her arm. The oxytocin drip, commonly known as "the pit. drip", is at present being used with uncritical abandon on a scale which can hardly be justified on the basis of genuine indications. Wrigley (1962) sounded rather like a voice crying in the wilderness when he concluded, in the large series which he quoted, that it is "questionable whether the

oxytocin drip saved the life of a single baby and it is certain that its employment never made labour more normal or more comfortable for the patient". What makes the matter worthy of serious thought is that accidents undoubtedly occur and the procedure cannot be regarded as totally safe. These hazards will be discussed later.

It would appear that sometimes the cervix is ripened if not dilated by the attempt and a high head may be encouraged to engage.

The recommendation to stay with the patient throughout administration is more important in fact for the maintenance of her morale than her physical safety. This last point is more important than commonly realised since a patient left alone, apparently at the mercy of a relentless and pain-producing drug whose administration she can lie back and watch but not control, is very liable to panic.

Uterine spasm can occasionally be intense and prolonged, sometimes for over ten minutes in the hyper-reactive case or where control has not been adequate, and the baby is in great danger from asphyxia. It may in fact be necessary to turn the patient quickly onto her left side and relax the spasm by chloroform administered by face mask.

It may be asked what other disadvantages are to be expected from the oxytocin drip. These are that it often fails to work in the cases where it is most needed, is frequently painful, is time-consuming and may alarm the patient. The danger of uterine tetanic spasm has been mentioned and patients vary enormously in their sensitivity to this drug. Under proper supervision, however, this should not occur. The other risk is that of uterine rupture for which faulty supervision may not be wholly to blame.

Contra-indications to Oxytocin Drip

The chief absolute contra-indication is grand multiparity because of the tumultuous precipitate labour which can follow even quite small quantities of dilute oxytocin drip. Even medical supervision at the time may not be sufficient to prevent a sudden disaster of this sort. In one of the patients in my own unit (a para 9), within a minute or two of setting up the oxytocin drip, cautiously administered, in standard dilution and in full view of the supervising medical attendants, the uterus "stood on its head" and ruptured. Within the following twenty minutes I had removed the uterus. The baby was already dead and the patient was so profoundly shocked, rather than exsanguinated, that she died some time later from renal failure which we failed to reverse. One such catastrophe alone must wipe out the alleged benefits of many hundreds of other cases so treated.

Because of this danger of uterine rupture I am chary of employing an oxytocin drip in cases of previous Cæsarean section, unless, by the opportunity of previous palpation from inside the uterus at a subsequent labour, I can be confident of the integrity of the scar.

Disproportion or sub-clinical varieties of it are common causes of inert labour and the oxytocin drip is not only likely to fail in such a case but may have damaging effects on both mother and baby. Where hydramnios is present it is reasonable to get rid of the over-distension of the uterus by amniotomy first, before using an oxytocin drip. Cases of transverse lie constitute other absolute contra-indications because of the obvious risks of early membrane rupture and cord prolapse. We are also opposed to its use in diabetic pregnancy because of the natural hazards to which the fœtus is heir in any case and which will not suffer any addition from this extraneous cause. Any pathology of the cervix involving scarring, for example following previous operation or repair, is a further contra-indication because of the risk of splitting. The effect of an oxytocin drip is on the whole to exaggerate the uterine pattern already existing in a given labour. For this reason a colicky type of behaviour is likely to be aggravated although the hypotonic type of inertia may be considerably benefited.

In cases of multiple pregnancy, there is much to be said for an oxytocin drip being kept running in the course of the second and third stages of labour at a very slow and judicious rate, particularly with triplets and quadruplets where the hazards of uterine inertia and consequent postpartum hæmorrhage are very considerable. Such a drip should not be taken down until the uterus is thoroughly well retracted at the end of the whole delivery.

One would naturally like to predict the chances of success from an oxytocin drip induction before inflicting the experience upon a patient in whom it subsequently fails. Smyth (1958) had described an oxytocin sensitivity test in which repeated injections of small quantities of oxytocin were given and their effect studied by tocography and an attempt was made to find a threshold thereby to oxytocin sensitivity. This idea has been considerably simplified by Eddie (1963), who dispensed with the tocodynamometer or other specialised apparatus. After suitable reassurance and relaxation an intravenous injection of dilute oxytocin solution is given into an arm vein with the operator using one hand for the injection and the other for palpating the uterus. Synthetic oxytocin (Syntocinon) 0·05 I.U. in 5 ml. of sterile water is used. The rate of injection is 1 ml. or 0·01 Units in one minute and the injection is stopped when the uterus contracts or when all 5 ml. of solution have been injected, whichever is the sooner. If a contraction occurs during the five minutes of the injection it is classed as positive. It is distinguished from Braxton Hicks contractions by the presence of pain. About two-thirds of the 154 tests on these lines were followed by amniotomy and the test was, therefore, used more as an indication of the likelihood of success following surgical induction. In 91 per cent of the cases in which the

test was positive labour supervened within 48 hours, where the full 5 ml. were injected. One would, however, expect to get this success rate in any case from all surgical inductions. The test was more significant, however, when the response was obtained to less than 0·03 units (3 ml.). A positive test at this level predicted a successful outcome to induction in 100 per cent of cases. We ourselves have tried to predict the likelihood of a successful outcome by the use of oxytocin snuff as a gauge of oxytocin sensitivity. I am not yet convinced of the value of these tests in clinical practice, however. One should not start on the induction road without wanting to induce labour and if one wants to induce labour, then one induces labour, and if the induction fails, one resorts without hesitation to more drastic measures to deliver the patient, but if one were inducing labour for social reasons or on grounds of convenience, then such tests might enable one to meddle with a clearer conscience.

Because of the misery of an intravenous drip in an otherwise well woman and the forced immobility which it involves, there has always been considerable interest in other possible routes of administration. Oxytocin is destroyed at once in the stomach, which makes the oral route useless and, as already mentioned, intramuscular and subcutaneous injections are futile or dangerous, or both, because of the complete unpredictability of the rate of absorption and destruction, but some of the mucous membranes are capable of absorbing oxytocin at a more even rate. At first the nasal route seemed an attractive alternative using oxytocin snuff and later a spray, which was found to be as safe as the intravenous route and almost as effective,[5] although it never achieved much popularity in this country. The introduction of buccal oxytocin was immediately accepted, however, and for a time it was hoped that it could replace amniotomy and surgical methods; but it was soon evident that it was no more effective as a medical induction than the old-fashioned methods, including the use of quinine which I remember in the 1930s. Only 67 per cent in one series[23] was successful and of the 33 per cent failures, 22 were successful after artificial rupture of the membranes. The present view is that except for cases of intra-uterine death or as a "trial of induction" in postmaturity (which we do not approve of) the greatest use for buccal oxytocin is following amniotomy for the induction of labour[19] The maximum dosage as recommended by the makers (Parke-Davis—Buccal pitocin) is to start with half a scored 200 unit tablet, i.e. 100 units for the first two doses at half-hourly intervals and thereafter to increase hourly with each alternate half-hourly dose until a maximum of 600 units is being given at a time.

In other words, three hours after the start of treatment the patient is receiving the maximum half-hourly dose of 600 units. This dose, of course, is cut back long before the maximum level is reached if the

Dosage Scheme of Buccal Pitocin

Starting Point	100 units (½ tablet)
½ an hour	,, ,, ,,
1 hour	200 units (1 tablet)
1½ hour	,, ,, ,,
2 hours	400 units (2 tablets)
2½ hours	,, ,, ,,
3 hours	600 units (3 tablets)
3½ hours	,, ,, ,,
4 hours	,, ,, ,,
4½ hours	,, ,, ,,
5 hours	,, ,, ,,

uterine response is adequate and thereafter the dosage is adjusted accordingly. The total number of units given over such a five-hour course comes up to 4,400, but this must be regarded as an absolute maximum and, if no satisfactory result is achieved, the attempt can be regarded as having failed and unlikely to succeed if repeated the next day. The tablets take almost an hour to dissolve when placed correctly between the cheek and the outer border of the upper gums and if an unexpected over-reaction of the uterus occurs they can be spat out and the mouth rinsed. The effect will be abolished within the next fifteen minutes. Some patients have difficulty in not munching the tablets and swallowing them inadvertently and also they tend to accumulate in the mouth to an embarrassing extent, but these minor inconveniences are a small price to pay for the greater comfort and mobility of the patient. We certainly have used this method a great deal and have found it very acceptable, but it is an extravagant way of giving oxytocin compared with the minute quantities which are effective intravenously. All the hazards and precautions necessary with the use of intravenous oxytocin apply with equal force to the buccal route. No advantage whatsoever is gained in safety and the best method of all is undoubtedly the Sage pump technique already described, because the drug can be stopped instantly by switching off the pump. The indications and contra-indications remain exactly as before. The latter include fœtal distress, disproportion, malpresentation and grand multiparity, with the addition of severe pre-eclampsia, abruptio placentæ and the presence of a Cæsarean section scar in the uterus, in which oxytocin may only be given under the most carefully supervised and controllable conditions, if at all.

Attempts have been made to achieve equally satisfactory results with doses far short of the maker's recommended maximum. There is indeed much to be said for holding off buccal oxytocin after amniotomy for the induction of labour for a period of three hours, because

13 per cent of all cases will go satisfactorily into labour without the need for this drug.[20] Nothing is lost by this caution and a good deal gained, but in spite of a number of reports to the contrary our own feeling is in agreement with Ritchie and Brudenell that not much is to be gained by a more timid dosage. The important point is to recognise when a satisfactory level has been reached in accordance with the uterine response and thereafter not to exceed it. This requires high grade supervision.

Although it is said that an unripe cervix does not particularly matter, nor influence one's decision as to the desirability of induction, all of us, nevertheless, welcome a ripe and easily stretchable cervix with a well-applied presenting part.

Mechanical stimulation of the uterus.—Forceful stretching of the cervix is often effective, but produces shock and may cause a deep tear, and is not, therefore, recommended.

Safer by far is the sweeping of the membranes off the lower uterine segment with the finger. This is often done as a preliminary to other surgical methods of induction. It is most unusual to be unable to pass a finger through the cervix near term, and an anæsthetic provides better opportunities for thoroughness.

The remaining methods involve leaving foreign bodies in the genital tract and are now only of historical interest.

Artificial rupture of the forewaters.—This widely used method is not difficult nor is an anæsthetic necessary except in the nervous primigravida. A premedication with Omnopon and Scopolamine usually suffices. Because of the occasional need to employ anæsthesia, however, especially if the cord unexpectedly prolapses, or if acute fœtal distress is manifest, or if a "bloody tap" of major degree is encountered, it is a wise plan for the patient not only to have this minor operation in suitable surroundings, such as a proper obstetric theatre where Cæsarean section can be carried out, but she should come with an empty stomach. For this reason we aim to carry out all our elective surgical inductions before 12 noon. Quite apart from being safer, it is a lot kinder to the patient.

In the interests of asepsis the patient should be in the lithotomy position, full aseptic and antiseptic ritual must be observed and the bladder must, as usual, be empty.

The introduction of a speculum and gripping the cervix with a vulsellum is not as a rule necessary, and after passing a finger through the cervix and separating the membranes from the region of the internal os, a long toothed artery forceps is passed, by touch, alongside the finger in the cervix and the forewaters are "tweaked". Sometimes, because the head is applied closely to the membranes, no gush of liquor occurs, and it may be doubted whether the membranes have, in fact, been ruptured; a few fœtal hairs in the tips of

the forceps is evidence, of course, but the purpose of the operation is to drain off some liquor. By gently pushing up the head for half an inch with the finger through the cervix, the operation may often be more successful and intermittent displacement of the head and withdrawal of the finger may produce gushes until the desired amount of liquor has been withdrawn.

If a uterine contraction occurs, so much the better, but care must be taken neither to rupture the membranes nor to displace the head during one, in any case where the head is not deeply engaged, for fear of provoking cord prolapse, a disaster which in any event must always be excluded by examination at the end of the operation.

Rarely, it is not possible to pass a finger through the cervix, and blind stabbing with forceps is to be deprecated. Although there are many who would proceed to dilate it forcibly with dilators, the safer view is that the case is not suitable for surgical induction.

Occasionally some bleeding may occur, usually due to a minor degree of placenta prævia. With the forewaters already ruptured this is almost certain to cease in a minute or two, and only in cases of prolonged and serious bleeding will Cæsarean section be indicated. Finally, the fœtal heart should be auscultated to ensure that all is well.

Artificial rupture of the hindwaters.—The preliminary steps are the same as for the operation of forewater rupture and the same remarks about anæsthesia apply.

The Drew Smythe catheter is the instrument of choice, and it is introduced with the point of the stilette withdrawn and guided through the cervix by the sense of touch. It is slowly and gently passed between membranes (previously separated) and uterine wall directly posterior to the presenting part; occasionally a posterolateral insertion may serve better. On no account is any force to be used, nor is it necessary. When the whole of the distal curve of the instrument has been passed through the cervix the direction of thrust is altered by gradually lowering the handle until the shaft of the instrument is pressing backwards on the perineum. The tip is now safely pointing directly forwards and the stilette is pushed home. A small downward movement of the handle is now made and the moment of membrane puncture can usually be detected. The stilette is now withdrawn and the liquor is collected in a measuring jug (Fig. 1). An alternative instrument is a curved male metal catheter. This is introduced posteriorly or sometimes more laterally and then twisted in its long axis with a flick in order to puncture the amniotic sac. It does not enter the uterus as far as the Drew Smythe catheter and is therefore less likely to encounter placenta, but in my hands, at least, it fails more often to rupture the membranes. Removal of sixteen to

twenty ounces of liquor is generally sufficient and often one has to be content with less. As a rule, the success of the induction depends far more upon the period of gestation than the amount withdrawn.

Sometimes, on rupturing the membranes, only a small quantity of meconium-stained liquor is obtained. If the meconium is clearly fresh, i.e. turbid and "particulate" rather than old watery staining,

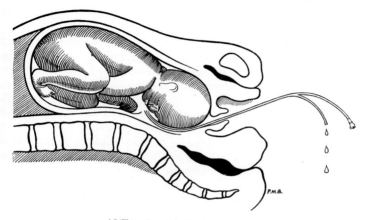

15/Fig. 1.—Hindwater puncture.

one should be very vigilant for further signs of fœtal distress and the fœtal heart should thereafter be checked every quarter of an hour. The fœtus is clearly near the end of its tether and as Leslie (1959) has pointed out, a prolonged labour of more than twenty-four hours is dangerous indeed for the fœtus. These cases come to a high operative delivery rate, either by Cæsarean section or forceps, on account of further evidence of fœtal distress, but one is reminded by Leslie of the higher incidence of fœtal abnormality in these cases and an X-ray should be taken while there is yet time to decide the issue.

Certain troubles may be encountered. The commonest is to be rewarded not by liquor but by frank blood, due either to encountering placenta or vasa prævia; a blood-stained ooze from the decidua is of no moment. When bleeding occurs the Drew Smythe catheter should be withdrawn, and if it does not stop readily, as indeed it usually does, the forewaters should be ruptured. In all such cases the blood passed must be sent forthwith to the laboratory to exclude fœtal hæmorrhage (see earlier). When the cervix will not admit a finger (a bad omen) and it is decided nevertheless to proceed, it is better to do so under direct vision with the help of a Sims' or Auvard speculum and a sponge forceps applied to the anterior lip of the cervix. With a tight or difficult cervix it is certainly much easier to rupture

the hindwaters by passing a Drew Smythe catheter than to rupture the forewaters.

The fœtal heart should be auscultated at the end of the operation. Irregularities and slowing of the rate are a warning that the child is not likely to stand the strain of prolonged delay in delivery.

Occasionally a fœtal hand may be felt alongside the head during surgical induction. It should be pushed out of reach, and provided the head settles well on to the cervix it is unlikely to give further trouble.

Induction by Intra-amniotic Injections

It has already been mentioned that paracentesis, even with a fine needle, of the amniotic cavity may be followed by labour even when this is not intended. Bengtsson (1962) described the method of inducing therapeutic abortion in women between the 16th and 24th week of pregnancy by injecting hypertonic 20 per cent saline into the amniotic cavity. This injection produced a sharp fall in blood progesterone levels and incidentally he noted that if systemic progesterone was given before the hypertonic saline injection the onset of labour might be delayed for up to two days or more. Bengtsson reckoned that the hypertonic solution destroys placental function and removes the progesterone "block". Œstrogens now given are effective in initiating the abortion process.

Because of the destruction of placental function this method of induction, of course, is reserved for cases of intra-uterine death or gross fœtal abnormality, as fœtal survival is not involved. The use of hypertonic glucose[25] has now been abandoned after a series of impressive disasters, including clostridial infection of the uterine contents and pressure-induced amniotic fluid embolism. Our own practice is to eschew intra-amniotic injections because of their unacceptable hazards as described in the chapter on abortion.

INDICATIONS FOR SURGICAL INDUCTION

Whenever there are indications for medical induction, one should as a rule be prepared to acknowledge them for surgical induction as well, and failure of the one method should be followed by an attempt at the other. If one is not prepared to carry out this sequence, one is logically bound to admit that the grounds for interference were in the first place inadequate. To prescribe a medical induction which does not succeed and then to leave the patient to solve the problem for herself is both bad obstetrics and bad psychology, and repeated medical inductions are no better. Such treatment betrays a mind not sufficiently made up or one that has not the courage of its convictions. Intra-uterine fœtal death is the only absolute exception to this rule.[18]

For this reason the indications for inducing labour whether by surgical or non-surgical means are grouped together, and are either for maternal or fœtal interests or more commonly for a combination of both.

The indications come under two headings:

(1) Obstetrical conditions.

(2) Certain medical conditions aggravated by pregnancy.

Obstetric Indications

(1) Pre-eclamptic toxæmia. Both fœtal and maternal interests are at stake, but are often not mutually compatible, so that the choice for the moment of induction requires judgment.

(2) Eclampsia, which is not followed by the onset of spontaneous labour within forty-eight hours, demands induction of labour as the patient is sitting on a volcano.

(3) Previous history of large babies. The tendency is for birth weights to increase in successive deliveries. No child is the better for being more than nine or ten pounds at delivery and the mother is appreciably worse off.

(4) Postmaturity. The risks of this to the baby are generally acknowledged, but mistakes are very frequently made in assessing its degree or significance and the case should be carefully reviewed. As Wrigley (1958) pointed out, "there is no such thing as an exact date for delivery, any more than there is an exact height or weight for a person," and he took into account, in assessing postmaturity, the amount of liquor relative to the fœtal bulk on repeated examination by the same observer.

The older the patient the more seriously should postmaturity be taken and the more readily should labour, after term, be induced (Baird, 1957).

(5) Recurrent intra-uterine fœtal death. This peculiar entity, said to be due to placental insufficiency, may, by the warning history, provide an opportunity to forestall disaster by shrewd or lucky timing.

Grouped into this class come cases of dysmaturity or the "small for dates" baby. A great deal of interest is focused on this vexing problem and is dealt with in a later chapter, but much effort, and possibly ingenuity, are being devoted to the assessment of intra-uterine well-being, including growth rates as measured by sonar, in order to detect when fœtal growth comes to a standstill and thus to determine the optimum moment for elective induction and delivery. An absence of maternal weight gain throughout pregnancy is often a pointer towards the possibility of dysmaturity.

(6) Cases of mild disproportion. On the whole induction is best

reserved for multiparæ, in whom the risk of inertia is much less and whose obstetrical prowess can be assessed from the history of previous deliveries. In any case, it is not to be done without full clinical assessment of the pelvis and, if possible, X-ray pelvimetry.

(7) Severe hydramnios producing marked pressure symptoms may call for relief. Abdominal paracentesis with a lumbar puncture type of needle may be tried in the hope of prolonging pregnancy, but the amniotic cavity usually fills up rapidly again if labour is not already provoked and in the end deliberate induction is likely to be indicated. The danger of accidental hæmorrhage following artificial rupture of the membranes in these cases has already been described.

(8) Monsters. The prolongation of pregnancy is profitless and undesirable. It is better to deliver a small monster than a large one, and, on grounds of humanity as well, pregnancy is better terminated. The back-door escape, however, of Cæsarean section is closed should labour subsequently become inert, and it is as well to bear this risk in mind and meet it to some extent by deferring induction until after the 36th week, by which time it is more likely to succeed.

(9) Certain cases of placenta prævia in which the placenta is situated clear of the margins of the internal os and in whom a sufficient degree of maturity has been reached to make the risks of prematurity less than those of recurrent bleeding. It need hardly be pointed out that forewater rupture is the only method to consider, as it alone will reduce the chances of further antepartum hæmorrhage and the operation should be performed in an operating theatre and under anæsthesia.

(10) Rh factor iso-immunisation cases. The degree to which a fœtus is affected with hæmolytic disease *in utero* can now be determined by amniocentesis and spectrophotometry of the liquor amnii. In moderately or severely affected cases, where pregnancy has already reached the 34th week, induction of labour and delivery of the child in spite of prematurity is safer and more likely to be successful than intra-uterine transfusion, which is reserved for cases that have not yet reached this degree of maturity. The object of the induction is to get the child delivered so that it is available for exchange transfusion after birth and the timing will depend upon the likely severity of the disease.

(11) Breech presentation provides a controversial point, particularly with extended legs. With the addition of every pound to the baby's weight over seven pounds, the fœtal mortality begins to climb with increasing steepness, and there is much to be said for inducing labour if the child's size is already reckoned to be approaching that figure. In any case, however, labour should not be induced before the 37th week, as the aftercoming head would be too vulnerable. Naturally, attempts at external version will have been made

previously. The choice of method is debatable, but Drew Smythe catheter induction is not only feasible but preferable, as it prevents a dry labour. Whichever method of membrane rupture is employed, the risk of cord prolapse is minimal with a deeply engaged presenting breech.

(12) Intra-uterine death of the fœtus which is radiologically proven is only a relative indication for induction. Spontaneous labour will always start eventually, but the patient can often be spared some very wretched weeks of waiting if labour is induced. Surgical methods, as already stated, cannot be too strongly condemned, but drug induction is both safe and usually efficacious.

(13) Hyperemesis with signs of ketosis appearing in late pregnancy, particularly in a multipara, occasionally betokens some acute toxæmic process which is generally ill-understood. Not only should the ketosis be urgently combated with intravenous glucose saline, but labour should be induced forthwith. Many of these cases have hiatus hernia.

(14) Icterus gravidarum may be another grave sign of obstetrical toxæmia and has a bad prognosis. Pregnancy must be terminated promptly.

General medical diseases which may indicate induction.—(1) Chronic nephritis. Pregnancy has no known beneficial effects whatever on the healthy kidney, and where renal function is already damaged the effects of pregnancy vary between bad and disastrous. If only maternal indications were at stake all such pregnancies should be terminated whenever and as soon as the diagnosis of chronic nephritis is established and the patient should be sterilised. Mild cases, however, may reach the later months of pregnancy, and in the almost certain knowledge that no future pregnancy is likely to fare better, if as well, it may be justifiable to gamble for a few extra weeks in the baby's interests. Induction has a limited field, however, mainly restricted to the multiparous, and Cæsarean section and sterilisation there and then, or subsequently, are generally preferred. Such decisions and the timing of intervention are among the most difficult in midwifery.

(2) Hypertension. The effects of pregnancy are, as a rule, harmful here as well, but the position is far less clear cut than in the case of chronic nephritis. Much will depend upon the condition, if known, before pregnancy started, the period of gestation at which hypertension appeared, the rate at which it develops, whether or not other signs of pre-eclamptic toxæmia are superimposed, the age and parity, and many such factors. The risks to the baby of prematurity have to be weighed against those of intra-uterine death, and the longer the hypertension is allowed to operate the more likely is the mother to be handicapped with a high blood pressure for the rest of her life. In-

duction of labour, therefore, plays a very large part in the management of these cases.

(3) Diabetes. Whether or not pre-eclamptic toxæmia is added to this complication, induction of labour is often called for to forestall intra-uterine fœtal death, which is a very real risk, and to obviate delivery of an oversized yet premature child of less than usual resilience to the stresses of labour. Wherever possible we try to induce labour by amniotomy between the 36th and 37th weeks of pregnancy since the danger of intra-uterine death rises steeply after this period.

(4) Recurrent pyelitis betokens structural alterations in the upper urinary tract which are likely to become permanent if neglected, and the possibility must be borne in mind of more deep-seated urological pathology which prolongation of pregnancy is likely to aggravate.

(5) Chorea gravidarum. This complication is sometimes so severe or difficult to control that pregnancy may have to be terminated by Cæsarean section. In the later weeks, however, induction of labour may suffice.

(6) History of bleeding in earlier pregnancy. As Lennon (1957) said, "Placental damage, once sustained, is irreversible and fœtal survival depends upon the amount of residual functional placental tissue and the fœtal maturity". For this reason (which applies even more commonly to pre-eclamptic toxæmia) we very readily induce cases who have threatened to abort earlier in pregnancy and we are very reluctant to allow them to become postmature for fear of intra-uterine fœtal death.

In broad and general principles, however, non-obstetrical diseases are served no better by induction than by awaiting spontaneous delivery at term, for induced labour is, as a rule, no kinder to mother or child and occasionally demands its own price.

CONTRA-INDICATIONS TO INDUCTION OF LABOUR

Under the following circumstances the induction of labour is absolutely contra-indicated:

(1) Disproportion which is more than borderline. It must have been made abundantly clear already that such treatment is little short of wanton folly rewarded with a high failure rate, a prohibitive fœtal mortality and the likelihood of maternal morbidity.

(2) Where pregnancy has not yet reached the 34th week—except in cases of established eclampsia—firstly, because the onset of labour may be dangerously long in starting, and, secondly, because the risks of prematurity are too high; there is, however, one exception in the case of gross fœtal abnormality associated with hydramnios which is producing symptoms.

(3) Where the lie is other than longitudinal, for obvious reasons.

(4) In cases which have previously been subjected to Cæsarean section on account of contracted pelvis or who have failed in a previous trial of labour for disproportion.

(5) Where a tumour occupies the pelvis.

(6) Cases of cardiac disease are exposed to the additional hazards of subacute bacterial endocarditis at the best of times and surgical induction is likely only to increase them, especially if there is subsequent delay in completing delivery, since there is no such thing as an aseptic surgical induction. Usually induction is not necessary in these cases anyway as they tend not to go postmature and spontaneous labour is usually expeditious.

(7) Elderly primigravidæ with malpresentation are better delivered by Cæsarean section without more ado.

Lastly, it is reiterated that surgical induction cannot be too strongly condemned when the fœtus is known to be dead.

The above is categorical teaching more or less throughout the world, but at the time of writing it has come to my notice that Professor Townsend of Melbourne, at the 5th World Congress of Gynæcologists and Obstetricians in Sydney (which, for health reasons at the last moment, I could not attend), produced a paper holding the exactly opposite point of view and strongly recommending that the membranes should be ruptured in any case of intra-uterine death after the 20th week of gestation and active steps taken to promote delivery by the use of a determined oxytocin infusion. He produced a series of 40 cases so treated without disaster and claimed that the method eliminated psychological stress for the patient and reduced the hazard of hypofibrinogenæmia.

It is the view of my more conservative colleagues that the chances of developing hypofibrinogenæmia are no more than 25 per cent and that if it does occur the patient may not necessarily bleed but that 8 g. of fibrinogen should be at the ready to cope with any bleeding, ante- or postpartum. Delivery itself should prevent recurrence of hypofibrinogenæmia but in the unlikely event of it not ensuing, following blood loss, the further microcoagulation and loss of more fibrinogen can be prevented by heparin. This in turn should be reversed by protamine sulphate within an hour before delivery or before any form of surgery. It is only very rarely necessary to have to go through all these therapeutic steps, which however are trivial compared with a surgical induction which misfires and rewards one with only a few spoonfuls of turbid liquor amnii at amniotomy (Fig. 2).

RESULTS OF INDUCTION

Even before labour starts, cases of pre-eclamptic toxæmia often show some temporary improvement after rupture of the membranes

and the blood pressure tends to drop so that eclampsia may, for a few hours, be less imminent; the respite is, however, only brief, and must not encourage a relaxation in vigilance; nevertheless, it may suffice, particularly in the multipara.

Other immediate effects before the onset of labour are the relief of pressure symptoms from hydramnios and the control, as a rule, of antepartum hæmorrhage in cases of lateral placenta prævia.

The penalties are reflected in an increased fœtal mortality and maternal morbidity rate, but it is hardly fair to blame induction for these without taking into account the indications for which it is done.

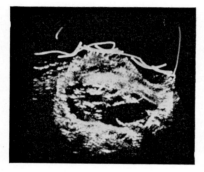

15/Fig. 2.—Ultrasonogram, in longitudinal section, of retained intrauterine dead fœtus due to Rh-hæmolytic disease at the 28th week of gestation, the size of uterus being no more than 20 weeks.

Note: Thick Rhesus placenta in the upper part of the picture, i.e. anteriorly and the relative scanty amounts of liquor (black areas).

The deformed, dead fœtal head is partially seen lower right of picture.

Induction-delivery interval.—This is now being recorded in an increasing number of maternity reports of various institutions and gives a good indication of the success of induction methods in securing their objective, namely, the onset of labour; what it fails to do, however, is to show up how much of this interval is spent in the course of a prolonged labour and this information is not so easy to come by. An I.D.I., to give it its usual abbreviation, of sixty hours, for example, may represent forty-eight hours of waiting and twelve of expeditious labour, or twelve hours of waiting and forty-eight of an inert and possibly dangerous first and second stage, and it is felt that this latent period should be included in these tables.

Where the latent period exceeds forty-eight hours in the case of medical induction or high puncture of membranes with a Drew Smythe catheter, it is probable that the induction was not responsible for the onset of labour contractions. In the case of forewater rupture this is less true, of course, because the continued seepage of liquor continues to operate in stimulating the uterus.

It may be considered a paradox that rupture of the forewaters is used as a method of induction on the one hand and yet, on the other, spontaneous early rupture of the membranes often presages a prolonged first stage. The difference in mechanism can be explained in

that, in the latter, the membranes may have ruptured early because the presenting part does not fit snugly in the lower uterine segment, as, for example, in occipito-posterior positions which, of themselves, cause inertia.

When labour does not start within forty-eight hours of induction, the operation then is usually considered as having failed, and there is an increasing tendency to regard this as an indication for lower segment Cæsarean section, to prevent uterine infection from gaining a firm foothold which would prejudice the same operation carried out at a later date, and, as Govan (1962) has shown, histological evidence of placentitis is demonstrable in one hundred per cent of cases with an I.D.I. of 48 hours or more. The baby suffers most from such infection and may be born with an established intranatal pneumonia.

To perform Cæsarean section because induction has failed and because of the threat of intra-amniotic infection is an extreme but perfectly logical point of view, and is the only prudent line to take if the indications for induction were sufficiently pressing in the first place. It is when inductions of convenience are undertaken that trouble, on the rare occasions when it occurs, is particularly galling. I have heard D'Esopo talking of "delivery by appointment" by means of elective induction, but I note that he is careful to restrict the practice to supernormal cases, parous women, with the head well engaged and the cervix already 2 cm. dilated.

TABLE V

SURGICAL INDUCTION 1960–62
(Glasgow Royal Maternity Hospital)
3,104 Surgical Inductions of Labour
i.e. 17·25 per cent of all labours

of which

8·2 per cent = 255 patients *undelivered* at 48 hours, and
5·1 per cent = 160 patients *not in labour* at 48 hours;
of these 160 patients:

23 Cæsarean section (14·4 per cent)
6 Breech deliveries
19 Forceps or vacuum extractions
112 Spontaneous deliveries

―――

160

―――

Our own results in what we regard as genuinely indicated inductions are shown in Tables V and VI, but here we are dealing not with normality but with abnormality.

TABLE VI

160 FAILED SURGICAL INDUCTIONS

Oxytocin drip	42	
of whom spontaneous delivery .	29	
Infected clinically	33	(20 per cent)
Perinatal loss	21	(13 per cent)
Perinatal loss due to infection .	6	

Manly (1956) recorded that 10 per cent of his patients in whom induction had been carried out were still undelivered after 72 hours. It is agreed that the amount of liquor withdrawn bears little relation to the induction delivery interval. The "ripeness" of the cervix as a prognostic factor is also very variable although one is discouraged by a cervix which is like a long, rigid and unyielding spout. If a finger cannot be passed through the cervix, it is probably better to desist for the time being.

A cervix displaced far backwards towards the hollow of the sacrum [what Cocks (1955) has aptly described as the "sacral os"] augurs even less well for spontaneous vaginal delivery.

Now, if one were to perform Cæsarean section on all women who failed to go into labour within some arbitrary period following surgical induction, e.g. 48–72 hours, one would be guilty indeed of an unnecessarily high section rate. The following alternatives are now open:

1. Take a cervical swab for bacteriological culture and antibiotic sensitivity testing and do nothing further.

2. Set up an oxytocin drip in addition.

3. Rupture the membranes again if liquor has ceased to drain. This is likely to increase morbidity.

4. Cæsarean section.

The choice will depend upon the urgency of the case and on the original indications for which labour was induced.

The shortest induction-delivery intervals occur, as expected, again on average, in the postmature cases, and whether the cervix appears clinically to be ripe or not, the I.D.I. is about twice as long following high puncture as after forewater rupture.

As an omen for successful induction, whatever figures may suggest, it is the common experience of all of us that a well-taken-up and effaced cervix, with a thin lower uterine segment and a deeply engaged vertex, all these, together with a uterus which demonstrates its irritability on palpation, betoken a stage well set for labour and delivery. It is unlikely that the added stimulus of artificial rupture or puncture of the membranes will fail to trigger off the processes of labour.

In conclusion, then, let one's reasons for inducing labour be carefully and honestly weighed, let the circumstances be favourable, and let the Rubicon be crossed with no lingering glances behind.

REFERENCES

1. BAINBRIDGE, M. N., NIXON, W. C. W., SCHILD, H. D., and SMITH, C. B. (1956). *Brit. med. J.*, **1**, 1133.
2. BAIRD, D. (1957). *Brit. med. J.*, **1**, 1061.
3. BARR, W., and GRAHAM, R. (1967). *Postgrad. med. J.* Suppl. **43**, 101.
4. BENGTSSON, L. P. (1962). *Lancet*, **1**, 339.
5. BORGLIN, N. E. (1962). *Acta obstet. gynec. scand.*, **41**, 238.
6. COCKS, D. P. (1955). *Brit. med. J.*, **1**, 327.
7. D'ESOPO, A. (1963). Obstetrical and Gynaecological Assembly of Southern California, Los Angeles.
8. DONALD, I. (1961). *Practitioner*, **186**, 549.
9. EDDIE, D. A. S. (1963). *Brit. med. J.*, **1**, 723.
10. GOVAN, A. D. T. (1962). Personal Communication.
11. LENNON, G. G. (1957). *Proc. roy. Soc. Med.*, **50**, 793.
12. LESLIE, D. W. (1959). *Brit. med. J.*, **2**, 612.
13. McCALLUM, M. F., and GOVAN, A. D. T. (1963). *J. Obstet. Gynaec. Brit. Cwlth.*, **70**, 244.
14. MACVICAR, J., and HOWIE, P. W. (1967). *Lancet*, **2**, 1339.
15. MANLY, G. A. (1956). *Lancet*, **2**, 227.
16. MATHIE, J. G., and DAWSON, B. H. (1959). *Brit. med. J.*, **1**, 1162.
17. MAYES, B. T., and SHEARMAN, R. P. (1956). *J. Obstet. Gynaec. Brit. Emp.*, **63**, 812.
18. MITCHELL, A. P. B., ANDERSON, G. S., and RUSSELL, J. K. (1957). *Brit. med. J.*, **1**, 611.
19. RITCHIE, J. M., and BRUDENELL, J. M. (1966). *Brit. med. J.*, **1**, 581.
20. RITCHIE, J. M., and BRUDENELL, J. M. (1967). *ibid.*, **1**, 608.
21. RUSSELL, J. K., SMITH, D. F., and YULE, R. (1956). *Brit. med. J.*, **2**, 1414.
22. SMYTH, C. N. (1958). *Lancet*, **1**, 327.
23. SPENCE, D. N., and CHALMERS, J. A. (1964). *Lancet*, **1**, 633.
24. THEOBALD, G. W., KELSEY, H. A., and MUIRHEAD, J. M. B. (1956). *J. Obstet. Gynaec. Brit. Emp.*, **63**, 641.
25. WOOD, C., BOOTH, R. T., and PINKERTON, J. H. M. (1962). *Brit. med. J.*, **2**, 706.
26. WRIGLEY, A. J. (1958). *Lancet*, **1**, 1167.
27. WRIGLEY, A. J. (1962). *Lancet*, **1**, 5.

CHAPTER XVI

DISPROPORTION

THE art of obstetrics is more often travestied in the name of disproportion than in any other instance. The prediction that cephalopelvic disproportion will adversely influence labour, as well as the assessment of its extent and the treatment with which the problem is met, are more than matters of mathematical measurement and demand a skill and experience which no textbook can provide. With modern radiological technique it is possible nowadays to measure up the pelvis in all sorts of planes, and yet the fact that trial of labour is so frequently instituted is acknowledgment enough of the inadequacy of these scientific aids.

The dynamics of labour are more important than the mechanics, and the efficacy of uterine contractions, the capacity of the fœtal head to mould and the stamina and the temperamental resilience of the patient contribute more to the outcome of labour in the minor and commoner types of disproportion than the pelvic measurements themselves. An appreciation of the mechanism of labour in disproportion is, therefore, essential.

In this chapter only vertex presentations will be considered, for the delivery of malpresentation with contracted pelvis hardly comes into the realm of good obstetrics. Nevertheless, restricting our consideration to the four vertex positions, it must be acknowledged straight away that occipito-posterior positions have a particularly adverse effect.

Successful delivery will depend in large measure upon good uterine contractions. Unfortunately these are often lacking. To an almost similar extent, an attitude of good flexion on the part of the fœtus is essential. Flexion is the essence of normal labour. In flexion, after all, we come into this world and bent up with old age we go in flexion to our graves; flexion is the alpha and the omega—the beginning and the end!

Poor flexion causes poor pains and poor pains aggravate poor flexion. It is altogether a depressing combination. The mechanism of labour has been studied with much detail and ingenuity, and all sorts of models, which are imaginative masterpieces, have been produced to illustrate it. Caldwell, Moloy and D'Esopo have also studied the mechanism of labour by means of radiology but, when all is said and done, difficult labour boils down to an attempt on the part of Nature to force a large foreign body through a somewhat in-

adequate orifice. The size of the foreign body, that is to say the baby's head, is a major consideration, yet this is one of the more uncertain factors.

In about 1959–60 I noticed that two echo blips were obtainable from the fœtal head *in utero* by means of a standard ultrasonic flaw detector used in industry to reveal deep-seated defects in metal structures. My then ward sister (now matron) was quick to employ it as a means of identifying the presentation in doubtful cases before my grand rounds. The two blips, as shown in the diagram of Fig. 1,

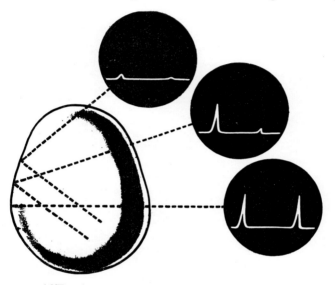

16/Fig. 1.—ULTRASONIC BIPARIETAL CEPHALOMETRY.
In the lowest diagram the biparietal diameter is revealed by the simultaneous appearance of two huge echo blips on a cathode ray screen because both reflecting surfaces are at right angles to the beam of ultrasound. In the other two diagrams above these conditions do not apply.

depend upon the fact that the echoes only return to the probe (applied to the abdominal surface through a film of olive oil to secure acoustic coupling) when the incident beam of ultrasound strikes the fœtal skull surfaces at right angles.[5] Both sides of the fœtal skull can only thus reflect squarely and simultaneously if the beam lies along either the biparietal or the occipito-frontal diameters, i.e. the true diameters of the elliptical fœtal skull and not a chord of the ellipse. The biparietal diameter is easily accessible, usually lying antero-posterior, whereas the occipito-frontal is less accessible and anyway is much larger and unlikely to be confused.

The parietal eminence is searched for by palpation and the ultra-

sonic probe is then applied in this region and rocked about until both blips from the near and far walls of the fœtal skull show up simultaneously on a cathode ray screen. It was a logical sequence of this discovery to relate the distance between the two blips to the actual distance between the parietal skull bones, in other words, the biparietal diameter. Willocks and Duggan, of my department, have

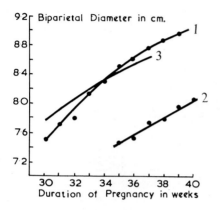

16/Fig. 2.—BIPARIETAL GROWTH CURVES *IN UTERO*.

(1) A normal curve. (2) A case of placental insufficiency. (3) A baby of a diabetic mother with normal growth curve and delivered at 37 weeks.

16/Fig. 3.—BIPARIETAL GROWTH CURVES *IN UTERO*.

(4) Demonstrates the reduced growth rate as term is approached. (5) A case of postmaturity. (6) Intra-uterine death resulting in macerated stillbirth (Willocks, 1963).

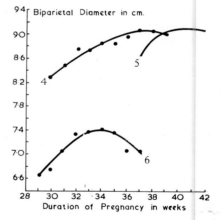

since developed the technique to a high degree of accuracy, of the order of a millimeter, and have observed the continued rate of growth of the fœtal skull in the last weeks of pregnancy (Figs. 2 and 3). This is a very simple technique (from the patient's point of view) and only takes a few minutes without even moving her from her bed. We believe that its use will become more general as it is better known.

More recently another member of my department, Stuart Camp-

bell, has refined the technique still further by identifying the fœtal head and its exact attitude in two dimensions with sonar, thus identifying the biparietal diameter pictorially beyond all shadow of doubt and usually demonstrating the midline echoes from the falx as well. Then switching the signals from the ultrasonic probe onto my A-scan apparatus, in one dimension as before, very accurate measurements, often to half a millimetre, can be made using electronic cursors as devised by Duggan.[23]

That the head enlarges in the last weeks of pregnancy there can be no doubt. Chassar Moir reckons that the biparietal diameter increases by about 2 mm. each week before birth, and Glass (1956), who measured 100 fœtal skulls by weekly radiocephalometry, in the last four weeks of pregnancy found an average increase in diameter of over 1 mm. per week. There is, therefore, bound to be a significant difference in the size of head between the 38th week and the 42nd week of gestation. Now, moulding can reduce the biparietal dimension by a quarter of an inch or more (6–7 mm.), but such gross degrees are not compatible with the child's safety and it is not desirable that moulding should cause more than a reduction of 4 mm. In a clear-cut case of disproportion, therefore, it is not fair to the child to rely upon moulding to secure its delivery, except perhaps in the case of the flat pelvis, which demands moulding in only one meridian.

Disproportion at the brim is often partly countered by the mechanism of asynclitism, whereby the lateral rocking of the head presents a slightly diminished diameter, namely, the subparieto-superparietal diameter of $3\frac{1}{2}$ inches (9 cm.), as compared with the biparietal diameter of $3\frac{3}{4}$ inches (9·5 cm.). There are two sorts of asynclitism. The commoner is the anterior variety, also known as Naegele's obliquity, whereby the anterior parietal bone presents predominantly so that the sagittal suture lies nearer the sacrum. This is a favourable mechanism. The other type is the posterior asynclitism, also known as Litzmann's obliquity, in which the posterior parietal bone presents, thereby placing the sagittal suture closer to the pubic symphysis. This is an unfavourable mechanism and augurs very badly for spontaneous delivery if it persists.

Disproportion at the outlet is a definite entity and is dealt with more fully later. One of the most important features here is the width of the subpubic arch and the acuteness of the subpubic angle. A narrow arch and angle cause a great waste in the antero-posterior dimensions of the outlet because the head can only emerge by passing farther back, with detriment to the maternal pelvic floor. Greater forces in delivery are therefore necessary in these cases and outlet difficulties are far more often responsible for extreme moulding and elongation of the head than brim dystocia.

The mechanism of successful internal rotation of the fœtal head may be hampered by the presence of disproportion, but even more commonly is this fault due to uterine inadequacy. The various types of contracted pelvis, however, profoundly influence the mechanism of labour, and these individual aspects will be discussed presently.

When to Suspect Disproportion

It is naturally a part of good antenatal care that major degrees of contracted pelvis should be evaluated long before the patient reaches term. Nowadays, the main problem is confined to the lesser degrees and border-line cases. A fœtal head deeply engaged within the pelvis during the last four weeks of pregnancy practically rules disproportion out of court, for there is no finer pelvimeter than the fœtal head, but where satisfactory engagement of the head is not present, disproportion is one of the numerous diagnostic possibilities.

Certain general features are worth taking into account in forming an early impression. The stature of the patient is relevant, and although quite small women very often have good obstetrical pelves, any woman whose height is less than 5 feet should have an accurate assessment of the pelvis made during pregnancy, and if she is a primigravida, radiological pelvimetry may be indicated. The size of shoe worn also supplies some general indication of bony stature, and contracted pelvis in a woman of medium height or over is rather unlikely if the shoe size is greater than 5. A history or the stigmata of rickets are now rare in this country, but the problem is certainly more common overseas. Deformities of the lower extremities, if congenital or contracted in early youth, should always raise a suspicion of pelvic asymmetry, and spinal deformities are likewise significant. Beware of the primigravida with the pendulous abdomen. This is often due to the inability of the head to find room for itself in the pelvis.

The primigravida is a dark and untried horse, and a proper clinical assessment at least, of the pelvis, should never be omitted during pregnancy. The multipara, however, can supply information of priceless value, and the history should take note not only of the weight of the baby but the duration of labour, the extent of perineal damage, the degree of moulding at birth, the readiness with which the child breathed and the maturity at the onset of labour. A history of previous stillbirth or neonatal death should be very carefully inquired into, as a contracted pelvis might have been responsible. Nevertheless, a successful vaginal delivery in the past does not always guarantee a repetition next time, because successive babies tend to be larger and, in rare instances, the actual capacity of the

pelvis may be diminished, especially in high degrees of parity, by partial subluxation forwards of the sacral promontory. The factor of uterine inertia, however, seldom complicates the issue in multi-parous labour, although "delayed labour" in a multipara should make one think of the two likely possibilities of unsuspected brow presentation or unsuspected disproportion.

External pelvimetry has now been abandoned by all except the most old-fashioned of us who have time for such tomfoolery. The figures so obtained are inaccurate and valueless, the external conju-gate most of all. A thorough vaginal examination has remained a vitally important source of information ever since Smellie first measured the diagonal conjugate digitally, and the advent of X-ray pelvimetry in no way dispenses with the need for it. Vaginal examina-tion is often misleading if sought in early pregnancy, and the opti-mum time for digital assessment is at the 36th week of pregnancy, when the soft tissues are sufficiently dilated to facilitate it. This should be a routine practice in all primigravidæ except those already under observation for antepartum hæmorrhage.

An appreciation of the mounting hazards of exposure to ionizing radiations, which are now known to be genetically cumulative and possibly a factor in malignant disease in childhood (M.R.C. Report 1956 and Stewart et al., 1956), has made nonsense of the statement which once originated across the Atlantic that every bride should have her pelvic measurements inscribed on the inside of her wedding ring! Court Brown et al. (1960, however, checked the fate of over 39,000 live-born babies of mothers subjected to abdominal or pelvic irradiation in pregnancy between 1945 and 1956 in London and Edinburgh and found only nine to have died of leukæmia by 1958 against an expected natural incidence of more than ten. Lewis (1960) likewise in a smaller series at Queen Charlotte's Hospital actually found more cases of childhood leukæmia among the controls than in those whose mothers had been irradiated antenatally!

Radiopelvimetry is reserved for cases in which the information sought is vital, for example in forthcoming breech delivery and in which satisfactory measurements may not have been obtainable by clinical methods. Our caution in rationing diagnostic radiology in pregnancy, however, must not be allowed to expose the baby or mother to even greater risks through neglecting to assess mechanical difficul-ties in labour. In spite of pelvimetry and every conscientious effort to assess disproportion, one is still sufficiently uncertain of the likely out-come to invoke trial of labour to resolve the doubt. Unfortunately, even a trial of labour often fails to answer the question. Gibberd, in the course of his Canadian lecture tour, in a piece of brilliantly analy-tical criticism, pointed out from a series at Guy's Hospital that, where-as the prediction that the pelvis would prove adequate was wrong in

only 1 out of 650 cases, the diagnosis of pelvic inadequacy remained still unproven in about half the cases submitted to trial of labour because for one reason or another the trial could not be carried through to a full and final verdict.

It is to Munro Kerr that modern obstetrics largely owes the direction of its attention to the ability of the foot to fit the shoe or the head to fit into the pelvis, and, whatever other aids to diagnosis we may invoke, above all there remains the cardinal observation—Is the head engaged or is it not, and, if not, can it be made to do so?

Causes of a High Head at Term

The commonest cause is posterior position of the occiput. This is often associated with some degree of deflexion, which must rank as the second commonest cause. In multiparous pregnancy likewise the head may be late in engaging and in fact may occasionally not do so until labour is well advanced. In all three instances, however, it should be possible to push the head into the pelvis by manipulation. There is a growing tendency, even in Glasgow, to ignore the possible significance of a high head at term in the primigravida and I am constantly deprecating the attitude which, translated in Glaswegian dialect, amounts to "Hoots to a high head." It must, of course, colour one's attitude towards forthcoming labour and how vigorously it is to be pursued, but above all it calls for a thorough clinical assessment—no bad thing!

A full bladder or, it might be added, even a half-full bladder, should never be forgotten as a cause of high head at examination.

Mistaken maturity might be mentioned here as a spurious cause, the head being high simply because the patient is not so far on in pregnancy as her alleged dates would suggest.

A high angle of inclination of the pelvic brim discourages engagement. It occasionally operates singly, but is more commonly associated with compensatory lordosis of the spine, and pendulous abdomen, with or without this bony anomaly, may discourage the head from engaging. Sometimes a high head is found which cannot be pushed into the pelvis because that is already occupied by the presenting part of another twin. This mistake is easier to make than one would imagine.

Hydramnios, besides being a cause of unstable presentation, is not uncommonly a cause of high head. The mechanism is obvious. No case, however, associated with hydramnios should be simply dismissed on that account, but should be examined radiologically for fœtal abnormality or to exclude multiple pregnancy.

Now, and only now be it noted, is disproportion mentioned. Naturally disproportion may be due to a contracted pelvis with a

normal-sized baby or to an over-sized baby without pelvic contraction. Of the latter, hydrocephalus constitutes an extreme example.

Lastly, there may be an adventitious obstacle to engagement of the head in the form of placenta prævia or the presence of pelvic tumours, such as a fibroid or an ovarian cyst within the pelvis. The above is a large list to consider, and it has been given as far as possible in the order of probability if not of importance. Notwithstanding the above, however, there are some cases, usually fairly muscular girls, in whom no adequate explanation presents itself. It is as though the whole uterus, including the lower uterine segment, tended to ride high. In such cases disproportion is hard to exclude, and only the events of labour will provide evidence in retrospect.

Before proceeding to an account of the assessment of disproportion, mention should be made of a syndrome which, though not common, may, if recognised, give advance warning of difficult labour associated with disproportion. I refer to what is known as the dystocia dystrophia syndrome.

Dystocia Dystrophia Syndrome

These patients are of a definite type which is worth recognising, and Williams (1942) gave a very good account of 62 observed cases. The syndrome was recognised by Horner, but it was De Lee who gave it its clumsy though descriptive name. Characteristically, the patients are of stocky build, somewhat bull-necked with broad shoulders, short thighs and a tendency to obesity. Added to the above attributes there may be a male distribution of hair, and the hands are stubby, with the middle three fingers of approximately the same length. The bony structure of the pelvis tends towards the android type, which often gives rise to deep transverse arrest of the head in the cavity and difficulties at the outlet. The dimensions of the vagina are skimpy, notably in the vaginal vault, and the cervix is small. There may be a family history of dystocia.

It is not surprising that these patients are rather subfertile and often do not conceive until late middle age. Their subfertility may be reflected in irregular menstruation, and spasmodic dysmenorrhœa is common. Having conceived, they have an appreciable tendency to abort. Over half of Williams' cases developed pre-eclamptic toxæmia and the incidence of eclampsia is higher. More than two-thirds of them become postmature.

Labour starts indifferently with the head often high, and in the majority of cases occipito-posterior in position, the membranes rupture early, and labour drags on inertly. The average duration of labour in Williams' cases was over 50 hours and more than two-thirds of his patients had either an occipito-posterior position or a transverse arrest of the occiput at the time of eventual operation.

Not one of his cases had a spontaneous delivery. The perineum is rigid, and this, together with the combination of a large postmature baby and an android type of pelvis, often makes rotation and forceps delivery a difficult undertaking.

Their response to induction of labour is usually so unsatisfactory, because of uterine inertia, that it is very doubtful if it is worth performing in these cases. Finally, they complete the unsatisfactory obstetrical picture by lactating very indifferently.

ASSESSMENT OF DISPROPORTION

Pressing the Head into the Brim

An attempt is first made to push the head into the brim, and many methods are employed to execute this manœuvre, but because of the resistance of the abdominal muscles and the oblique tilt of the plane of the brim, normally 60° from the horizontal, many of these methods are often unsatisfactory. Sitting the patient up and then palpating is a poor method, because either it is impossible, in this position, for the patient fully to relax her abdominal muscles or the abdominal wall overhangs the area above the symphysis pubis and intererfes with the examination. The use of the standing position is little better and increases the angle of pelvic brim tilt, so that it becomes more difficult to push the head into the brim.

My own method is to keep the patient lying on a couch with the knees not fully raised but fairly widely separated, the head being supported by a pillow. Standing on the right of the patient and using the third, fourth and fifth fingers of both hands, the head is gripped at sinciput and occiput. It will be noted that both index fingers and both thumbs are still free. One of the index fingers, usually the left, now reaches over and identifies the position of the top of the symphysis pubis. The thumbs are then pressed backwards against the parietal eminence. A complete grip of the head is thus obtained and its relationship to the symphysis pubis is fully appreciated (Fig. 4). Now, and not before, an assistant applies his hands to the baby's breech and presses the whole child towards the pelvis. At the same time the thumbs which are applied to the parietal eminence press downwards and backwards while the fingers on sinciput and occiput can observe what is happening and the index finger of the left hand is kept as before at the upper margin of the symphysis pubis. If the head is mechanically capable of engagement, it can now be steered into the brim with the thumbs and the whole movement can be fully appreciated. Often the head can be unmistakably pressed well down into the pelvis by this method.

Equivocal terms like "engaging" should never be used. Either a head is engaged or it is free, and if it is free it can either be made to

engage or it cannot, and students or candidates who use the term engaging are trying to hedge and get the best of both worlds and deserve no credit. Only one definition of engagement is acceptable, namely the biparietal diameter has passed the plane of the pelvic inlet or brim.

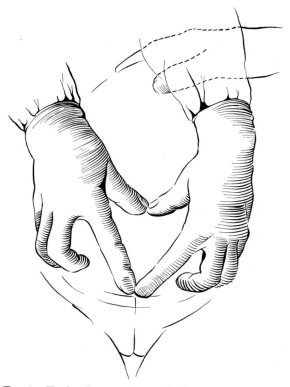

16/FIG. 4.—Testing for engagement. Assistant presses on breech.

The term "fixed" is often used as though it were synonymous with "engaged". It should not be used, because this is by no means always the case. A head can be fixed in the brim but still be too large to pass through it, or may be deep in the pelvis and so small in relation to pelvic size that it is anything but fixed. A good simile is the case of the egg and the egg-cup. Most eggs will sit fixed in the brim of the egg-cup, but disproportion clearly exists, whereas a bantam's egg is easily engaged within the egg-cup and is not fixed.

If the head cannot thus be pressed into the pelvis a vaginal examination should be performed. After the 36th week, this should be made

with proper aseptic and antiseptic ritual. It is true that any pathogenic organisms introduced into the genital canal through careless technique will probably disappear within a few days, but one cannot at this stage of pregnancy be certain that labour might not presently ensue, hence the need for proper precautions.

The Vaginal Examination in Apparent Disproportion

Everything possible must be found out at this examination and nothing should be allowed to interfere with its thoroughness, because it is undesirable to have to repeat it later. To this end it is worth admitting the patient to hospital, at least for the day. She is shaved and properly prepared, an enema is given, and the bladder is emptied. The nervous patient may require an anæsthetic, but usually a powerful sedative is all that is necessary. It is our practice to take them to the Labour Room, and just before the examination to give an injection of up to 100 mg. of pethidine with 0·4 mg. of scopolamine

The patient is now placed in the lithotomy position and after swabbing down and painting is properly draped. The resistance of the pelvic floor is noted and then the presenting part is identified and the state of the cervix observed. The fingers are now gently but firmly pressed onwards until the sacral promontory is reached. In the lithotomy position and under the influence of the drug there should never be any difficulty in reaching the sacral promontory. With the help of sterile callipers, the depth of insertion of the fingers in reaching the promontory is accurately measured. It is a good plan for the operator to know exactly the distance between the tip of his middle finger and the crease of the metacarpophalangeal joint of the index finger. In this way the diagonal conjugate is assessed.

Using the traditional Munro Kerr method and with the help of an assistant pressing upon the fundus of the uterus, an attempt is now made to push the head into the pelvis on top of the fingers lying along the diagonal conjugate. The thumb of the examining hand is swept over the front of the symphysis pubis and feels for overlap. This often needs quite a good manual stretch, as it may be difficult sometimes for the thumb to reach far enough. If the head can be pushed down to the level of the ischial spines, what the Americans call "zero station", brim disproportion can be excluded. If it cannot, the thumb notes the degree of overlap. In first-degree overlap the parietal bone lies flush with the anterior surface of the symphysis pubis (Fig. 5). This amounts to about a quarter of an inch of overlap, and, given good contractions and a favourable position, the chances are that the head will go through. If, however, the head is felt by the thumb to overhang the symphysis pubis, second-degree overlap is diagnosed. The outlook then for vaginal delivery is very poor.

Unfortunately, the assessment is not as simple or cut and dried as most descriptions, including the above, would infer, and there are certain snags, the chief of which is that although the pelvis seems large, the diagonal conjugate above reproach and the head of no more than reasonable size, yet it is still impossible to push the head

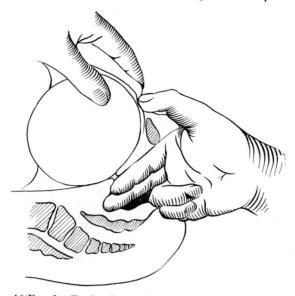

16/Fig. 5.—Testing for overlap. (Munro Kerr method.)

down to the level of the ischial spines. One may rightly feel certain that there is no question of disproportion, although the Munro Kerr test has failed, and in all honesty it has to be admitted that one sometimes comes away from the examination with doubts far from resolved.

In the normal pelvis the diagonal conjugate should measure not less than $4\frac{3}{4}$ inches (12 cm.), but this measurement alone is not enough. The examination is not complete without further observations. The finger should be swept round the inside of the pelvic brim and an estimate made of its shape, particularly the fullness of curvature of the anterior portion. Any tendency to "beaking" suggests an android type and diminishes the *effective* lengths of the antero-posterior diameters. The length of the symphysis pubis should also be noted. An unfavourable sign is the impression of great pelvic depth which one gets with the android pelvis and with cases of high assimilation. The angle of inclination of the pelvic brim is also noted; the steeper the angle the less favourable the prognosis. The fingers

are now swept around the side walls of the pelvic cavity in order to detect any tendency to convergence. The prominence of the ischial spines and the depth or width of the sacro-sciatic notches can be easily assessed, and the finger is now swept down the anterior surface of the sacrum, noting any false promontories, irregularities, straightness, angulation and general roominess of the sacral bay. The sacrococcygeal joint is tested for mobility and finally completion of the examination involves an estimate of the outlet. The sub-pubic arch should comfortably accommodate the backs of two fingers. It should be in the shape of the Norman arch rather than the Gothic. The length of the descending pubic rami is also observed and, using the fingers of both hands, an estimate of the sub-pubic angle is made. The normal angle is somewhere between 80° and 85°. It will be noted that we distinguish between sub-pubic arch and sub-pubic angle, although as a general rule an acute angle tends to go with a narrow arch and vice versa. Lastly, with the patient still in the lithotomy position, the intertuberous diameter can be very satisfactorily assessed with the knuckles. Obstetricians should know the width of their four knuckles. Depending on the size of one's hand, either the knuckles of the first inter-phalangeal joints can be used or the knuckles of the clenched fist, which appears to be a more stable measurement. The examination thus conducted is of priceless value, and properly carried out with a co-operative patient can yield almost as much information as a whole set of X-rays. It is an examination which calls for good patient handling. Gentleness is essential, as the patient is likely to be frightened by the general ritual of the labour theatre. A running commentary must, therefore, be kept up with the patient throughout and there must be no hesitation in explaining what is going on and reassuring her on every good point noted. This is very important, because if the patient once suspects that she is mechanically incapable of delivering herself the subsequent outcome of labour is prejudiced from the first.

Measurements of the Normal Pelvis

A consideration of the pelvic diameters in three planes will suffice namely the plane of the brim, the cavity, and the outlet. There are one or two observations to be made before giving the traditional list. Firstly, the true conjugate may be of less relevance than the obstetric conjugate. The latter is measured from the inner margin of the upper part of the symphysis pubis to the nearest point of the sacrum, which often lies below the actual promontory. In certain cases the difference may be as great as half a centimetre, and since the head must negotiate this smaller diameter it should, in such cases, be separately noted. The transverse diameter of the brim is usually

taken as the widest measurement, but, particularly in the android type of pelvis, this diameter lies rather closer to the sacral promontory and is not fully available in labour. It is, therefore, worth noting what is known as the available transverse diameter. This latter measurement is made transversely at mid-distance between fore and hind pelvis.

Traditionally the normal true conjugate has been given as $4\frac{1}{4}$ inches or 10·8 centimetres, but it is now generally recognised that the correct figure should be $4\frac{1}{2}$ inches (11·45 cm.).

The average value of the obstetric conjugate varies from 11·2 to 11·8 centimetres. The transverse diameter of the brim varies from 12·6 to 12·9 centimetres (5–$5\frac{1}{8}$ inches) (Chassar Moir). The interspinous diameter is 10–10·8 centimetres (4–$4\frac{1}{4}$ inches).

One cannot draw a hard and fast line of demarcation at which contracted pelvis is categorically diagnosed. The shape of the pelvis and the angle of inclination must also be taken into account. Disproportion, however, in a given pregnancy occurs when delivery cannot be safely accomplished because of a reduction in one or more measurements of the bony pelvis. The average biparietal diameter is $3\frac{3}{4}$ inches or 9·5 centimetres. A diameter of 9·6 centimetres represents a fairly large head. If any of the diameters in any of the three planes measures less than 4 inches (10·15 cm.) one can fairly safely state that contracted pelvis exists. The decision as to the method of delivery is discussed later. A true conjugate, however, of $3\frac{1}{2}$ inches (8·9 cm.) or less represents gross pelvic contraction, and a baby small enough to negotiate such straits is often too fragile to do so in safety.

Clinical examination of the pelvis will only produce an estimate of the true conjugate by inference from measuring the diagonal conjugate. This is generally accepted as being half an inch greater than the true conjugate; in other words, in normal cases, practically 5 inches (12·6 cm.) but this difference is by no means standard, and in order to obtain really accurate measurements one has to resort to radiology. Intra-vaginal measurements taken with callipers have not even been discussed; they are difficult to make, uncomfortable to the patient and too inaccurate to be of much use.

Radiology, in the case of the maternal pelvis, has brought to obstetrics almost as much as it has to orthopædic science. The fact that it may be abused is no reflection upon radiology but rather upon the clinician who lacks sufficient common sense and clinical judgment to make intelligent use of it. Chassar Moir dismissed the fear that more radiology would lead to unnecessary intervention by saying that this will only occur when bad radiology is combined with bad obstetrics. The generation which prefers stethoscopes to chest X-rays in dealing with pulmonary tuberculosis is not quite dead. There is a counterpart in obstetrics. Proper clinical examination of

the pelvis, however, must never be omitted simply because X-rays are available. Both sources of information should be studied, for one is complementary to the other. We will now review what radiology has to offer in the study of disproportion. A fuller description of the technical aspects of radiological pelvimetry by Dr. Ellis Barnett will be found at the end of this chapter.

X-ray Pelvimetry

Not only can the pelvis be very accurately measured by modern techniques, but the general shape and type of the pelvis are revealed, and this is almost as important as actual measurements. The relationship of the head to the pelvis can also be studied and, in certain cases, progress of labour can be observed. To some extent bony dystocia can also be forecast, at certain levels other than the brim, and this knowledge may be helpful in modifying the conduct of a difficult labour.

Of all the available views, a lateral X-ray taken in the erect position is unquestionably the most valuable. The following is a list of the points to be observed and the information which can be obtained from a lateral X-ray:

1. The relation of the head to the pelvic brim.
2. The angle of inclination of the pelvic brim.
3. Posterior position of the occiput.
4. Angulation of the fœtal neck; this is likely to occur when occipito-posterior position is combined with a high angle of pelvic inclination. It is an unfavourable sign because it indicates some misdirection of the uterine thrust, the components of whose force tend to be directed in front of the symphysis pubis instead of downwards into the cavity of the pelvis.
5. The measurement of the true conjugate.
6. A false promontory, if present.
7. The measurement of the obstetrical conjugate if different from the true conjugate.
8. The shape of the sacrum and the fullness of the sacral bay. A straight sacrum or one with a reverse curve is unfavourable.
9. Measurement of the sacral angle. This is the angle subtended by the true conjugate and the anterior surface of the first two pieces of the sacrum (Fig. 6). It is an observation of the greatest importance and is not sufficiently stressed in current teaching. The angle is normally greater than 90°, in which case it can be confidently predicted that a head which has once negotiated the brim will find its passage easier thereafter. On the other hand, a sacral angle of less than 90° suggests funnelling, and labour is likely to become more difficult as it proceeds.

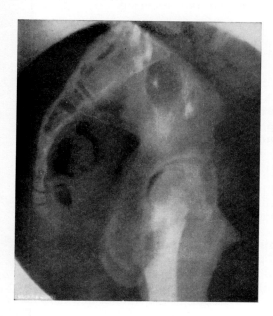

16/Fig. 6 (*a*).—Acute
sacral angle.

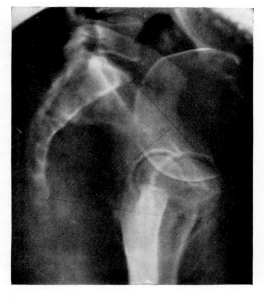

16/Fig. 6 (*b*).—Obtuse
sacral angle.

(By courtesy of Dr.
J. W. McLaren.)

10. The number of pieces in the sacrum, indicating the possible presence of an assimilation pelvis. High assimilation, i.e. incorporation of the fifth lumbar vertebra in the sacral body, is an unfavourable sign.

11. The width and depth of the sacro-sciatic notch. The notch should be wide and fairly shallow in the good pelvis.

12. The antero-posterior measurement of the outlet.

13. The relationship of the sacral attitude to the pubis and descending rami. The latter should be nearly parallel to a line joining the sacral promontory and the sacral tip. Convergence in a downward direction is an unfavourable sign.

To obtain all the above information the picture must be very well taken and properly centred. The heads of the two femora and the acetabular margins should be superimposed upon each other or at least very nearly so.

The brim view is also valuable because, apart from the actual measurements, antero-posterior, oblique and transverse, which it furnishes, its shape largely indicates the type of pelvis. Unfortunately, as pointed out by Dr. Ellis Barnett later, this involves a much higher exposure to radiation. A discussion of the features and influences upon labour of the various genetic types will follow presently. The outlet view is on the whole somewhat less important, as much of the information can be obtained by clinical means.

Types of Contracted Pelvis and their Influence on Labour

Attempts have been made, notably by Caldwell and Moloy, to classify the types of female pelvis, whether or not contraction is present. Their classification is now more generally accepted than that of Thoms. The pelvic type becomes much more important when contraction in any of the diameters is present. Now, Caldwell and Moloy have defined four generic, parent types applicable, more or less, to the majority of women. In rough figures the type frequency is as follows: gynæcoid 50 per cent, android 18 per cent, anthropoid 26 per cent, platypelloid 5 per cent. None of these types is pathological unless any of the diameters are substantially reduced below average. The following are the characteristics of each (Fig. 7).

Gynæcoid.—The brim is well rounded and there is a good, full curvature of the fore pelvis. The maximum transverse diameter does not lie far behind the mid-point of the true conjugate, with the result that the area of the hind pelvis is only somewhat less than that of the fore pelvis (Fig. 8a). The cavity of the pelvis is almost the segment of a sphere and there is no convergence of the side walls. The ischial spines are not prominent and the sacro-sciatic notches are relatively wide and shallow in a vertical diameter. The sacral bay has a full and

even curve. The sub-pubic arch is normal in shape and the sub-pubic angle is not less than 85°, while the descending pubic rami are short and slender. The sacral angle exceeds 90°.

Android.—This is more like a triangle with the base towards the sacrum. The fore pelvis is beaked rather like the bows of a ship, and the maximum transverse diameter of the brim intersects the true conjugate very close to the sacrum so that the area of the hind pelvis is only a fraction of that of the fore pelvis (Fig. 8*b*). Because of the beaking of the latter the fœtal head is unable to make use of much of the fore pelvis area and has to pass at some distance posterior to the

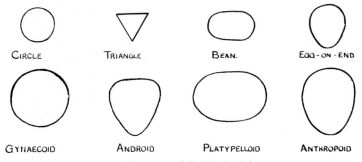

CIRCLE   TRIANGLE   BEAN.   EGG-ON-END

GYNAECOID   ANDROID   PLATYPELLOID   ANTHROPOID

16/FIG. 7.—Diagrams of Caldwell-Moloy types.

symphysis pubis. The side walls of the pelvis tend to converge downwards, the ischial spines are often prominent and the sacro-sciatic notches are narrow and deep in a vertical direction. The length of the symphysis pubis is greater than usual, the sub-pubic arch tends towards the Gothic, the sub-pubic angle is definitely acute and the descending pubic rami are long and thick. The head in its passage to the outlet is not able to make use of much of the sub-pubic space, and therefore has to emerge farther back. The angle of brim inclination is steep and the sacral angle is less than 90°.

Platypelloid.—This is the flat type of pelvis. The transverse diameter is very much larger than the antero-posterior diameter and the sacral promontory tends to encroach upon the area of the hind pelvis (Fig. 8*c*). The cavity tends to be more roomy than usual, the side walls of the pelvis diverge downwards, the sacral angle is greater than 90°, the sacrum may be somewhat flattened in its upper portions with a rather sharp curve forwards near its tip. The sacro-sciatic notches are very wide and shallow in a vertical direction and the ischial spines are not prominent. The symphysis pubis is not deep, the sub-pubic arch is wide and the sub-pubic angle is in excess of 90°. The outlet diameters are consequently increased.

Anthropoid.—In this type the brim has an antero-posterior dia-

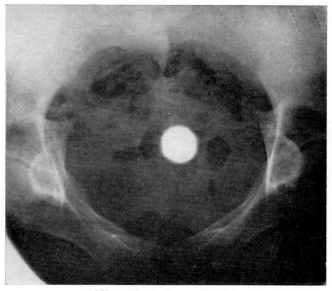

16/Fig. 8 (a).—Gynæcoid pelvis.

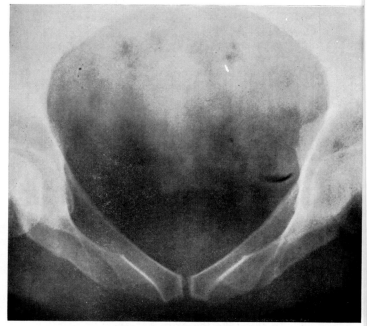

16/Fig. 8 (b).—Android pelvis.

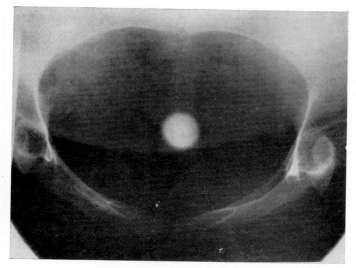

16/Fig. 8 (c).—Platypelloid pelvis.

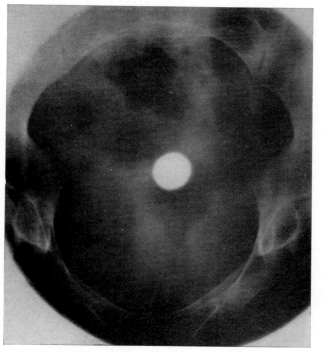

16/Fig. 8 (d).—Anthropoid pelvis.
(Figs a, b, c & d by courtesy of Dr. J. W. McLaren.)

meter which exceeds the transverse, giving it an oval appearance. The maximum transverse diameter may intersect the true conjugate fairly near its mid-point, providing a reasonable ratio between the areas of fore pelvis and hind pelvis, but the normal engagement of the head in the occipito-transverse position is discouraged (Fig. 8d). The cavity and outlet have no gross distinguishing characteristics.

The pelvic types are not as pure as the above description would suggest, and there are all manner of subdivisions, for instance a woman may have a gynæcoid hind pelvis and an android fore pelvis and all sorts of combinations may occur in the different straits. When contraction is present, however, the pelvic type may materially influence the mechanics of labour. The small gynæcoid pelvis, which used to be called the small round or justo minor pelvis, provides a tight fit the whole way. The mechanics are those of normal labour calling for increased expulsive forces if delivery is to be achieved, and extreme degrees of flexion of the fœtal head will be required. The android type of contracted pelvis is one of the most treacherous and may easily be missed on clinical examination alone. What makes it more dangerous is that the clinical estimate of the diagonal conjugate may show no reduction, and indeed the true conjugate may be normal but, as already hinted, much of this length is wasted in the narrowness of the fore pelvis. Even when the head has safely negotiated the brim it meets increasing difficulties in the cavity because of funnelling, so that labour may come to an obstructed halt at a later stage with the head tightly wedged, unable to rotate and incapable of advancing. When it reaches the outlet the head meets even greater trouble. Extreme moulding may cause it to appear at the vulva long before the main bulk of the skull vault has properly reached the pelvic floor. Because of the need to pass farther back from the symphysis, the perineum and other maternal soft tissues are subjected to increased stress and damage may be extensive. There is only one compensation in difficult labour with a contracted android pelvis, namely that the narrowness of the fore pelvis provides a protective arch for the bladder neck and its supports, so that damage in the form of subsequent stress incontinence or pressure necrosis of the bladder neck, resulting in vesico-vaginal fistula, is less likely to occur in this type of disproportion than in other types.

The anthropoid type of pelvis, when contracted, discourages transverse engagement of the head, so that it engages either occipito-anterior or occipito-posterior. Should the latter occur, long internal rotation is not likely to take place and a persistent occipito-posterior position results. Under these circumstances it may be unwise to attempt to rotate the head to the occipito-anterior position in order to deliver with the forceps, and these cases are better delivered in the unreduced position, namely, face to pubis.

The contracted platypelloid type of pelvis influences labour in a manner similar to the rickety flat pelvis. Here the difficulties are mainly confined to the brim, where most of the pressures of engagement are borne on the sacral promontory and on the back of the symphysis pubis, to the great detriment of the bladder neck, which lies between two bony millstones. If there is uterine obliquity and the occiput happens to lie on the same side as the obliquity, the parietal eminences may get held up on the brim and cause the head to become deflexed, even resulting in a secondary face presentation. Indentation of the cranial bones by the sacral promontory may occur, and even a depressed fracture may in rare instances be caused. Asynclitism is often a necessary mechanism, as has been explained earlier. Chassar Moir has shown by means of a simple model, consisting of a wire hoop and child's balloon, that, for a given circumference, a head will more easily negotiate a contracted flat pelvis than a small round brim.

Once the head has passed the brim, all is relatively plain sailing, although internal rotation may occur late because of the usually flattened sacrum. Outlet dystocia is most unlikely.

CLASSES OF PELVIC DEFORMITY

Firstly, there are those which are due to diseases affecting the skeletal system as a whole. Of these, rickets is the principal offender. Not only may it produce stunting in growth, with general contraction, but the characteristic deformity is flattening of a type which exaggerates the worst features of the platypelloid pelvis, inasmuch as the sacral promontory may bulge so far forward as to give the brim a reniform shape (Fig. 8e).

Secondly, the pelvis may be deformed as a result of disease in one of the lower limbs contracted in childhood or of congenital origin. Examples are poliomyelitis, congenital dislocation of the hip, tuberculous arthritis of the hip, serious injuries and talipes. The woman who comes into the antenatal clinic with a severe limp requires a careful investigation of her pelvis.

Thirdly, there may be abnormalities of the spine. Scoliosis is often associated with disease affecting the lower extremities, and in these cases there may be pelvic asymmetry.

Kyphosis is important, particularly in relation to its site. A high dorsal kyphosis is usually offset by a compensatory lordosis, so that the pelvis is not altered in shape, although one must mention other obstetric considerations, such as the reduced distance between xiphisternum and symphysis pubis which may make a transverse lie inevitable for want of room in the abdominal cavity. A kyphosis

situated low down in the spinal column may, for like reason, encourage a pendulous belly. The outlet tends to be contracted in the latter instance, but these cases often go into premature labour so that the baby may be small enough to be delivered by the vaginal route.

There are two types of assimilation pelvis, the high and the low. In the former, the last lumbar vertebra is incorporated in the body of the sacrum, thus not only increasing the sacral length but placing

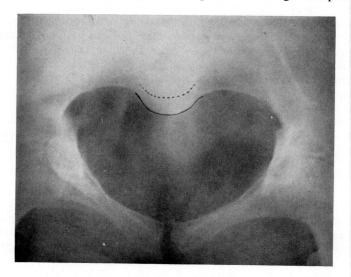

16/Fig. 8 (e).—Flat pelvis with marked encroachment of the sacral promontory.
Probably due to rickets.
(By courtesy of Dr. Ellis Barnett.)

the sacral promontory at a higher level than normal. This has the effect of steepening the angle of pelvic inclination and reducing the sacral angle well below 90°. It may be a potent cause of dystocia. In the low assimilation pelvis only four pieces comprise the body of the sacrum and there are no obstetrical disadvantages (Fig. 9).

Every undergraduate student remembers the freak pelves of Nægele and Robert. They are mainly of museum interest and only a very few cases of the latter have been recorded. In the Nægele pelvis one sacral ala is not properly developed, resulting in profound asymmetry (Fig. 10). In the Robert pelvis the condition is bilateral.

Spondylolisthesis, too, is rare, though less so. The lumbar spine is subluxated forward on the sacrum, thus reducing the antero-posterior diameter of the brim. In grand multiparity something akin to this process may occur.

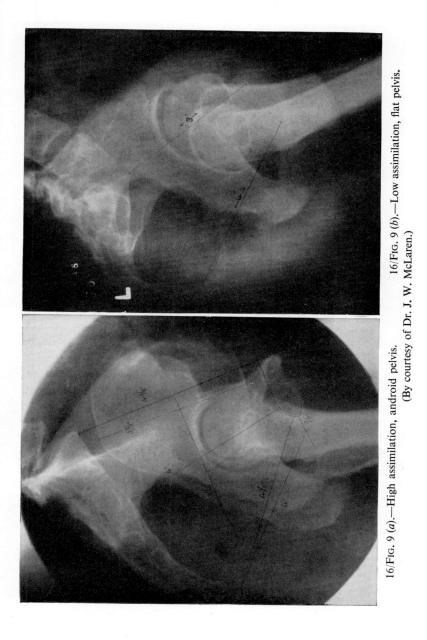

16/Fig. 9 (a).—High assimilation, android pelvis.　16/Fig. 9 (b).—Low assimilation, flat pelvis.

(By courtesy of Dr. J. W. McLaren.)

481

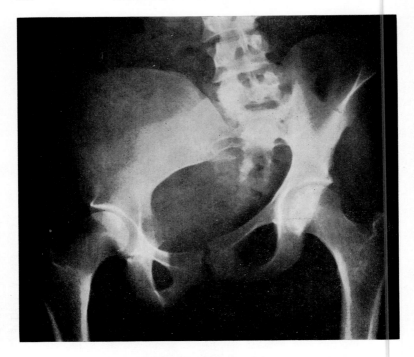

16/Fig. 10.—Nægele pelvis.
(By courtesy of the late Dr. G. W. Garland.)

Osteomalacia, very rare in this country, produces a three-cornered-hat type of pelvis.

Lastly, to complete the list, deformities of obstetrical significance may result from pelvic fractures, chondroma and osteoma.

OUTLET CONTRACTION

There are those who, like Hawksworth, do not believe in the existence of outlet contraction as an entity. They state categorically that if a head can be got through the brim it can be got through the outlet. I agree, as far as my own experience goes, but I have seen cases in the hands of very able colleagues where this has not been so. The above sweeping statement is technically true, but the price paid for vaginal delivery may be very high indeed. Unfortunately, the price is paid by the baby, who may suffer considerable cerebral damage, and the mother, whose soft parts may never be the same again. The amount of traumatic force which may have to be em-

ployed in delivering such cases with forceps can reduce the art of obstetrics to brutish barbarism.

The diagnosis of contracted outlet is often wantonly made in order to explain difficulties encountered in forceps delivery, which are more often due to faulty technique or a tight pelvic floor, and this diagnosis is one of the commonest with which patients are admitted to hospital after a failed attempt at forceps delivery. (In the majority of such cases the cervix is found to be not fully dilated, hence the difficulty.) Nevertheless, the condition undoubtedly occurs, although it is uncommon. The contracted android pelvis is likely to provide more instances than any other.

An examination of the outlet is a part of the routine assessment of the pelvis during the antenatal period. Firstly, the distance between the ischial tuberosities is estimated with the knuckles and it will often be found that in early pregnancy this transverse diameter is apparently contracted. In the majority of cases, however, the loosening up of the pelvic joints during pregnancy causes some widening before term. The importance of the sub-pubic arch and sub-pubic angle has already been mentioned. The antero-posterior diameter of the outlet is measured from the bottom of the symphysis pubis to the tip of the sacrum. Freeth maintains that if this measurement is found to be less than 4 inches (10 cm.), outlet contraction can be accepted as definite on clinical grounds. It is not difficult to make accurate measurements of the pelvic outlet without X-ray pelvimetry, but outlet views are well worth obtaining if there is any doubt. The information may be of vital importance to the conduct of labour. For instance, trial of labour is not applicable if the pelvic outlet is in doubt, because the true state of disproportion will not be apparent until very late in labour.

One may be reluctant to plan abdominal delivery simply because X-ray pelvimetry indicates a contracted outlet. It is in these cases that, having made a very full vaginal examination, preferably under anæsthesia, there is something to be said for allowing the patient to proceed inlabour. If all seems well and the second stage of labour is reached fairly easily, one may proceed to what is now referred to as a trial of forceps should further progress come to a halt. If it now appears that forceps delivery will be difficult and hazardous, it is far better to resort to Cæsarean section at this stage than to blunder on, doing irreparable damage. Injudicious force, besides injuring the baby, may even dislocate a sacro-iliac joint or disrupt the symphysis pubis.

The other alternative when faced with outlet obstruction is to resort to symphysiotomy. Needless to say, if the baby is unquestionably dead, perforation is the treatment of choice rather than a strenuous forceps delivery with the fœtal head intact. Perforation makes a surprising difference to the ease with which the head can be

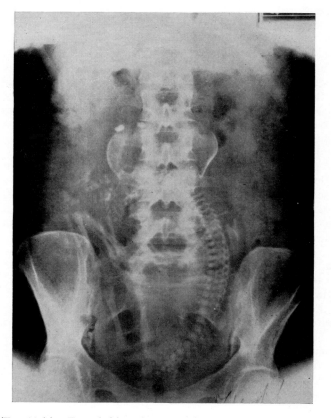

16/Fɪɢ. 11 (a).—Extended breech presentation, not apparently abnormal.

delivered. Only in rare instances should it be necessary to resort to
more destructive procedures, for only the gross types of contraction
justify them and should have been noted long ago.

In remote parts of the world where antenatal care is not available, gross degrees of contraction may first be encountered late in
labour, and cephalotripsy and cranioclasm still have their place in
the neglected and seriously infected case. There are, nowadays, few
obstetricians in this country who have much experience of these
ghastly operations, and, considering the good conditions under
which they work, the patient is probably better off with a lower
segment Cæsarean section than shocked, exsanguinated, lacerated
and bruised by the prolonged piecemeal delivery of a dead and
infected child's body. Things should never have been allowed to
come to this pass.

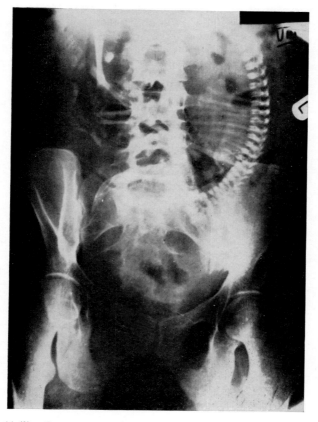

16/FIG. 11 (*b*).—Same case as Fig. 11*a* 5 weeks later. Gross hydrocephalus has developed, although the vertex now presents.

(Fig. 11 *a* and *b* by courtesy of Miss Lois Hurter.)

Hydrocephalus

The commonest indication for craniotomy these days is hydro-cephalus. Since the hydrocephalic fœtus commonly presents by the breech, the treatment is straightforward, because the aftercoming head is easy to tap. By pulling downwards on the neck, the head is safely stabilised and perforation in the sub-occipital region is simple. Alternatively, a metal cannula can be pushed up the spinal canal from below in order to draw off the cerebrospinal fluid. This is an even easier matter when there is associated myelocele, but otherwise the method has no advantage over perforation.

When the hydrocephalic fœtus presents by the head (as occurred

in 68 per cent of Feeney and Barry's 304 cases), treatment is less simple; for one thing, the head is above the brim and, for another, it is often difficult to stabilise its position; the cervix may not dilate very readily, thus increasing the hazards of perforation, and great care has to be taken in inserting the perforator that the points do not slip off at glancing incidence and damage maternal tissues. The head can also be slowly decompressed from below by inserting a lumbar puncture needle through a fontanelle. This does not kill the baby. There is an alternative method of tapping the hydrocephalic head through the anterior abdominal wall, after catheterising the bladder, but this is not without its risks and free bleeding may be started up if one is unlucky enough to strike a large blood vessel.

TREATMENT OF DISPROPORTION

We have already considered the plight of the patient and her doctor when disproportion is diagnosed only late in labour. It is part of the essence of modern obstetrics that the diagnosis should have been gone into before labour ever starts. Under these circumstances one has the choice of three methods: elective Cæsarean section, trial of labour, and induction of premature labour.

ELECTIVE CÆSAREAN SECTION

This is the method of choice for all cases in which the degree of pelvic contraction is gross. In fact, there is no reasonable alternative. Any pelvis with a true conjugate of less than $3\frac{1}{2}$ inches (9 cm.) is severely contracted, and a normal-sized baby cannot be reasonably expected to negotiate the diameters in safety. True, some women with such pelves, especially of the flat variety, are capable of delivering themselves vaginally, but the amount of moulding called for constitutes a serious risk. A small and premature infant might theoretically fare better, but the softness of the skull and the well-known liability to intracranial hæmorrhage in premature infants more than offsets the advantage of reduced size.

If borderline disproportion is present in the elderly primigravida, the only prudent thing to do is to deliver her by Cæsarean section. Her obstetrical future is too short to justify doing otherwise.

All malpresentations which cannot be corrected by external version, if associated with contracted pelvis, indicate elective Cæsarean section. There can be no trial of labour, for example, in a breech presentation. The verdict would come too late.

Major degrees of contraction of the outlet also call for Cæsarean section, for reasons above stated.

INDUCTION OF PREMATURE LABOUR

Theoretically this would be an ideal method of meeting the problem if only one could be completely certain of the degree of disproportion, if one could guarantee effective uterine action, if any method of surgical induction were both certain and safe, and if there were no penalties to prematurity. Alas, it is just on these very matters that this solution may let us down. In the cases in which this line of treatment appears to have been successful it has to be admitted that the absence of moulding of the fœtal skull seriously questions the original need for intervention. In other words, in the cases in which it succeeds it is hard to be certain that it was necessary and in the cases where it fails the results may be disastrous. The penalties of a long induction-delivery interval have already been dealt with in the chapter on induced labour, and one's hand is often forced in these cases into performing Cæsarean section, an operation which is prejudiced in advance in spite of antibiotics. Moreover, there must always remain the suspicion in these cases that if the patient had been left strictly alone and not induced she might have delivered herself spontaneously.

The indications, therefore, for induction must be very clear cut, and primigravidæ are as a rule unsuitable because, obstetrically speaking, they are unknown quantities and the fœtal mortality may be as high as 20 per cent.

The only cases generally accepted as suitable for induction are those in whom disproportion is no more than borderline and in whom a history of a previous delivery is available on which to assess the patient's obstetrical prowess. In the fit multigravida, therefore, who has had, for example, difficulty in delivering herself of an 8-pound baby because of disproportion, there is a very strong case for inducing labour prematurely next time.

One might well be tempted to try to get the best of both possible worlds by surgically inducing the patient near term when the disproportion is only of a very minor degree, in the hope of securing vaginal delivery before further enlargement of the fœtal head renders it difficult. In doing so one makes also the mental reservation that a trial of labour will be conducted and resorts to Cæsarean section at the first sign of trouble or arrest of progress. This procedure is undoubtedly becoming more popular but is questionable. It smacks of meddlesome interference, and labour is sufficiently likely to be inert as a result of the induction to prevent the subsequent trial from being a fair one.

TRIAL OF LABOUR

Trial of labour dates from about 1925. Because we cannot yet foretell how well a patient with disproportion will surmount her

difficulties, a wait-and-see policy is adopted. This is not as casual as it sounds, for these labours are conducted with great vigilance and with full facilities in the background for the safe performance of Cæsarean section. It goes without saying that a patient should not be aware of one's mental processes and above all that the trial should be conducted without ceremony.

This practice has conferred many benefits to date. Firstly, it has reduced the rate of Cæsarean sections electively decided upon. Secondly, it has eliminated an enormous amount of unwarranted and injudicious induction, and thirdly, a successful trial of labour practically guarantees a woman's obstetrical future. It is not without its disadvantages, however, chief of which is that it often proves nothing and, as Gibberd has pointed out, trial of labour may become a test not of disproportion but of readiness of the cervix to dilate, and in half the failures disproportion remains unproven because Cæsarean section had to be undertaken on account of uterine inertia or fœtal distress. In Gibberd's series the cervix was less than half dilated at the time when Cæsarean section was performed in nearly 70 per cent of these cases at Guy's between 1934 and 1950. In other words, more trials fail because of ineffectual contractions than because of proven disproportion. Good contractions, after all, are worth half an inch of true conjugate.

Another disadvantage is that the fœtal mortality is higher than would be the case with elective Cæsarean section, and death from intracranial hæmorrhage after trial of labour serves only to condemn it in retrospect. The maternal morbidity rate is also raised, but nowadays this is a less serious consideration. Not the least of the disadvantages is the fact that when a woman fails in a trial of labour she has now to face a major surgical operation, demoralised, disappointed, dehydrated, frightened and, at least potentially, infected.

Trial of labour is definitely not applicable to quite a large number of cases, as follows:

1. The elderly primigravida.
2. Cases of malpresentation.
3. Where there is outlet contraction.
4. In the presence of pre-eclamptic toxæmia or hypertensive disease.
5. Where any cardiac or pulmonary lesion or other relevant medical disease complicates pregnancy.
6. If the true conjugate is less than $3\frac{1}{2}$ inches (9 cm.), because, in such cases, the prospects of success are too remote.
7. If a genuine previous trial of labour has failed.

Trial of labour should on no account be conducted outside a hospital which is not only well equipped but, and this is more im-

portant, is properly staffed so that the case can be adequately watched.

Conduct of the Trial of Labour

For the trial to have maximum validity the onset of labour should be spontaneous and not induced. Everything should be done to preserve the membranes intact for as long as possible. In respect of duration, the trial only commences from the time of membrane rupture. Up to this point the mother and baby are hardly at risk, but from now on the condition of both must be frequently observed and the rate of progress estimated. As long as the head remains not engaged the patient should be nursed in bed, and no enema should be given once labour has started for fear of provoking rupture of the membranes.

As soon as the membranes rupture the patient must be examined to exclude prolapse of the cord. Often the head will now be found to have engaged in the pelvic brim and this is a good moment to assess its position. A fluid balance chart should be maintained, bearing in mind that the longer dehydration can be staved off, the later will maternal distress appear.

There are two criteria of progress:
1. The progressive descent of the presenting part.
2. The progressive dilatation of the cervix.
Either singly or together denotes progress.

Nowadays the tendency is to shorten trials of labour in order to reduce the risks to the fœtus. It is useless to set an arbitrary time limit to the duration of the trial after the membranes have ruptured. Various authorities have recommended periods ranging from two to seven hours, but the case should be judged on its own merits and account taken of the rate of progress, the general condition, the patient's fortitude and the state of dilatation of the cervix so far achieved. The onset of fœtal distress calls for prompt intervention. There should be no hesitation in using intrapartum radiography in the case that is not going well. A lateral view, erect if possible, is particularly important, but features to note are any evidence of fœtal abnormality as this will discourage the employment of Cæsarean section, signs of moulding of the fœtal head (Fig. 12), the level of the head and its attitude, e.g. occipito-posterior and unfavourable factors such as inclination of the head on the neck. The decision to operate is better taken early rather than late.

The conduct of labour with disproportion in the case of the African woman presents an altogether different set of problems. For one thing the African pelvis is extraordinarily shallow so that the head may bulge at the vulva before the biparietal diameter has yet passed the brim and uterine inertia is very unusual. The chances of

having to face a really difficult forceps operation are usually prevented either by spontaneous delivery due to tumultuous pains and a more or less physiological type of autosymphysiotomy or the clamant need for a Cæsarean section with the established threat of obstructed labour. In the European woman the position is far less clear cut.

In many ways the most difficult cases are those in which a midcavity forceps operation becomes necessary after a long and difficult first stage. Having gone so far one is reluctant to turn back, but vaginal delivery may be secured at too high a price, especially to the baby, and a difficult forceps operation of this nature may be almost as dangerous to the baby as internal version and breech extraction.

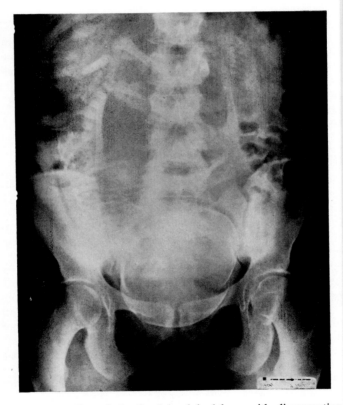

16/Fig. 12.—Moulding of the fœtal head in labour with disproportion. An intrapartum X-ray taken after 18 hours with the membranes ruptured, with strong contractions and without advance during the last 12 hours. Maternal height 4 ft. 11 in. Cervix 4 cm. dilated. Delivered by lower segment Cæsarean section. Birth weight 9 lb. 6 oz. Postnatal pelvimetry indicated a true conjugate of 10 cm. with a small gynæcoid pelvis with contracted outlet.

This is a task for the skilled obstetrician only, and if the forceps delivery threatens to prove very difficult, Cæsarean section, even at this late stage, may be the wiser course. In such cases forceps delivery should only be attempted on an operating table in an operating theatre equipped for Cæsarean section so that there need be no hesitation in proceeding to abdominal delivery. If in doubt, section is safer than savagery with forceps.

Hawksworth, in an impressive paper, came out strongly in favour of trial of labour in cases of uncomplicated disproportion, and analysed a series of 124 such trials. It is clear that the trials were pushed to considerable length, because no fewer than 16 of these cases had labours lasting more than 72 hours, 95 had operative deliveries of whom 58 reached full dilatation, and 37 did not. Forty-one per cent of his cases failed in their trials and came to Cæsarean section. The results, as far as maternal and fœtal survival go, are excellent, but it will be noted that, in spite of pushing the trial as far as skilful observation would allow, the failure rate is very high and many of these women laboured in vain. One cannot afford to be so impressed by survival statistics that one ignores the patient's subjective experiences, and to many women a long and unsuccessful labour evokes the firm resolution "never again".

The institution of trial of labour may easily encourage slovenly clinical assessment of the patient, on the argument that there is time enough to start worrying when the patient fails to make progress in her delivery. Nothing could be more deprecated than to subject a woman wantonly to an ordeal which has no reasonable prospect of rewarding success. It is not only bad science, it is bad doctoring. Furthermore, one's attitude to the labour itself should take into account every available feature, including the capacity of the cavity and the outlet. If one were only concerned with the problem of brim dystocia, as in the rickety flat pelvis, one could afford to be less punctilious in the safe knowledge that once the true conjugate was negotiated all would be well.

Trial of labour, therefore, just as much as induction of premature labour for disproportion, calls for scrupulous attention to every detail and the employment and intelligent use of every diagnostic aid. There is, after all, little credit in seeing the head negotiate the brim only, thereafter, to wreck the outcome in the course of a difficult forceps delivery. With foreknowledge of the lower pelvic straits one may well be influenced to curtail a trial of labour which at an earlier stage is not promising well.

Trial of labour may be the best that we can do under the circumstances, but it is a confession of our present-day ignorance and its failure a reproach to our scientific knowledge. Chassar Moir and his like are pioneers, whatever their results, in their attempts to make a

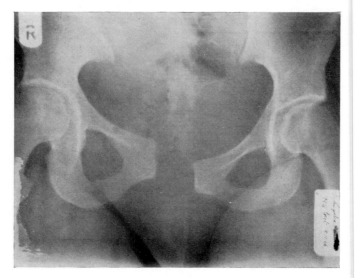

16/FIG. 13 (a)

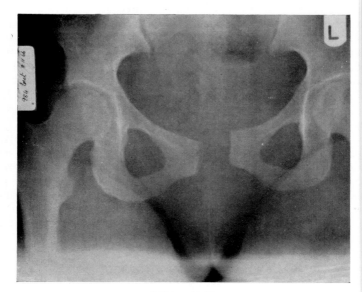

16/FIG. 13 (b)

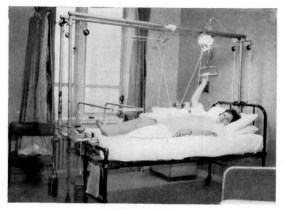

16/Fig. 13 (c)

16/Fig. 13.—Pelvic osteoarthopathy.

(a) Patient standing on right leg.
(b) Patient standing on left leg.
(c) Pelvic girdle maintained in a felt sling support during puerperium.

scientific forecast of the course of labour, and their work points the way to research in the future which may yet make an anachronism of trial of labour, so that obstetricians may one day refer to it as trial by ordeal.

Pelvic Osteoarthropathy

This interesting condition though not normally associated with disproportion had best be described here. As a result of the hormones of pregnancy, particularly "relaxin or progesterone," the joints of the pelvic girdle loosen up resulting sometimes in an abnormal separation and mobility at the symphysis pubis. The patient begins to feel considerable pain in her back and tenderness over the symphysis in the last month of pregnancy and the gap between the two halves of the pubis can sometimes be so wide as to be easily palpable. The diagnosis is not difficult to make provided it is thought of and can be confirmed by getting the patient to stand out of bed, first on one leg and then on the other, while the examiner's fingers palpate the symphysis pubis. The level of the two halves of the symphysis will be found to alter in relation to each other as the patient shifts her weight from side to side and the diagnosis can be further confirmed by X-ray (Fig. 13). The treatment is to put the patient to bed on a mattress with a hard board underneath it, which will greatly relieve her discomfort. She has, after all, a more or less physiological

symphysiotomy and labour is not usually complicated, but the condition may persist for some weeks after the puerperium and great care should be taken not to subject the pelvic girdle to undue strain by encouraging too early ambulation, particularly without adequate support from strapping and binders. In extreme cases it is best to make a felt sling for the whole pelvis suspended by pulleys and weights from a Balkan beam (Fig. 13c). In the case shown here this had to be maintained for three weeks before the patient could be comfortably got out of bed. Fortunately in the postnatal weeks the pelvic girdle becomes more stable.

SAFETY ASPECTS OF RADIOLOGICAL PELVIMETRY

by ELLIS BARNETT, F.F.R., D.M.R.D.
Radiologist, Royal Maternity and Women's Hospital, Glasgow

The possible radiation hazard in obstetrics is still regarded as a major consideration in the selection of cases for radiological pelvimetry. Radiologists are acutely aware of the dangers of excessive radiation, and since the initial report by Stewart *et al.* in 1956, radiological techniques generally have been analysed with reference to radiation protection and reduction of dosage to the patient. In this respect also, further attention has been paid to X-ray apparatus and emphasis placed upon accurate coning down of the X-ray beam to cover only the essential area, the use of faster films and X-ray screens, and the application of various protective shields. In addition, increased filtration of the X-ray beam ensures that only the hard (that is, more penetrating) radiation reaches the patient.

The latest report of the Adrian Committee (*Radiological Hazards to Patients*, H.M. Stationery Office, 1960) summarises the present attitude and makes certain recommendations. In view of the great importance of this subject not only in obstetrics but in medicine generally, the reader is strongly recommended to study this report. However, several extracts relevant to obstetrics are recorded below for general guidance.

"Our survey has shown that in the present circumstances, the dose to the gonads from any X-ray examination is small in comparison with that considered by the Medical Research Council to be acceptable to the individual, without causing any undue concern on behalf of himself or his offspring."

"Pregnant women should be subjected to pelvimetry only after thorough clinical examination by an experienced obstetrician. The full radiological examination is necessary for only a small proportion of primigravidæ, and very few multigravidæ, but once decided upon, the examination should be very thorough. Of the four projections in common use—erect lateral, antero-posterior, subpubic arch and outlet, and supero-inferior or inlet—the last named presents by far the

highest dosage to both the maternal ovaries and the fœtal gonads, and should be omitted whenever possible." In support of this are the figures recorded for the average gonad doses in milliroentgens per exposure to the fœtal gonads and maternal ovaries during radiological pelvimetry, as listed below.

Projection	Dose	
	Maternal Ovary	Fœtal Gonads
Antero-posterior	460	630
Lateral	577	535
Subpubic arch and pelvic outlet	670	140
Supero-inferior pelvic inlet or Thom's	992	2,242

Most radiologists agree that the supero-inferior or Thom's view (Fig. 14) should now be avoided wherever possible, in view of the greater dose particularly to the fœtal gonads. The antero-posterior view of the pelvis is an acceptable alternative to the Thom's view,

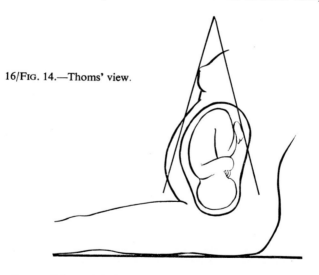

16/Fig. 14.—Thoms' view.

although the shape of the pelvic brim cannot be as readily appreciated due to foreshortening. There is evidence to show that using the antero-posterior view with very accurate coning of the X-ray beam by means of triple lead diaphragms, the dose to the fœtal gonads is reduced to a negligible level (Fig. 15). Should the Thom's brim view be deemed necessary in a particular case, the radiation to the fœtal and maternal gonads can be reduced by placing a lead disc of suitable

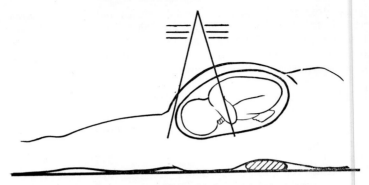

16/Fig. 15.—Reducing X-ray dosage of fœtal gonads.

size in the path of the primary beam and close to the X-ray tube. The resultant film will show only the bony pelvis, the pelvic cavity being obscured (Fig. 16).

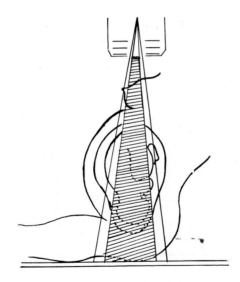

16/Fig. 16.— Thoms' brim view, with masking off of fœtus by means of a lead disc.

The Technique of X-ray Pelvimetry

It must be emphasised at the outset that in radiological pelvimetry the consideration of pelvic shape is just as important as the calculation of certain linear measurements. Pelvic shape is discussed elsewhere (see pp. 475–482).

The basic views of the maternal pelvis used for the purpose of pelvimetry are:

1. Erect lateral view (Fig. 17).
2. Outlet view (Fig. 18).
3. Antero-posterior view (Fig. 19).
4. Thoms' brim view. For the reasons already stated this view should be avoided wherever possible.

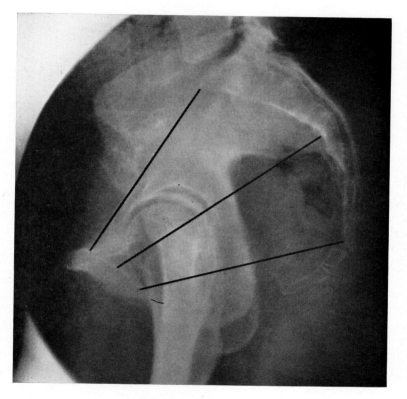

16/Fig. 17.—Erect lateral view.

In the X-ray department of The Royal Maternity Hospital, Glasgow, the first three views indicated above are used when a full pelvic assessment is desired. But the erect lateral film is without a doubt the most important, and if only a limited examination is necessary this is the view of choice, for very often cephalopelvic disproportion can be appreciated or excluded as far as the inlet and mid-pelvis are concerned, by examination of this film even without measurements.

P.O.P.—17

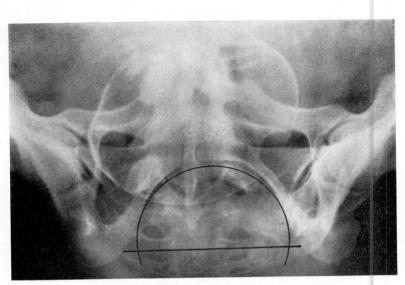

16/Fig. 18.—Outlet view.

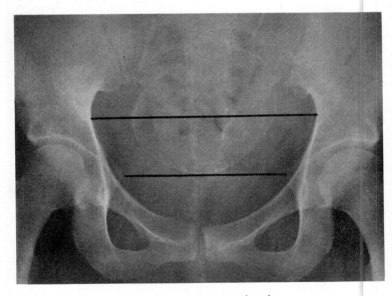

16/Fig. 19.—Antero-posterior view.

Nevertheless, whenever possible, we prefer to evaluate the pelvic capacity more completely.

Having obtained the three basic views of the pelvis, certain pelvic diameters are measured on the films and corrected for magnification by the simple geometric problem of comparison of similar triangles as shown in Fig. 20. The thickness of the X-ray table (HB) is fixed, and

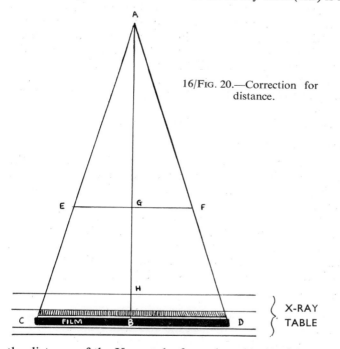

16/FIG. 20.—Correction for distance.

the distance of the X-ray tube from the table (AH) is also kept constant. Thus the only variable is the distance of the diameter in question (EF) from the table top, that is, the distance (GH), and this will of course vary with the thickness of the patient. For the lateral view, we measure the distance between the natal cleft and the top of the X-ray table, whereas for the antero-posterior view the pubis to table-top distance is determined. The outlet film is taken in such a position that no measurement on the patient is necessary, as will be discussed.

Various authorities utilise different pelvic diameters. We use the following combination of pelvic diameters (Figs. 17, 18 and 19).

From the lateral film:

1. The available (obstetric) conjugate diameter of the inlet, which is a line joining the upper limit of the posterior wall of the symphysis pubis just where it starts to curve forwards, to the nearest point on

the sacrum. The posterior extremity often, but not necessarily, coincides with the sacral promontory.

2. The antero-posterior diameter of the mid-pelvic cavity, which is taken as a line joining the middle of the posterior wall of the symphysis pubis to the middle of the anterior surface of the third piece of the sacrum.

3. The antero-posterior diameter of the lower strait. (This diameter is often referred to as the antero-posterior diameter of the outlet, but strictly speaking it is not in the plane of the outlet, therefore the term lower strait is recommended.) This is a line joining the lower limit of the posterior wall of the symphysis pubis just where it starts to curve forwards, to the first sacrococcygeal joint, thus taking into account the occurrence of partial or complete fusion of the coccyx to the sacrum.

4. Measurement of the sacral angle (see p. 472).

From the antero-posterior film:

1. The transverse diameter of the inlet, which is taken at the widest transverse diameter which can be measured on the film.

2. The bispinous diameter, which is a line joining the tips of the ischial spines.

Blair Hartley has shown that the transverse diameter of the inlet and the bispinous diameter lie respectively $\frac{2}{3}$ and $\frac{1}{3}$ of the distance of the symphysis pubis from the table top, with the patient supine. Thus having measured the pubis to table-top distance on the patient, the correction factors for these diameters can be readily calculated.

From the outlet film:

This view is taken with the patient sitting directly on the film, and bending as far forwards as possible, the abdomen lying between the separated thighs. Thus the positioning of the patient for this view brings the transverse diameter of the pelvic outlet and also the inferior ischio-pubic rami into close relationship to the film. Therefore, using a sufficiently great tube to film distance, the magnification will be negligible. To allow for the soft tissues overlying the ischial tuberosities we take the transverse diameter of the outlet as a line joining the medial margins of the descending rami at a level 1 cm. above the tips of the ischial tuberosities.

The average measurements recorded by Ince and Young (1940) in a survey of 509 cases are as follows:

INLET

True Conjugate	=	11·83 cm.
Transverse	=	13·06 cm.
Posterior Sagittal	=	4·87 cm.
Area	=	121·30 sq. cm.

LOWER STRAITS
    Pubo-sacral   =   11·97 cm.
    Intertuberous   =   10·90 cm.
    Ischial bispinous   =   9·95 cm.

The sub-pubic angle can be measured by joining the two extremities of the transverse diameter of the outlet to a point at the lower border

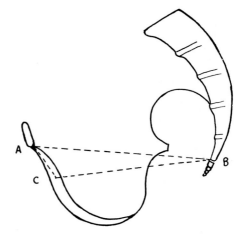

16/FIG. 21.—Available antero-posterior diameter of lower strait.

AB = Antero-posterior diameter of lower strait.

AC = Waste space of Morris.

CB = Available antero-posterior diameter of lower strait.

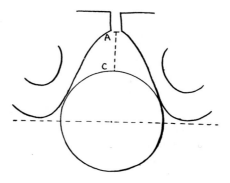

of the pubic symphysis, but we feel that this angle is of little practical value, as it does not allow for the curvature of the descending ischio-pubic rami. It is much more important to assess the capacity of the sub-pubic arch and to determine the extent to which the average fœtal head can utilise the space available. This is done by determining the Waste Space of Morris. A circle 9·3 cm. in diameter is applied to the outlet film between the descending rami. This will give a practical

indication of the extent to which the average fœtal head can utilise the arch. Morris (1947) considers that the head, moulded in the attitude of flexion, approximates closely to a cylinder with the biparietal, sub-occipito-bregmatic, and occipito-frontal diameters more or less equal. The diameter of this cylinder at term may be taken as 9·3 cm. Normally the distance between the lower border of the symphysis and the circumference of the circle is not more than 1 cm. and the coronal diameter of the circle should be at least 1 cm. in front of the ischial tuberosities. Obviously if the waste space is large the antero-posterior diameter of the lower pelvic strait as measured on the lateral film is false for practical purposes, as the head cannot fully utilise the whole of this diameter, which must therefore be adjusted and the *available* antero-posterior diameter of the lower strait be determined as shown in Fig. 21. The only measurement of the fœtal head which is thought to be measurable with sufficient accuracy on routine views is the biparietal diameter as measured on the erect lateral film when the head is presenting in the occipito-transverse position, and is not deviated to either side in the antero-posterior view.

REFERENCES

1. CALDWELL, W. E., and MOLOY, H. C. (1939). *Amer. J. Roentgenol.*, **41,** 305, 505, 719.
2. CALDWELL, W. E., MOLOY, H. C., and D'ESOPO, D. A. (1935). *Amer. J. Obstet. Gynec.*, **30,** 763.
3. CAMPBELL, S. (1966). Personal communication.
4. COURT BROWN, W. M., DOLL, R., and HILL, A. B. (1960). *Brit. med. J.*, **2,** 1539.
5. DONALD, I., and BROWN, T. G. (1961). *Brit. J. Radiol.*, **34,** 539.
6. DONALD, I., MACVICAR, J., and WILLOCKS, J. (1962). *Proc. roy. Soc. Med.*, **55,** 637.
7. DOUGLAS, L. H., and KALTREIDER, D. F. (1953). *Amer. J. Obstet. Gynec.*, **65,** 889.
8. FEENEY, J. K., and BARRY, A. P. (1954). *J. Obstet. Gynaec. Brit. Emp.*, **61,** 652.
9. GIBBERD, G. F. (1952). Eighth Annual Meeting of Society of Obstetricians and Gynaecologists of Canada, June 6th.
10. GLASS, D. T. (1956). *J. Obstet. Gynaec. Brit. Emp.*, **63,** 251.
11. GOLDBERG, B. B., ISARD, H. J., GERSHON-COHEN, J., and OSTRUM, B. J. (1966). *Radiology*, **87,** 328.
12. HARTLEY, J. B., and FISHER, A. S. (1955). *A Plan for Radiography in Obstetrics*, 2nd edit. Manchester: United Manchester Hospitals.
13. HAWKSWORTH, W. (1952). *Proc. roy. Soc. Med.*, **45,** 527.
14. INCE, J. C. H., and YOUNG, M. (1940). *J. Obstet. Gynaec. Brit. Emp.*, **47,** 130.
15. LEWIS, T. L. T. (1960). *Brit. med. J.*, **2,** 1551.
16. MOIR, J. C. (1946). *J. Obstet. Gynaec. Brit. Emp.*, **53,** 487.

17. MOIR, J. C. (1947). *J. Obstet. Gynaec. Brit. Emp.*, **54**, 20.
18. MORRIS, W. I. C. (1947). *Edinb. med. J.*, **54**, 90.
19. M.R.C. Report (1956). *The Hazards to Man of Nuclear and Allied Radiations*. London: H.M. Stationery Office.
20. STEWART, A., WEBB, J., GILES, D., and HEWITT, D. (1956). *Lancet*, **2**, 447.
21. WILLIAMS, B. (1942). *J. Obstet. Gynaec. Brit. Emp.*, **49**, 412.
22. WILLOCKS, J. (1963). M.D. Thesis, Univ. Glasgow.
23. WILLOCKS, J., DONALD, I., DUGGAN, T. C., and DAY, N. (1964). *J. Obstet. Gynaec. Brit. Cwlth.*, **71**, 11.
24. WILLOCKS, J., DONALD, I., CAMPBELL, S., and DUNSMORE, I. R. (1967). *J. Obstet. Gynaec. Brit. Cwlth.*, **74**, 639.

CHAPTER XVII

PROLONGED LABOUR

"O, that a man might know
The end of this day's business ere it come!
But it sufficeth that the day will end,
And then the end is known."
SHAKESPEARE, *Julius Cæsar*, Act V, Sc. 1.

A LABOUR which is unduly prolonged is likely to give rise to one or more of three types of distress, namely maternal, fœtal or "obstetricians' distress". Of the three the last may be easily the most dangerous! These cases tax clinical judgment, often to the limit, and then a second opinion, come freshly on the scene, is worth a lot. In hospital practice this is usually automatic, but in domiciliary work importuning relatives may easily distract judgment already wavering in the cause of plain humanity, with the result that intervention is often prematurely, ill-advisedly or unnecessarily undertaken.

There is no doubt that any patient labouring for more than 48 hours is worth transferring to hospital on that ground alone. In the case of multiparæ more than 24 hours of labour is sufficient to indicate transfer to hospital. Here at least a more objective attitude is easier to adopt, more minute supervision is possible and facilities for dealing with the complications are immediately available.

Any labour which lasts for more than 36 hours is to some extent abnormal, but in order to exclude border-line cases it is the practice of most hospitals to restrict their classification of prolonged labour to cases exceeding 48 hours. The terms uterine inertia, either primary or secondary, are often loosely used, but they signify little appreciation of what is actually going wrong. If even half as much research had been undertaken into uterine function, both normal and abnormal, as has been expended upon the mechanical aspects of the pelvis and birth canal, the position today might be less unsatisfactory in a subject which, next to pre-eclamptic toxæmia, provides the most serious gaps in obstetric science. A brief reference must therefore be made to the present-day conceptions of uterine function, both normal and abnormal.

UTERINE FUNCTION

An adequate study of this cannot be made by observation and palpation alone, and various tocographic techniques have been used which fall into two main classes: (*a*) external, (*b*) internal.

An example of the former is the guard-ring tocograph (Fig. 1) devised by Smyth (Nixon and Smyth, 1957). A flat perspex plate is applied to the abdominal wall, turning the area covered into a flat surface. In the middle of this plate there is a hole about one inch in diameter through which a "button plunger" projects from a fairly stiff leaf type of spring. Two strain gauges are bonded to the leaf spring, one above and one below and form two of the resistances of a Wheatstone bridge circuit. Any change of pressure within the uterus

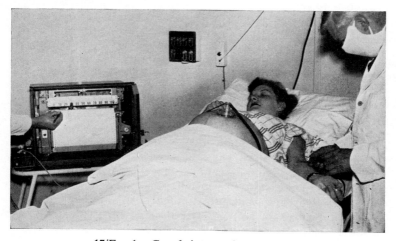

17/Fig. 1.—Guard-ring tocodynamometer.
(By courtesy of Dr. C. N. Smyth.)

is transmitted to the button plunger moving in the central hole of the perspex plate and thus the leaf spring is subjected to stress which increases the tension on one strain gauge and at the same time relaxes it on the other, thus altering their electrical resistances in opposite directions. This unbalances the Wheatstone bridge, the electrical imbalance so induced being proportional to the distorting mechanical force. By suitable amplification very stable (i.e. free from drift) records can be made.

Good records of the patterns of uterine activity can thus be obtained, as indeed they also can by careful clinical palpation, but it is less certain that absolute intra-uterine pressure measurements can be made by this means as there is some evidence that the figures given are affected by the pressure with which the apparatus is applied to the abdominal wall, and the thickness and natural resistances of this wall presumably play a part too.[15] The method, however, has the great advantage that it subjects the patient neither to risk of infection nor to discomfort.

Of the internal methods, one of the oldest, and dating from the last century, is the use of a tambour inserted between the membranes and the uterine wall. At the same time similar tambours can be placed either in rectum or bladder to record the amount of expulsive force due only to intra-abdominal pressure. The disadvantages of internal methods are of course the risks of sepsis due to the presence of a foreign body. The pressures in the tambours can be simply registered by a U-tube manometer. A tidier and better method is to insert a fairly large polythene tube into the amniotic sac by means of a Drew Smythe catheter introduced at the same time as performing induction of labour by hindwater rupture. The polythene tube is connected to an electromanometer.

To be able to pick up and record the electrical action currents of the uterine muscle during labour would be ideal but is technically extremely difficult, as I soon learnt myself, due to the enormous amount of interference from neighbouring voluntary muscle and cardiac activity.

The internal method described above only gives a picture of uterine activity as a whole with the resultant pressures achieved, and Caldeyro and his colleagues (1950) have made interesting observations by combining external and internal methods. They have shown that in normal labour there is good synchronisation of activity and have also detected asynchronism and other anomalies in abnormal labour.

The pacemakers of the uterus are believed to be situated in the region of the tubal ostia, from which waves of activity spread synchronously downwards. In the colicky type of uterus there may be ectopic pacemakers. The above workers have found the following characteristics of satisfactory uterine action:

1. There are large rises in intra-amniotic pressure exceeding 24 mm. of mercury.

2. There is fundal dominance as compared with the strength of mid-zone activity and the lower segment shows minimal action.

3. There is good synchronisation.

4. The wave pattern is regular

5. There is good relaxation of the uterus between contractions as demonstrated by a satisfactory resting base-line of intra-amniotic pressure. In normal labour this amounts to no more than 5–6 mm. Hg but in hypertonic and colicky types of uterine action the "resting" pressures may exceed 15–20 mm. Hg and in fact may remain dangerously above the pain threshold level.

This last observation is of particular importance, because of the need for utero-placental circulation to recover its volume between contractions. The interference with effective uterine blood flow caused by uterine activity has been well demonstrated by Wright et al. (1958) who studied the clearance rates of radiosodium injected into the

away. The presence of the fœtus in these cases now stimulates an irritable uterus like a foreign body and causes it to apply itself to the fœtal contours, producing a condition which I remember the late Kenneth Bowes graphically describing as the "hug-me-tight" uterus.

Constriction rings in the first and second stage of labour only occur with ruptured membranes. They resemble the "hug-me-tight" uterus in many ætiological respects, but represent areas of intense local hyperactivity. The ring usually forms round some indentation in the fœtal surface, most commonly round the neck, and the junction of the upper and lower segments is one of the more usual sites. A constriction ring can seldom be diagnosed by abdominal examination and is only found when the hand is inserted to ascertain the cause of delay. We prefer the term constriction ring to contraction ring, although the two are synonymous and in no way to be confused with the retraction ring of Bandl, of which more anon under "obstructed labour". Because polarity is deranged the lower segment is not thinned out nor stretched in cases of constriction ring and there is no danger of uterine rupture from labour obstructed due to this cause. Attempts to deliver the fœtus forcibly past the ring only make it clamp down the more viciously. Fortunately, the condition is reversible, but only with the lapse of time, generous sedation with morphia or deep anæsthesia. Amyl nitrite and adrenalin have a transitory effect in reducing the spasm and are sometimes useful in the course of operative delivery. Asymmetrical uterine activity is mainly recognised with the help of methods such as those of Reynolds. One theory is that the two halves of the Mullerian system may act out of step with each other with the production of pain and contraction mainly to one side. This is a state of affairs which can happen particularly in cases of imperfect Mullerian fusion, for example in the septate uterus.

Cervical dystocia.—This not very common condition comes into a subcategory of its own. Occasionally it results from some structural abnormality of the cervix of acquired origin as a result, for example, of fibrosis and scarring following cervical cautery, trachelorrhaphy or amputation. In other instances the cervix may be poorly developed and incapable of ready dilatation or there may be an excess of fibrous tissue within its substance. In labour, cervical dystocia may also represent another variety of incoordinate uterine action. In any case, a mechanical obstruction is offered to delivery. This is situated at the external os, which presents to the examining finger an unquestionably hard, leathery and undilatable rim. The presenting part is well applied to the cervix, and the other forces of labour have usually driven it low into the pelvis. In these cases full dilatation of the cervix can only be achieved at the expense of tearing, and occasionally annular detachment of the cervix results. It is an im-

portant condition to recognise in labour, because not only does it account for the delay in the first stage and for the patient's pain, which may be very great, but also because of the likelihood of extensive damage.

A somewhat similar condition occasionally occurs in which the os becomes displaced upwards and behind the leading surface of the presenting part so that there is a tendency for the anterior wall of the lower segment to sacculate, since the cervical canal is out of the line of thrust (sacral os). If the bony fit of the pelvis is a tight one, necrosis may occur, and the presenting part may side-track the cervix and burst its way through the lower segment into the vagina. A similar mechanism may occur posterior to the cervical canal, and as a rule the rent above the external os does not subsequently heal and can be found at later examinations. I had one such case with a large posterior aperture into the uterine cavity who, presumably as a result of it, suffered subsequently a series of very bloody abortions.

False labour.—Normally a patient is not painfully aware of uterine activity until the commencement of labour, but this is not invariably so. Before being certain that labour has started, the cervix, too, should show at least some sign of dilating. I once had a patient who had apparently agonising uterine contractions throughout the last eight weeks of pregnancy. She repeatedly turned up at a nursing home where she was booked for her confinement, but there was no sign whatever of cervical dilatation until she reached term, whereupon she delivered herself spontaneously and without trouble. Subjectively at least she had been in the first stage of labour for two months.

Cases of postmaturity have often demonstrated a short period of false labour round about term, and such a history may be of help in deciding if a case is in fact postmature. It is often difficult to decide whether a patient is in true or false labour and overnight observation is usually necessary. The injection of morphia 15 mg. (gr. $\frac{1}{4}$) helps to distinguish the two conditions. Morphia will seldom stop true labour but is effective in false.

MATERNAL AND FŒTAL MORTALITY

Nature and time are unreliable allies (Jeffcoate, 1961). The mortality rate for both mother and baby is roughly quadrupled in prolonged labour. It is difficult to compare the figures of different workers because of the adoption of differing standards, and many cases of prolonged labour are not due purely to uterine functional faults, so that catastrophe may, for example, arise from underlying causes such as neglected malpresentation or disproportion, or may be due to accidents following the treatment adopted for those con-

ditions. Jeffcoate (1952) quoted a maternal mortality of roughly 1 per cent and MacRae in his series found a maternal mortality of 0·4 per cent as compared with an overall maternal mortality at Queen Charlotte's Hospital in the same period of 0·12 per cent. He made the interesting observation that two of the three maternal deaths followed Cæsarean section which, in his opinion, had been undertaken too late. The commonest causes of maternal death in these cases are sepsis, hæmorrhage and shock as a result of ultimate intervention.

The fœtal death-rate rises with the duration of the first stage of labour and the time which has elapsed since the membranes ruptured, the last factor being particularly important. The curve climbs very slightly in the first 48 hours but thereafter steepens, and after 72 hours the fœtal outlook becomes very steadily worse. It is somewhat futile, however, to take figures in this respect too literally if all cases of prolonged labour are lumped together. A true picture can only be obtained by segregating the cases of hypotonic inertia from those of hypertonic activity and assessing the role of any underlying and ascertainable causes. The chief causes of fœtal death are intrauterine asphyxia, tentorial damage and intracranial hæmorrhage and intranatal pulmonary infection in which the baby is born with an already established pneumonia.

ÆTIOLOGY

There must, of course, be a cause for everything, but in the case of inertia it is frequently not apparent. Primiparity is the most constant factor, for it is essentially a condition of primigravidæ, 96 per cent of MacRae's cases, for example, being pregnant for the first time. The multiparous uterus, faced with mechanical difficulty, sometimes fights it and ruptures in the process. The primiparous uterus nearly always responds with inertia in the first instance and becomes inco-ordinate. Sepsis then follows as a matter of course. The influence of age has been somewhat overrated in the past, but the important point to remember in this respect is that the effects of prolonged labour are increasingly significant. Likewise, early rupture of the membranes has been traditionally held to be a cause, but this is no longer generally believed, and it would certainly seem poor logic to induce labour by invoking one of the reputed causes of inertia.

Overdistension of the uterus, either from twins or hydramnios is another accepted cause of inert labour, but this is only partially true. Admittedly the uterus will function to better mechanical advantage if excessive quantities of liquor are drained off, and in the case of twins the first stage is rather more commonly prolonged. To some extent, the babies being each smaller than a single fœtus, their size compensates for the mechanical effects of uterine overdistension.

Breech presentation has also been impugned, but in the frank breech with extended legs the presenting part acts as an efficient cervical dilator and prolonged labour is not common. Indeed, prolonged labour in cases of breech presentation should not be allowed to occur and our present practice is to regard any breech labour lasting more than 20 hours with considerable mistrust and calling for quite definite reasons why Cæsarean section should *not* be performed to reduce the fœtal casualty rate. Grand multiparity is dangerously accepted by some as a cause, the supposition being that much of the uterine wall is infiltrated with fibrous and elastic tissue. It is a safe rule, however, to regard all cases of delayed labour in multiparæ as being possibly due to an undiagnosed brow presentation, until this has been excluded by very thorough vaginal examination. Fibroids, too, are blamed for inertia, but the majority of cases so complicated encounter no such difficulties, at least in the first stage of labour, and it is possible that the attendant's interest in the patient's fibroids may contribute much to her anxiety. Uterine hypoplasia is also quoted as a cause by people who are more ready to guess than to think. This is obviously nonsense, or how else could the uterus have carried a pregnancy right up to term, and if anybody can diagnose uterine hypoplasia at 40 weeks' gestation he must be either a magician or a poet. Hormonal imbalance has also been postulated, but only in a nebulous and as yet unsubstantiated way.

So far we have chiefly considered many of the traditional views which cannot be taken very seriously, and we feel much more inclined to agree with MacRae who, with refreshing honesty, stated that in 82·4 per cent of his series the inertia appeared to be idiopathic. There are, however, certain ætiological factors of great importance which should be considered in all cases of prolonged labour. Chief among these is disproportion, and failure to recognise it may lead to disaster.

Of all the malpresentations and malpositions the occipito-posterior position is the most important in prolonging labour, though there is here some admixture of cause and effect, since a lively uterus will soon deal with poor rotation of the occiput. The other malpresentations, save the extended breech, operate as obvious causes in prolonging labour and demand recognition and treatment in their own right. Beware particularly of undiagnosed brow presentation and minor degrees of hydrocephalus.

Any cause of a badly fitting presenting part in the lower uterine segment deprives labour of one of its most important mechanical stimuli. Placenta prævia must be included under this heading. Congenital abnormalities in the uterus very occasionally cause inertia, but in many cases labour runs a perfectly normal course, so that the condition is not even suspected.

There are certain general types of patient who tend to labour badly and the dystrophia dystocia syndrome is an extreme case in point. This has been dealt with more fully in the chapter on disproportion. The association of obesity and inert labour is common experience, and in these cases there is often also a family history of prolonged labour, so that it would appear that the endocrine make-up of the patient is important in a general sense.

Postmaturity is not infrequently associated with long and difficult labour. At least a part of the reason for this is mechanical because of the hardness and slightly increased size of the fœtal head. Cause and effect here are mixed together since postmaturity besides discouraging brisk labour may, itself, be the result of disordered uterine activity. The older the patient the more sinister does the combination become.

The injudicious use of powerful drugs can often be rightly blamed for holding up labour. Nobody would expect a patient, who was kept continuously under a deep anæsthetic, to deliver herself smartly, and to a lesser extent the same argument must apply to the too early administration of "knock-out" drugs.

Let us never forget the full bladder and the full rectum, particularly the former. Not only are uterine contractions reflexly inhibited, but it is quite astonishing how even a moderately filled bladder can discourage deep engagement of the presenting part.

The question of inertia following induction of labour has been dealt with in the chapter on induced labour. It is a matter of some importance and readily incriminates the use of injudicious interference of this sort.

As has already been said, in the majority of cases the prolongation of labour cannot be explained under the above headings, and we now tend to fall back upon possible psychological causes. Anxiety and fear have been so largely accepted as causes that the science of obstetrics has become cluttered up with much speculative theory and it is difficult to sort out the wheat from the enormous quantity of chaff. All women facing labour do so with some degree of fear, some reacting more outwardly than others; but a patient can be frightened into labour just as well as she may be reputedly frightened out of it. Thunderstorms are terrifying to many people and in most induce a state of some sort of excitement, but midwives are usually extra busy at these times. A woman who has previously had a horrifying labour has extra reason to fear the next. Many, in fact, from fear decline to embark on further pregnancies. On this basis inertia ought to be more common amongst multiparæ than in primigravid patients. But the reverse is the case. It might be argued, however, that the fear of the unknown is more potent than fear of the known, but the professional torturers of history do not appear to

have worked on this principle, and they should know! A repetition of an unpleasant experience is often worse than the original incident and lowers one's threshold to further stimuli of that nature. The contrary argument that patients may become habituated to the pains of labour is of course nonsense. Surely the explanation of the differences in suffering and the length of labour between the primigravida and multipara lies in the fact that anatomically the two women differ. The multipara has had her cervix stretched in a previous labour, and it is suggested that, since this stretching is always accompanied by some degree of structural damage to the cervix, some type of modified local sympathectomy has been achieved by nature.

Much specious argument has been expended in explaining prolonged labour in terms of psychological aberrations and, as a result, all manner of therapy has come into vogue ranging from hypnosis to simple reassurance, the latter being obviously desirable without invoking scientific justification. Patients who can be bothered and who have the time can, according to taste, sit around relaxing, breathe Yoga fashion, or romp about in the gymnasium of a department of physiotherapy training their muscles. The cardiac case, who does not get this training, is seldom inert. All this huge and varied fabrication is based on the observation that the course of labour can be modified by the patient's mental state. This is too obvious to need further elaboration, but the methods of dealing with the matter have often little basis in science and are probably less effective than frank witchcraft and certainly less picturesque. A patient's reactions to her condition are on the whole more important than the condition itself, and if these reactions can be modified, as it is agreed they indeed can, so much the better. The patient who trusts her doctor and has healthy insight into the processes through which she is going, co-operates in her labour in the comforting knowledge that she will not be asked to bear more than is reasonably necessary and no scheme of antenatal preparation for labour, however elaborate or grotesque, can be accepted as a substitute for confidence between the doctor and his charge.

MANAGEMENT OF PROLONGED LABOUR

It goes without saying that any operative cause present such as, for example, disproportion, should be looked into and carefully evaluated and the treatment modified appropriately, but in the large so-called idiopathic group there is much to be done.

General care.—Everything should be done to stave off, for as long as possible, the onset of maternal distress in the hope of delivery being completed before one's hand is forced into operating.

Now, the signs of maternal distress are chiefly those of dehydration and ketosis. The lower the fluid intake, therefore, the sooner will labour dehydrate the patient. Until recently it was commonly taught that no opportunity should be lost of encouraging the patient to drink adequate quantities of fluid such as sweetened drinks flavoured with fruit juices. Unfortunately the very patient most in need of fluid and carbohydrate is also the one least likely to benefit from such treatment. At best she will vomit most of it and at worst she will merely accumulate it by the pint, unabsorbed, in her hypotonic stomach and upper intestine, where it lies treacherously in wait to be vomited back if, and when, a general anæsthetic has to be given. She will then be lucky indeed if she does not aspirate some of this deadly and copious vomit. We now regard fluids by mouth as dangerous in prolonged labour because of this risk, and unhesitatingly prefer the intravenous route to combat dehydration and ketosis. Hawkins and Nixon (1957) reported that in labour lasting longer than 24 hours, plasma specific gravity rises with the loss of plasma water before clinical signs of dehydration are manifest. After 48 hours, plasma potassium and chloride levels fall. They attribute this to hypersecretion of the adrenal cortex and suggest that the lower potassium level contributes to the uterine inertia and prolongation of labour. More electrolyte balance studies are clearly indicated.

The signs of maternal distress are a dry tongue, a rising pulse above 100, later a rising temperature and in advanced cases a hot, dry vagina, with possibly some purulent secretion. The urine becomes increasingly concentrated and scanty, and presently, if the patient is vomiting and has achieved only a very unsatisfactory carbohydrate intake, acetone, albumin and sometimes red blood corpuscles appear. Acetone in the urine, in any appreciable quantity, is an indication for the setting up of an intravenous drip. The customary solution for infusion is 5 per cent glucose, but in our own practice, where only the best is still not quite good enough, we have gone over to the use of lævulose which can be given in any desired concentration, up to 50 per cent even, without damaging the vein walls and causing thrombosis. There is no point, however, in giving such high concentrations in a patient who is already dehydrated and therefore needs fluid as well, although the only disadvantage of giving too much is that there is urinary spillage before this carbohydrate can be properly made use of. An infusion rate of 0·75 g. of lævulose (e.g. Lævosan) per kg. body weight per hour up to 2 g. per kg. body weight can be given over prolonged periods. Alternating with the lævulose solution, an infusion of Ringer's solution is much to be preferred to the traditional normal saline because the former contains a far more representative set of much needed electrolytes, including potassium. Two litres of such intravenous therapy can make a most astonishing difference to a

patient's wellbeing and often to the progress of her labour. The treatment of maternal distress apart from the treatment of the cause is not surgery but judicious intravenous therapy.

If there is any doubt about the patient's ability to empty her bladder completely, there should be no hesitation in catheterising, since it often takes very little urine in the bladder to hold up labour. The modern objections to catheterisation, on the ground that the urinary tract may be infected thereby, are less pressing in maternity units than in gynæcological or general wards where the bacterial population is much more dangerous. Nevertheless, it is worth noting Linton and Gillespie's recommendation to instil some antiseptic jelly such as chlorhexidine into the urethra a minute or two before passing the catheter. Our own practice is to instil 50 ml. of a pure 1 in 5,000 solution of chlorhexidine and leave it in the bladder at the end of catheterization.[14] The aseptic technique too should be above reproach and sterile gloves should always be worn. Wet, slimy hands are a bacteriological insult to any bladder. Provided the head is engaged an enema should be given, but this should be withheld if it is above the brim once labour has started, because the longer the membranes can remain intact the better. The patient can be up and about during the day, provided the head is engaged, but she should remain in bed if malpresentation is present because of the risk of cord prolapse. Vaginal examinations should be kept to a minimum and rectal examination usually suffices.

In all cases where labour lasts for more than 24 hours a high vaginal swab should be taken for bacteriological culture. The use of prophylactic antibiotics, without first demonstrating the bacteriological need for them, is to be deprecated; all the more reason, therefore, to obtain a report on the culture from the genital tract early rather than late. While awaiting identification and sensitivity results from the bacteriologist, a bactericidal antibiotic with a broad spectrum is worth starting in all cases where infection is especially to be feared or thought likely. Cephaloridine is particularly suitable and the fact that it has to be given by injection, because it is inadequately absorbed after oral administration, is no disadvantage in labour because gastric and intestinal absorption are capricious anyway. Intramuscular injections of 500 mg., or in more serious cases of 1 g., every 12 hours will maintain an effective dose level in the blood. Most Gram-positive and many of the Gram-negative organisms encountered in prolonged labour are sensitive to cephaloridine. Sensitive organisms include staphylococci, streptococci, including *Str. viridans*, the clostridia, coliforms and *Proteus*. This drug is capable also of crossing the placental barrier in an effective concentration and will remain in the baby's serum for many hours, thus helping to protect it from infection. The drug works its way round to

the liquor amnii in adequate concentration in two or three hours after administration. Some such antibiotic should be given in all cases where the maternal pyrexia is already 99·4°F. or more, when the membranes have been ruptured in labour for more than 24 hours, in cases of maternal heart disease and diabetes, and where there is established evidence of genital tract infection.[2, 3]

The fœtal heart should be observed at regular intervals, and certainly as soon as possible after the membranes rupture. Fœtal distress has to be taken very seriously in these cases, as there is a limit to the number of hours that a baby will survive in its presence. Some obstetricians, with remarkable sang-froid, will hang on though the baby passes meconium for as much as 24 hours before it is delivered, but this is taking a very real risk, and usually fœtal distress, especially demonstrating marked slowing of the heart below 100 or irregularity of beat, indicates Cæsarean section within the next hour or two. A fœtal heart is just about ready to stop by the time its rate has dropped to 80 beats a minute, and particularly if it is irregular as well. One seldom has the opportunity of hearing one much slower before noticing its absence altogether and I cannot recall a fœtal heart rate as low as 60.

FOETAL DISTRESS

The term Fœtal Distress covers a number of ugly realities of which hypoxia is only one, albeit the chief one. Other contributory factors in fœtal distress are antecedent subnutrition in the uterus due to placental inadequacy for a very large variety of causes, including partial separation, mechanical stresses in labour, intra-uterine infection and the action of drugs. Our methods of assessing the baby's wellbeing or the reverse before birth are extremely crude and depend mainly on observation of the fœtal heart rate and the passage of meconium. A combination of slowing and irregularity is the most serious, while slowing alone to below 120 beats a minute is significant, and below 100 a minute more sinister. Fœtal tachycardia above 160 may provide an earlier warning of trouble to come.

Alterations in the fœtal heart rate are therefore not necessarily due to hypoxia but to other causes and so-called fœtal distress does not necessarily mean fœtal hypoxia. It is often thought that unexpected death before delivery is due to inadequate fœtal heart monitoring, but this is not necessarily so. Nevertheless one has to recognise three mains classes of cause in fœtal bradycardia. One is caused by head compression and the slowing is related to the contractions both in timing and severity. The second variety involves cord compression which is more variable in its relationship to the contractions and may produce a type of vasovagal response in the baby. Both these classes

affect the bowel by vagal stimulation and consequently meconium is passed. In the third and more difficult class of uteroplacental insufficiency, which may be aggravated by oxytocin, there is sometimes a more delayed type of slowing in relation to the uterine contractions.

The clinical observations leading up to the diagnosis of fœtal distress do not sufficiently distinguish between the three types mentioned above, of which the last mentioned is probably the most treacherous because fœtal death may occur with less warning.

An interest in the biochemistry of fœtal distress may contribute more both to the understanding and treatment. Fœtal acidosis in labour may be of two types, namely, metabolic and respiratory, of which the metabolic is the commoner and more serious and it is to some extent related to maternal acidosis which usually appears during the last two hours of labour.[44] Measurements of base excess, the metabolic component of the acid base balance, may indeed indicate fœtal acidosis and imminent fœtal distress and it is possible to reduce both maternal and fœtal acidosis by the administration of sodium bicarbonate in standard solution of 155 mEq. per litre. Running the infusion rate at about 2·5 ml. per minute up to 6 ml. per minute is the recommended dosage.[44] As an alternative to maternal blood studies in labour, attempts have been made to determine the acid-base status of the amniotic fluid as an indicator in assessing the threat of intra-uterine asphyxia, but this has been found not to tally with the true maternal state in labour.[45] In the assessment of fœtal distress, therefore, it must be obvious that the only accurate method is to look at the fœtal blood itself and herein lies the importance of Saling's work.[46] One of the amazing compensatory factors in fœtal physiology at birth is the ability of the central nervous system, and in fact the baby as a whole, to survive quite prolonged periods of hypoxia by resorting to anærobic metabolism which is many times less efficient then standard ærobic metabolism of carbohydrates but adequate to sustain life. Anærobic metabolism depends upon an adequate supply of glycogen, an increasing amount of which is laid down in the tissues, notably the liver and myocardium, as term and the stresses of labour approach. The brain stores no glycogen and is dependent upon an active circulation of glucose derived from glycogen to keep it alive. Tissue glycogen is broken down first to lactic acid and then in the presence of oxygen converted to pyruvic acid. When anærobic metabolism occurs because of the lack of oxygen, the lactic acid is not thus converted and an assessment of the lactic/pyruvic acid ratio gives an index of anærobic metabolism. It will be seen therefore that a prolonged period of hypoxia will use up glycogen to a more deadly degree than a brief episode of fœtal distress late in the second stage. This accounts for the ready response of the latter type of case to resuscitation at birth even though the baby is coated with thick,

fresh meconium, whereas the baby who has been chronically deprived of oxygen, and therefore in the ultimate of glycogen (without which there is no life), may die with far less dramatic warning.

Amnioscopy

No death without defæcation. This would appear to be the basis of Saling's theorem that the threat to fœtal life can be foreseen by observing meconium in the liquor amnii. Although this is not invariably the case, nevertheless the association of meconium and asphyxia, or perhaps in the more important negative sense of fœtal health and clear liquor, is sufficiently common to make observation in the liquor thoroughly worth while. I have frequently been infuriated by juniors who rupture the membranes in the course of vaginal examination in labour and give as their excuse that they wanted to see if there was any meconium in the liquor. There is now no such excuse for this mischievous habit because the liquor can be viewed through the intact bag of forewaters by means of one of Saling's conical amnioscopes.

The sight of clear liquor with flakes of white vernix floating within it is certainly reassuring that all for the moment is well. As long as a finger can be got through the cervix it is possible to introduce one of these amnioscope specula which are conical and have an obturator rather like that in a proctoscope. The sight of clear liquor may encourage one to hold off inducing labour because of suspected placental inadequacy, particularly in association with postmaturity for example. I have found that the use of the lithotomy position is by no means invariably necessary; in fact in the apprehensive patient and particularly in the case of one not already in labour, the full left lateral Sim's position is much less distressing. Whichever position is used it is important to protect the sensitive lower anterior vaginal wall from pressure. Therefore it is recommended that after inserting two fingers in the vagina to protect the subpubic region and turning the palmar surfaces of the fingers backwards, the amnioscope should be introduced with the pressure directed onto the perineum. In this way the point can be guided into the cervical canal with very little discomfort. If the liquor looks meconium loaded it is a simple matter to rupture the membranes there and then under direct vision.

Fœtal blood sampling.—This can be undertaken at any stage of labour after the membranes are ruptured; again my own preference is for the left lateral position, although the lithotomy position is more commonly employed. The technique has been fully described by Morris and Beard.[33] The speculum is applied to the fœtal caput which is wiped clean with small swabs, for which purpose dental swabs are admirable, and the area under review is then sprayed with ethyl chloride in order to make it hyperæmic and to "arteriolise" the

capillary blood as far as possible. The skin is painted with a little silicone jelly to encourage the formation of a proper globule of blood on puncturing it, and then a stab is made with a guarded knife whose blade projects beyond the holder no more than 2 mm. Very often one fails to draw blood adequately and an attempt to make a small linear incision is defeated by the scalp moving with the knife. The lower the head in labour, the easier is this manœuvre to carry out. Once a drop of blood forms at the puncture site it is aspirated carefully into a heparinised plastic tube. It is important to obtain an unbroken column of blood within this tube especially if it is proposed to undertake Pco_2 measurements. Sometimes bleeding is embarrassingly persistent from the scalp and the only method of stopping it is to apply continued pressure. The blood sample should be examined as soon as possible, preferably within a matter of minutes and the first observation is the fœtal pH. Admittedly a low figure may not be abnormal if much of this is due to maternal acidosis.[4] On the other hand a pH above 7·25 indicates that the baby is not in severe fœtal distress even before undertaking further micro-Astrup measurements of fœtal acid-base status.

A very extensive experience has been obtained in Queen Charlotte's Hospital which the rest of us throughout the country are now belatedly following up, because it is quite clear to all that far too many Cæsarean sections are being unnecessarily undertaken for a diagnosis of fœtal distress, which the baby refutes by crying lustily at birth. There was indeed a marked reduction in the Cæsarean section rate, purely for fœtal distress, at Queen Charlotte's Hospital, from 49 cases in 1964 to 26 in 1965, and it has now become unusual to perform the operation for clinical signs of fœtal distress if the pH is within normal limits.[5, 6] However, where the fœtal pH is low and particularly if it is less than 7·20, the evidence of fœtal asphyxia must be regarded as overwhelming and further studies are immediately required. For instance, the difference between the maternal and fœtal base deficit at birth provides a striking index of the degree of asphyxial depression. Studies of pH alone, however, are often not enough and certainly will not distinguish between a respiratory and metabolic acidosis, the latter indicating a more prolonged stage of asphyxia, which, presumably because of the drain on glycogen stores, amongst other things, is the more serious of the two. The usual procedure in this country is to estimate Pco_2, standard bicarbonate and base excess by the micro-Astrup technique in order to help in the above differentiation, but Saling and Schneider[48] equilibrate the fœtal blood sample with carbon dioxide at a tension of 40 mm. of mercury in order to assess the metabolic component of the acidosis. They claim a very significant reduction in perinatal death rate since introducing amnioscopy and fœtal blood sampling in Berlin, and it appears

that the severity of fœtal acidosis is not necessarily related to the degree of fœtal bradycardia. In the first few minutes after birth acidosis is likely to be even worse and the possible association of severe and prolonged degrees with subsequent neurological damage is worth bearing in mind.

It is clear that neither fœtal blood sampling nor fœtal heart monitoring are by themselves complete as methods of detecting fœtal distress early. Fœtal life may indeed be saved occasionally by securing prompt delivery when fœtal distress is genuinely assessed, but even more often mothers will be subjected to fewer unnecessary Cæsarean sections.[52]

A more critical attitude has been expressed from the United States where, in a much smaller series,[37] no predictable relationship could be found between the subsequent condition of the baby at birth and the pH as determined in labour, and it has been said that there is no critical pH level to indicate definite fœtal danger, nor that the findings are in themselves sufficiently reliable to indicate immediate delivery.

I have often complained that the fœtus lives behind a veritable Iron Curtain and, whatever the ultimate truth of this matter, I cannot help feeling that anything which tells us more about what is going on inside the uterus is too important to ignore.

Pain Relieving Drugs

It is important to ensure a satisfactory night's sleep for the patient in the hope that on the morrow she will wake fresh and more likely to continue expeditiously with her labour. The drugs available to secure this are of great variety, and much will depend upon the stage of labour already achieved and the amount of the patient's pain.

The majority of mortals faced with the ordeal of severe pain need, and therefore deserve, drugs of one sort or another to make it tolerable. If psychoprophylactic methods could eliminate the need for pain relief by drugs, labour itself would undoubtedly benefit and the baby would be spared the depressant effects upon its centres, which all such drugs, in some degree, are bound to inflict. The performance of the uterus throughout labour and particularly in the third stage would likewise be more physiological. Everything, unfortunately, has its price and nothing in this world can be got for nothing. Drugs are no exception, since none is wholly without penalty and no drug yet devised can ever be both harmless and effective at the same time.

As far as possible, however, such drugs should conform to the following criteria:

(*a*) They should effectively relieve pain.

(*b*) They should not cause fœtal asphyxia.

(c) The course of labour should not be adversely affected and in particular the ability of the uterus to maintain retraction should in no way be undermined.

(d) Elimination should be rapid in order to prevent accumulation.

(e) The safety margin should be wide and there should be no undesirable side-effects.

All the above is asking too much.

Sedatives

The best that can be said for sedatives is that they are harmless. They may, in the very early stages of labour, encourage the patient to have a ration of sleep before labour really gets under way and this is useful in the nervous patient, who then has a chance to wake up some hours later with labour convincingly established. Varying mixtures of potassium bromide, chloral hydrate and tincture of opium have enjoyed popularity amongst midwives for generations. The traditional "Mother's Mist." is some variant of the following:

R

Potassium bromide	15 gr.
Chloral hydrate	30 gr.
Tincture of opium	℥ 15
Chloroform water to 1 fluid oz.	

Hypnotics

These, of which the barbiturates form the most important group, have no effect in raising pain threshold but allay anxiety and may promote sleep. Only the short-acting drugs of this class should be employed, such as Seconal (quinalbarbitone) or Amytal (amylobarbitone) or Nembutal (pentobarbitone) in doses of up to 0·2 g. The longer-acting barbiturates may seriously depress the fœtus at birth. Unfortunately the baby's respiratory centres are extremely susceptible to barbiturates, particularly in prematurity and unfortunately, as Roberts has constantly pointed out, these undesirable effects may persist for quite a few days after birth, the baby remaining sleepy with sluggish reflexes, disinclination to feed and with a fall in body temperature. As for labour itself, the woman becomes unco-operative and is the more likely to require assistance in the second stage on that account. These drugs have the further effect of depressing maternal respiration as well which is undesirable, particularly in a patient who may subsequently require general anæsthesia.

Basal Narcotics

These are more potent and the safest is undoubtedly paraldehyde, since it does not cause much respiratory or circulatory depression. Between 70 to 80 per cent of the drug is destroyed within the body

(Levine *et al.* 1940) and the remainder is excreted through the lungs, so that all within range suffer the smell which, to the majority of people, is most unpleasant. It is much too hateful to take by mouth, but it used to be traditional practice to give it per rectum, in doses of up to 8 drachms until a ghastly accident in the southeast of England occurred in which a nurse misread the prescribed "drachm" sign and interpreted it as "ounces" and killed the patient. This route is messy and uncertain, especially as the patient is liable to return some of it before it is all absorbed leaving one in doubt about how much the patient has retained. The best way to give paraldehyde is by deep intramuscular injection (although some give it intravenously in eclampsia). The dose by intramuscular injection is from 5 to 10 ml. and the injection must be deep or considerable pain and, later, an abscess may be caused. If it was not for its smell this drug would undoubtedly be used more, since it does not interfere with uterine action and produces considerable lethargy and quite a deep sleep. Unfortunately its action is not very prolonged and the patient may be clamouring for further relief at the end of three hours.

Tribromethanol (Avertin) is somewhat more useful than paraldehyde and has no objectionable odour. My impression is that it is much less likely to be returned when given per rectum, which is the route of administration. The dose is 0·075 g. per kilo of body weight. It is hardly ever used nowadays purely and simply for the relief of pain since we have better agents than the basal narcotics to hand and its use is mainly restricted to cases of eclampsia or the imminent threat thereof. The precautions for testing with congo red before administration are as outlined in the chapter on eclampsia.

Glutethimide, a rapidly acting non-barbiturate hypnotic and effective sedative with minimal side-effects, is much favoured by some (Abbas, 1957), but I have not used it myself. Oral administration of 500 mg. early in labour is reputed to reduce the amount of pethidine subsequently required.

Narcotics

Pethidine (Demerol) is 1-methyl-4-phenyl piperidine-4-carboxylic acid ester hydrochloride and is every bit as effective as morphine in relieving pain. There is probably no drug which can produce addiction quite so fast as pethidine, it is said even within twenty-four hours, and it is for this reason that its use is almost wholly restricted to relieving the pain of dying or of child-bearing, neither of which can be described as constantly recurring conditions or providing the setting for addiction. Pharmacologically pethidine is analgesic, sedative and anti-spasmodic. One hundred mg. of pethidine should be reckoned as the equivalent of 10 mg. (gr. $\frac{1}{6}$) of morphine and therefore the usual 100 mg. dose is too small to alleviate the pains of strong

labour. Even when given in larger doses, and one can safely go up to 200 mg., pain relief is likely to be much more satisfactory if scopolamine is given at the same time.[20] By using Scopolamine the dosage of pethidine can be reduced.

Pethidine would appear to be less likely to cause third stage uterine atony than morphine but its effects on the fœtal respiratory centre are just as bad. Some patients vomit repeatedly after morphine whereas pethidine seldom produces this undesirable side-effect.

Labour should be well established before pethidine is given in order to allow one the opportunity to assess a patient's likely analgesic needs and to avoid "shooting one's bolt" too soon. Certainly the os should be showing signs of dilatation, preferably over two fingersbreadth in a primigravida and up to this amount in a multipara. Pethidine 100 mg. can then be combined with scopolamine 0·4 mg. (gr. $\frac{1}{150}$) intramuscularly. This will give some yardstick of the patient's responsiveness to pethidine. Some may require nothing further for four hours or more, in others higher doses may later have to be given. Normally one would expect to have to give the second dose at about three-quarters dilatation of the cervix and 150 mg. of pethidine alone at this point may suffice. One has to remember that the effect should preferably have worn off by the end of the second stage so that the baby will not require special resuscitation. The primigravida is likely to need at least two injections of pethidine unless labour is very expeditious. If it is prolonged she will need many more, but it is better to give repeated doses than doses which are too large.

Pethidine can be given intravenously, but in reduced dosage and very slowly over a few minutes, because of the sudden respiratory depression which intravenous injections produce. This route should be reserved for acute cases such as the multipara who insists on bearing down before full dilatation. The intravenous dose of pethidine should not exceed 50 mg. and scopolamine 0·4 mg. may, with advantage, be added, but less may suffice. Apart from sudden respiratory depression, rapid intravenous injection may produce dizziness, nausea and vomiting of a very unpleasant degree, hence the need to give the injection slowly, preferably diluted in at least 10 ml. of saline.

A study of respiratory minute volumes in newborn infants has been made by Roberts and Please (1958) and Roberts et al. (1957), using a trip spirometer (Donald and Lord, 1953), and they have found that pethidine, even in average doses, is capable of reducing these volumes, particularly during the first few hours of life. Fortunately we have antagonist drugs in the form of nor-allylnormorphine (nalorphine) and levallorphan. If 1 mg. of such an antagonist is combined with 100 mg. of pethidine the analgesic effect is considered to be little if

anything diminished and the respiratory depression of the infant is very markedly reduced. Roberts *et al.* considered that in some patients the addition of levallorphan actually enhanced the analgesic effect. Intramuscular doses of pethidine 100 mg. premixed with levallorphan 2 mg. were studied by Bullough (1959) and the effects compared with those of pethidine alone and mixtures of pethidine and nalorphine. In spite of the small dose of pethidine, analgesia was good in over three-quarters of the cases and nearly 90 per cent of the babies cried within sixty seconds and required no resuscitative treatment; in fact, none in the series required stimulants, intubation nor other methods, such as the now out-moded intragastric oxygen, nor were the operative delivery or postpartum hæmorrhage rates increased.

Nalorphine is available combined with pethidine in suitable dosage as indicated above and marketed as Pethilorfan. Where this precaution has not been taken earlier in labour, nalorphine can be administered to the mother during the second stage to counteract the narcotic effect on the baby's respiratory centre and the dose intravenously for this purpose is 5 to 10 mg. Most of us, however, prefer to await the arrival of the baby to see if nalorphine is even necessary. Given intravenously into the umbilical vein in a dose of 0·2 to 0·5 mg. it will immediately correct the depressant effects of not only pethidine but morphine, Omnopon, heroin and the other drugs of this class, but it is useless against other pain-relieving drugs and, if given either unnecessarily or in excessive dosage, may of itself produce excessive cerebral stimulation of the baby or more likely a severe respiratory depression which may be very hard to counteract.

Amiphenazole is another drug which is antagonistic to morphine and pethidine and has a special selective action on respiratory depression due to drugs of the morphine class. Holmes (1956) described its use in association with morphine in a series of cases to whom large doses of the latter were counteracted by 30 mg. of amiphenazole. Our own practice is to use morphine or Omnopon or heroin very seldom late in labour, but we rely upon pethidine and counteract its effects upon the baby, if necessary, with nalorphine. Pentazocine (Fortral) is reputed to have a pethidine type of action as regards pain relief because less crosses the placenta into the fœtal circulation and it is less addictive. The suggestion has been made that it might be a more suitable drug to use in labour. My personal experience of it is so far limited to relieving pain in cases of inoperable gynæcological cancer.

Morphine will always have a place in the relief of pain in labour, although it has been largely replaced by pethidine. Of its power to elevate the pain threshold there can be no doubt, producing relaxation, apathy, lethargy and sleep. The patients often wake up from it without any appreciation of the hours of suffering which they have

been spared and I can recall my singular lack of gratitude for it in periods of great pain in my own life. Morphine, of course, in common with drugs of this class and power, besides depressing the respiratory centres of the baby, has the characteristic disadvantages of encouraging uterine atony, which, in the third stage, can be positively dangerous, and, occasionally of inducing vomiting in the patient; nevertheless, many labours, inert because of anxiety and tension on the part of the patient, are paradoxically hastened by the mental apathy which morphine induces.

Heroin, like morphine, is a useful drug with similar applications. The dose can be varied between 10 mg. ($\frac{1}{6}$ gr.) and 2·5 mg. ($\frac{1}{24}$ gr.). The usual dose is 5 mg. ($\frac{1}{12}$ gr.). Like morphine it depresses respiration in the mother as well, but its analgesic action is both rapid and profound, and in prolonged difficult and colicky labours the drug is unquestionably of very great value.

Tranquillisers

These have more to offer in the control of pain in labour than would at first have been expected. Amongst their many pharmacological properties, which have been described as vagolytic, sympatholytic, sedative and anti-emetic, their greatest use in labour is their undoubted power of potentiating the activity of a number of drugs acting upon the central nervous system, i.e. anæsthetics, hypnotics and analgesics. The common tranquillisers used in obstetrics are chlorpromazine (Largactil) and promazine (Sparine). An example of the use of this synergistic action is provided by Lacomme et al. (1952) who devised a "lytic cocktail" which consisted of an infusion of 500 ml. of pyrogen-free glucose saline containing 50 mg. of chlorpromazine and 100 mg. of pethidine, the drip being run fairly rapidly until the patient showed signs of pain relief when the drip rate was cut back to 30 to 50 drops per minute and subsequently adjusted according to her needs. Another method of administering tranquillising drugs is the injection of a combination of:

> Pethidine   100 mg.
> Chlorpromazine   50 mg.
> Promethazine   50 mg.
> Distilled water to 20 ml.

Of this solution 2 to 3 ml. may be given intravenously when labour is established and repeated as necessary intramuscularly.

In our own practice we prefer promazine to chlorpromazine, having had one very troublesome case of jaundice which was attributed to the latter. The danger of agranulocytosis has also to be borne in mind. Promazine, on the other hand (Sparine), has proved of the

greatest value and would appear to have a very high safety factor. Given slowly by intravenous injection in the form of Sparine 50 mg., pethidine 50 mg., and hyoscine 0·4 mg. (gr. $\frac{1}{150}$) even the most hysterical and colicky type of patient "keels over" in a few seconds and may sleep for several hours without apparent respiratory depression and may thereafter be found to be at full dilatation of the cervix or nearly so within that time. Nevertheless, behaviour may be unpredictable and the patient should be constantly supervised after such treatment. The hyoscine is most likely to be responsible for this and more often nowadays we inject 50 mg. of Sparine intravenously first, observe the effect, and reinforce it, if necessary, within half an hour with 100 mg. of pethidine intramuscularly. The combination is certainly most useful.

Promazine hydrochloride (Sparine) is a member of the phenothiazine group of drugs and is regarded as one of the least toxic members of this family. Besides its useful anti-emetic effects it reduces the amount of pethidine required by potentiating the latter's analgesic effect and although inducing relaxation and even sleep between injections, does not interfere with the physiological course of labour. It is also safe even in premature labour, since there is no foetal respiratory or circulatory depression.

Thrombophlebitis is a very rare complication after intravenous injection, but is most easily avoided by diluting the Sparine with saline and avoiding concentrations higher than 25 mg. per ml. Such an injection should also be made very slowly.

Promazine is believed to be safer than chlorpromazine as far as the foetus is concerned since the phenothiazine, which has been detected in the urine of babies whose mothers have been given the latter, has not been found in either foetal blood or urine after promazine, even though it has been given intravenously and Pollock et al. (1960) doubt if Sparine crosses the placental barrier in significant amounts. Experiences in our own unit with this drug have been reviewed by MacVicar and Murray (1960) and our favourable view of this drug continues to this day.

Tachycardia sometimes occurs but would appear to be the only noteworthy side-effect from Sparine. The course of labour is not slowed up, but rather the reverse. So far we have not observed any untoward effect on the baby, nor upon its respiratory centre at birth. The happy property of this drug would appear to be its ability to induce a state in the patient of unawareness of her present miseries, a sort of "medical leucotomy". In our view Sparine is one of the most important drugs to have been introduced into obstetrics since the discovery of pethidine.

On the whole we tend to distrust polypharmacy in labour and combinations of drugs should be used sparingly. However, not only

may Sparine potentiate the analgesic properties of pethidine but Phenergan (25 mg. by injection) is also useful.

One should always bear in mind the possible effects of any drugs used on subsequent general anæsthesia. Although Sparine is unlikely to produce a hypotensive effect in the customary thiopentone/relaxant/nitrous oxide/oxygen technique, a severe fall in blood pressure may occur if halothane is used; in any case an unpopular anæsthetic because of its encouragement of atonic postpartum hæmorrhage. Promazine however should not be used if spinal or epidural anæsthesia is in the offing.[11, 16] A reminder here could profitably be given that anæsthetists should always be informed of all drugs administered before his advent, so that he may be on the look-out for rare cases of untoward interaction between the drugs and subsequent anæsthetic agents.

Sedatives and analgesic drugs should be used very sparingly in cases of hypotonic inertia and mainly reserved to ensure, if necessary, a good night's sleep, but in the hypertonic types these drugs can be used far more liberally, where, by allaying the patient's anxiety and fear, quite apart from relieving her pain, they may have the para-doxical effect of accelerating the course of labour.

INHALATION ANALGESICS (SELF-ADMINISTERED)

These all have the advantage of rapidity of effect and reversibility on discontinuing the administration. Ever since Queen Victoria had the pains of childbirth relieved by intermittent whiffs of chloroform (narcose à la reine) this method of analgesia has never lost ground.

Chloroform may be dead but it will not lie down. In all the years of anæsthetic history nothing has yet been found quite so handy, unobjectionable and effective in domiciliary practice. Unfortunately coroners take a very hard view of its use in spite of the great skill and safety achieved with it by an older generation of obstetricians. Its free vaporisation in a Junker inhaler greatly increases the safety of administration as compared with the drop-on mask technique, as dangerous concentrations are avoided thereby and it takes quite a lot of hard bag-squeezing to produce real anæsthesia with a Junker machine.

Chloroform becomes dangerous when there is much adrenaline being secreted by the patient, where administration is prolonged, when induction is repeated several times and when the patient has a period of apnœa and a dangerously high concentration is allowed to accumulate under the mask for the patient suddenly to inspire, but these objections cannot apply to self-administration techniques. Chloroform undoubtedly depresses uterine activity and may increase the incidence of postpartum hæmorrhage and since it crosses the

Epidural Analgesia

This works on the same principle as the older caudal analgesia which it has now more or less superseded. As before, the epidural space is entered and a fairly large volume of anæsthetic agent is injected to involve particularly the sensory roots. In the case of caudal analgesia the epidural space was approached through the sacral hiatus and the sacral canal, a difficult, dirty and hazardous route. A soft, malleable catheter was introduced, through which a fine nylon catheter was passed further in, through which an intermittent or continuous drip of anæsthetic solution could be fed. Occasionally the malleable catheter got into some strange places and I remember one case, many years ago, who did not walk properly for three months.

Better by far is our present practice of continuous epidural analgesia, in which the space outside the dura mater is approached through the lumbar region of the back as in lumbar puncture, but care is taken not to penetrate the dura. The epidural space is identified by the "loss-of-resistance-technique". A blunt tipped plastic catheter is then advanced into the epidural space, the needle is withdrawn and the catheter is connected to a sterile syringe filled with 2 per cent lignocaine with 1/200,000 adrenaline added. This syringe is sealed inside a transparent polythene bag and strapped to the abdominal wall so that further injections can be given without the need to scrub up or endangering asepsis. The dose varies with the height of the patient, from 6 to 9 ml. i.e. 120 to 180 mg. of lignocaine, although more may have to be given if the anæsthetic is continued for operative delivery. For the same reasons prilocaine should not be used because the accumulation may cause methæmoglobinæmia. The technique is certainly one for the practised anæsthetist because of the occasional complications which may ensue. Common amongst these is hypotension which can occasionally be severe. It is undoubtedly aggravated by the supine position in which the patient may be lying and the first step is to turn her onto her side. The intravenous injection of methoxamine 3 mg. may restore a normal blood pressure but may cause fœtal bradycardia and it is probably better to lower the head of the patient's bed. Doing so benefits the maternal cerebral circulation but does very little for the placental circulation. Cases that readily develop hypotension are perhaps better off without persisting in this technique. Another complication is the puncture of an epidural vein, which of course must be recognised before the injection is proceeded with. Toxic effects from lignocaine are unlikely if the dose is kept below 250 mg. at each injection. Attention will have to be paid to the bladder because the patient less readily voids her urine spontaneously. The diagnosis of full dilatation is only likely to be made by vaginal examination as the patient is unlikely to want to bear down and for

this reason too over 90 per cent of cases have to be delivered by either forceps or Ventouse. Continuous epidural analgesia is no contra-indication to an oxytocin drip but cases so treated must be supervised with extra care.

The needle for introducing the plastic catheter into the epidural space is appreciably thicker than the ordinary lumbar puncture needle and therefore the effects of accidental puncture of the dura mater are very much more serious in the form of post-operative headache and I have had a case in which this very distressing symptom persisted for three weeks and necessitated nursing in the flat or head-down position. This accident was presumably due to leakage through the puncture hole of cerebrospinal fluid.

Another troublesome phenomenon is that of tachyphylaxis in which the patient seems to get relief lasting for shorter and shorter periods, sometimes as little as 40 minutes, and requires repeated top-up injections. Where each injection is liable to be complicated by a hypotensive reaction it is better to recognise defeat early on and cut one's losses. Failure to do so may result in serious degrees of fœtal suboxygenation. I am now inclined to think that this phenomena is likely to be even more serious in the case of twins, whose placental circulatory demands are correspondingly greater. An additional reason, however, for contra-indicating epidural analgesia in twin delivery is possible difficulty with the delivery of the second because of a uterus which is overactive and is said to clamp down too soon after the delivery of the first.

Notwithstanding all this, epidural anæsthesia has a most important part to play in the management of inco-ordinate uterine action, quite apart from its great uses as a single shot anæsthetic for difficult instrumental deliveries. The relief of the patient is quite astonishing to witness. She more or less grins her way through labour and we are always prepared to consider the advisability of this type of analgesia after 24 hours of labour in primigravidæ, provided the case is other-wise obstetrically normal. One has plenty of time now to correct maternal acidosis and to give the cervix every chance to dilate; another advantage to be reaped is the excellence of uterine retraction in the third stage so that blood lost from the episiotomy usually exceeds that from the placental site.

Once the patient has been given the treat of epidural analgesia, however, her attendants are absolutely committed to complete delivery during the course of that anæsthetic, because the patients take it very hard to be exposed to the unaccustomed pain of the late first stage of labour if the anæsthetic is allowed to wear off. There is obviously a limit to the desirable length of time for maintaining epidural analgesia and we are certainly reluctant to allow the business to go on for more than 30 hours and usually much less. It

follows that one must be prepared to deliver either by forceps or by Cæsarean section within that time according to the degree of dilatation achieved.

This account is full of cautionary remarks which are reason enough for not using this type of analgesia indiscriminately; in fact with careful selection combined with enthusiasm for the method the incidence of epidural analgesia at the Queen Mother's Hospital, Glasgow, is just over 4 per cent of all labours (Moir, personal communication).

Counter irritation and distraction.—An interesting method of which we have a limited experience is the use of what is called "white sound". This is a curious noise involving a wide spectrum of frequencies producing a resultant sound rather like the continuous noise of a wave breaking upon a beach made up of fine pebbles. This weird continuous noise is mixed up with good music, such as a Schubert quartet. The first time I used this instrument the expensive part of it, namely the Hi-Fi recording of the quartet, was not available, only the curious noise, so we abandoned culture for the moment and supplied the more practical element via headphones to a patient who was making very heavy weather of her first stage and suffering uncontrollably with each contraction. For hours thereafter she grinned her way through each contraction and said it was "smashing", but she still came to Cæsarean section that evening for total lack of progress. I do not think the Schubert would have made much difference. Dentists are known to find this method helpful, especially with children who take less kindly than most of us to assaults in the dental chair, but I doubt if we are yet in a position to say that the same beneficial effects cannot be more simply produced by the judicious use of pain-relieving drugs.

Abdominal decompression.—The problem of painful, prolonged and troublesome labour has been tackled by Heyns (1959) and his colleagues in Johannesburg by reducing the atmospheric pressure around the trunk from axillæ to thighs. A cage is placed over the abdominal wall rather like a foot cradle on an ordinary hospital bed and over this is placed a plastic polythene suit enclosing the trunk. The patient controls the suction pressures by operating a valve herself and a gentle and partial vacuum induced in the system lifts the abdominal wall forwards and removes its embarrassing effect upon uterine activity. In the primigravida with a particularly strong abdominal wall, failure to relax may, it is believed, discourage the contracting uterus from assuming an efficient and spherical shape and may also force it backwards against the vertebral column into an unfavourable axis. This exaggerates the adverse factors in occipito-posterior positions. Theoretically this seems a very good idea and it has been claimed that the course of labour may be much expedited

by allowing the uterus to assume the most efficient shape and position by removing the inhibiting influence of a tense abdominal wall. Apart from encouraging labour, pain was also reckoned to be alleviated. Later on Heyns *et al.* (1962) postulated that this kind of treatment could be applied twice daily for half-hour periods throughout the last trimester of pregnancy as well as during labour, in order to improve placental circulation and therefore fœtal oxygenation.

The claims of the Johannesburg workers have been investigated by Loudon (1961) in Edinburgh. He came to the conclusion that the beneficial effects were to some extent attributable (personal communication) to the interest of those handling the apparatus and conducting the experiment, which may indeed be a sad reflection on the hunger for care which women in labour experience in our hospitals.

Psychoprophylaxis.—The late Grantly Dick Read developed almost a cult for the easing of childbirth's miseries by mental as well as physical relaxation. By now generations of labouring women have acknowledged benefit from this type of brain-washing which was more readily accepted in the United States than in this country. In somewhat similar fashion a psychoprophylactic preparation for childbirth is more popular and acknowledged on the other side of the English Channel. At a meeting of the Natural Childbirth Trust in London in March, 1961, Dr. Pierre Vellay of Paris described his methods of psychoprophylactic preparation, continuing the work of Lamaze who is said to have derived his technique from Russian methods. He claimed that 35 per cent of all deliveries by this method are completely painless, in 63 per cent there is tolerable pain and in only about 5 per cent is there a total failure. Dr. Vellay attributes painless childbirth so achieved to a combination of the correct conditioned reflexes, adequate training exercises and successful human relations. Where psychiatric probing reveals disturbance, the services of a "psychosomatician" are called in, but to judge by the report of this meeting, in 80 per cent of cases pregnancy and labour are sufficiently normal for obstetrician and midwife to suffice and this should make those of us who practice this branch of medicine feel a little better! He said that 30 per cent of all women in France are delivered by this method of psychoprophylaxis. The fees charged for the course, which consists of some lectures, a visit to the obstetrical unit and a film, etc., are refunded by the Securité Sociale. He claims that it is possible to deliver a woman with forceps without any need for anæsthesia. At this same meeting Dr. Lee Buxton, after a study of thirty-three obstetrical units in Europe and the United States, found more than twenty different methods of psychological preparation for childbirth and he suggested that if we were to look for a common denominator in all these methods it might be the personality or enthusiasm of the person conducting the labour, or

even the kindness, competent humanity and care given by someone trained to give it. I wonder if this is not just part of the essence of good doctoring and whether it might not be as well to abandon some of the grandiloquent phrases which tend to suggest that doctors hitherto have not known how to understand, succour and comfort their patients. The subject is an emotive one and a large number of women have been so greatly helped by modern psychoprophylaxis that it deserves a better account than I can give. Accordingly Dr. Alan Giles of Stobhill Hospital, Glasgow, who has great experience of it has kindly supplied an essay on psychoprophylaxis at the end of this chapter.

Specific treatment.—Unfortunately we do not have a very satisfactory choice at our disposal, which is not surprising considering the imperfection of our knowledge of pathological uterine behaviour. The exhibition of œstrogens, for example, even in huge dosage, is more or less useless.

Continuous epidural anæsthesia would be ideal if it were not for the technical difficulties, the need to steer the case continually until delivery is completed and the almost invariable need to complete delivery with the forceps, since the patient so treated is incapable of bearing down. To be effective the level of anæsthesia should reach up to D.12 in order to block the sympathetic innervation of the uterus. Spinal anæsthesia is too dangerous to consider and cannot easily be maintained for more than a few hours.

A constriction ring, if present, may be temporarily relaxed by the inhalation of two capsules of amyl nitrite, but the effect is very transient, and its only use is in the course of operative delivery.

We come therefore to our main standby, namely oxytocin. This is not without its dangers, and it should not be used in the presence of any of the varieties of hypertonic inertia. Unfortunately, it is in just these hypertonic cases that the need for treatment is most clamant. In so far as oxytocin works at all, it works by accentuating the pattern of uterine activity already present, in other words, small regular contractions tend to become large regular contractions, hence its great use in hypotonia; but where the uterine tone is already increased, and where the contractions are ill co-ordinated, these very factors are quantitatively rather than qualitatively modified, with the result that, in the presence of incoordinate action, the onset of both maternal and fœtal distress is likely to be precipitated. The injudicious use of oxytocin during labour, therefore, involves danger of asphyxia to the fœtus if the nature of the anomalous uterine activity is not first accurately assessed and the effects of the drug scrupulously controlled by observation. The use of intermittent subcutaneous injection of pitocin has, in the past, not always been fraught with the danger one would expect, simply because it is a

highly inefficient method of administration and it is very doubtful how much of the drug injected actually reaches the uterus in active form. For the pharmacological effect to be fully felt the administration should be by the intravenous route, whereupon minute quantities of the drug produce a large and immediate response.

If therefore oxytocin is to be used at all in the management of the first stage of labour, it should be included in an intravenous drip solution in the strength not exceeding 5 units per litre of glucose in water. The rate of the drip is cautiously started at first and worked up to 10 drops per minute and the effect constantly observed. From now on uterine activity can largely be steered by controlling the rate of the drip, but it is imperative that this treatment should be under continuous control. Provided the doctor is prepared to sit with the patient and observe each contraction the method is safe.

By using hyaluronidase, oxytocin can be effectively given and sufficiently rapidly absorbed by the intramuscular route.[21] Oxytocin, 10 units, is added to a pint of normal saline and given by slow continuous drip (about 8–12 drops per minute) deeply into the vastus lateralis muscle of the thigh. 1,000 Benger units of hyalase in 1 ml. of saline is injected into the distal end of the rubber tubing and effectively promotes rapid absorption for the next 3 or 4 hours when a further 1,000 units of hyalase can be added. This is a very handy method and not only spares a vein but leaves the patient's arms and hands free.

As an alternative to the oxytocic drugs acting directly upon the uterus the search continues for drugs which, instead of stimulating, modify uterine activity through its nervous control. In the U.S.A. reports have appeared of Sparteine sulphate as a drug capable of safely cutting short the early or latent phases of labour, especially after induction, because of its mildly oxytocic action. In labour already in progress Plentl et al. (1961) recommend hourly intramuscular injections of 150 mg. and found that three such doses sufficed in 90 per cent of patients. There were no increased hazards noted for mother nor baby. The drug is not recommended in cases of cephalopelvic disproportion or when there is a scar in the uterus.

Operative treatment.—Decisions here may be very difficult. In the first place, the presence of intact membranes is a gift horse which should not readily be looked in the mouth. Few things annoy me in the conduct of prolonged labour by my junior colleagues as much as "rupturing the membranes on examination", sometimes even referred to as "R.O.E."! Done for a reason, which should be stated, is excusable, but from clumsiness—intolerable. Their artificial rupture may help in hypotonic inertia provided the cervix is more than half dilated, but the need for this intervention in many cases is not very great. Where one of the hypertonic states exists, rupture of the membranes, whether spontaneous or artificial, in no way improves

the behaviour of the uterus, and brings in its train a series of risks which had been better postponed.

The application of Willett's forceps or, at further stages of dilatation, the use of the obstetric forceps with a continuous light-weight traction has been used in the past, even by me. An admirable ladder of ascending infection is thereby supplied, and this line of treatment has only historical interest. The Ventouse (vacuum extractor) comes into a different category and may resolve a lingering first stage most satisfactorily. To use it, as I have, in a case of labour lasting more than four days because of indolent hypotonic inertia with the cervix still only four fingersbreadth dilated and to have the patient quietly and successfully delivered without hæmorrhage or other mischief within the next half hour, is an experience sufficient to convince the most stubborn (see Chapter XVIII).

The indications for operative intervention are chiefly those of fœtal distress, maternal distress or the arrest of all further progress in labour over the course of a reasonable period of observation, such as 12 hours. The nature of the interference will largely depend upon the stage of cervical dilatation and the position of the fœtal head. Where the cervix is more than three-quarters dilated and the pelvis is roomy, it is often possible by digital manipulation to push the cervix above the maximum diameters of the presenting part and to deliver with forceps. This is an operation calling for considerable skill, but is certainly preferable to applying the forceps without first stretching the cervix over the fœtal head and relying upon brute force to deliver, a procedure which is shocking both physically and æsthetically. The Ventouse nowadays makes a better and safer delivery of this sort.

Often, after reaching full dilatation at last the patient may be too exhausted by her first stage to achieve spontaneous delivery in the second, and MacRae noted that the forceps rate was no less than 68·9 per cent in his series of cases of prolonged labour. He found incidentally that the postpartum hæmorrhage rate was as high as 12·5 per cent. It will be seen, therefore, that there are certain hazards to vaginal delivery "at any price".

Though largely replaced by the Ventouse, incision of the cervix is worth considering but only in a very few cases, and this procedure should be reserved for the rare instances of cervical dystocia with the head low within the pelvic cavity. Duhrssen's incisions consist of a series of short nibbles round the posterior margin of the cervix, but it is often more effective to make a frank cut. O'Sullivan recommended cutting the cervix to a depth of half an inch on each side at nine o'clock and three o'clock, but it is probably safer to keep away from the mid-lateral area and incise at eight o'clock, six o'clock and four o'clock. There is one technical snag about this, namely each cut

should be completed in one bite, because the V-shaped gap in the cervix which it makes is immediately flattened out and cannot again be identified, so that a second bite taken in the same region is unlikely to coincide with the original cut. The cervix must now be pushed up over the head, especially in front. O'Sullivan performed this operation with only analgesia instead of anæsthesia, and the patient could sometimes now be left to proceed to spontaneous delivery. Where, however, a general anæsthetic has been used, one is more or less obliged to proceed to forceps delivery rather than face the prospect of having to induce a second anæsthetic should spontaneous delivery not occur.

Provided the head is very well applied to the cervix there is usually surprisingly little bleeding from incising it, but the cases must be very carefully selected and the following conditions must be present:

1. The head must be very deep, preferably on the pelvic floor.
2. The cervix must be at least 3 fingers dilated.
3. There must be no suspicion of contraction of the bony outlet.
4. The cervix must be tightly and thinly stretched over the head.
5. Contractions, though weak, must be regular in nature.

It will be seen, therefore, that the operation is quite unsuited to the colicky type of uterus. In any case very profound shock may be caused, mainly because of the traction which is felt upon the imperfectly prepared lower uterine segment before full dilatation and only exceptionally can this be regarded as the operation of choice.

It has been traditionally stated that Cæsarean section has only a limited use in cases of inertia and prolonged labour, and statements to this effect were made more than once at a meeting of the Royal Society of Medicine devoted to this subject in 1948. Nothing could be a greater travesty of the truth, and Nixon at this same meeting sensibly pointed out that it was safer to perform Cæsarean section in many cases, as being less traumatic than securing vaginal delivery at the cost of much tissue tearing and bruising. There are two criteria of progress in labour, namely progressive dilatation of the cervix and progressive descent of the presenting part. As long as either is present labour can be said to be progressing, but if neither criterion is satisfied in the course of 12 hours the question of Cæsarean section arises, if not sooner. The universal use of the lower segment operation together with the exhibition of antibiotic drugs, where indicated, has made this outcome of labour a far preferable method to brutish delivery before the completion of the first stage. While deploring the indiscriminate use of abdominal delivery in these cases, the plea is here made for Cæsarean section a little too early rather than too late. Our own experience in Glasgow and the ultimate method of delivery are summarised in Table VII.

COMPLICATIONS

It is not enough nowadays to confine one's view of results merely to maternal and fœtal survival. Such a narrow view will come soon to be condemned as neo-Georgian. The maternal morbidity rate rises according to the duration of labour, particularly from the time the membranes rupture, and MacRae found that 43·2 per cent of cases in his series had puerperal pyrexia, of whom a third were

TABLE VII

PROLONGED LABOUR—OVER 48 HOURS

(Glasgow Royal Maternity Hospital)

1960–62

309 Primigravidæ
74 Multiparæ   383 Cases

Outcome	Primipara	Multipara		
Spontaneous vertex delivery .	. 113	39	152	40%
Breech	9	2	11	
Forceps	133	18	151	40%
Ventouse	16	7	23	6%
Cæsarean section. . .	38	8	46	12%
	309	74	383	

19 *Stillbirths*
    Accidental hæmorrhage 3
    Intra-uterine infection 5
    Hydrocephaly 4
    Postmaturity 3
    Asphyxia 4

3 *Neonatal deaths*
    Intra-uterine infection 2
    Breech delivery 1

Perinatal mortality 57 per thousand.

judged to be due to urinary infection. It is probable that the repeated need to catheterise in prolonged labour contributes to this. MacRae further noted that the morbidity rate was 100 per cent for those who came to Cæsarean section. One of the greatest risks of operation, whatever its nature, lies in the anæsthetic. These patients are sometimes in poor shape, often dehydrated, ketosis may be marked and their stomachs are treacherously full, so that vomiting easily complicates the induction of anæsthesia.

Among the sequelæ one must consider the prospects for future labours and the attitude of the patient towards embarking upon

further pregnancies. Jeffcoate pointed out the significant fact that of those who were ultimately delivered by Cæsarean section almost half avoided further pregnancies, and of those who were delivered by forceps the percentage who remained voluntarily sterile was only a little less. This is a point of no mean importance. The outlook for future labours is usually satisfactory provided on the previous occasion vaginal delivery was achieved whether by forceps or not, but the repeat Cæsarean section rate remains very high, especially if the cervix did not reach more than half dilatation.

OCCIPITO-POSTERIOR POSITION

Occipito-posterior positions, because of their frequent adverse effect upon the length of labour, deserve consideration here on their own. About 10 per cent of all vertex presentations occupy posterior positions at the onset of labour, but in about four-fifths of these labour is not much affected. The other 20 per cent in rough figures require some form of intervention.

On average, labour is prolonged about $3\frac{1}{2}$ hours in primigravidæ and about $1\frac{3}{4}$ hours in multiparæ.

The occipito-posterior position, though common, cannot truly be regarded as normal. There are many reasons for the normal occipito-anterior position, among which are the respective curvatures of the maternal lumbar and fœtal spines. Clearly it is more suitable for these curvatures to lie in parallel than with their convexities opposed, and if, as happens in occipito-posterior positions, these curvatures are opposed, it is easy to see how a deflexed attitude of the fœtus results. Furthermore, in the erect posture there is more room anteriorly for the curvature of the fœtal back. A lesser factor is the position of the placenta, since the foetus tends to face it *in utero*, and it is known that the placenta is more commonly sited on the posterior wall than on the anterior, though the difference is not great enough to account for the frequency of occipito-anterior positions.

Most cases of O.P. malposition are usually unexplained. Occasionally a pendulous belly allows so much room posteriorly for the fœtal back that an anterior position is not necessarily encouraged, but these cases suffer no trouble from this cause.

If the head should engage in an anthropoid type of brim with the occiput posterior in the first instance there is, of course, reason enough for its unwillingness to negotiate the relatively narrower transverse strait by long internal rotation, and these cases often prefer the shorter rotation into the hollow of the sacrum.

The well-known military attitude so often seen in a tight uterus signifies a state of deflexion, but it would be hard to say whether this was a cause or effect of occipito-posterior position.

A flat pelvis, with uterine obliquity towards the same side as the occiput, encourages deflexion of the head after the manner of producing a secondary face presentation (which constitutes an extreme example), and this may be a minor ætiological factor. Lastly, some

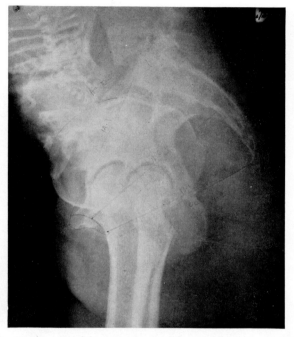

17/Fig. 2.—Persistent occipito-posterior position, two hours in second stage of labour after 26 hours in the first stage. Note moulding and extension of head. Delivered Caesarean section. Birth weight 4 kg.

(By courtesy of Dr. R. A. Tennent.)

cases are attributed to primary brachycephaly which shortens the lengths of the lever from the frontal region to the atlanto-occipital joint and therefore reduces its effective moment in flexing the head.

Quite apart from the generally accepted need for long internal rotation of the occiput through three-eighths of a circle (which will depend both on really adequate uterine contractions and pelvic roominess), the mechanism of labour is adversely affected in many other ways. The axis of uterine thrust, for one thing, transmitted from the fundus through the fœtal vertebral column tends to operate at a mechanical disadvantage, because it is out of alignment and not at right angles to the pelvic inlet (Fig. 2). The steeper, therefore, the angle of inclination of the pelvic brim the more serious does this factor be-

come, so that on taking a radiograph there will often be observed a marked lateral angulation of the fœtal neck (Fig. 3). The forces necessary to drive the head deeply into the pelvis are often misdirected and therefore misspent.

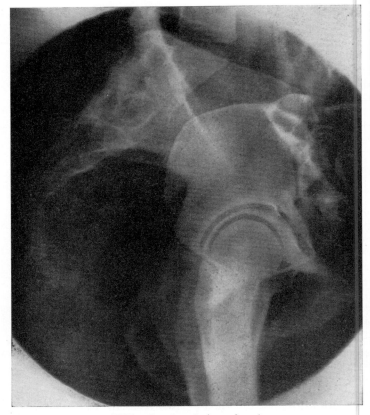

17/Fig. 3.—Angulation of neck.

Now, in the multipara with her more lax abdominal wall the uterine body sags farther forward, so that the direction of uterine thrust through the fœtal spine more nearly approaches the direction of engagement. This partly explains why occipito-posterior positions seldom inconvenience the labouring multipara.

The deflexed head presents an ovoid rather than a sphere to the lower segment and therefore tends to fit badly, so that poor pains result from inefficient stimulation. The forewaters are not plugged off efficiently by the presenting part during uterine contraction and

the membranes rupture early so that rotation is somewhat discouraged as a result.

If deflexion is marked, the occipito-frontal diameter of 11·3 cm. (4½ inches) may present instead of the sub-occipito-bregmatic, and mild cases of deflexion present with the sub-occipito-frontal measuring 10·25 cm. (4 inches). This is a common cause of high head at term. If both fontanelles remain at the same level, in what is called by some authorities the median vertex position, the head, in its descent through the pelvis, inadequately presents the vertex to the gutter mechanism of the pelvic floor, which is therefore unable to choose which variety of internal rotation to encourage. Transverse arrest of the head then results. As long as transverse arrest remains uncorrected, the patient is incapable of delivering herself, and the head usually sticks in the mid-cavity at a level at which about one pennyworth of scalp or caput can be seen on separating the labia.

Occasionally the posterior fœtal shoulder may get caught on the wrong side of the maternal vertebral column and this, too, discourages internal rotation.

When the occiput remains posterior, its mechanical pressure backwards towards the rectum is very liable to give the patient the desire to bear down and push before full dilatation, and it is very common indeed for the onset of the second stage to be prematurely diagnosed by the attendant. As a result, the patient may be urged to push with her pains, all to no purpose, so that, after the lapse of a statutory period, delay in the second stage is diagnosed and preparations are made for forceps delivery which might not have been necessary if the patient had not been encouraged to exhaust herself with fruitless efforts prematurely.

If labour proceeds to face to pubis delivery, it is obvious that greater diameters must ultimately distend the vulval outlet. Maternal lacerations are therefore more common, and the narrower the sub-pubic angle happens to be the worse will be the damage to the pelvic floor.

A narrow sub-pubic angle presents a less attractive escape gap to the presenting part, so that, particularly in the android type of pelvis. the condition of deep transverse arrest of the head persists. Similarly, a poor sacral bay favours transverse arrest.

It is not surprising, therefore, that the operative delivery rate is high. Of those cases who start labour with the occiput posterior, approximately 63 per cent deliver themselves spontaneously with the occiput anterior, about 14 per cent have spontaneous face to pubis deliveries and the remaining 23 per cent require operative delivery. The frequent need for episiotomy is obvious, and the technique and pitfalls of manual rotation of the occiput and forceps delivery are described in the chapter on forceps.

Because of the increased length of labour and the greater need for operative intervention maternal morbidity is naturally higher. The fœtal mortality is higher and is not usually less than 8 per cent in cases requiring rotation and forceps. The jam-pot type of moulding which is characteristic of the persistent occipito-posterior presentation is particularly unfavourable from the point of view of tentorial damage because of the extreme elevation of the falx cerebri which it entails.

It would not be an exaggeration to say that occipito-posterior positions and transverse arrest of the head account for more second-stage trouble than all the rest put together.

OBSTRUCTED LABOUR

This should never be encountered in modern obstetric practice, for it can only result from woeful neglect. Only the briefest summary will therefore be given. Its causes include disproportion, brow presentation, persistent mento-posterior position, shoulder presentation and impacted breech. One of two possible sequences of events must now take place. Either the uterus will give up the unequal struggle and become inert from exhaustion, the patient ultimately dying of sepsis, or, more commonly, the contractions come more fast and furious until the uterus relaxes not at all between pains. This tetanic condition of the uterus is called tonic contraction. The upper segment has retracted fully at the expense of the lower segment which is stretched to the limit and beyond. The junction between the two segments is represented by a ridge, Bandl's ring, which rises higher in the abdomen usually at an oblique angle. The patient's condition is desperate. Pain is continuous and very severe, the uterus is hard and so tender that palpation of the fœtus is impossible. The maternal pulse is rapid, usually over 120 per minute, and may be thready. The temperature is raised and all the signs of dehydration are present, including a dry, dirty tongue, a hot, dry vagina, and highly concentrated, scanty urine containing albumin, acetone, blood and casts. Uterine rupture is imminent, and most commonly occurs through the posterior wall of the thinned-out lower segment. The baby is of course already dead from asphyxia, and unless very prompt and skilful treatment is immediately available the mother, too, is well on her way to the next world. Of all obstetric deaths it is probably one of the most terrible, and in underdeveloped countries often made worse by attempts outside to bring about delivery.

PSYCHOPROPHYLAXIS
by ALAN M. GILES,
B.SC., M.B., CH.B., D.P.H., F.R.C.O.G., F.R.C.S. (Glas.)

Psychoprophylaxis is a psychological method of antenatal preparation designed to prevent, or at least to minimise, pain and difficulty

during labour. The pregnant woman is taught how to use her natural brain processes to her advantage.

The method is based on the work of the neurophysiologist Pavlov. Applying the principles of his experiments, the Russian obstetricians, Platonov, Velvosky and Nicolaiev, evolved the method at the same time as Dr. Grantly Dick Read was developing his ideas on "natural childbirth". Read stated that fear produced tension and tension produced pain. He advised relaxation during a contraction. The Russians did not agree with Read. On the contrary, they advocated activity, both mental and physical, during labour. In 1951 Dr. Lamaze, a French obstetrician, visited Russia and saw women, trained in psychoprophylaxis, deliver without pain. On his return to Paris he and Dr. Vellay adapted the Russian method for use in the Western world. The method has now spread to some 44 countries.

Childbirth is surely the greatest physical act performed by woman, and it can also be a great emotional experience. The physical and the psychological aspects cannot be separated. For most women labour is a time of apprehension, of fear and agony, but this need not be so. As a result of suitable antenatal preparation the majority of women can have a labour that is easy and painless, or almost painless, and can actually enjoy the labour and experience a sense of fulfilment. It can be postulated that the basic sensations from the contracting uterus are those of tightness and that these sensations are interpreted by the brain as pain, only when there are added factors due to emotion or to previous conditioning. The Russian obstetrician Nicolaiev[58] states that it is necessary to reshape the mind of the woman who has come to believe that pain in labour is inevitable. Nicolaiev reshaped the woman's mind by a process of deconditioning and reconditioning. To this method of antenatal preparation was given the name psychoprophylaxis—prevention by use of the mind.

Vellay[57] describes the method as verbal analgesia. During the training period words are used not only to cancel previously acquired conditioned reflexes, which will be harmful, but also to build up favourable reflexes, which will come into play during labour.

As psychoprophylaxis is based on the use of Pavlovian principles, it would be pertinent to consider them in some detail. Basic reflexes are inherited and are therefore present from birth. They are essential to survival and form permanent nerve pathways, so that a given stimulus produces a constant resultant activity. In one example, the sight and smell of food results in salivation. But most reflexes are acquired and are the result of experience and environment. They are the conditioned reflexes. The classic example was described by Pavlov. As a result of repetitive training the dog came to associate the ringing of the bell with food. A new nerve pathway was developed—a conditioned reflex—so that, in the absence of food, the sound of the bell produced

salivation. In human beings, conditioned reflexes are the physiological basis of man's activities. Most of his daily actions are dependent on conditioned reflexes. A previously experienced situation presents itself and he responds appropriately. Constant repetition strengthens a reflex. Disuse weakens it.

Pavlov described a second way in which a conditioned reflex can be established. That is by the use of speech—the second signalling system. By listening to speech or by reading the printed word, man can establish a conditioned reflex to a given stimulus or complex of stimuli without ever having experienced the stimulus. He learns how he should react to a given situation. For example, a child can be taught that a bull is a dangerous animal. Repetition of the fact establishes a conditioned reflex, bull—danger. Years later the boy finds himself in a field with a bull. The sight of the bull is the signal and the result is the realisation of the presence of danger. This, in turn, calls into play a defence mechanism preparing the boy for flight. The sight of the bull produces dramatic changes in body function, varying from increase in heart rate to ischæmia of the skin. Man is constantly being conditioned by this second signalling system. He listens; he learns; he filters information; he absorbs and assimilates. He develops prejudices and preconceived ideas. On this fact is based the principles of advertising, propaganda, and all forms of teaching, etc.

In this way many women become conditioned to expect pain and difficulty during labour. The conditioning probably begins at puberty. The attitude of the girl's mother may produce a favourable or an unfavourable impression. One mother may describe menstruation as a bit of a nuisance and say that childbirth is a time of happiness and may praise the joys of family life. She creates a favourable impression. Another mother may describe her own dysmenorrhœa and painful labours. This mother has started the formation of an adverse conditioned reflex. In the years between puberty and pregnancy the girl gathers information from many sources—from her schoolmates, from her older sisters. She overhears gossip about pregnancies and births. The information is absorbed by her brain and creates a conditioned reflex. The information may be favourable—descriptions of happy and normal births. But, on the other hand, it may be of tragedies, of sickness in pregnancy, of long difficult labours, of stillbirths and deaths, and fœtal abnormalities and, above all, of pain. Some of the expressions used to describe the birth process are unfortunate. The word "labour" itself conveys an impression of unpleasantness, and many still use the word "pain" when they should say uterine "contraction." The conditioning continues during the patient's pregnancy and even during her labour. In the labour room the attitude of the staff is of prime importance. An unguarded word may increase a patient's fears and apprehension. The patient's personality and her

intelligence undoubtedly play a part. The introvert is more likely to absorb adverse information.

As a result of her experience and environment during the years before her pregnancy, during the antenatal period, and even during her labour, a patient is conditioned favourably or unfavourably. If unfavourably, the reflex will be—signal—contraction of the uterus, result—pain and difficulty. If the patient has pain in labour then fear, apprehension and tension appear. A defence mechanism may be called into play. Release of adrenaline may cause ischæmia and spasm of the uterus, and result in even more intense pain. The patient may attempt to reject the cause of the pain, i.e. the contractions of the uterus—and so may prevent the normal increase in tempo of the labour and the normal increase in strength of the contractions. The result is often a long and painful labour. The pain of patients in labour is usually treated by giving strong analgesics and tranquillisers.

During training in psychoprophylaxis the patient is deconditioned and reconditioned by the use of speech and by detailed education. Again and again it is stressed that the uterus is a muscle similar to that of the bowel. That when a skeletal muscle or smooth muscle contracts, pain is not usually felt. The sensation should be that of tightness. But if the muscle is in spasm, as during indigestion, pain will be felt. The woman is asked to feel her own painless Braxton Hicks contractions. In the last few weeks of pregnancy she proves to herself that the uterus can contract without pain. A patient, who has had a painless labour, is introduced to the class and asked to describe her experience. By persuasion and constant repetition the woman is made to accept that the uterus can contract painlessly. A new conditioned reflex is produced, contraction of uterus—tightness. Furthermore, the woman is taught that the contractions of the uterus dilate the cervix and that the quicker the cervix dilates the shorter will be the labour. She is persuaded to welcome the onset of the next contraction and to hope that it will be strong. A new conditioned reflex is built up, signal—contraction of uterus, result— welcome tightness. The conditioned reflexes at play during labour are even more complex than described but the principles involved are the same.

Another neurophysiological principle was described by Pavlov. Arriving at the brain are large numbers of stimuli. Some process of selection is necessary to prevent mental chaos. If man did not have a power of concentration and selection, he would not be able to carry out any continuous action but would be frequently diverted by the arrival of new stimuli at the brain. This selection is effected by the balance of two nervous processes—positive excitation and negative excitation (or inhibition). The arrival of a stimulus at the cortex produces a positive excitation which tends to diffuse but is contained

by a process of inhibition. It is further contained by the action of inhibition from other areas of excitation. The end effect of these conflicting processes is selection and concentration on one centre of activity eliminating other secondary activity. This is the principle involved in the use of counter-irritation. The patient tends to select and concentrate on the new stimuli eliminating or diminishing the original pain stimuli. On the same principle is based the use of "white sound".

It is possible to use this principle during labour. A woman's active participation in her labour can inhibit stimuli from the uterus—can eliminate pain. In psychoprophylaxis the woman is required to be active—both mentally and physically. By this alertness and activity the patient's brain is flooded with stimuli which tend to crowd out, to minimise the stimuli from the uterus. The sensation of tightness is therefore lessened and any tendency for the tightness to become pain is reduced and delayed. In an attempt to make the stimuli from the uterus secondary, the patient is instructed to select and concentrate on some extraneous activity during the contraction. An untrained patient, feeling pain during the contractions, tends to concentrate on the sensations from the uterus. She will be relaxing on her bed. During the contraction she will close her eyes—unfortunately stopping all light stimuli—and she will hold her breath—reducing stimuli from her chest. She concentrates on the painful contraction of the uterus making it seem more intense. The trained woman is taught to concentrate on her breathing, on knitting, reading or watching television. By this concentration the woman makes the stimuli from the uterus secondary and so reduces their effect. Man has this power of concentration and selection. For example, toothache may disappear when the sufferer is engaged in an interesting conversation. In the old days patients used to scrub the floor as a distraction during the first stage of labour.

Pavlov states that an inhibition can be conditioned. That is, a signal can be made to cause inhibition or suppression of a previously expected effect. When Pavlov sounded a low note the dog's salivation was inhibited. Using the second signalling system, a reflex can be built up inhibiting stimuli from the uterus. The patient is told that if she performs a certain action during a contraction it will prevent her from feeling pain. By repetition we build this up into a conditioned reflex which will inhibit sensation from the uterus. In psychoprophylaxis the woman is taught to breathe in a definite pattern.

The psychoprophylactic method of preparation is based on the following principles described by Pavlov. 1. Man is constantly being conditioned by experience and environment. 2. Conditioned reflexes can be established by the use of speech. 3. Old reflexes can become weak and new reflexes can be established. 4. The effect of one group

of stimuli on the brain can be diminished by the inhibitory effect of other stimuli. 5. By a process of selection and concentration on stimuli from one source, stimuli from another source can be made secondary. 6. Inhibition of stimuli can be conditioned. In addition there are many other points which contribute to the success of the method, e.g., the patient is taught to relax the levator ani muscles while contracting the diaphragm and rectus muscles during the bearing down effort. Contraction of the levators would resist descent and might cause perineal tears. She is taught how to direct the bearing down effort into the pelvis by raising her head and shoulders. Education is detailed. The *Birth Atlas* is used in teaching the anatomy and physiology of pregnancy and labour. Much time is spent in discussing in detail everything that happens from admission procedures, conduct of the first stage, to the actual delivery. The patient is told exactly what each procedure will be and why. A tour of the labour room and introduction to the labour room staff is arranged. Fear of the unknown is, as far as possible, removed. The patient develops faith in the method, confidence in the staff and, most important, faith in her own ability. Psychoprophylaxis is made a discipline.

In the training programme described by Vellay of Paris, the main emphasis is placed on the lectures which are really a form of psychotherapy. Throughout the lecture course there is constant repetition of the general principles, thus deconditioning and reconditioning the woman's mind. The Pavlovian principles involved are described using many simple examples which the patient can understand. An appeal is made to her intelligence. Intelligence is not synonymous with education or culture. The less intelligent patient may prove easy to train because she has absorbed less adverse information and because she may develop faith more easily.

The exercises described by Vellay are few and are simple, and are used mainly as a vehicle for the psychotherapy. It is accepted that the only effective muscle working during the first stage is the uterus and that there is no known method of excercising it. Some of the exercises are training for the bearing down effort. The main exercise is the practice of the shallow breathing which will be carried out during the contractions of the first stage of labour. This breathing drill acts in several ways. As the patient is required to practise it every day she has therefore to think about the method daily. During the actual uterine contractions in labour, this breathing acts as a distraction on which the patient concentrates. During the training period the practice of the shallow breathing effects the conditioning of an inhibition. The patient comes to believe that by breathing during the contraction she will not feel pain. And lastly, instead of holding her breath, as do many woman during a contraction, the trained woman

ensures a continuous absorption of oxygen from her lungs during labour.

The degree of success of the method is dependent on many factors. There is the ability and willingness of the patient herself to learn and carry out the detailed practice. The quality of the teaching is of great importance. The teacher should be someone with a full knowledge and experience of midwifery. Order of preference would be doctor, midwife, physiotherapist. Probably a team of all three would be ideal. The personality and teaching ability of the individual would obviously influence the choice of personnel. There is no place for lay teachers, even although their enthusiasm and motives are beyond question. The conduct of the staff during the patient's labour is another important factor which can contribute greatly to the chance of success. The staff must understand psychoprophylaxis. They must supervise the patient's breathing, they must encourage her to be mentally and, up to a point, physically active. The labour lounge should be specially designed to provide interest and distraction. Sleep should be discouraged and hypnotics should not be given routinely. If the patient's brain is sleepy, the stimuli from the uterus will become primary. The atmosphere in the labour room should not be that of a busy casualty department. The staff should be kindly and firm but not sympathetic, and there should be no suggestion of preparing the patient for an ordeal to come. The patient who is going to have an easy labour does not require sympathy. The patient's faith may be lightly held and can easily be upset by sceptical doctors or midwives. If the patient does experience pain she should be given an analgesic. The patient herself is the best judge of her need and should be consulted. She should not be given drugs routinely because she is in strong labour. It is obvious that the presence of untrained patients having pain will lessen the trained patient's chances of success.

Some patients prove difficult to decondition and, in spite of training, will have long and painful labours. It is often possible to forecast the result and to give these women supplementary training. Such a patient could be taught the principles of psychoprophylaxis while she was in a true hypnotic state. If the patient fails, she is naturally disappointed but at Stobhill Hospital there has not been a case who was psychologically upset. On the contrary, most of these women study the method more intensely during their next pregnancy and often succeed then.

The husband should be allowed to be present if he and his wife so wish, and if the geography permits, but he must attend special lectures and must aid his wife at her daily practice. He can be a definite support to her during labour. It can be argued that the unity of the family can be greatly strengthened if the husband shares the experience of childbirth.

There are many forms of antenatal preparation. The simplest is the reassurance given by the doctor or obstetrician at the patient's routine antenatal visits. Many of the methods place the main emphasis on complicated exercises. The choice of words used by the teachers is more important than the actual exercises, accounting for differing success rates found throughout the country. Many of the "relaxation class" teachers have absorbed some of the principles of psychoprophylaxis but do not feel competent to discuss brain function and conditioning in detail. They still concentrate on exercises. Whatever the method used, the most important factor is the "psychotherapy" and the ability of the teacher to get it over to the patient.

Psychoprophylaxis is a definite discipline, combining the necessary psychological conditioning and simple exercises, the meaning and purpose of which can be readily understood by patients, physiotherapists, and not least by midwives and doctors.

REFERENCES

1. ABBAS, T. M. (1957), *Brit. med. J.*, **1**, 563.
2. BARR, W., and GRAHAM, R. (1967). *Postgrad. med. J.*, Suppl. **43**, 101.
3. BARR, W., and GRAHAM, R. (1967). *J. Obstet. Gynaec. Brit. Cwlth.*, **74**, 739.
4. BEARD, R. W., and MORRIS, E. D. (1965). *J. Obstet. Gynaec. Brit. Cwlth.*, **72**, 496.
5. BEARD, R. W., MORRIS, E. D., and CLAYTON, S. G. (1966). *J. Obstet. Gynaec. Brit. Cwlth.*, **73**, 562.
6. BEARD, R. W., MORRIS, E. D., and CLAYTON, S. G. (1967). *J. Obstet. Gynaec. Brit. Cwlth.*, **74**, 812.
7. BULLOUGH, J. (1959). *Brit. med. J.*, **2**, 859.
8. CALDEYRO, R., ALVAREZ, H., and REYNOLDS, S. R. M. (1950). *Surg. Gynec. Obstet.*, **91**, 641.
9. CLELAND, J. G. F. (1933). *Surg. Gynec. Obstet.*, **57**, 51.
10. COOPER, K., and MOIR, J. C. (1963). *Brit. med. J.*, **1**, 1372.
11. DOBKIN, A. B., KEIL, A. N., and WONG, G. (1961). *Anaesthesia*, **16**, 160.
12. DONALD, I., and LORD, J. (1953). *Lancet*, **1**, 9.
13. DONALD, I., KERR, M. M., and MACDONALD, I. R. (1958). *Scot. med. J.*, **3**, 151.
14. DONALD, I., BARR, W., and MCGARRY, J. A. (1962). *J. Obstet. Gynaec. Brit. Cwlth.*, **69**, 837.
15. DUGGAN, T. C., LAUGHLAND, A. W., and MACGREGOR, J. (1966). *Lancet*, **1**, 488.
16. DUNDEE, J. W., and MOORE, J. (1962). *Brit. J. Anaesth.*, **34**, 247.
17. HAWKINS, D. F., and NIXON, W. C. W. (1957). *J. Obstet. Gynaec. Brit. Emp.*, **64**, 641.
18. HEYNS, O. A. (1959). *J. Obstet. Gynaec. Brit. Emp.*, **66**, 220.
19. HEYNS, O. S., SAMSON, J. M., and GRAHAM, J. A. C. (1962). *Lancet*, **2**, 289.

20. HINGSON, R. A., and HELLMAN, L. M. (1956). *Anesthesia for Obstetrics* Philadelphia: J. B. Lippincott Co.
21. HOLMES, J. M. (1955). *Lancet*, **1**, 870.
22. HOLMES, J. M. (1956). *Brit. med. J.*, **2**, 765.
23. JEFFCOATE, T. N. A. (1961). *Lancet*, **2**, 61.
24. JEFFCOATE, T. N. A., BAKER, K., and MARTIN, R. H. (1952). *Surg. Gynec. Obstet.*, **95**, 257.
25. LACOMME, M., LABORIT, A., LE LORIER, G., and POMMIER, M. (1952). *Gynéc. et Obstét.*, **4**, No. 3, bis.
26. *Lancet* (1961). Report "Training for Childbirth", **1**, 765.
27. LEVINE, H., GILBERT, A., and BODANSKY, M. (1940). *J. Pharmacol. exp. Ther.*, **69**, 316.
28. LINTON, K. B., and GILLESPIE, W. A. (1962). *J. Obstet. Gynaec. Brit. Cwlth.*, **5**, 845.
29. LOUDON, J. D. O. (1961). *Current Medicine and Drugs*, Vol. **1**, No. 10, p. 1. London: Butterworth & Co.
30. MACRAE, D. J. (1949). *J. Obstet. Gynaec. Brit. Emp.*, **56**, 785.
31. MACVICAR, J., and MURRAY, M. H. (1960). *Brit. med. J.*, **1**, 595.
32. MOIR, D. D., and BISSET, W. I. K. (1965). *J. Obstet. Gynaec. Brit. Cwlth.*, **72**, 264.
33. MORRIS, E. D., and BEARD, R. W. (1965). *J. Obstet. Gynaec. Brit. Cwlth.*, **72**, 489.
34. NIXON, W. C. W. (1948). *Proc. roy. Soc. Med.*, **41**, 313.
35. NIXON, W. C. W., and SMYTH, C. N. (1957). *J. Obstet. Gynaec. Brit. Emp.*, **64**, 35.
36. O'SULLIVAN, J. V. (1948). *Proc. roy. Soc. Med.*, **41**, 312.
37. PAUL, W. M., GARE, D. J., and WHETHAM, J. C. (1967). *Amer. J. Obstet. Gynec.*, **99**, 745.
38. PLENTL, A. A., FRIEDMAN, E. A., and GRAY, M. J. (1961). *Amer. J. Obstet. Gynec.*, **82**, 1332.
39. POLLOCK, G. B., SPITZEL, J. J., and MASON, D. J. (1960). *Obstet. and Gynec.*, **15**, 504.
40. REICH, A. M. (1951). *Amer. J. Obstet. Gynec.*, **61**, 1263.
41. ROBERTS, H. (1948). *Brit. med. J.*, **2**, 590.
42. ROBERTS, H., KANE, K. M., PERCIVAL, N., SNOW, P., and PLEASE, N. W. (1947). *Lancet*, **1**, 128.
43. ROBERTS, H., and PLEASE, N. W. (1958). *J. Obstet. Gynaec. Brit. Emp.*, 33.
44. ROOTH, G. (1964). *Lancet*, **1**, 290.
45. ROOTH, G., and SJÖVALL, A., (1966). *Lancet*, **2**, 371.
46. SALING, E. (1962). *Arch. Gynäk.*, **197**, 108.
47. SALING, E. (1964). *Geburtsh. u. Frauenheilk.*, **24**, 464.
48. SALING, E., and SCHNEIDER, D. (1967). *J. Obstet. Gynaec. Brit Cwlth.*, **74**, 799.
49. SMYTH, C. N. (1957). *J. Physiol (Lond.)*, **137**, 3 P.
50. SMYTH, C. N., and WOLFF, H. S. (1960). *Lancet*, **2**, 412.
51. TAFEEN, C. H., FREEDMAN, H. L., and HARRIS, H. (1966). *Amer. J. Obstet. Gynec.*, **94**, 854.
52. WOOD, C., LUMLEY, JUDITH and RENOU, P. (1967). *J. Obstet. Gynaec. Brit. Cwlth.*, **74**, 823.

53. WRIGHT, H. PAYLING, MORRIS, N., OSBORN, S. B., and HART, A. (1958). *Amer. J. Obstet. Gynec.*, **75**, 3.

PSYCHOPROPHYLAXIS

54. BONSTEIN, I. (1958). *Psychoprophylactic Preparation for Painless Childbirth.* London: Wm. Heinemann Med. Bks.
55. CHERTOK, L. (1959). *Psychosomatic Method in Painless Childbirth.* Oxford: Pergamon Press.
56. LAMAZE, F. (1958). *Painless Childbirth. A Psychoprophylactic Method.* London: Burke Publishing Co.
57. VELLAY, P. (1959). *Childbirth Without Pain.* London: Hutchinson & Co.
58. VELVOVSKY, I., *et al.* (1960). *Painless Childbirth Through Psychoprophylaxis.* Moscow: Foreign Languages Publishing House.

CHAPTER XVIII

TECHNIQUE AND PITFALLS OF INSTRUMENTAL DELIVERY

THE development of the obstetric forceps dates from the discovery made by one of the members of the Chamberlen family around A.D. 1600, since when innumerable modifications and improvements have been made right up to our own time. The fascinating history of this aid to delivery is well dealt with in certain of the larger text-books, such as that of Greenhill-DeLee, and Munro Kerr and Chassar Moir's *Operative Obstetrics*. It will not be discussed at length here; suffice it to mention a few of the landmarks of major importance.

The original forceps had no pelvic curve, and this introduction is attributed to Levret in Paris during the first half of the eighteenth century. This was a major advance. It was Smellie who first used the forceps for the after-coming head in breech delivery. Even the introduction of the pelvic curve only partially obviated the difficulties of high forceps application, and in 1877 Tarnier conceived the idea of axis traction employing a principle not far dissimilar from that of the modern Milne Murray forceps. The principle of axis traction at once made possible a more satisfactory pull in conformity with the curvature of the birth canal with an associated decrease in the amount of force necessary, thus sparing the maternal tissues to say nothing of the fœtal head, because it is consequently possible to resolve the forces of traction into their more appropriate components and to pull in the correct direction. In the case of a brim or high cavity application the only alternative to axis traction is the use of Pajot's manœuvre, in which the same resultant effect is attempted by pressing downwards on the shanks of the blades at the same time as traction is exerted (Fig. 1). This manœuvre, incidentally, was introduced before the discovery of the principle of axis traction and is far cruder. Nowadays the importance of axis traction is dwindling, as the high forceps operation is only rarely performed in sound obstetric practice.

Neither axis traction nor the use of Pajot's manœuvre, however, dealt adequately with the usually associated problem of the malrotated head, and to Kielland must go the honour of making the greatest single advance in forceps design, since when little of major importance has come on the scene.

Functions of the Obstetric Forceps

The chief of these is to supply traction in cases in which the unaided expulsive efforts of the mother are insufficient to effect a safe delivery in time. The second function is that of rotation, and this can only be guardedly mentioned, for, with the exception of Kielland's forceps, which are designed and eminently suitable for the purpose, rotation of the fœtal head with forceps, whether by Scanzoni's manœuvre or any other diabolical practice, is very questionable. The third function of the forceps is to provide a protective

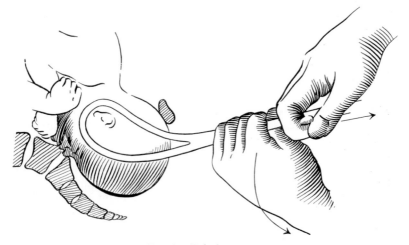

18/Fig. 1.—Pajot's manœuvre.

cage for the head from the pressure of the maternal parts, an advantage which is most noticeable in the case of the after-coming head in breech delivery. In the latter case the forceps properly handled can prevent uncontrolled and too rapid delivery of the head with all its dangers of sudden decompression.

Lastly, the forceps to some extent decreases the transverse diameter of the head by compression, but in so doing increases the vertical diameter. Only where a perfect cephalic application has been achieved is this hypothetical function an advantage, and compression achieved between face and occiput, for example in a thoroughly bad application, is likely to be nothing less than lethal.

Types of Forceps

Time was when many obstetricians, as part of their climb to fame, designed a new type of obstetric forceps to suit their fad or fancy, and

space will not be wasted here in enumerating them. Quite apart from variety in design, Rhodes (1958) has drawn attention to the not inconsiderable discrepancies by different manufacturers in the measurements of allegedly the same design of forceps. A certain haphazard development, too, has led to no very clear idea of what the measurements should be and amongst other recommendations Rhodes suggests that the distance apart of the tips should be 3·0 cm. the widest distance between the blades 9·0 cm., the blade length 16·0 cm. and the radii of cephalic and pelvic curves 11·25 and 17·5 cm. respectively.

Only three main types will be considered (Figs. 2, 3 and 4). Of all the varieties of axis traction forceps that of the Milne Murray type is one of the best, because the traction rods are applied to the bases of the fenestræ, which is the point at which the traction should be applied and where the hinging is most necessary. There is also the further advantage that the degree of flexion of the head can be independently controlled by the main handles of the instrument. There are innumerable varieties of long curved forceps, such as those which can be used with and without their axis traction attachments, and individual preference and training must determine the choice.

The second main group consists of the short curved forceps, such as the Wrigley pattern, which by their lightness and generous cephalic curve are ideal when the head is on the perineum. These beautiful little instruments are worth their weight in gold and can be applied with delicate ease and with the minimum of anæsthesia; they are kindness itself to both the baby's head and maternal soft parts.

The third main class is Kielland's forceps or some variation on this basic type which, with their sliding lock and peculiar shape, can, in practised hands, make wizardry of a difficult forceps delivery of the badly rotated head. I would be content to go through the rest of my obstetrical career with no forceps other than a pair of Kielland's and a pair of Wrigley's.

The Shute parallel forceps[38] looks like a very useful instrument although I have only occasionally used it myself. Its main feature is the special screw back which ensures that the shanks, though separated, are always parallel and the compression of the fœtal head is both controlled and limited by the screw-lock mechanism (Fig. 5).

CONDITIONS WHICH MUST OBTAIN FOR FORCEPS DELIVERY

A legitimate indication must be present. This is mentioned first, because many of the troubles in obstetrics are due to interference which is either unwarranted or premature or both. The further indications will be dealt with presently.

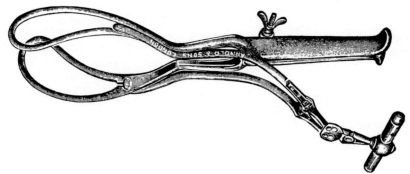

18/Fig. 2.—Milne Murray axis traction forceps.

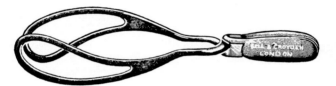

18/Fig. 3.—Wrigley's forceps.

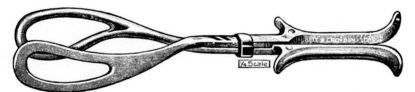

18/Fig. 4.—Kielland's forceps.
(Figs. 2, 3 & 4 by courtesy of John Bell and Croydon.)

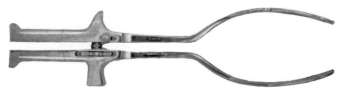

18/Fig. 5.—Shute parallel forceps.
(By courtesy of Down Bros., Mayer and Phelps.)

Delivery must be mechanically feasible. By this is meant that there should be no insuperable bar to delivery because of disproportion. While one can arrive at a very reasonable estimate of the size of the patient's pelvis, the same cannot be said about the size of the baby's head without very specialized techniques, but if it is deeply engaged in the pelvis then, clearly, its diameters must be less, at least, than those of the brim and mid pelvic straits. This does not necessarily mean that in every case no further mechanical difficulty may be encountered, although outlet contraction with a good-sized brim is very uncommon. As a general rule, vaginal delivery can be completed in any case in which the head passes satisfactorily through the brim, but occasionally it may be achieved only at a severe price. Estimates of the true conjugate are a guide, but no more, to the feasibility of forceps delivery, because the strength of uterine contractions and the capacity of the head to mould cannot be forecast. Nevertheless, in any case in which the true conjugate is less than $3\frac{3}{4}$ inches (9·5 cm.), the prospects of safe vaginal delivery must be carefully questioned.

The presentation must be suitable. The only presentations applicable are vertex presentations, face presentations where the chin is anterior, never when it is posterior, and the after-coming head in breech delivery.

The position of the head must be known, not only in respect of its level, but the degree of rotation and flexion must be accurately assessed before the forceps is applied. To apply the forceps blindly to a malrotated head, particularly one arrested in the transverse position, can play havoc with the baby.

The cervix must be fully dilated. The words "or nearly so" are often added, but have given rise to more trouble in forceps delivery than all the other difficulties put together. Often on examining the patient before applying the forceps a fringe of cervix can be felt, and it may appear that the cervix is so near to full dilatation that the head may be eased past it. Now there is all the difference in the world between a cervix which is fully dilated and one which is not quite so, and it is easy to be deceived about the practicability of forceps delivery there and then. Even though it appears that the cervical rim can be pushed over the maximum diameters, traction on the forceps can only mean traction on the lower uterine segment with its neighbouring rich nerve supply in the bases of the broad ligaments. A profound degree of shock is the not uncommon reward, and the cervix is almost bound to suffer more damage, in the form of a lateral split, than is usually foreseen. This state of affairs is commonly encountered in occipito-posterior positions where the patient shows, to all outward appearances, the signs of being fully dilated and is therefore encouraged to bear down. No advance of

the head occurs, however, and after the lapse of an hour or two signs of maternal distress may develop and preparations are made for forceps delivery. The situation presently develops all the ingredients of a shambles. With the patient now anæsthetised, one is faced with the unwelcome alternatives of either delivering her through an incompletely dilated cervix, with all its attendant risks, or of calling off the anæsthetic and leaving her to continue her labour until she is unquestionably in the second stage. If at this point fœtal distress is already established, one may have to choose the former alternative or perform Cæsarean section. In other respects the latter is by far the safer course, although at the time it may appear the less humane. The original mistake, of course, was in diagnosing full dilatation prematurely. True, a rectal or a vaginal examination without an anæsthetic may have been made originally, but the mis-diagnosis may be made because the cervix was not reached by the examining finger. This is a sequence of events which is so often encountered that there is a strong case for not interesting oneself in the moment of full dilatation until the head is on the pelvic floor and the patient is bearing down of her own compulsive volition. If this rule were more frequently followed, the premature application of the forceps before full dilatation would be very much less common and disasters thereby avoided.

To add the obstetrical crime of forceps delivery before full dilatation, simply because one has been mistaken about the cervix in the first place, is seldom justifiable; nevertheless, from time to time circumstances arise in which the risks of such a delivery have to be taken advisedly. This is a task only for the experienced operator. In the majority of cases the situation should not have been allowed to arise. The application of the Ventouse before full cervical dilatation is much less of a crime, and may have to be undertaken deliberately.

The patient must be suitably anæsthetised. The modern preference is for local analgesia whenever practicable, i.e. in the vast majority of cases (see later). Obstetrical anæsthesia is an art in its own right and is full of treachery, especially as the patient's stomach is often full. Induction should be smooth and quick, so that the patient is steered past the risks of asphyxia which is even more damaging to the baby than to the patient herself. Thereafter a light plane of anæsthesia should be maintained. The first plane of the third stage is the ideal level, as uterine activity is thereby less likely to be affected.

The bladder and rectum must be empty. The former is the more important of the two; nevertheless, either of them, when not empty, can reflexly hold up progress in labour and attention to them may often remove the apparent indications for forceps. Even more important is the danger to which a full bladder is exposed in forceps

delivery. An empty bladder is very much less vulnerable. The passage of a catheter, therefore, before applying the forceps is a routine necessity. Because the head is jammed tightly against the symphysis pubis it may often be difficult to insert a catheter. This demands not the use of greater force but a slight elevation of the head to overcome the obstruction of the urethra. The catheter should be passed a fair distance inside and if no urine is at first withdrawn it may be necessary to pass in half of its length. This is because the lower part of the bladder may be empty due to compression by the fœtal head. Suprapubic pressure should be applied not only in the midline but on both sides of it in order to tap every available drop of urine.

Uterine contractions should be present. Not only do they indicate the likelihood of the uterus retracting suitably after the extraction of the child, but any contribution to expulsive force which the uterus can supply reduces by that amount the traction force necessary with the forceps. In most cases a contraction is reflexly stimulated as soon as the forceps is pulled upon. To deliver in the presence of complete uterine atony is to invite one of the worst-known varieties of postpartum hæmorrhage.

Lastly, the membranes should have been already ruptured. This is less important, because delivery is perfectly possible with intact membranes, but the point is that this very fact alone may be the cause of delay and their deliberate rupture may remove the apparent indication for forceps.

LOCAL ANALGESIA VERSUS GENERAL ANÆSTHESIA FOR FORCEPS DELIVERY

There can be few greater therapeutic insults offered to a woman in labour than inexpertly administered anæsthesia. A formidable collection of unhappy reminiscences has convinced me that obstetrical anæsthesia is no job for the occasional anæsthetist and unsupervised junior house officers. The only reason why chloroform once enjoyed a peculiar reputation for safety in parturient women was its relative rapidity of induction before vomiting occurred and the fact that general practitioners used it with the patient lying on her side for forceps delivery in the left lateral position, thus incidentally reducing the risks of inhaled vomit.

It would be an exaggeration to say that anæsthetists, today, kill more mothers in labour and babies than obstetricians, but careful reading between the lines of maternal mortality reports will far more often implicate anæsthetic accidents than the statistics would suggest. Parker (1954 and 1956) reckoned that aspiration of inhaled vomit was responsible for 4 per cent of maternal deaths occurring in

Birmingham and this may be an understatement as post mortem proof is often lacking. It is not the large chunks of solid matter that may be aspirated that cause the trouble as a rule, though they can be dangerous enough, but the highly irritant brown fluid, often made more deadly with glucose, copiously regurgitated and sucked deeply down the bronchial tree, far beyond the reach of even bronchoscopic suction, which is not only lethal but may leave little trace unless the patient survives for more than a day and long enough for the bronchiolar reaction to be demonstrable at necropsy.

Mendelson (1946) differentiated two types of case following aspiration of vomit; the obstructive group due to solid particles of food and the "asthmatic" type which is the commoner danger in obstetrics and whose importance is now better recognised. At the time of induction or recovery from inhalation anæsthesia vomiting occurs, but it is often not realised at the time that foreign matter has been aspirated. For a variable period up to a few hours the patient's condition may at first appear to be satisfactory but presently cyanosis, dyspnœa and marked tachycardia with hypotension develop. A type of pulmonary œdema sets in together with bronchospasm sometimes and progressive collapse usually. Death may occur within 12 hours in the worst cases and sometimes in 4 or 5 days if an aspiration bronchopneumonia supervenes.

Fortunately, in the majority who survive and whose perilous adventures do not find their way into maternity reports, recovery would appear to be complete. Treatment consists of oxygen and antibiotics. Digoxin is often given but usually fails to control the tachycardia.

Intravenous aminophylline (250 mg.) may be tried if bronchospasm is evident. Bronchoscopic suction is usually disappointing and one feels remarkably helpless when faced with this clinical picture. I have seen a patient die within a few hours, chattering and excited to within an hour or two of death, with deep cyanosis which an oxygen tent affected not at all and an uncontrollable tachycardia. There had been no hæmorrhage but the antecedent labour had been prolonged.

It has been suggested by Hausmann and Lunt (1955) that the underlying pathology is an acute adrenal failure and they appear to have had some success with intravenous hydrocortisone started immediately (100 mg. given within 4 hours in a 5 per cent glucose drip). If hypotension is very severe, noradrenaline should be added to the drip (e.g. Levophed 2–4 mg. to the half litre) and the drip regulated around 10–20 drops per minute according to very frequent blood-pressure readings.

Clearly, this is an ugly complication of operative delivery which it is worth going to great lengths to prevent. The patients, after all, are unpremedicated and often in poor metabolic shape before anæsthe-

sia, quite apart from their full stomachs. Some anæsthetists empty the stomach first by passing a stomach tube—probably the safest course, but by no means wholly effective. Holmes (1956) induced severe vomiting by the intravenous injection of apomorphine and follows this up with atropine, but neither method can be a comfortable experience for a patient already demoralised in the second stage of labour. Coleman and Day (1956) recommended the routine use of cuffed endotracheal tubes but, with inexperienced anæsthetists, the damage may be done before the tube is passed, or after it is withdrawn.

The problem is further aggravated by the fact that few labour ward beds can be rapidly tilted into the head-down position should vomiting occur and far too many labour wards are without efficient mechanical suction instantly available. In order to minimise the hazard of acid aspiration we make it an invariable rule now to give 14 ml. ($\frac{1}{2}$ an ounce) of standard magnesium trisilicate mixture by mouth immediately before all general anæsthetics and when there is abdominal distension in prolonged labour we pass a stomach tube as well. The effects of the magnesium trisilicate mixture last for up to two hours by way of neutralising the gastric contents.

Quite apart from the more dramatic risks of obstetric anæsthesia enumerated above, there must also be remembered the effects upon the baby in addition to those of accidental asphyxia.

All anæsthetics not only put the mother to sleep, but the baby and the uterus to some extent as well.

Finally, if one counts up all the anxious time one has spent awaiting the arrival of a suitable anæsthetist, it is small wonder that modern local analgesia has been welcomed on an increasing scale.

It is now the practice in my unit to use local analgesia, if possible, in all forceps delivery in which the vertex presents, the only absolute contra-indications being eclampsia and cases for trial of forceps (see later), in which the possibility of Cæsarean section as an alternative is being considered. Even the "hysterical" patient can usually be talked into co-operation, if necessary with the help of intravenous promazine (Sparine) 50 mg. Furthermore, we now prefer to train our junior residents in the techniques of forceps delivery having first effected local analgesia, since a bad or rough application cannot be made without protest from the patient and less traction effort is required because of the contribution which the patient and her uterus can be encouraged to make in delivering the head. In fact, forceps delivery under local analgesia is not only safer for the mother, but the lively condition of the unanæsthetised babies proclaims it as the method of choice. The popularity of low spinal or saddle block anæsthesia, or more often epidural anæsthesia, which is so widespread in the U.S.A. is less widely shared in the United Kingdom. Our own

reasons for preferring pudendal nerve block are its simplicity, its great safety and, not least, the fact that the patient retains her expulsive reflexes and is able to contribute to the delivery and reduce the traction effort with forceps. Notwithstanding all the above I was interested to find out from our own hospital figures that general anæsthesia was used as often as 29·8 per cent of all anæsthetics for forceps delivery and that epidural anæsthesia was used for a further 9 per cent, leaving only 61·2 per cent of all forceps deliveries conducted under pudendal block.

Technique of Local Analgesia

Lignocaine hydrochloride (Xylocaine 1 per cent) or, as an alternative, prilocaine (Citanest 1 per cent) have proved, in our experience, the most useful agents yet tried. They are remarkably nontoxic and complications are rare, and are only likely to follow accidental intravenous injection or frank overdosage. Allergy has not been reported, but dizziness and collapse may occur if a large quantity of the drug rapidly enters the circulation. Hypotension may require a pressor drug such as methyl amphetamine during the immediate emergency and if it persists 100 mg. of hydrocortisone should be given by drip infusion. Convulsions may be controlled by intravenous thiopentone. Such accidents are very unlikely in standard dosage which gives a good duration of analgesia sufficient for most forceps operations and repair of episiotomy thereafter. Its "spreading power" is so great that the use of hyaluronidase is unnecessary; in fact, by increasing the rate of diffusion, hyaluronidase proves a nuisance by shortening the duration of anæsthetic effect.

Perineal Infiltration

Local infiltration of the perineum is all that may be necessary for the performance of episiotomy and very low outlet forceps or the application of the Ventouse at the end of the second stage. Indeed, if the fœtal head is very low it may be impossible to reach the ischial spines for the purpose of pudendal nerve block without hurting the patient. It is also sufficient for most perineal repairs. The technique is very simple. Using a long, fine needle, on a 20 ml. syringe, 10–20 ml. of 1 per cent lignocaine is injected fanwise, from a point in the midline at the fourchette. If possible it is as well to insert a couple of fingers into the vagina first to put the perineal tissues on a slight stretch.

Premedication—for delivery under local analgesia.—The best premedication of all is a thoughtful and careful explanation to the patient of what one is about to do, explaining the help that is about to be offered for her baby's sake as well as her own and securing her intelligent co-operation. A conversational patter maintained

throughout with the patient will often suffice for even apparently hysterical patients. It is here particularly that the rapport established between doctor and patient in the course of good antenatal care begins to reap its dividends. However, the situation on the psychological front may have been allowed to get out of control before operative intervention is contemplated. In these cases we have found intravenous injection of Sparine, as described in the previous chapter, of great help. There are all manner of variants on this theme and Coxon (1961) recommends a premixed solution of pethidine, levallorphan and promethazine intravenously so that tne patient receives for every stone (6·5 Kg.) body weight 10 mg. of pethidine, 0·125 mg. of levallorphan and 2·5 mg. of promethazine intravenously. A ten-stone woman (65 Kg.) would, therefore, receive a slow injection of 100 mg. of pethidine, 1·25 mg. of levallorphan and 25 mg. of promethazine. This is given about 10 minutes before the patient is placed in the lithotomy position and draped.

Pudendal Nerve Block

The only apparatus required is a 20 ml. syringe and a fine needle at least five inches in length. The aim of the injection is to place the solution around the internal pudendal nerve as it passes into the ischio-rectal fossa adjacent to the ischial spine. In actual practice the spread of effect of lignocaine makes up for indifferent technique to a most comforting extent. It will be remembered that this nerve leaves the pelvic cavity above the pelvic diaphragm through the lower border of the sacro-sciatic foramen and, in company with the pudendal artery, winds round the outer surface of the ischial spine and then enters the ischio-rectal fossa below it. At any distance thereafter it may give off inferior hæmorrhoidal and perineal branches before it goes on to reach the clitoris. Quite a small quantity of local anæsthetic, therefore, placed in the strategic position near the inferior and outer border of the ischial spine will achieve a wide field of anæsthesia.

There are two methods of placing this injection and for both a one per cent solution of lignocaine or prilocaine without adrenaline or hyaluronidase is recommended. The older and now dying method is to inject via the ischio-rectal fossa. For this purpose a weal is first raised on either side at a point midway between the ischial tuberosity and the anus. A finger is then placed in the vagina and the ischial spine identified. The ischial spine is aimed for with the needle and the finger in the vagina helps to guide it just below its inferior border. The plunger is withdrawn to make sure that a vessel has not been entered and a solution of 10 ml. of lignocaine is injected on each side. A further 5 ml. can be placed just medial to the ischial tuberosity in order to block an aberrant inferior hæmorrhoidal nerve and finally 5 to 10 ml. can be

injected under the greater part of the length of skin covering each labium majus, in order to block any filaments from the ileo-inguinal nerve. In actual fact this latter procedure is seldom necessary. It will be noticed that the total dose now given does not exceed 40 to 50 ml. of one per cent lignocaine which is well within the safety limit. It used to be my practice to infiltrate the perineum first with about 15 ml. in order to make the examination and the palpation of the ischial spines more comfortable for the patient and also to cover up any deficiencies in technique. Such is the spreading power of lignocaine, however, that even a reasonably approximate approach to the ischial spine on the point of emergence of the pudendal nerve is sufficient to produce an efficient block and the extra dosage in the perineum is not usually necessary. The makers of lignocaine advise restricting the total volume administered to no more than 50 ml. of one per cent solution, although I have often exceeded this dose. The anatomical details of the technique have been well illustrated by Gate and Dutton (1955). If one is less confident of this technique and wishes to fall back on larger quantities of solution it is better to use a half per cent strength, which is also quite effective, rather than increase the dose.

The second method of achieving pudendal nerve block, and one which we increasingly favour, is by the transvaginal route as graphically described by Kobak et al. (1956), and by Huntingford (1959). This technique provides the shortest possible route to the nerve and would seem to be the last step in the evolution of pudendal nerve block. A six-inch, seventeen-gauge spinal needle is recommended, together with a 20 ml. syringe. The index and middle fingers of one hand, held in apposition, reach for the ischial spine. If there is difficulty in palpating it because it is not prominent, the sacro-spinous ligament can be felt as a ridge converging on it. The shaft of the needle can be placed in the groove between the two fingers and the needle and is thus made to penetrate the vaginal skin just below the ischial spine. The direction of the needle is now altered so that it is parallel with the table on which the patient is lying. This will take the point of the needle slightly behind the spine and after aspiration to ensure that a blood vessel has not been entered, a very accurately placed injection is possible. If blood is aspirated it is better to withdraw the needle and reinsert it slightly more to the midline to avoid the vessels.

This technique involves the intravaginal use of two fingers and it is very easy to puncture the glove with the needle tip.

The method which Huntingford recommends is slightly different and involves guiding the needle to the tip of the ischial spine by the index finger of one hand with the thumb of the same hand flexed on the shaft of the needle. When the needle point is at the tip of the

P.O.P.—19*

ischial spine, it is advanced about 0·5 cm. to bring it over the sacro-spinous ligament, then, by bending the point of the needle by firm pressure with the index finger against the resistance of the thumb on the shaft the sacro-spinous ligament is penetrated and following aspiration for blood, as before, the injection is made deep to the sacro-spinous ligament.

At this point mention should be made of the Iowa trumpet. I was introduced to this delightful instrument by Dr. Edwin McDaniel of Thailand and I am very grateful to Dr. Dan S. Egbert of Fort Dodge, Iowa, for sending me one for my own use. It consists of a guide for a 5-in. needle which can only project a few millimetres beyond a blunt bulbous tip. At the proximal end of the guide is a ring for the thumb, while the finger can be placed over the bulbous tip which is guided onto the lower tip of the ischial spine before the long needle is passed through it and inserted in the usual fashion.[8] The use of this instrument makes child's play of pudendal block anæsthesia and secures an accurate placing of the anæsthetic solution and therefore anæsthesia is almost immediate. This can be verified by asking the patient to draw in the anus which she should now be unable to perform because of levator paralysis, also needleprick in the region of the anus produces no response from the external sphincter. The pelvic floor becomes very much slacker after pudendal block has been achieved, thereby facilitating operative procedures and examination even before episiotomy. The duration of anæsthesia is seldom less than thirty minutes, sometimes more, and can easily be extended by further injection later when it wears off, but it is adequate in most cases for the subsequent repair of an episiotomy and for many cases of manual removal of the placenta, if a general anæsthetic for this operation is not immediately available. My own enthusiasm for pudendal block using the Iowa trumpet may to some extent be conditioned by the fact that I usually put in some local perineal infiltration as well and there are some who have suggested that the efficacy of pudendal block simply depends upon the perineal infiltration alone.[36] This I do not believe because the forceps operation under perineal infiltration alone is seldom a painless affair.

One of the arguments against using adrenaline with lignocaine, apart from the fact that it is unnecessary, is that there is danger of sudden ventricular fibrillation if the patient at the same time has trichloroethylene, for example, from a self-administering inhaler.[24] If any form of self-administered inhalation anæsthetic is required because of a partially unsuccessful pudendal block, then the 50/50 nitrous oxide and oxygen mixture as delivered by the Entonox apparatus would be the most suitable.

The ensuing operation calls for great finesse. By careful reassurance of the patient, careful timing of movement, slow and deliberate gentle-

ness and attention to the direction of pull, it is possible to slip on the forceps blades and deliver the head with less pain and discomfort for the patient than a normal spontaneous delivery in a primipara. Smellie must have worked with such delicate touch on far less suitable but unanæsthetised patients in his day and we would do well to remember his example.

Not least of the advantages of a well-conducted delivery under pudendal block analgesia is the lively interest and co-operation of the patient in what is her greatest hour.

To exploit the technique of this method to the full one must become familiar with the use of Kielland's forceps, since rotation of the head is best done with this beautiful instrument. Manual rotation requiring the half hand, or more often the whole hand in the vagina, may require general anæsthesia.

Local analgesia was successful in 94 per cent of all types of forceps delivery in Scott and Gadd's series (1957) and in 84 per cent of all cases of delivery by Kielland's forceps, although a supplementary injection of chlorpromazine ($12\frac{1}{2}$ mg.) and pethidine (100 mg.) was necessary in a minority of cases (where we would use promazine).

Scott uses a proper operating table with the patient's buttocks overhanging the edge, in order to facilitate the application of the anterior blade of Kielland's forceps in the direct method of application (see later). These workers have shown the traction forces applied by the use of a dynamometer attached to the handles of the Kielland's forceps, and they class as moderate traction forces of from 35 to 50 lb. and 70 lb. as severe, above which level damage to the baby's head is likely.

Epidural Anæsthesia

Well executed pudendal nerve block is so efficient that the fuller type of anæsthesia produced by the epidural route is seldom called for in the case of operative vaginal deliveries. Nevertheless, where it is necessary to remove pain completely or in cases where the possibility of proceeding to Cæsarean section is being considered in the event of failure to deliver by the vaginal route, there is much to be said for inducing epidural anæsthesia in the first place. Continuous epidural anæsthesia has already been discussed at some length in the previous chapter on prolonged labour. The disadvantage is that the patient can contribute nothing, or practically nothing, to her own delivery by voluntary bearing down efforts because of her temporary paraplegia, and most of the forces to achieve delivery have to be applied through the instrument used. Nevertheless, this technique enjoys very great popularity in the United States and deservedly so. In competent hands it provides a most excellent and safe anæsthetic,

particularly from the baby's point of view. The technique is as follows: the patient lies on her left side with the legs moderately flexed and the shoulders parallel. There should be no attempt to flex the spine unduly since this stretches the dura and also reduces the capacity of the peridural space. After infiltration of the skin in the midline between either the 2nd and 3rd or 3rd and 4th lumbar vertebræ, a fairly large bore needle with a sharp stilette (similar to a 16-gauge Tuohy needle) is inserted, keeping constantly in the midline, and advanced until the tough ligamentum flavum is encountered. The latter is the important structure which indicates the correct progress of the needle, and as the needle goes beyond this tough medium there is a definite sense of release conveyed through the needle to the operator. Attempts to inject fluid or air whilst the point of the needle is still in the ligament result in a rebound of the piston, whereas, when the point is in the peridural space the syringe empties easily. The hanging-drop technique may be employed to estimate the progress of the needle. It is essential to appreciate the dangers of inadvertent intrathecal injection, since the introduction of such a large volume of fluid into the subarachnoid space would cause the most severe complications, if not death. Therefore, after ascertaining the inability to withdraw cerebrospinal fluid, a test dose of 2 ml. is advisable, followed by a pause of about 5 minutes to check for the development of somatic anæsthesia. If the test proves negative, it should be followed by a further injection of about 20 ml. A fairly large pillow beneath the head and shoulders of the patient will ensure that the analgesic fluid will extend caudad and thus include the sacral nerves; so essential in vaginal deliveries. The solutions used are the same as in caudal blocks, again preferring lignocaine or prilocaine, 1 per cent, or 1·5 per cent without adrenaline. Slow injection is desirable, as this minimises the likelihood of hypotension.

It is interesting to compare the blood loss at forceps delivery carried out under different types of anæsthesia and this has been investigated at the Queen Mother's Hospital by Moir and Wallace (1967) in 214 consecutive and unselected mid-cavity forceps deliveries in which episiotomy was performed at the same time. The estimation was carried out by the hæmoglobin extraction dilution technique using the Perdometer apparatus into which were fed all gowns, gloves, swabs and in fact almost every drop of blood lost at delivery, into a sort of washing machine containing a solution which extracted the hæmoglobin and passed the washing fluid of known volume through a photoelectric mechanism, adjustment having been previously made for the patient's known hæmoglobin. The amount lost was very much greater than expected whatever the anæsthetic, a fact which no longer surprises me, but the mean loss was found to be 518 ml. under general anæsthesia, 412 ml. under pudendal block and only

276 under epidural analgesia, much of the latter coming from the episiotomy wound.

INDICATIONS FOR FORCEPS DELIVERY

It has for long been customary to think of the indications in terms of faults in forces, passages and passenger, but this generalisation needs qualifying. Agreed the forces may be inadequate ; nevertheless they should be present. With regard to faults in the passages, the only genuine indication in this class is undue resistance to delivery by maternal soft tissue. Bony disproportion is not a proper indication; in fact it may be a positive contra-indication. Faults in the passenger are more usually due to malrotation and deflexion than anything else, and it will be seen that this classification of indications is far too incomplete and misleading to be any longer acceptable. It is, therefore, better to class the indications for forceps as maternal, or fœtal, or both.

Physical maternal distress is indicated by a dry tongue, a rising pulse, a variable degree of pyrexia, and in extreme cases by hotness and dryness of the vagina. Of these the dry tongue is the most important. No woman in the second stage of labour with a clean moist tongue can be genuinely regarded as physically distressed however heavily she appears to be weathering her labour. In other words, dehydration is a part of the mechanism of maternal distress, and the urine likewise shows increasing specific gravity and, in advanced cases, may contain appreciable quantities of albumin and acetone.

In certain general maternal conditions the threat of maternal distress becomes an indication since its frank development cannot be tolerated, for example cases with cardiac lesions, pulmonary tuberculosis and thyroid disease associated with dyspnœa. In eclampsia, likewise, at full dilatation forceps delivery is indicated in both maternal and fœtal interests, and one could extend the list indefinitely. The fœtal indications are mainly those of asphyxia or the threat thereof. Unfortunately the signs of fœtal distress are only clinically apparent when fœtal asphyxia is already advanced and irreparable damage may already have been done.The Saling method of fœtal blood sampling during labour has already been dealt with in the previous chapter and this would appear to be the best available means at the moment of assessing the gravity of apparent fœtal distress. As it is, the only clinical aids are the changes observed in the fœtal heart rate and its rhythm and the passage of meconium in cephalic presentations, this last being a very serious sign. During a powerful uterine contraction the fœtal heart often slows because of the temporary restriction in blood supply to the placental site, but

its rate should be immediately restored as soon as the contraction wears off.

The first cardiac sign of fœtal distress is acceleration of the heart rate above 160 beats to the minute. This is an irritative phenomenon, may be very short lived and is often missed. Thereafter the child's vasomotor centres become depressed and the fœtal heart is slowed. A rate below 120 per minute is suggestive, and if it falls as low as 100 is a definite indication of fœtal asphyxia. Irregularity of the fœtal heart is an even more definite sign. Faintness of the fœtal heart is often regarded as a further sign but, being a purely subjective observation, is less reliable.

There are additional fœtal indications in which the threat of fœtal asphyxia is so definite as to constitute an immediate indication for delivery. Instances of such are prolapse of the cord at full dilatation and eclamptic seizures in the mother. A further very significant sign of fœtal asphyxia is the appearance of violent convulsive movements of the baby indicating that it is literally in its death throes.

Of course, to apply the forceps to the head of a distressed fœtus is to increase its distress somewhat further. Nevertheless, it is safer to deliver it forthwith than to leave the original conditions of asphyxia still in full operation. A baby *in utero* will not withstand genuine distress for very long. In such a delivery everything possible must be done to spare further trauma to the baby's head and an episiotomy is obligatory.

Failure to advance is an accepted indication, but it must be qualified in the light of the nature of the uterine contractions. Although a duration of the second stage of 2 hours is regarded as a more than adequate maximum, midwifery cannot be run according to the clock, and in some cases of hypotonic uterine inertia the patient may be regarded simply as performing a perfectly normal delivery but in a slower gear. In these cases, in the absence of fœtal and maternal distress, labour can safely be allowed to continue normally. More commonly, however, it is apparent that the patient's own expulsive forces are not enough of themselves to effect delivery and in these cases failure to advance becomes a genuine reason for operating long before the elapse of two hours; in fact lack of progress in spite of good contractions for an hour calls for action. In any case of doubt a vaginal examination should be made and the reason for the delay may then become more apparent. An occipito-posterior position or a head which is not rotated from the transverse position will in many such cases be found to be the real cause.

INCIDENCE OF FORCEPS DELIVERY

This varies very widely from one institution to another and from one obstetrician to another, even though the maternal morbidity

hand laterally alongside the head and, holding the left blade of the forceps between finger and thumb of the left hand, lightly to steer it directly alongside the baby's head. In this manœuvre the handle of the forceps blade starts above the symphysis pubis and parallel to the right inguinal ligament on the patient's right and swings down in an arc towards her left (Fig. 8). The left half hand is now inserted alongside the baby's head and the manœuvre repeated with the other blade held as before but in the right hand. Correctly applied, the locks should come easily together and the handles should be very little separated. The other standard method is to insert the left hand into the vagina in front of the hollow of the sacrum and to introduce each blade in turn posteriorly first, then manipulating it round to the side of the baby's head. The blades should lock comfortably and easily as before.

Difficulty may be experienced in applying the blades. This is no indication for the use of more force, which should, anyway, never exceed the power which three fingers can apply, and it indicates rather the need for re-examination. If the cervix is not fully dilated, one may fail to apply the forceps simply because the point of the blades is being pushed into one of the vaginal fornices. The most common source of difficulty, however, is due to the fact that the head has not been properly rotated with the occiput anterior. Under these circumstances the locks may fail to come together or the handles may appear to be widely separated. This assuredly denotes a faulty application and demands re-examination, correction of the malposition and applying the blades again. Cramming the forceps together by brute force is only to be deplored. Sometimes failure to lock the blades is due to the fact that they have not been introduced far enough, and it is a common mistake for beginners to hold the handles too far forward, which prevents the proper insertion of the blades. A correct cephalic application advertises itself by the ease with which the handles come together. In this position the blades lie along a line joining the chin and junction of the posterior and middle thirds of a line joining the anterior and posterior fontanelles.

Manual Rotation of the Occiput

This is a very necessary part of the forceps operation in which the occiput is not already anterior. It requires a certain amount of knack and at times can be very difficult. During its performance two objectives must not be forgotten, namely to maintain as far as possible a good degree of flexion and to avoid undue displacement upwards of the head. If the head escapes above the brim it may be reluctant to engage again in its new position, so that one is faced with the alternatives of a high forceps application, an internal

version and breech extraction (very hazardous) or Cæsarean section. Some upward displacement is inevitable in order to facilitate manual rotation, but its degree should, as far as possible, be controlled. In the case of R.O.P. and R.O.L. positions, it is usual to use the left hand and vice versa so that the movement of forearm and wrist is one of pronation (Fig. 9). The rotation of the head should be accompanied by rotation of the trunk by manipulation of the baby's anterior shoulder *per abdomen*, and one should not be content with less than over-correction to a few degrees on the opposite side of the midline in order to ensure against the malposition recurring. Beware of using too much lubricant as it will make the grip too slippery. One of the great advantages of the use of Kielland's forceps is that rotation can be completed with the minimum of displacement

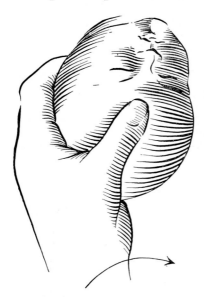

18/Fig. 9.—Manual rotation of head in R.O.P. position.

of the fœtal head and these forceps prevent the malposition from recurring. Often, too, the head is more easily rotated at a lower level in the pelvis than can be achieved by the hand. This will be discussed more fully later.

An alternative method of manual rotation is to pass the fingers up over the baby's face, thus improving flexion, and to rotate by supinating the arm, using the right hand in R.O.P. positions and the left hand for L.O.P. positions. Sometimes it suffices to reach up no further than the anterior fontanelle, using the pressure of the ulnar border of a finger on the fontanelle margin to achieve rotation. The sacral promontory sometimes prevents full rotation by getting in the way of the sinciput. The remedy is to displace the head a little farther upwards, but a hand must, at the same time, be applied to the abdomen to control the displacement and to push the head down into the pelvis again when the sinciput can be negotiated into the opposite parasacral bay.

The deliberate employment of manual rotation of the head before full dilatation of the cervix, in order to expedite a first stage which is dragging on from three-quarters dilatation, is usually a waste of time

since delivery cannot yet be completed with forceps and the malposition is likely to recur. It occasionally happens, however, that one may be examining a patient under anæsthesia in order to determine the cause of delay, in which case an attempt at manual rotation is justifiable. Under these circumstances the Ventouse may prove the most suitable instrument, being less likely to damage the cervix.

Traction Difficulties

The difficult forceps operation must presently become as much of an anchronism as cranioclasm and cephalotripsy. A mother's pelvic tissues, may, with luck, recover. A child's brain may not. The amount of force which can be justified in pulling on the forceps should not exceed that which can be applied by the forearms alone. Using an axis tractionometer (with a spring scale) Wylie (1963) reckoned that forces exceeding 70 Kg. inflicted too great a risk of injury to justify further attempts at vaginal delivery.

Whether the standing or the sitting position is employed is a matter of personal taste, but, on the whole, better control is obtained with the latter. In either event there are few things more distressing to mother, baby and onlookers than a powerful man applying his weight, aided by the pressure of his feet up against the bed, to extract the child. Such force is clearly misapplied and therefore both unnecessary and harmful. One has only to compare the bearing down pressures which the patient in normal labour exerts to deliver herself (pressures which amount to not much more than 200 millimetres of mercury), and the immense force which is sometimes injudiciously employed. Clearly in such instances something is wrong. Either the case is not suitable for forceps delivery or a proper cephalic application of the forceps is lacking. Thirdly, the case may be one of undiagnosed persistent occipito-posterior position, or brow presentation, or perhaps traction is being made in the wrong direction, usually too far forwards, so that the back of the maternal symphysis is taking the brunt of the operator's effort, to the lasting detriment of intervening structures, particularly the bladder neck and its supports. The direction of the birth canal should be remembered in relation to the station of the baby's head, so that in high mid-cavity positions the direction of pull is somewhat downwards and backwards, gradually levelling out as the head descends and finally turning upwards and forwards as the occiput stems round the symphysis pubis (Fig. 10).

If, therefore, with reasonable traction no advance is made, attention should be directed to the possibility that traction is being exerted in the wrong direction or that the occiput is directed posteriorly or, again, the cephalic application of the blades may be faulty. Only when one has considered these possibilities should one consider the less likely diagnosis of contracted outlet. In all the above in-

stances, except the first, re-examination is called for after removing the blades. This is far better than pressing on to the very death (of the baby)!

Another disconcerting accident associated with forceps traction is the slipping off of the blades. This is most injurious to both mother and child. The commonest cause of this is the undiagnosed persistent occipito-posterior position, in which instance the forceps obtain

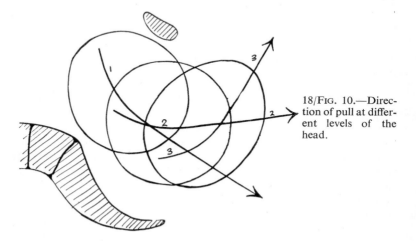

18/Fig. 10.—Direction of pull at different levels of the head.

a far less secure grip of the head. The other cause of the blades slipping off is an oblique or antero-posterior application over the baby's occiput and face.

Lastly, an appreciable degree of vaginal bleeding may appear at this stage of the operation, which can be very worrying, especially since, delivery not being completed, it is not possible to find its source and deal with it. It usually originates from a split in the vaginal wall or an internal tear of the perineum and usually ceases as delivery proceeds.

If traction is made in association with a uterine contraction, the amount of force necessary is by that much reduced. Fortunately, as soon as pulling starts, a reflex contraction is usually evoked. Steady but intermittent and convincing pulls should be made, and the locks should be eased open a little between whiles, in order to relieve the baby's head from continuous compression. As soon as the resistance of the pelvic floor is met it is customary nowadays to perform episiotomy, and there is much from the baby's point of view to commend this practice, inasmuch as it reduces the wear and tear upon the baby's head.

Towards the final point of forceps delivery, traction is being made

more or less directly upwards, and care should be taken to control the force used in order to minimise the extent of perineal damage. As soon as the head is crowned, the forceps should be removed, whereupon the delivery of the head can be slowly completed by extension as in the conduct of a normal second stage.

Vaginal bypass in the form of Cæsarean section is infinitely preferable for the baby and often for the mother too than difficult forceps delivery and evidence of cerebral damage has been noted in 18·7 per cent of quite a large series of cases in which difficulty was experienced in the course of mid-cavity forceps delivery.[40] This is sufficient to condemn difficult forceps delivery in retrospect. In this series the main factors appear to have been some degree of contracted pelvis, especially with a flat sacrum and restriction of the cavity associated with transverse arrest or posterior position of the occiput. This naturally raises the question of trial of forceps. By this is meant the application of forceps with the mental reservation that should the operation prove difficult there should be no hesitation in removing the blades and resorting forthwith to Cæsarean section, for which preparations have been fully made in advance. To undertake a proper trial of forceps, therefore, it is mandatory that the operation not only finishes but starts in a properly equipped operating theatre. It is our practice at the Queen Mother's Hospital to carry out all obstetrical operations, even the simplest, under full surgical conditions in an operating theatre, but very few units are thus generously equipped and if a patient happens, as is likely, to be in what is euphemistically called a forceps delivery room, the business of removing her into an operating theatre, commonly on a different floor (and even in one place where I worked across a snow-covered courtyard) is so daunting as to discourage one from resorting to Cæsarean section and trying yet again another good hard pull. This is certainly not trial of forceps. I have done enough "bathroom obstetrics" in my life to know that the best judgments are only made under the best conditions and preparedness in every physical and geographical sense for Cæsarean section is an indispensable ingredient of a true trial. Successful trial of forceps indeed is most rewarding, but an unsuccessful trial terminating in Cæsarean section is an unpleasant business for mother, baby and obstetrician. All the more need therefore for a full pre-operative assessment. Trial of forceps is like lion taming. It is not the sort of exercise one would willingly undertake in expectation of failure.

Face-to-pubis Delivery with Forceps

Unwittingly performed, because of missed diagnosis about the position of the child's head (and we have all from time to time made this mistake), the head is liable to pop out suddenly with extensive

damage to the perineum, unless prophylactic episiotomy has been performed. This, too, is one of the cardinal causes of a third-degree tear. Nevertheless, in certain cases it is preferable to deliver in the unreduced P.O.P. position deliberately, provided care is taken to prevent the forceps from slipping off or the head from suddenly popping out. With a generous episiotomy, made in advance, this method is preferable to manual rotation under the following circumstances:

1. If the head is already bulging the perineum and the patient has only failed to deliver herself spontaneously face-to-pubis at the last stage of the head's descent.

2. In cases of marked anthropoid shape of the pelvis. In this instance the rotation of the head would involve negotiating the narrower transverse diameter so that it becomes neither necessary nor wise.

3. In cases of prolonged and dry labour, in which the uterus is so closely applied to the baby's body that it is impossible to rotate it in conformity with the rotation of the head.

It can be argued with some justification that in cases in which the occiput lies directly posterior one should accept this as an indication for proceeding with face-to-pubis delivery, since the pelvis in such cases must be either anthropoid in type or roomy enough to have allowed the head to have rotated into this position so there is now no indication for turning it. Furthermore, the mechanics of moulding are better not disturbed at this late stage.

The position is altogether different in the more commonly met cases of transverse arrest of the head or where the occiput lies obliquely posterior. These cases must be rotated.

Incidentally, the jampot moulding in occipito-posterior position so often described in textbooks is rather uncommon. More often a lop-sided oblique moulding occurs in conformity with the oblique or transverse position of the baby's head, and even in the full face-to-pubis position one more often sees the moulding of extreme flexion which exaggerates to a depressing degree the apparent vertical length of the baby's forehead, before the eyebrows can be made to appear from under the symphysis pubis.

Forceps to the After-coming Head

It is a mistake to regard the use of forceps as the last resort in dealing with the difficult delivery of the head in a breech delivery, because, by now, it may be too late. The forceps should be sterilised and available in advance, especially in the case of primiparous breech delivery, so that there need be no delay in applying. In the first place, the head should be brought as low down as possible by hanging the body of the child downwards until the occiput lies up

against the back of the symphysis pubis. An assistant then raises the legs of the child so as to lift the body out of the way. The forceps blades are applied on either side of the baby's head from underneath its body, that is to say on its ventral aspect (12/Fig. 2). An episiotomy should, of course, have been made already. A great advantage of the forceps in these cases is that the head can be gently extracted and its rate of delivery accurately controlled. Unfortunately, it is not possible to perform this operation without the help of a second pair of hands to lift the body of the child.

Forceps in Face Presentation

It is essential that the chin be already fully rotated to the front before the forceps is applied, except, of course, in the case of the Kielland's forceps which may be used for the rotation of the face. An episiotomy is absolutely essential in these cases, and traction should at first be continued somewhat downwards and backwards in order to maintain the fullest possible extension of the head until the chin unquestionably clears the bottom of the symphysis pubis. Thereafter, the head is delivered by flexion. In this sort of delivery the forceps blades should be applied with the handles rather farther forward than in the case of the vertex deliveries, so that when traction is made in the correct direction, as above, any attempt by the head to become flexed will be thereby discouraged.

FAILED FORCEPS

In recent years the emphasis upon certain causes of failure to deliver with forceps, notably cases of disproportion, has shifted, largely as a result of antenatal care. Miller in 1927 found that there was an incidence of 17·6 per cent of cases of failed forceps amongst a series of 500 emergency admissions to hospital, and of these the cause of failure was disproportion in no less than 40 per cent, of which 7 cases had outlet contraction. In 1928 he published a series of 558 cases of failed forceps collected from Edinburgh, Glasgow and Manchester. The causes were listed as follows:

Disproportion with flat pelvis predominating	221	(outlet contraction 14)
Constriction ring	6	
Occipito-posterior positions . . .	161	
Face presentation	12	(5 persistent mento-posterior)
Brow presentation	8	
Hydrocephalus	8	
Breech	2	
Shoulder	2	
Ovarian tumour	2	
Locked twins		

Furthermore, in no less than 151 cases there was no evidence of disproportion and the head was in normal position, and it was probable that the failure was due to premature intervention originally.

A very different state of affairs was described many years later by Freeth (1950), who enumerated 100 cases of failed forceps between the years 1941–48 from the Birmingham Maternity Hospital. Three-quarters of these cases were primigravidæ, and persistent occipito-posterior position and transverse arrest of the head accounted for no less than 50 per cent, while the cervix was not fully dilated in 20 per cent. There were 5 cases of contracted outlet, 4 of hydrocephalus, and odd cases of face and brow presentation, constriction ring, ovarian cyst and septate vagina made up the remainder. Freeth also made the interesting observation that 29 per cent of the cases were apparently more than two weeks overdue.

The difference between Miller's figures and those of Freeth is very striking in the much smaller importance of disproportion as a cause in more modern times. It will be noted that in both series hydrocephalus was by no means a minor factor, and slight degrees of this abnormality constitute a serious pitfall. Without a previous X-ray, such a diagnosis is not always easy to make, especially when the characteristic separation of the sutures has been obliterated by the forces of labour. When a case is sent in from outside by a doctor, who has failed to deliver a patient with forceps, he usually attributes his difficulty to a contracted outlet, but in a significant majority of cases the patient, on being examined in hospital, is found either to be not fully dilated or to have a fœtus in a malrotated position. With regard to the former diagnosis I often suspect that the doctor outside has been unjustly blamed for applying the forceps before full dilatation of the cervix; sometimes the cervix, I am sure, shuts down after a failed attempt, much as a constriction ring may form. It is inconceivable that the doctor could have inserted the blades without accepting this hypothesis in cases where the cervix is found to be only half dilated or less.

We once received an interesting call from a general practitioner to take over a case of failed forceps and he explained on the telephone that this case was rather different inasmuch as the main difficulty had not been in putting the forceps on but in getting them off. On inquiry as to where the forceps were at the moment he replied that they were still inside the patient and that the patient was already in a waiting ambulance. He then requested, with some urgency, that we return his forceps after recovery, a point on which we quickly reassured him that this was indeed our invariable practice. A few minutes later, however, he rang again in a much more cheerful voice to state that he had had a brainwave and had given the patient an injection of 10 units intramuscularly of oxytocin and that the patient had promptly

delivered herself of baby, forceps and all. He apologised for having troubled us but stated with some satisfaction that he had got his forceps back.

There is a special type of failed forceps which is not uncommon in hospital practice and follows what has been apparently a successful manual rotation of the occiput. In these cases the head has escaped above the brim and has become deflexed. It is also less likely to re-enter the brim in the antero-posterior position unless the pelvis is of gynæcoid or anthropoid shape or of huge diameters, in which case it should not have been necessary to displace the head so far in the first place. When this accident occurs, a high forceps application is far more dangerous, and also less likely to succeed, than performing internal version forthwith, with its equally serious dangers of fœtal death and uterine rupture. The other alternative of proceeding straightway to Cæsarean section is better employed in the interests of the child.

Parry Jones (1952) summarised the causes of difficulty in forceps delivery under the headings of maternal and fœtal. He listed the maternal causes as follows:

1. Cervix not fully dilated.
2. Disproportion.
3. Generalised tonic contraction of the uterus.
4. Constriction ring.
5. Non-dilatability of the paravaginal tissues.

Fœtal causes he listed as follows:

1. Malposition.
2. Deflexion.
3. Large baby.
4. Shoulders impacted at the brim.

In spite of all these lists which various writers have produced, there is no doubt that premature intervention with forceps is responsible for a far larger number than the figures indicate. A patient is often diagnosed as being fully dilated because of her desire to bear down and because the cervix is not palpable on rectal examination or vaginal examination without an anæsthetic. This is common, particularly in occipito-posterior positions. Then, after two hours of ineffectual pushing, it is decided to apply the forceps because of failure of the head to advance. Now, at any time during this last two hours the patient may, in fact, have become fully dilated and the second stage has not lasted anything like as long as estimated. The result is that less moulding can have occurred and intervention is undertaken far sooner than one would have contemplated had the time of full dilatation not been mistaken. It is a

mistake to interest oneself in the duration of the second stage as measured by the clock, and a patient should be encouraged to use her best efforts only when the head is actually seen to be on the pelvic floor. In this way much premature maternal distress will be avoided and there will be fewer cases of unnecessary or too early application of the forceps, with resulting failure in a proportion of cases.

MORTALITY AND THE RISKS OF FAILED FORCEPS

Earlier reports, such as those of Miller and Feeney, show a thoroughly depressing mortality rate both for mothers and babies. The principal causes of death are shock, sepsis, uterine rupture and postpartum hæmorrhage, while the persistent ill-health which may follow cannot even be approximately assessed. Miller long ago reckoned that 50 per cent suffered from impaired health and quoted a maternal mortality of 10 per cent (54 cases), of which 37 died as the result of sepsis. In a different series he reported 17 deaths out of 88, a mortality of 19 per cent. Feeney (1947), in reporting 121 cases of failed forceps in Dublin, and adding a further 225 cases from the literature, found a maternal mortality of 11 per cent, but only the complicated cases were included in these figures, so that the maternal mortality was correspondingly exaggerated.

The institution of the Flying Squad and the more effective use of chemotherapy and antibiotics, together with the present availability of blood for transfusion, has enormously improved this depressing picture, and Freeth (1950) found a maternal mortality of 2 per cent. Cæsarean section after a failed forceps delivery is now nothing like so hazardous as formerly.

The improvement in fœtal mortality is nowhere near so satisfactory. In Miller's series fœtal mortality was 64 per cent and in Freeth's series in 1950 it was still as high as 34 per cent, excluding cases of hydrocephalus. Three major factors contribute towards these bad results both for mother and child. Firstly, the condition which originally caused the failure to deliver with the forceps, secondly, the repeated intervention to which the patients are inevitably subjected, with its attendant risks of sepsis and shock, and thirdly the need which is often present for the repeated induction of anæsthesia. In this last respect chloroform is especially dangerous, and even the pre-operative use of a 10 per cent glucose infusion does not provide adequate protection.

Undoubtedly a certain percentage of cases of failed forceps never needed the operation in the first place, and it is therefore interesting to review the outcome. Miller, for instance, reported that in 78 cases in the disproportion group, subsequent spontaneous delivery or low forceps delivery finally occurred, indicating that intervention, even

although there was disproportion, had been premature. In Freeth's cases 62 per cent were delivered with the forceps, no less than 17 per cent had a spontaneous delivery, 8 per cent had internal version and 6 per cent were delivered by Cæsarean section, while craniotomy and breech delivery made up the remainder. The lesson to be learned from all this is that one should never ignore or transgress the indications for forceps delivery nor flout the conditions which must be present before attempting it. To be wrong in the selection of one's cases is bad enough, and to fail, having put one's hand to the plough, only makes matters many times worse.

Trial of forceps, advisedly undertaken, however, comes into a completely different class. Here, one recognises all the difficulties in advance and has made due preparations for them. Such an operation must be undertaken on an operating table, in a properly equipped operating theatre with an anæsthetist in attendance. The decision to abandon the forceps and to proceed to Cæsarean section must not be regarded as a matter of "failed forceps" but as an enlightened step in recognition of the hazards, particularly to the baby, of persisting with vaginal delivery.

KIELLAND'S FORCEPS

This really wonderful instrument makes possible a true cephalic application, regardless of the station of the head, which is impossible with the usual long curved forceps types without prior rotation. The Kielland's forceps achieves this objective by interrupting the pelvic curve at the commencement of the shanks, which are bent backwards at a slight angle with the blades. The other important feature is the sliding lock which caters for varying degrees of asynclitism. The Scanzoni manœuvre in the case of the malrotated head is so crude by comparison with a rotation with Kielland's forceps that it does not really merit description.

Those who have once mastered the technique of using Kielland's forceps are enthusiastic, and most of the criticism comes from ignorant or prejudiced sources. The argument has even been advanced in one major undergraduate teaching hospital that Kielland's should never be used because the students might get the wrong idea and be encouraged later on to try using it themselves when they entered practice. If this argument had anything in it, students who were destined for general practice ought never to see a hysterectomy or any other major surgical procedure. This is not to deny the instrument is tricky and is not for the occasional obstetrician. House surgeons should be taught carefully how to handle it, preferably with local analgesia (see earlier), by seniors who are well practised, for, in inexperienced hands, there are undoubtedly pitfalls which

we will now review. This is an argument for learning to use the instrument correctly rather than for condemning it out of hand.

Risks of Kielland's Forceps

Because of the sliding and therefore unstable lock, considerable damage can be done to vagina and cervix and occasionally lower uterine segment if the blades are not correctly applied in the first place. Under these circumstances the points tend to rise away from the baby's head and, in the course of rotation, can lacerate the maternal tissues. The bladder may thus be injured and give rise to a vesico-vaginal fistula from direct laceration or from pressure necrosis. Spiral tears of the vagina are reported in addition to tears of the cervix, and the lower uterine segment can be ruptured especially in the classical method of applying the anterior blade. Parry Jones mentions other risks, which, however, are not peculiar to Kielland's, but may occur with any forceps delivery, for example, dislocation of a sacro-iliac joint, fracture of the terminal part of the sacrum, separation of the symphysis pubis and injury to the nerve trunks of the sacral plexus.

Risks to the baby are considerably reduced by the use of Kielland's forceps, because far less compression to the fœtal skull can be achieved across the fulcrum of the sliding lock than with the usual forceps. Moreover, the ability to obtain an accurate cephalic application enormously lessens the strain upon the tentorium cerebelli. Facial abrasions and depressed fractures of the skull are no more likely with this than with any other forceps. One risk, however, must be mentioned, and that is the trapping of the cord or possibly the baby's hand if the classical method of application of the anterior blade is used. Prolapse of the cord is regarded as one of the risks, but it is considerably less than with high upward displacement of the head in order to achieve manual rotation.

There is undoubtedly a tendency to cause more damage to the perineum with Kielland's forceps, mainly because of the angle of the shanks, but this can be minimised by an episiotomy which in any case should always be carried out in conjunction with Kielland's forceps delivery because the perineum is very liable to get in the way of the shanks and may prevent the proper application of the blades.

Method of applying Kielland's Forceps

It is best to perform episiotomy first since this facilitates the application of the blades. There are three methods—classical, wandering and direct. The classical method was mainly introduced for the high forceps operation with the head not properly engaged, and has now been largely discarded because of the modern abandonment of this operation. However, it merits description. The anterior blade is ap-

plied first between the baby's head and the symphysis pubis with the concavity of the cephalic curve directed upwards. In order to decide which of the blades is the anterior one it is a good rule to assemble the forceps in front of the patient before applying them, so as to obtain the correct orientation of the position which they will occupy once they have been inserted. Needless to say, in this assembly, the concavity of the pelvic curve is directed towards the child's occiput, whose position is already known following proper examination. The anterior blade is then slipped in "butter side upwards". It is essential to use only finger-light force, and no attempt must be made to rotate it butter side downwards until it has been pushed in far enough. It is not until the more or less rounded junction of blade and shank is lying between the baby's head and the symphysis that it will be safe or even possible, without force, to rotate it (Fig. 11).

KIELLAND CLASSICAL METHOD

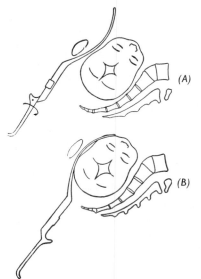

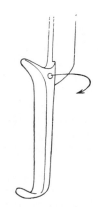

18/Fig. 11 (a).—The position of the blade before rotation (A); the position of the blade after rotation (B).

18/Fig. 11 (b).—The direction knob lies on the same side as the pelvic curve. Rotation of the blade is carried out towards the same side.

When the blade has been pushed in far enough, it will be found that the shank is pressing against the posterior vaginal wall. With very gentle and careful manipulation the blade is now turned through 180° on its long axis, so that the pelvic concavity is turned against the convexity of the fœtal skull, and to make matters simpler

there is a small knob on the handles which points in the direction in which the blade should be turned. Some difficulty may be encountered in this manœuvre, the commonest being due to the tight application of the fœtal head against the top of the symphysis pubis. Now it goes without saying that unless a finger can be inserted between the head and the symphysis pubis, a blind attempt to force the forceps blade in this area is not justified and another method of application is to be preferred. The higher the head, however, the less likely is this difficulty to operate and the more applicable the classical method.

Another common cause of failure is that the blade has not been inserted far enough, in which case the fault will be advertised by the fact that the handle instead of sloping downwards towards the perineum is more horizontal than it should be.

Occasionally a constriction ring may prevent the insertion and proper rotation of the blade, and lastly the child's anterior shoulder may get in the way. If difficulty is encountered, force must on no account be used to overcome it, but as a rule it is surprising how easily the blade slips round. It is at this point that there is always the chance that a loop of cord may get caught as the blade is pulled back home to engage upon the head.

With the head in the transverse position and the blade correctly applied, the handle should be sloping somewhat downwards and a little to the side of the midline on the opposite side to the baby's occiput. If an assistant can now steady it at this point so much the better. The posterior blade is now applied, and in many ways it is the more difficult of the two, because the point of the blade often bumps up against the sacrum and it appears impossible to negotiate the sacral promontory. The secret is not to use more force, but to depress the handle which is usually being prevented by the perineum. It is this fact which makes an initial episiotomy so valuable in order to assist one in drawing the perineum backward and out of the way. If, in spite of drawing the perineum well back and depressing the handle, the obstruction of the sacrum is still felt against the tip of the blade, more room may be found slightly to one or other side of the midline.

The wandering method is the one most generally applicable. It is usually recommended that the anterior blade be applied first, but this is optional, and personally I prefer to start with the posterior blade. The same technique with the posterior blade is followed, but in this case it is easier because the other blade is not now taking up room nor is it in the way. Again, it is a common mistake not to slide the blade in far enough. When correctly applied (and it is a good plan to aim for the baby's ear), the handle is sloping somewhat downwards towards the floor and a little towards the opposite side to which

the occiput lies. The anterior blade is now applied laterally directly over the baby's face guided by two fingers. By very careful manipulation of the handle and with two guiding fingers, the blade is gently "jilled" through a quarter of a circle around the periphery of the pelvic cavity, until it matches up with the posterior blade (Fig. 12). Carried out this way it will now be found, in the case of the right occipito-lateral position, that the handles will have to be crossed on each other for the locks to meet, but this can always be easily and gently done. With the occiput to the left the handles do not have to be crossed over. As the locks engage the shanks should, of course, be in line with each other, and it will now be noticed that one blade is farther in than the other. In other words, the head is nearly always in a position of some degree of asynclitism. This is gently corrected by the sliding lock.

The direct method of application is used when the head is very low or very small, since there is not enough room otherwise to apply both blades directly without one of the above manœuvres.

Above all, always remember to keep the handles well down. Failure to observe this is responsible for more difficulties with Kielland's forceps than any other fault.

Rotation of the Head

Having corrected any asynclitism with the help of the sliding lock, the mobility of the head within the pelvis is cautiously assessed with the forceps and a gentle attempt is made to rotate it. Only finger force should be used. If it appears that the head cannot be rotated in its present position, it is a good plan to draw the head down a little in the uncorrected position and to try again, and if this fails to push it up slightly and repeat the attempt at a slightly higher level. In this manner, by carefully feeling one's way and always keeping the handles well down, the safest level at which to rotate the head can be determined, the safest being that at which least force is necessary. The sense of control of the head has to be experienced to be believed. Lastly, it is a wise precaution to desist from attempts to rotate the head while a contraction is in force.

Traction with Kielland's Forceps

The direction of pull is largely determined by the direction in which the handles are pointing. This is somewhat downwards (more so than with ordinary forceps) until the occiput appears behind the symphysis. On no account must the handles be raised, even so far as the horizontal, until this point is reached. At no time do the handles rise so high as in the case of the ordinary long curved forceps.

As soon as the now rotated head is pulled well down on to the pelvic floor, a light low forceps of the Wrigley pattern may be

applied in the place of the Kielland forceps, in order to spare the perineum additional damage, but this is a refinement which is hardly necessary, and with care in the direction of pull at the outlet the operation can be completed with Kielland forceps with great finesse.

There can be few operations in all midwifery so satisfying as a correctly performed delivery with the Kielland forceps, especially under local analgesia only. See Figs. 13–19.

BONY CONTRACTION OF THE PELVIC OUTLET

Sometimes contraction of the outlet is not discovered until in the course of a forceps operation. This is a regrettable but nevertheless occasional fact. The subject is dealt with more fully in the chapter on disproportion, but we must consider here the steps to be taken when, having applied the forceps, it is clear that a serious degree of bony obstruction exists.

There are three alternatives now before us: the most commonly practised is to deliver the child with forceps by brute force. This is highly deplorable. It has been said that in practically every case the head that will pass through the brim can be got through the outlet. True, but at a fearful price sometimes which is borne both by mother and baby. It is in these cases that symphysiotomy comes into its own. The operation is not difficult and makes a tremendous difference to outlet difficulties. Few people in their senses, who had foreknowledge of outlet contraction, would plan to deliver the case by forceps and symphysiotomy as an elective decision, and Cæsarean section would be preferred.

The third alternative is to remove the forceps and proceed to Cæsarean section forthwith. Craniotomy is only to be considered if the baby is unquestionably dead. There is no doubt that either Cæsarean section or symphysiotomy is vastly preferable to the first method of brute force, in which not only may the child be seriously damaged or killed, but the mother's sacro-iliac joints may be dislocated, her bladder and its supports traumatised, and her pelvic floor damaged beyond reasonable hope of adequate repair.

SYMPHYSIOTOMY

This is an operation which has never been popular in this country nor in the United States. It is by no means new, and has had brief vogue from time to time during the last few hundred years. The alternative of pubiotomy has been if anything consistently less popular. Much of the unpopularity of these operations has been earned through faulty selection of cases. As a method of treatment of brim disproportion it is quite unsuitable, and its only indications

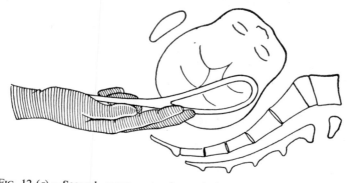

18/Fig. 12 (*a*).—Second movement of wandering. The internal fingers rest behind the fenestration, ready to push the blade anteriorly.

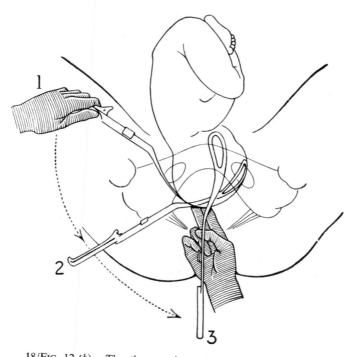

18/Fig. 12 (*b*).—The three main movements of wandering.

(Figs. 11 and 12 from *Kielland's Forceps* by courtesy of Dr. E. Parry Jones and Butterworth & Co.)

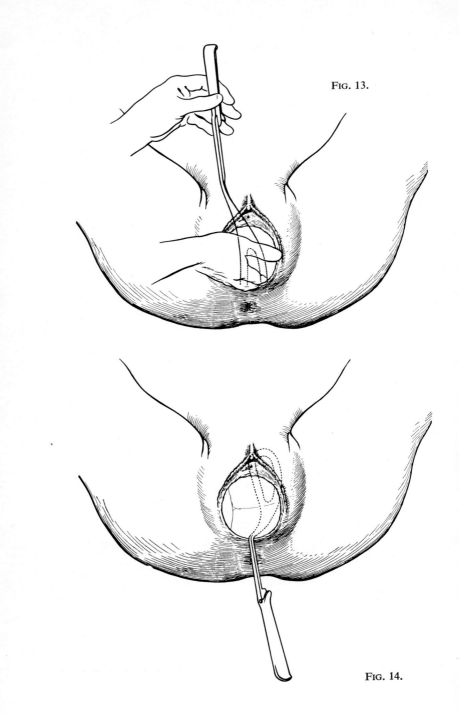

FIG. 13.

FIG. 14.

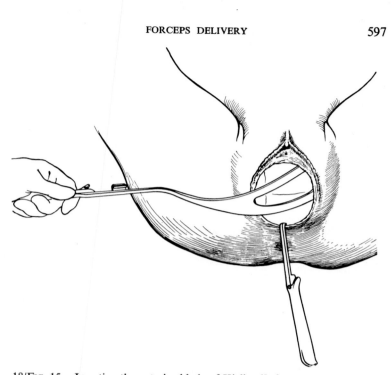

18/FIG. 15.—Inserting the anterior blade of Kielland's forceps over the face.

are in cases of outlet disproportion late in labour or in the case of immovable malposition of a deeply placed fœtal head. The cases, therefore, for which it is considered are usually those of android, funnel-shaped pelvis.

In primitive communities, as Seedat and Crichton (1962) have shown, there is still a place for symphysiotomy since many patients disappear into the bush and insist on being delivered at home next time and the theory is that a patient who has had a symphysiotomy will fare better and more safely in a subsequent delivery than one who has had a previous Cæsarean section. From the point of view of uterine rupture and catastrophic death a long distance from medical aid this may be true, but in other respects the matter may be regarded as open to some argument. A further reason given is that the high infant mortality rate makes repeated delivery by Cæsarean

18/FIG. 13 (*see opposite*).—Applying the posterior blade of Kielland's forceps in a case of transverse arrest with the occiput to the right.

18/FIG. 14 (*see opposite*).—The posterior blade of Kielland's forceps when properly placed points the handle somewhat downwards and laterally.

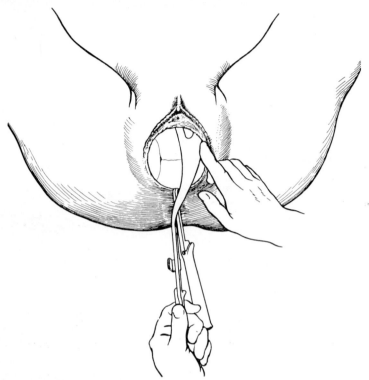

18/FIG. 16.—"Wandering" the anterior blade into position. Note how the handles will have to be crossed over in R.O.T. positions for the lock to engage.

section hardly worth while. This too is debatable by civilised standards, but Seedat and Crichton had a large series of 505 cases in Bantu women without maternal mortality and with only ambulatory difficulties in 16 cases and stress incontinence in a further 5, a truly remarkable record. In the following year (Crichton and Seedat, 1963) they published details of 1200 cases in Natal with 4 instances of vesico-vaginal fistula and 12 of vestibular together with sometimes urethral tears, all of which were successfully repaired and for which the antecedent pressure necrosis was more of a factor than the operation itself. The situation is very similar in Nigeria where symphysiotomy is commonly employed in the management of disproportion.[5] Since so large a proportion of the world's population live under conditions which these workers describe it would be wrong for those of us who practise in more fortunate communities to dismiss the importance of this operation.

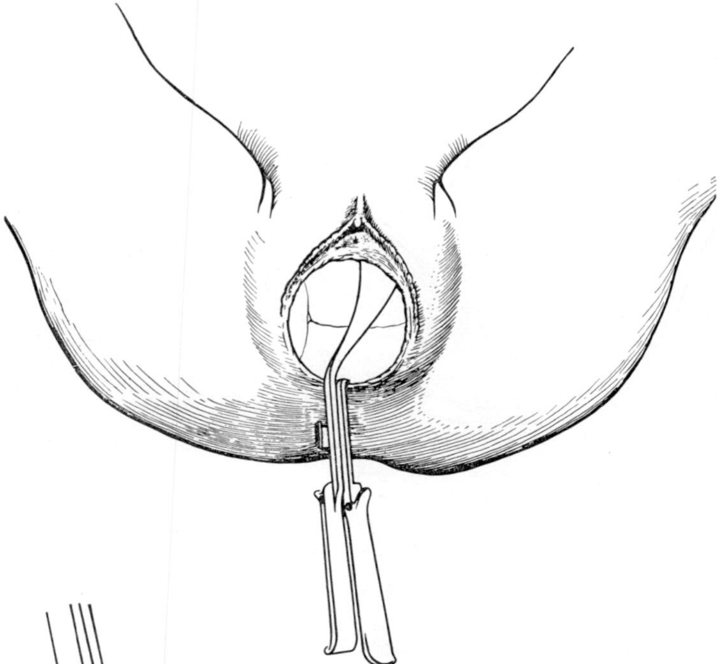

18/Fig. 17 (*above*).—The Kielland's forceps immediately after application and before correction of asynclitism. Note the position of the handles, sloping somewhat downwards and laterally to the side away from the occiput.

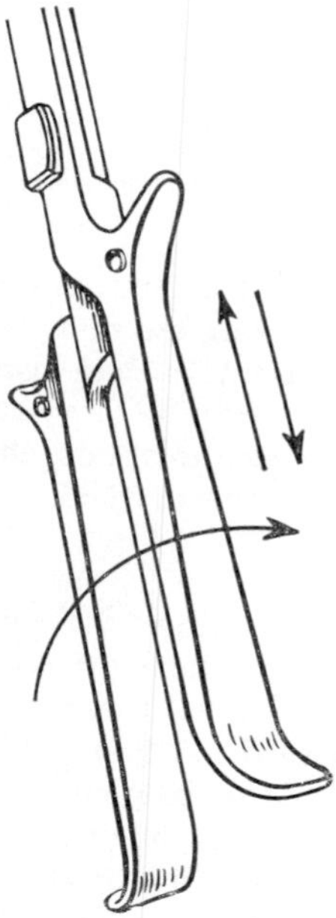

18/Fig. 18.—Correcting asynclitism and rotating from occipito-transverse to occipito-anterior position.

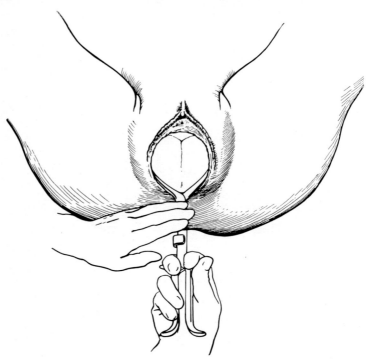

18/FIG. 19.—Traction and Pajot's manœuvre applied to the Kielland's forceps.

Pubiotomy is usually performed by inserting a Gigli saw behind the pubis to one side of the midline and severing the bone. It is on the whole a more traumatic and vascular procedure than symphysiotomy.

Technique of symphysiotomy.—There are two methods, the open and the closed, the latter being the more usually described, although the former has had a vogue in Dublin.

In the closed method a subcutaneous approach is made with a long solid scalpel, the incision being placed just above the symphysis pubis. The blade of the knife is then inserted on the flat close against the front of the symphysis pubis and then turned through a right angle so that the cutting edge faces backwards. A finger is kept in the vagina so as to get a better idea of what is happening and the symphysis is divided from before backwards through the greater part, but not all, of its thickness. The legs are removed from the lithotomy poles and held by assistants who, by pressing on the trochanters and abducting the thighs, produce a distractive force which

slowly tears the remaining fibres of the posterior part of the symphysis pubis. The finger in the vagina is able to appreciate this, and a separation of no more than 1 inch to $1\frac{1}{2}$ inches is allowed. The transverse diameters of the outlet are immediately increased and thereafter delivery is facilitated.

It is a good plan always to insert a fairly stiff catheter into the bladder before starting the operation and to use the finger in the vagina to displace both the urethra and the bladder neck laterally well to one side of the symphysis before cutting it. An alternative to the above closed method is to work from behind forwards and from above downwards, introducing the knife behind the symphysis pubis at its upper border and keeping strictly to the midline. Probing with a needle may occasionally be necessary to identify the joint. Unless spontaneous delivery follows quickly it is becoming increasingly common now to complete the delivery with the Ventouse.

The open method is favoured by Barry in Dublin. Here the mons is incised vertically in the midline, bleeding points are secured and the front of the symphysis pubis is exposed to direct vision. The linea alba is incised, and a finger is inserted from above behind the symphysis pubis together with a narrow-bladed scalpel whose cutting edge is directed forwards so that the symphysis is severed from behind forwards. The same precautions are taken about holding the legs and controlling the amount of separation achieved. The operation tends to convert the dimensions of the outlet into a transverse oval, so that if Kielland's forceps is now applied to a transversely arrested head, it is often better to extract it in the unreduced position.

Fibrous union always occurs and the pelvic girdle nearly always regains its former stability, so that locomotion is not interfered with. During the puerperium the pelvis is supported by strapping or binders and the legs are usually bandaged together, but for the first few days there is often considerable œdema which may provide some nursing trouble, especially in catheterisation. The patients seem to suffer remarkably little pain.

It is true that the bladder or its supports may be injured in such cases, but this is not the direct result of operative technique, more often being due to the delivery which follows after the protective bony arch supporting the bladder has been robbed of its supporting properties as a result of severance. At the completion of the operation a large speculum is inserted and a very careful search made for any signs of splitting or tearing of the anterior vaginal wall. It goes without saying, therefore, that the manipulation with the forceps after symphysiotomy must be carried out with extra care. One of the very great advantages of symphysiotomy is that the pelvis remains permanently enlarged, so that subsequent deliveries are likely to be much easier. In a city like Dublin, where high degrees of parity are common,

this is a factor of some importance, as it helps to eliminate the need for repetitive Cæsarean section with all its penalties.

In Figs. 20a, b and c will be seen pelvimetry radiographs taken before and after symphysiotomy in a case which Barry demonstrated personally to me on a visit to Dublin. Although there is a small permanent increase in the transverse measurements, much of the benefit likely to appear in subsequent labours will be due to the ease with which the symphysis pubis will "open up" for the occasion.

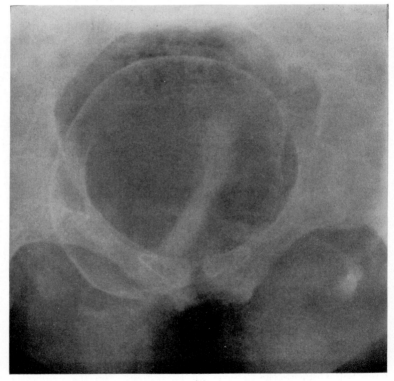

(a)

18/Fig. 20.

(a) Contracted pelvis before symphysiotomy. True conjugate 10·8 cm. Transverse 11·5 cm.

(b) (opposite). Outlet view before symphysiotomy.

(c) (opposite). Same case after symphysiotomy and delivery of healthy baby weighing 7 lb. 12 oz. delivered in the unreduced transverse position with Kielland's forceps. Transverse diameter 11·8 cm. Separation at symphysis pubis 1·6 cm.

(Figs. a, b and c by courtesy of Dr. A. P. Barry.)

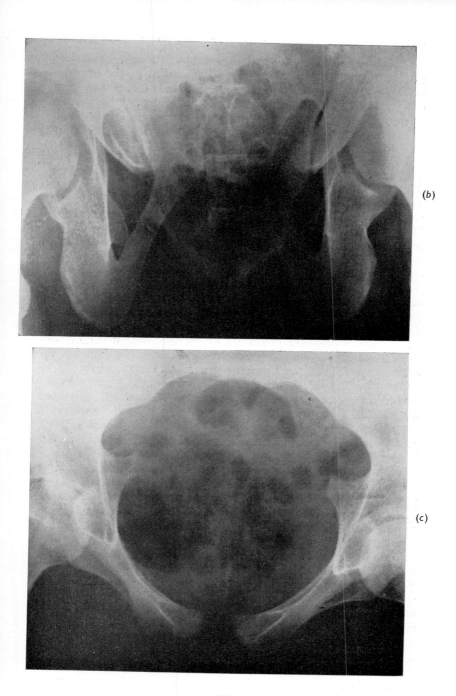

(b)

(c)

On this side of the Irish Sea, however, obstetricians are inclined to prefer repeated Cæsarean section for contracted pelvis, since they prefer to inflict a soft tissue injury on abdominal wall and uterus than a skeletal injury on the pelvic girdle, a prejudice perhaps but a natural one!

THE VENTOUSE (Vacuum Extractor)

The idea of delivering a baby's head with the aid of suction is by no means new but it is generally accepted that Sir James Young Simpson in Edinburgh was the first to produce an apparatus which actually worked and successfully achieved delivery. Malmström's modern vacuum extractor differs only in detail and refinement from Simpson's suction tractor of 1849, of which Simpson produced a number of variants. The idea had doubtless arisen from the old practice of cupping. Chalmers (1963) in his historical review recounts the pithy phrase of Neil Arnott, another Scot, who envisaged such a machine and observed that the tractor seemed "peculiarly adapted to a purpose of obstetric surgery, namely as a substitute for steel forceps in the hands of men who are deficient in manual dexterity whether from inexperience or natural ineptitude." Such an attitude of prejudice reinforced by the less efficient materials of the last century have possibly been responsible for the delay of over a century before the true merits of vacuum extraction came to be accepted in Europe. Interest certainly waned in the method until Malmström, with very much better design and materials, produced the present Ventouse which is now gaining a much more rapid acceptance. The most violent criticism of the Ventouse nearly always comes from people who have the least experience in using it, commonly none at all.

Simpson's cup with its incorporated piston and barrel must have been difficult to apply to a head not well down in the pelvis and was probably ineffective for pulls of more than a few kilograms, but the Malmström cup (Fig. 21) does not rely upon leather or rubber contact with the scalp but from the interesting shape of the metal cup and its flange which, following on the gentle building up of the vacuum by means of a very well made pump, allows the skin of the scalp and the induced caput succedaneum to "unfold" inside the cavity of the cup practically obliterating the potential space within it and forming the well-recognised "chignon" (Fig. 22). This secures an extremely satisfactory and atraumatic grip of the scalp without affecting the underlying structures of skull bones and brain.

Malmström's modern instrument has gained popularity throughout Western Europe and, in fact, in Professor Snoeck's department in Brussels, which I visited in 1961, I observed that this instrument had completely replaced the obstetric forceps since 1958, without any

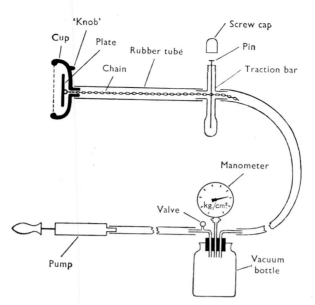

'Knob'

Cup

Plate

Chain

Rubber tube

Screw cap

Pin

Traction bar

Manometer

Valve

kg./cm².

Pump

Vacuum bottle

18/FIG. 21.—The Malmström cup.

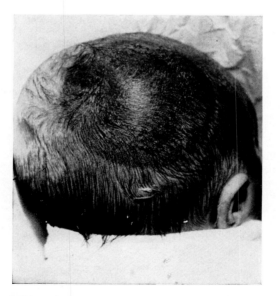

18/FIG. 22.—"Chignon" caused by the Ventouse. It has usually disappeared within a few hours and leaves a discoloured mark which fades within a week.

(By courtesy of Dr. R. J. Fothergill, Dr. J. A. Chalmers and the Editor, *Practitioner*.)

increase in the Cæsarean section rate. It was first taken up in this country on a large scale by Chalmers and Fothergill (1960) who reported very favourably upon it in a series of 100 cases, and since then have gone from strength to strength, with a progressive incidence of vacuum extraction and fall in overall fœtal mortality.[4]

Glasgow Royal Maternity Hospital. First 132 cases

TABLE VIII

ANÆSTHESIA FOR VACUUM EXTRACTOR

General anæsthetic	.	.	.	15 (11·4%)
Pudendal block	.	.	.	102 (77·3%)
Local infiltration of perineum	.	.	8 (6·1%)
Inhalational analgesia	.	.	.	4 (3·0%)
No anæsthetic	.	.	.	3 (2·2%)

132

TABLE IX

FAILURES WITH VACUUM EXTRACTOR

Total 26 (19·7%)

Delivered by Cæsarean section	.	.	.	2
Delivered by Forceps	.	.	.	24

V.E. produced full dilatation of cervix in	.	7
Failure due to faulty technique in	.	.	9
Failure due to unsuitable case in	.	.	10

TABLE X

INDICATIONS FOR VACUUM EXTRACTOR

Prolonged first stage	15 (11·4%)
Fœtal distress in first stage . . .	15 (11·4%)
Accidental hæmorrhage in first stage .	1 (0·75%)
Prolonged second stage . .	65 (49·2%)
Fœtal distress in second stage .	20 (15·1%)
Severe pre-eclampsia in second stage .	4 (3·0%)
Cardiac disease in second stage .	6 (4·5%)
Brow presentation in second stage .	1 (0·75%)
Brow and prolapsed cord in second stage	1 (0·75%)
Compound presentation (hand and head) in second stage	1 (0·75%)
Breech presentation in second stage .	1 (0·75%)
Twins in second stage . . .	2 (1·5%)

132

We, ourselves, have now acquired a considerable experience with it and our present use amounts to about 20 per cent of instrumental deliveries. Naturally the most comprehensive evaluation of indications and results comes from Sweden—its country of origin.[27]

Description of instrument.—A self-explanatory diagram is shown in Fig. 21. The most important part, of course, is the interestingly shaped cup already mentioned. Traction on this is achieved not through the rubber tubing which maintains the vacuum, but through a plate attached inside the cup to a chain that lies inside the lumen of the tubing and is fixed by a pin which is part of the assembly of the traction bar. A suction bottle with accurate vacuum gauge and a very well made pump, together with a bracket for hanging on the side of the bed, complete this fundamentally simple equipment. There is also an efficient vacuum release valve. Vacuum pressures are recorded in kilograms per square centimetre, a designation which my much-forgotten arithmetic is incapable of translating into pounds per square inch, millimetres of mercury, or any of the better-recognised terms of measurement. Below is a table designed to provide an idea of the suction used.

PRESSURE CONVERSION TABLE

Kg./cm.^{2}	lb./in.^{2}	mm. Hg
0·1	1·422	73·56
0·2	2·844	147·11
0·3	4·266	220·67
0·4	5·688	294·22
0·5	7·110	367·78
0·6	8·532	441·34
0·7	9·954	514·89
0·8	11·376	588·45
0·9	12·798	662·00
1·0	14·220	735·56

Technique of use.—There are certain rules which should be followed if the best results are to be obtained. The first of these is to use the largest possible cup. There are four sizes and if the cervix is fully dilated, or anywhere near so, the largest cup can nearly always be applied. If the head is already bulging the perineum, local infiltration only with 1 per cent lignocaine will suffice, but usually we employ pudendal block the technique of which has been described earlier. General anæsthesia may be used but, on the whole, it is not favoured because the function of the Ventouse is simply to lead the head out with the help of the patient's own expulsive efforts and her active co-operation is much to be desired. I would liken the operation to leading a horse through a gate; one steers the animal out by its ead but the major propulsive power is supplied by its own muscles.

This differs very much from the principle of forceps delivery under general anæsthesia, where much greater tractive efforts have to be applied.

Having induced pudendal nerve block the perineum is retracted with two fingers of one hand and the cup inserted with the knob, for reference, pointing towards the baby's occiput. The cup is pressed up against the baby's scalp and it is said to be best if it can be placed as near to the lambda as possible, but my own practice is to apply it to the most dependant and accessible part of the scalp, even over the parietal eminence in cases of transverse arrest of the head. This can be quite useful as will be seen later. One should at this stage ascertain, as far as possible, that no vagina or cervix has been included within the rim of the cup and an assistant is now asked to work the pump for a few strokes until a vacuum of 0·2 kilograms per square centimetre is registered on the gauge. Now is the time to make a proper check to ensure that no cervix or vagina has been included because there is just enough suction to maintain the cup in position. It is surprising how easy it is to include a bit of cervix and I have done so twice. Very careful palpation right round the rim of the cup is necessary to exclude this. If cervix or vagina is included in the cup it is difficult to achieve a stable vacuum and a hissing leak will almost at once be heard when traction is applied; also no advance whatever will occur, so the mistake will be very readily recognised on further examination or on the cup pulling off. The crescent of included cervix looks a little dusky as a result of being included but I have not seen any harm result from it. With the cup properly applied the longer one can take in building up the vacuum the more satisfactory will the artificial caput inside the cup become. If one is in a great hurry, because of fœtal distress for example, the vacuum can be built up in two or three minutes, but a much less satisfactory grip of the head is obtained and with all the patience in the world we prefer to spend at least eight minutes in building up the vacuum of 0·8 kilograms per square centimetre, which is what we usually employ. During this period the patient can be kept in intelligent conversation and full time is allowed for the pudendal block to take effect.

I have deliberately sought to measure the traction forces which can be applied before the cup pulls off the scalp. For this purpose I waited, and had to wait a long time, for a fresh stillbirth which occurred in a case of hyrdops late one Saturday afternoon. I hurriedly made in my workshop a sort of miniature lavatory seat to fit the baby's head exactly, wedged the head into this "brim" and applied the Ventouse in the standard manner. I then rigged the whole thing up in the mortuary so that weights could be applied directly to the Ventouse in increasing amounts and at 23 lb. the vacuum broke and the cup came

off. This is a very much smaller force than is usually applied with forceps as has been described earlier and constitutes one of the great safety factors in this operation.

As soon as the vacuum has been built up properly traction can begin, preferably synchronously with a uterine contraction, although as soon as pulling starts, of course, the uterus contracts in sympathy. Malmström recommended and indeed it is the usual practice to pull at right angles to the plane of the cup, but in order to do this the perineum has to be pulled well back with two fingers of the other hand in the vagina, but I have found it useful, especially in cases of malrotated head, to pull in different directions about 10 degrees off this perpendicular axis, watching the cup and any of the head that is visible to see if movement or rocking or any type of rotation looks like taking place. It will be appreciated that in cases of transverse arrest of the head the cup, if applied to the most dependant and accessible part of the scalp, may be over the anterior parietal eminence, or partly so, in which case the slight pulling off axis may swing the head most impressively and rotate it into the occipito-anterior position. Sometimes this does not occur until the head has come further down on the pelvic floor, but this technique demonstrates most beautifully the mechanics of spontaneous labour which has simply failed because the expulsive efforts of the uterus and patient have been inadequate hitherto to achieve what the assistance of the Ventouse now brings about so easily. It is certainly most interesting to see an occipito-posterior rotate with the help of the Ventouse almost spontaneously under the influence of the gutter mechanism of the pelvic floor. This operation involves no displacement of the head and is the nearest thing to physiological normal delivery that can be achieved. The forceps, after all, tends to fix and determine the position of the head at the will of the operator. The Ventouse allows the head to come the way it wants to, even sometimes face to pubis, and this is one of the most delightful features of the operation.

The warning hiss that the vacuum is about to break and the cup come off can usually be taken as an indication either that one is pulling too hard (and to one who has been used to forceps it takes a lot of discipline to restrict one's tractive efforts to what is suitable for the Ventouse), or else it is because maternal soft parts have been included within the rim, thus calling for re-examination. If the cup does come off no great harm is done. One of my patient's commented, "What was that?" The cup can be immediately reapplied over the same chignon as before, but it is a bad thing to do so more than once and one should consider alternative methods of delivery. There is a temptation to use the cup for screwing the head round, but this is not to be recommended as it tends to abrade the scalp. Less than half a dozen pulls with contractions will indicate the likeli-

hood of success and one should be able to have a fair idea within twenty minutes whether to persist or not.

Our own failure rate, Table IX, was depressingly high at first. The 132 cases quoted in these tables date to the beginning of 1963, since when, of course, our experience has considerably enlarged. Unfamiliarity with the instrument was mainly responsible and, to some extent, bad selection of cases.

The direction of pull is largely determined by what looks most rewarding and since adopting this principle the success rate has improved enormously.

The vacuum is released as soon as the head is crowned and delivery is then completed in the normal way. The indications for the use of the Ventouse are listed in Table X. The great indication, of course, is for the hypotonic case in the absence of mechanical disproportion who hangs fire at about four fingers dilatation. We do not like applying the instrument at less than this degree of dilatation, not only because it is more difficult but for fear of damaging the cervix, although others are more bold in this respect. To deliver a woman within half an hour, after many days of tedious and unrewarding labour, is a very satisfying experience and much to be preferred to Cæsarean section or forceps. Willocks (1962) who, in my department, has used the apparatus more extensively than any of us, has listed the following major indications:

1. To deliver some cases of fœtal distress occuring late in the first stage of labour.

2. To complete delivery in some cases of uterine inertia late in the first stage.

3. As an alternative to trial of forceps in some multiparæ in whom second-stage delay is associated with deflexion and malposition of the fœtal head at the pelvic brim or high in the pelvic cavity.

4. To rotate and deliver the head in many cases of occipito-transverse and posterior positions.

He also adds that the Ventouse may be used instead of forceps in the second stage and I agree that it makes a very pleasant alternative to the simple low forceps operation. I had the gratifying experience of delivering one of my own staff midwives with the Ventouse after an hour and a half of profitless second staging and her comment after delivery was, "I am so glad I managed it all myself". She did not even know at the time that she had been delivered with the Ventouse. I wonder if one could say the same even for the easiest of low forceps operations and I felt this was tribute indeed to the gentleness of the method.

One talks of trial of forceps with all preparations in the foreground rather than in the background for Cæsarean section if the trial fails. The same principle can be applied, particularly before full dilata-

tion, in the case of the Ventouse and we call it the "Ventouse Cæsarean section sequence". In actual fact, as our tables show, the Ventouse nearly always succeeds and the need for Cæsarean section does not, therefore, arise, but one of my colleagues in Glasgow has referred to it in derisory terms as "the suck it and see". I would agree however with the statement[10] that every high vacuum extraction must initially be regarded more or less as a trial of Ventouse, which, if failure occurs, should be followed immediately by Cæsarean section. There is a natural temptation to follow a failed vacuum extraction, with suspected disproportion, by the application of forceps, but if these two fail, the baby and the mother are now in poor shape and whenever I have gone through the whole miserable sequence of failed Ventouse, failed forceps, and ultimate Cæsarean section I have much regretted not having gone straight to section without an intervening attempt at forceps. The cumulative effect of all three methods is something which I do not wish to encounter again.

Hazards.—The literature is already replete with grisly accounts of sloughing scalps, intracranial hæmorrhages, cephalhæmatomata, depressed fractures of the skull, death and destruction, which accord ill with our own experience and that of colleagues of mine in other centres who have acquired a proper experience of the instrument. All this has helped to fan the prejudice of reactionary obstetricians, some of whom have argued fiercely with me and with apparent intelligence and then finally confessed that they had never even seen the instrument used or had certainly not attempted to use it themselves. Tradition dies hard and midwives of both sexes are often remarkable for their conservatism. Huntingford (1961) produced a very depressing account but on an extremely small series of cases and by our standards would appear to have made much more prolonged and possibly determined efforts to deliver than we would have attempted. Our own rule is to review the suitability of the case for delivery by this method if success does not appear to be likely within twenty minutes and certainly the delivery must be completed within about forty-five minutes of the application of the cup. Otherwise one is obviously asking for trouble. Nowadays one would think very seriously before tugging away at a baby's head with forceps for more than three-quarters of an hour and might be justified in considering Cæsarean section as a less traumatic method of delivery, particularly from the baby's point of view, and the same philosophy should apply to the Ventouse. We do not now talk about brute force in obstetrics but we still practice "brute forceps". Fortunately one cannot employ force with the Ventouse because it simply pulls adrift from the scalp. Theoretical objections have been raised that the vacuum applied to the scalp increases the incidence of intracranial hæmorrhage, by what mechanism is not clear. Snoeck, in fact, worked out that intra-

cranial stress and the risk of hæmorrhage were much less with vacuum extraction than with forceps delivery. After all this is simply a form of skin traction as employed in orthopædic surgery and the point of application of force is at the point of attachment of the scalp in the region of the base of the skull.

We have become much interested in the occasional phenomenon of scalp hæmatoma which may be so serious as to require neonatal blood transfusion and at the time of writing have found in all three such cases that there was an association of hypoprothrombinæmia in the baby. Willoughby, our hæmatologist, reckons that the thrombotest is very low in 10 per cent of all babies, but that no harm results from this unless some hæmostatic insult is inflicted, in this case, the Ventouse. We therefore do thrombotest examinations on all cases of Ventouse delivery except those at very inconvenient hours of the night when we give vitamin K_1 prophylactically (5 mg.) and, of course, in cases of recognised hypoprothrombinæmia.

Our own perinatal mortality in the first 132 cases is 3 per cent and corrected for intra-uterine death, gross prematurity and fœtal abnormality the figure works out at 0·9 per cent, which can hardly justify condemning the operation as a lethal procedure. Lange (1961) in Denmark has compared a series of 480 cases of vacuum extraction delivery with 376 cases of forceps delivery and has concluded that the former involves less danger for the mother and infant than forceps, with a perinatal mortality of about half. He, too, considers the method more physiological.

Reference has already been made to the use of the Ventouse to complete delivery after symphysiotomy. The African pelvis is very shallow compared with the European and it is not uncommon for part of the head and caput succedanium to be visible at the vulva, with the biparietal diameter still nowhere near negotiating the pelvic brim. I am much impressed with the combined effects of symphysiotomy and Ventouse extraction from witnessing the procedure in Uganda, carried out under local anæsthesia with the whole matter finished and done with within a quarter of an hour. Since about a quarter of instances of uterine rupture in underdeveloped countries are in previous uterine Cæsarean scars, this would appear to be a thoroughly worth-while alternative in treatment.[14]

As might be expected, those who have used the instrument most are the most enthusiastic and even allowing for slight admixture of cause and effect I think the advent of the Ventouse should be regarded as a major advance in operative obstetrics. Delivery can be achieved with extreme gentleness and finesse and with a minimum of anæsthesia.

Let us never forget there is no such thing as a minor anæsthetic.

REFERENCES

1. BARRY, A. P. (1952). Personal communication.
2. CHALMERS, J. A. (1963). *J. Obstet. Gynaec. Brit. Cwlth.*, **70**, 94.
3. CHALMERS, J. A., and FOTHERGILL, R. J. (1960). *Brit. med. J.*, **1**, 1684.
4. CHALMERS, J. A. (1964). *Brit. med. J.*, **1**, 1216.
5. COX, M. L. (1966). *J. Obstet. Gynaec. Brit. Cwlth.*, **73**, 237.
6. COXON, A. (1961). *J. Obstet. Gynaec. Brit. Cwlth.*, **68**, 934.
7. CRICHTON, D., and SEEDAT, E. K. (1963). *S. Afr. med. J.*, **37**, 227.
8. EGBERT, E. S., KEETTEL, W. C., and LEE, J. G. (1960). *J. Iowa St. med. Soc.*, Aug., 499.
9. FEENEY, J. K. (1947). *Irish J. med. Sci.*, **1**, 190.
10. FJÄLLBRANT, B. (1964). *Gynécologie*, **157**, 161.
11. FOTHERGILL, R. J., and CHALMERS, J. A. (1961). *Practitioner*, **186**, 559.
12. FREETH, D. H. (1950). *Brit. med. J.*, **2**, 18.
13. GATE, J. M., and DUTTON, W. A. W. (1955). *Brit. med. J.*, **2**, 99.
14. GEBBIE, D. A. M. (1966). *Brit. med. J.*, **2**, 1490.
15. HAUSMANN, W., and LUNT, R. L. (1955). *J. Obstet. Gynaec. Brit. Emp.*, **62**, 509.
16. HOLMES, J. M. (1956). *J. Obstet. Gynaec. Brit. Emp.*, **63**, 239.
17. HUNTINGFORD, P. J. (1961). *Lancet*, **2**, 1054.
18. HUNTINGFORD, P. J. (1959). *J. Obstet. Gynaec. Brit. Emp.*, **62**, 26.
19. JONES, E. P. (1952). *Kielland's Forceps*. London: Butterworth & Co.
20. KERR, J. M. M., and MOIR, J. C. (1956). *Operative Obstetrics*, 6th edit. London: Baillière, Tindall & Cox.
21. KOBAK, A. J., EVANS, E. F., and JOHNSON, E. R. (1956). *Amer. J. Obstet. Gynec.*, **71**, 981.
22. LANGE, P. (1961). *Dan. med. Bull.*, **8**, 11.
23. McDANIEL, E. B. (1963). Personal communication.
24. MacGREGOR, W. G. (1966). *Lancet*, **1**, 147.
25. MALMSTRÖM, T. (1954). *Acta obstet. gynec. scand.*, **33**, Suppl. 4.
26. MALMSTRÖM, T. (1957). *Acta obstet. gynec. scand.*, **36**, Suppl. 3.
27. MALMSTRÖM, T., and LANGE, P. (1964). *Acta obstet. gynec. scand.*, **43**, Suppl. 1
28. MENDELSON, C. L. (1946). *Amer. J. Obstet. Gynec.*, **52**, 191.
29. MILLER, D. (1927). *Brit. med. J.*, **2**, 685.
30. MILLER, D. (1928). *Brit. med. J.*, **2**, 183.
31. MOIR, D. D., and WALLACE, G. (1967). *J. Obstet. Gynaec. Brit. Cwlth.*, **74**, 424
32. PARKER, R. B. (1954). *Brit. med. J.*, **2**, 65.
33. PARKER, R. B. (1956). *Brit. med. J.*, **2**, 16.
34. RHODES, P. (1958). *J. Obstet. Gynaec. Brit. Emp.*, **65**, 353.
35. SCOTT, J. S., and GADD, R. L. (1957). *Brit. med. J.*, **1**, 971.
36. SCUDAMORE, J. H., and YATES, M. J. (1966). *Lancet*, **1**, 23.
37. SEEDAT, E. K., and CRICHTON, D. (1962). *Lancet*, **1**, 554.
38. SHUTE, W. B. (1959). *Amer. J. Obstet. Gynec.*, **77**, 442.
39. SNOECK, J. (1960). *Proc. roy. Soc. Med.*, **53**, 749.
40. TENNENT, R. A. (1965). *J. Obstet. Gynaec. Brit. Cwlth.*, **72**, 872.
41. WILLOCKS, J. (1962). *J. Obstet. Gynaec. Brit. Cwlth.*, **69**, 266.
42. WYLIE, B. (1963). *Amer. J. Obstet. Gynec.*, **86**, 38.

CHAPTER XIX

RESUSCITATION OF THE NEWBORN

To breathe or not to breathe—that is the question.

The term asphyxia neonatorum explains itself, but behind this outward manifestation of inability to breathe lies a whole sea of troubles, much of which has not yet been properly fathomed and is now engaging much interesting modern research.

Perinatal mortality embraces all stillbirths, whether macerated or fresh, and all neonatal deaths within the first week of extra-uterine existence and when one looks through tables of such statistics, whether national or local, it is readily appreciated that one is confronted with a very wide range of reasons for a baby's refusal to breathe at birth or successfully to maintain respiration thereafter. One has to review the whole subject and efficacy of resuscitation of the newborn against this wide pathological background and in the past failure to do so has been responsible for the rapidly changing fashions in resuscitative techniques, which have varied through the years from the bizarre to the picturesque and only a few have been based upon sound scientific fact. The reasons for respiratory failure at birth, in fact, differ so widely and it is so difficult in the crisis of such an emergency to make a satisfactory differential diagnosis that it is not surprising that no set order of procedure has yet proved satisfactory, and treatment has to fall back upon the general lines of maintaining oxygenation of the heart and vital brain centres by one means or another until a more definitive diagnosis and treatment can be instituted.

Important though the business of resuscitation must be, it has to be recognised that one is often dealing with overwhelming pathology and that the clinician is often presented with a hopeless case from adverse factors which have been operating already before birth and against which his resuscitative techniques can only have a marginal value in reducing perinatal loss. Any major improvement in fœtal survival chances will come, not through radical changes in methods of resuscitation, but in the better control of the complications of pregnancy and labour and above all in the elimination of prematurity. Abnormal labour may indeed be bad for the fœtus, but abnormal pregnancy may be even worse.

The National Perinatal Mortality rate varies between 30 and 35 per 1,000, with intra-uterine asphyxia of all varieties as the commonest cause. Congenital malformations make up about a fifth of the

20 and 75 ml. as compared with the usual 15 to 20 ml. of resting tidal volumes later on in a normal baby. Crying may raise the figure to 130 to 160 ml.

The resistance of the lungs to expansion, that is to say the lung compliance, consequently improves so that there is a progressive and rapid fall in the amount of effort needed on the part of the baby to maintain respiration. This is very important when one compares the satisfactory æration achieved within a few minutes by a healthy vigorous baby with the respiratory difficulties associated with atelectasis and prematurity.

We have repeatedly demonstrated the reduction in respiratory effort required which accompanies progressive pulmonary expansion and have made simultaneous recordings of the increasing tidal airs which indicate a bigger ventilatory reward at the same time.

In order to establish this physiological train of events a flying start to respiration is very necessary. Even a premature baby, if it achieves this flying start, can expand its lungs to full radiological clarity within 2 hours and is thereafter most unlikely to develop the pulmonary syndrome of the newborn (Donald, 1954).

The causes of the onset of respiration are usually a combination of factors.

Firstly, the child finds itself in a state of acute anoxia due to the cutting off of the oxygen supply from the mother. In normal labour this occurs as soon as the head is born, at which time the placenta has probably started to separate and the placental site will have already undergone some retraction in any case. The head and face turn a livid blue at this stage, which is an encouraging indication of the state of the baby provided further delivery is not delayed beyond a minute or two, and if the chest is not too tightly wedged within the pelvic cavity, the baby will often cry forthwith.

As soon as it is born, the stimulus of anoxia is reinforced by innumerable afferent stimuli which crowd in on the baby's central nervous system from skin, muscles and joints. The process of birth must come as a rude and painful shock. In certain animals, the fœtus falls on to its snout, which acts as a very efficient receptor for such afferent stimuli.

The carotid sinus plays an important part. Its response depends upon both chemical and pressor receptors. A rise in blood pressure stimulates respiration in a manner not seen in animals in whom the carotid sinuses have been denervated experimentally, and these sinuses are important chemical receptor organs in oxygen lack. This sensitivity may exceed that of the respiratory centre itself.

In like manner breathing is markedly depressed by sinus denervation in animals. The accumulation of carbon dioxide also stimulates the respiratory mechanism, but only if it is functionally healthy and

not handicapped or depressed by antecedent anoxia, immaturity or cerebral compression.

Ætiology of Asphyxia Neonatorum

In the first place, the baby may lack the necessary equipment to start or to maintain respiration. This is particularly the case in very premature infants where alveolar development may not be sufficiently advanced. Such infants, for a time, may be able to oxygenate their blood by breathing with their bronchioli which are capable of respiratory distension, but they often die within a day or two from pulmonary atelectasis.

Secondly, the respiratory centre may not be sufficiently sensitive to normal stimuli because of immaturity, or it may be depressed by any condition causing a rise in intracranial pressure, by drugs and anæsthetics, and it may be damaged by previous anoxia so that a rising carbon dioxide level may reach lethal proportions before it can stimulate it.

Thirdly, blood circulation may be so reduced as a result of fœtal shock that the supply of oxygenated blood, even if available, is unable to reach the respiratory centre in sufficient quantity to revive it.

Lastly, mechanical factors may prevent blood oxygenation, as, for example, where the respiratory passages are blocked by the aspiration of foreign material, or when there is delay in delivering the after-coming head in breech presentation or serious difficulty in delivering the shoulders of a large baby.

Asphyxia before Delivery as a Cause of Asphyxia at Birth

This is perhaps the most important class of causes.

Anything which interferes with placental circulation may damage the vital centres and their responsiveness following delivery.

Separation of the placenta, whether normally situated or prævia, may be insufficient to kill the fœtus straightaway, but often causes either premature inspiration *in utero* or results in unresponsiveness at birth. The placenta which is prævia has the further risk of being compressed during labour by the presenting part.

Pre-eclamptic toxæmia, and especially eclampsia, subject the child to varying degrees of anoxia which may damage it beyond recall, and placental infarction, particularly the diffuse variety, may operate in like fashion.

Prolonged labour with the membranes ruptured exposes the child to mounting anoxia due to the progressive retraction of the placental site, in addition to intranatal pneumonia.

Cord accidents are occasional causes of antepartum asphyxia, due to compression or tight winding round the neck and, more unusually, from true knotting.

Any condition which precipitately lowers the maternal blood pressure reduces placental oxygenation, as for example in shock, or in antepartum hæmorrhage in which the effects of hypotension may be added to those of placental separation.

A fairly common predisposing cause is maternal asphyxia in the course of inducing anæsthesia, and the ideal general anæsthetic which is free from this risk has yet to be discovered. Vomiting often complicates induction of anæsthesia, especially in the labouring woman whose stomach has been liberally plied with fluids in the course of labour, and the effects of such asphyxia can be more disastrous to fœtus than to mother. Long after the latter appears well oxygenated following "induction asphyxia", the uterus, with its slow but plentiful circulation, remains a dusky colour, as can be seen at Cæsarean section after a stormy passage through the lighter planes of anæsthesia.

The signs of fœtal distress during labour are usually those of asphyxia *in utero* and resuscitation after birth is consequently prejudiced.

Of all the drugs which depress respiration at birth, morphia and its allied derivatives are the chief offenders and for that reason should not be given in the last four hours before delivery, and in the case of premature deliveries the safety interval is even longer. Pethidine is less dangerous in this respect, but is best withheld during the second stage. Roberts *et al.* (1957) found that pethidine given to the mother during labour reduced the minute volume of respiratory activity in the baby by 10–15 per cent for some hours after birth. Fortunately nalorphine can counteract respiratory depression due to morphia and pethidine.

The barbiturates also contribute to neonatal asphyxia and a study of the concentration levels of phenobarbitone in maternal serum and umbilical cord serum has shown that the levels are within 5 per cent of each other and that the rate of elimination from the blood of the newborn is slower than or equal to that in adults (Melchior *et al.* 1967). The baby therefore suffers just as much of a hangover as its mother and may well be in less of a condition to have to face it. Paraldehyde still remains one of the safest drugs in this respect.

All general anæsthetics have some influence on neonatal breathing, depending more upon the depth of maternal narcosis than on the particular agent; trilene, however, is reasonably safe though often inadequate as an anæsthetic. Nitrous oxide and air analgesia lowers the percentage oxygen saturation of the maternal blood and should not be continued in the presence of established fœtal distress.

Every acute attack of anoxia depletes the fœtal glycogen reserves and chronic hypoxia depletes them chronically. There is very little glycogen in the liver early in pregnancy, but the stores increase rapidly and according to Shelley (1961) having reached at term double the level of the adult liver these hepatic glycogen reserves fall, after birth, very rapidly to about one-tenth of their former value within three hours, thereafter rising gradually to adult levels within the next two to three weeks. The fœtal brain stores very little glycogen but uses glucose, often by anærobic metabolism, but it does require an active circulation to supply it with glucose carried in the blood, and this depends upon an active myocardium (Mott, 1961). The myocardium, to maintain efficiency and therefore an effective circulation to the brain, depends upon its own glycogen reserves and these too are depleted in hypoxia. This is one of the reasons for the feeble slow heartbeat of the severely distressed baby at birth. The resistance of the brain of the newborn to anoxia is due to its ability to metabolise glucose anærobically and this in turn is furnished by the glycolysis of the liver stores, but survival will depend upon how well the stores of glycogen in the myocardium last out (Stafford and Weatherall, 1960). Experiments on newborn animals in an atmosphere of nitrogen show that survival depends on myocardial glycogen and when this is finally depleted circulatory failure ensues. A compensatory mechanism may put off the evil moment here since no animal can maintain its body temperature in the presence of anoxia and cooling may prolong survival possibly by retarding the utilisation of cardiac glycogen, hence the case for hypothermia as a therapeutic measure, but if oxygen is supplied and reaches the circulation an attempt may be made to maintain temperature by using up the glycogen reserves and death may follow. It is known that a baby, if warm, can survive without food for many days, but if it is allowed to get too cold it may use up its reserves of carbohydrate in an attempt to maintain body temperature and may then die in a state of hypoglycæmia (Mann and Elliott, 1957).

The state of the glycogen stores within the body, and particularly within the myocardium, therefore greatly influence a baby's ability to withstand anoxia and since it takes many hours for myocardial reserves of glycogen to be built up again it can be seen that chronic deprivation or repeated shortages of oxygen are far more deadly than the dramatically acute fœtal distress which may occur late in the second stage and from which the baby in this latter instance may make a much more dramatic recovery regardless of the technique employed (Donald, 1963). The importance will, therefore, be appreciated of those factors capable of reducing stores of fœtal glycogen before or during birth and, therefore, the chances of survival, such as maternal malnutrition, placental insufficiency, es-

pecially pre-eclamptic toxæmia and intra-uterine hypoxia of all varieties.

The concept of "placental insufficiency" is frequently invoked to explain intra-uterine anoxia and the mechanism and extent are by no means predictable or discernible in a large proportion of cases, but when perinatal mortality occurs as a direct result of asphyxia during labour the cause is usually much more obvious. Dawkins and colleagues (1961), in analysing one hundred such deaths, found that only two had no recognisable ætiological factor and they noted that the major causes of intrapartum asphyxia were complicated vaginal delivery, premature separation of placenta and inadequate placental reserve, more than half the deaths occurring in association with maternal toxæmia. In fact when toxæmia was combined with postmaturity or difficult labour the hazards were greatly increased, but postmaturity in otherwise uncomplicated cases rarely caused fœtal death during labour.

Fœtal Conditions as Causes of Asphyxia at Birth

The presence of mucus, often tenacious, and thick meconium in the upper air passages is rightly often blamed, and although post-mortem examination does not, as a rule, reveal such foreign matter in significant amounts, it would appear imprudent at least not to take the simple steps of clearing it out. Liquor which is not thickened with meconium is probably innocuous, for respiratory movements of the baby normally occur for some time before the onset of labour, although they are not deep. In any case normal liquor is readily eliminated from the tract or absorbed. Mucus regurgitated from the stomach is an additional source of trouble and gastric aspiration is increasingly practised.

Intracranial hæmorrhage, howsoever caused, whether by the mechanical trauma of labour or by asphyxia, operates differently, and the baby's asphyxia is only one of the several manifestations of fœtal shock. Even in the absence of significant intracranial bleeding, cerebral œdema may act in the same fashion.

In prolonged and infected labour with the membranes ruptured, intranatal bronchopneumonia is not uncommon, and the baby, if born alive, shows a degree of asphyxia as a result, but in this instance it takes rapid and largely ineffectual shallow breaths, bringing the accessory muscles into play and showing signs similar to those of pulmonary atelectasis.

Very rarely congenital abnormalities such as laryngeal atresia may prevent the onset of respiration.

Above all, if labour is complicated by asphyxia, then any mucus, meconium or blood which may be aspirated as a result is bound to increase the handicaps of a respiratory centre already depressed.

PATHOLOGY

The immediate effects of asphyxia are those of venous engorgement, especially in the brain where the vessels have already endured much in the course of labour and whose walls may finally give way. If the tentorium cerebelli is torn the brain is at once flooded with blood, but moulding, by dragging the apex of the tentorium upwards, may sufficiently restrict venous flow to raise back pressure to the point at which smaller tributary vessels rupture, even though the tentorium is not actually torn.

Apart from the brain, venous engorgement and capillary hæmorrhages are likely to occur throughout the body, especially in the liver and under its capsule, in the lungs, suprarenals and heart muscle, where petechiæ (Tardieu's spots) are characteristically seen. There is arteriolar constriction and the circulation is reduced, particularly to the brain with its vital centres, including not only the respiratory but the vasomotor centre as well, which are soon paralysed so that the signs of shock are manifested.

In cases of asphyxia developing after birth Edith Potter and Rosenbaum describe an accumulation of cerebrospinal fluid which may not be noticed at autopsy unless the skull is carefully opened. This is more likely to occur after Cæsarean section and in premature infants. It is associated with atelectasis which may be secondary, and although it may be due to mechanical causes, such as the sudden removal of the child from intra-uterine pressure, it is more likely to be the result of anoxia. The increase in fluid and the resulting pressure from it is then likely to aggravate the child's respiratory difficulties.

The vicious circle is easily completed. Asphyxia begets vasomotor and respiratory depression, which in their turn cause further asphyxia until irreversible changes end in the child's death.

THE CLINICAL STAGES OF ASPHYXIA NEONATORUM

In the past it has been customary to describe two types, namely the blue and the white, but the former may merge into the latter, which is a stage of decompensation and failure; on the other hand, white or pallid asphyxia may present from the first, in which case it comes as an outward manifestation of profound fœtal shock, however caused.

Cases of white asphyxia would be more accurately described as grey. The point at issue, however, in the difference in colour of the two types, is the state of the peripheral circulation. In both, asphyxia may be profound, but good circulation in the skin is necessary for

lividity to show itself, and the better prognosis in the blue variety lies in the better circulatory state.

The signs of early asphyxia, then, are a full and powerful heart beat which is also slower than usual, a mechanism whereby oxygen may be to some degree conserved, and the skin is a dusky blue.

Later these signs give place to grey pallor, a weak apex beat and flaccidity. The worse the child's condition, the slower the heart beat and the first sign of recovery is its acceleration, which precedes improvement in skin colour. The lips have a dirty purple colour, the anal sphincter is toneless, the tongue tends to fall backwards and the jaw is relaxed. The vocal cords lie separated from each other in the paralysed position, so that intubation is not usually difficult, for the reflex tone of the glottis, in common with the other reflexes, has gone.

Respiration is for a time very shallow, punctuated with occasional gasps, but soon becomes very infrequent and finally stops altogether.

Within ten to fifteen minutes the changes are irreversible, and the longer it takes to oxygenate the baby and restore its failing circulation, the greater will be the damage to the brain cells, and it is only possible to speculate on the extent to which its intellect, for example, may be impaired, not to mention the grosser evidences of neurological injury which may originate in the hazards of delivery

In cases of intracranial bleeding vaso-motor tone is poor from the very beginning; the mechanism is different here and there is no livid stage. The prognosis is correspondingly less favourable.

Even though the immediate response to resuscitation may be satisfactory, there are cases which relapse some hours later and develop respiratory distress. Apart from cerebral irritation, œdema or compression, which is the commonest cause, a few of such cases must be attributed to the aspiration of foreign material. Now, the aspiration of liquor amnii at birth, although admittedly common, would not account for secondary atelectasis some hours later; it is therefore probable that regurgitation of mucus from the stomach occurs and, chiefly in the case of the weak or premature infant, some of this mucus may find its way into the respiratory tract. The observations of Gellis, Priscilla White and Pfeffer with regard to the stomach contents at birth, particularly after Cæsarean section, will be referred to later.

In classifying asphyxia neonatorum, it is now more commonly the practice to grade it according to its severity rather than the baby's colour. Attempts to evaluate and compare different treatments and to assess subsequent progress are usually defeated for want of an objective standard which can be employed by a number of observers at birth. The scoring system, however, devised by Virginia Apgar (1953) deserves note. In this method the condition is assessed exactly one minute after birth in respect of five features, namely heart rate,

respiratory effort, reflex irritability, muscle tone and colour, allowing a maximum score of two for each, as shown in Table XV. The advantages of such a system are its ease of application, the reduced chances of observer error and non-interference with, nor modification by, resuscitative techniques since the assessment has strictly to be made at a given age, in our practice at 120 seconds.

TABLE XV

THE EVALUATION OF THE NEWBORN INFANT (APGAR)

METHOD OF SCORING

Sixty seconds or more commonly nowadays 120 seconds after the *complete* birth of the infant (disregarding the cord and placenta) the following five objective signs are evaluated and each given a score of 0, 1 or 2. A score of 10 indicates an infant in the best possible condition.

Sign	0	1	2
Heart rate	Absent	Slow (Below 100)	Over 100
Respiratory effort	Absent	Slow Irregular	Good Crying
Muscle tone	Limp	Some flexion of extremities	Active motion
Response to catheter in nostril (tested after oropharynx is clear)	No response	Grimace	Cough or sneeze
Colour	Blue Pale	Body pink Extremities blue	Completely pink

TREATMENT OF NEONATAL ASPHYXIA

In these days of demarcation disputes it might be debated whose job it was to resuscitate the newborn. This, however, is a crisis which brooks no argument and the answer is quite simply "anyone present who is competent to cope". The need, therefore, to train obstetricians, anæsthetists and pædiatricians in standard resuscitative techniques, including particularly tracheal intubation, is obvious. It is only in larger units that all three categories of individual are likely to be present at the same time and only then in the more complicated cases. There is, therefore, some need to try and predict

the type of cases where skilled resuscitation will be needed. Prediction is important in order to indicate that a doctor who can give undivided attention to the infant should be present at the delivery of all these high-risk patients (Corner, 1962). Ideally these would include all operative deliveries, all cases of malpresentation, fœtal distress, twins, premature labour and in cases where the mothers appeared clinically to be "small for dates". The importance of obtaining a flying start to respiration has already been mentioned and, in fact, about three-quarters of all cases of respiratory distress syndrome have Apgar scores below six (see later) and some trouble at birth is nearly always present in the majority of cases who subsequently develop hyaline membrane disease. A baby apparently well at birth can, within two and a half minutes of complete apnœa, drop its percentage oxygen saturation dangerously and with it follows the inevitable acidosis, so that the pH of the blood falls at the rate of about 0·1 per minute.

The history of neonatal resuscitation reflects little enough credit on the knowledge or imagination of those practising it, and the baby has often had to demonstrate a will to survive capable of defeating the most determined assaults of its wellwishers. In the Old Testament the prophet Elisha had some success with mouth-to-mouth insufflation, but perhaps he was ahead of his time.

To William Smellie, Scottish obstetrician of the eighteenth century, the matter was simple enough. To make the baby cry it should be well whipped and have its nose rubbed with onions. I once came across an account from an eighteenth century combined textbook of Theology and Midwifery which recommended inflating the intestine with tobacco smoke, with clysters. A converted non-smoker, like myself, can only heartily endorse the suggested use of this insanitary and expensive habit. In the last century Schultze's method of swinging the baby above the head and causing it to jack-knife, so as to compress its chest, enjoyed a certain vogue and a very eminent obstetrician in Northern Ireland claims to have survived this form of resuscitation at his own birth. Buist in 1895 described his use of it to the Edinburgh Obstetrical Society in the following words, "Standing in a space cleared in the midst of a small room, whose other denizens were withdrawn into the corners, my feet planted well apart and arms extended I taught the neonatus to perform a series of grand circles, while the meconium distributed itself in trajectories for which the room and its inmates, including the physicians, formed a comprehensive recording surface." Just before the turn of the century subcutaneous injection of tincture of belladonna and whiskey was recommended, provided that it was Irish whiskey. Even when I was a student we were taught the value of rubbing the baby's gums with brandy, which the midwives were reputed to have flavoured with meconium in order to discourage inroads by a thirsty student body.

A list of the methods of artificial respiration which were taught even in my own day relied on the principle of elastic recoil of the chest wall as in adults but, of course, this phenomenon is not to be found in the shocked baby with unærated lungs. Now these techniques have given way to airway clearance and positive pressure lung inflation in a baby too ill to make its own respiratory efforts.

As Gibberd has long pointed out, three conditions must be satisfied:

1. The air passages must be patent.
2. A suitable atmosphere must be available.
3. Respiratory movements must be adequate.

One might add a fourth condition, namely blood circulation must be adequate to revive the vital centres with oxygenated blood. Nevertheless we must face the sober truth that if a baby has even half a chance to breathe it will take it and its ultimate fate, whether to live or whether to die, is largely determined before resuscitation even starts.

Clearance of airway.—If possible, before the first gasp is taken, the mouth, pharynx and nostrils should be cleared by suction.

The traditional mucus catheter is totally inadequate for the purpose. Quite apart from its inefficiency, it is a septic weapon, and the sight of a midwife pulling down her mask, holding the other end between her teeth and blowing down it to clear it before reinsertion makes a mockery of all the other aseptic precautions. MacRae (1962), however, has described a disposable mucus extractor which gets rid of these objections and which consists of a short plastic mouthpiece which can be passed into the mouth behind a face mask without touching it. The unit includes a trap and a whistle-tip catheter with a side eye in addition. I would have preferred one cut off square at the end as less likely to suck mucous membrane into the lumen. The extractor is supplied presterilised. In hospital practice suction should, of course, be mechanical, either by connecting to a water suction pump attached to a nearby tap, which is both simple and efficient, or in the case of modern units, to the suction pipes which have been built into all labour wards and nurseries. The end of the sucker must be of soft rubber to avoid damaging the pharyngeal mucous membrane.

It is particularly important to clear the pharynx as soon as the mouth is born in the case of the after-coming head in breech delivery, or as soon as the head is delivered in Cæsarean section, or in forceps deliveries. The ceremonial wiping of the eyelids can well wait until this far more necessary step has been taken.

As soon as the child is completely delivered it should be held up by the ankles with its back steadied against the front of the operator's chest. This leaves him a free hand with which to direct the end of the

sucker. The suction pressure should not exceed 2–3 inches of mercury (Figs. 1 and 2).

Now, and not before, the cord may be divided and the child may be handed to the midwife in the happy knowledge that the most important steps have already been taken.

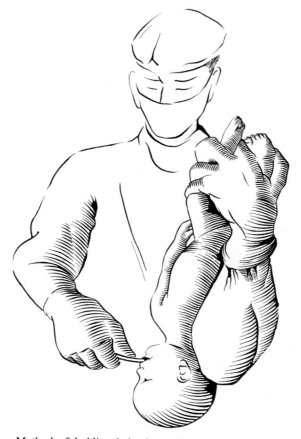

19/Fig. 1.—Method of holding baby immediately after delivery and sucking out pharynx.

The child is now laid, slightly turned to one side with the head downwards, in a warmed cot or tray inclined at about 20 degrees from the horizontal. The purpose of the head-down slope is to facilitate drainage of secretions and fluids and to discourage their aspiration, but once the pharynx and stomach have been properly emptied

by mechanical suction the baby will be the better off from being propped up and relieved of the embarrassing weight of the liver on its diaphragm.

Resuscitation trays can be improvised in which the portion supporting the head can be easily lowered to facilitate intubation, should it be necessary. The usual type of cot is not satisfactory, because the side at the head end gets in the way if a laryngoscope has to be used.

Should the child not show signs of spontaneous breathing within

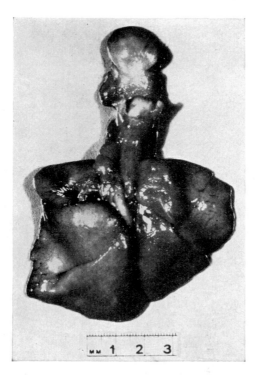

19/Fig. 2.—Mucus blocking glottis.

three minutes there should be no hesitation in clearing the glottis with the help of an infant's laryngoscope. Unfortunately, too many obstetricians are reluctant to familiarise themselves with the use of this instrument and tend to put off using it until the situation has become desperate and is made yet more desperate by unskilled hands.

If the glottic reflex is not present, the trachea should be intubated forthwith with a small curved soft plastic tube made specially for the purpose, for example close fitting plastic laryngeal tubes such as Warne's neonatal catheters. The point to remember is that if the child

is in any state to resent this manœuvre there is no need for it, and in the circumstances which call for it there is no difficulty in carrying it out gently and quickly.

Any mucus in the trachea can be sucked out now, and intermittent positive pressures of oxygen up to 35 cm. of water can be applied with the help of a manually operated rubber bag or some such device. The purpose of this is not to inflate the alveoli as might be expected, for in any case far higher pressures than this would be necessary, but the bronchial tree is thereby flooded with oxygen, some of which is directly absorbed; should the child take even a small breath, it can be certain of receiving a good concentration of oxygen of which it is in serious need. Should no improvement occur in a further few minutes, the outlook is grave indeed.

The value of intubation and the supply of oxygen by endotracheal catheter under positive pressure is now no longer questioned. It is only regretted that so few attending women in labour are sufficiently trained to employ it, and those in need of practice should use every opportunity afforded by fresh stillborn or dead babies. Unskilled attempts may do more harm than good. The technique has been minutely described by Barrie (1963) of which the following is a summary.

Tracheal intubation.—A nurse steadies the baby on its back on a resuscitation shelf or tray. The head is held in a slightly extended position. It is a great mistake to hyperextend the head. Holding the laryngoscope in the left hand the blade is passed over the back of the tongue until the epiglottis is seen. Now comes the slightly more difficult part of locating the glottis. If there is any mucus or debris lying about it should be aspirated now. The laryngoscope is then passed down further beyond and behind the epiglottis. Except in extreme degrees of flaccidity the expected triangular opening will not be seen but rather a dimple in the middle of a pinkish-coloured mound, which may open during a gasp. To get a good view, the tip of the laryngoscope blade has to hook under the epiglottis and lift it up against the root of the tongue. Barrie reckons as easier using the tip of the blade advanced into the space between the root of the tongue and the epiglottis (the vallecula) and raising the whole instrument so as to lift both structures forwards and thereby obtain a view. The position of the baby's head may have to be altered to achieve this. Suction is now applied to clear the airway and using the right hand an endotracheal tube is passed for 2 cm. into the trachea. Care must be taken not to displace the tube on removing the laryngoscope. An attempt may now be made by the operator's own lips, if necessary, to inflate the lungs or, better still, using an oxygen containing bag and a pressure gauge to see that undue pressure is not used. If the operator does his own puffing he will experience a charac-

teristic resistance described by Barrie as like inflating a balloon. Oxygen by a side tube introduced into the operator's mouth is a helpful idea. If the catheter has been introduced too far only one side of the chest will expand, usually the right, and the tube should be withdrawn. If the abdomen bulges instead of the chest, clearly one has introduced the catheter into the œsophagus instead of the trachea. A fine suction catheter should remove any mucus secretions lying about and the treatment thereafter continued with short, sharp puffs of oxygen using the manometer as a safeguard to limit pressures to no more than 35 cm. of water for as long as the child's colour can be maintained and the heart continues to beat. This period may exceed an hour and may still be followed by complete recovery. Pressures less than 30 cm. of water are unlikely to produce much visible chest expansion but higher pressures than this, if lasting more than a fraction of a second, may rupture alveoli, producing emphysema and areas of hæmorrhage in the lungs, or even pneumothorax (Fig. 3). This treatment, originally introduced by Gibberd and Blaikley in 1935, has stood the test of time better than most others, but clearly is not without its own dangers. Although a gasp is induced very frequently and the benefits of the immediately available oxygen within the bronchiolar system are dramatic, Cross et al. have also noted a marked apnœic response to lung inflation. As long, however, as the heart rate continues to accelerate or to maintain itself above one hundred beats per minute this method of artificial respiration will maintain efficient oxygenation for the vital centres. It is doubtful, however, if the alveoli are properly opened up without the presence of spontaneous inspiratory efforts which are necessary to bring about the circulatory readjustments already referred to within the pulmonary vascular tree, but the immediate benefit of endotracheal insufflation lies in oxygen absorption from the bronchi and bronchioles and a guarantee of an effective airway.

Difficulties of intubation are more often the result of faulty positioning of the child's head and lack of confidence on the part of the operator than anything else and certainly the manœuvre can be made easier by pushing back on the cricoid. This helps to close the œsophagus and is also useful in the course of mouth to mouth insufflation. Where for one reason or another endotracheal intubation cannot be carried out, an attractive idea has been suggested of using a rubber rat-tailed ear syringe and applying it, after clearance of the air passages, to one nostril while blocking the other and the mouth. Since the bulb has a capacity of about 60 ml. it is very suitable as a safe method of trying to inflate the air passages of the newborn. Again the trachea should be pushed backwards to help obliterate the œsophageal lumen and prevent the diversion of most of the air from the syringe bulb into the stomach (Lerman, 1967).

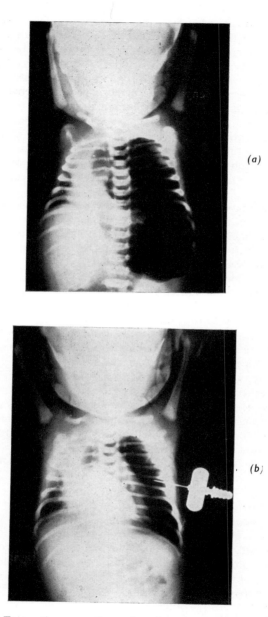

19/Fig. 3.—(a) Traumatic pneumothorax from intubation and positive pressure ventilation. (b) Pneumothorax relieved by prompt aspiration. Baby survived.

Since it so often happens that adequate skilled attention is not available at delivery, it is necessary to consider alternatives.

The old-fashioned method of standing in front of the fire, dangling the child by its ankles, may assist fluid to drain from its air passages and keep it warm, but to hold the child in this attitude for any length of time must greatly engorge the cerebral veins; moreover, the weight of the liver on the flaccid diaphragm discourages any inspiratory attempt.

Another method of securing an airway is to draw the tongue forwards with a tongue forceps. It used to be thought that intermittent tongue traction reflexly stimulated breathing but, apart from acting as an unpleasant afferent stimulus, no such anatomical reflex in fact exists.

There are now some very useful baby-size airways on the market and these may be used to deal with the sagging tongue.

A fine rubber catheter passed into the nasopharynx via a nostril, through which oxygen is slowly run, is a safe and moderately effective method.

Whatever method is used, gentleness of handling is the first essential. The child is in no need of afferent stimuli—its arrival into the outer world supplies these in plenty and its inability to respond to them is due to something pathological. Slapping, pinching, spraying with ethyl chloride, anal dilatation and other such primitive measures are no more sensible than striking a match to show a blind man down a flight of stairs.

As soon as possible, the child should either be wrapped up in a warm blanket or placed in a warmed oxygen cot and in either case left in peace.

Immersion in a tub of warm water has now gone out of fashion because no one has yet devised a satisfactory method of doing so with the head tilted downwards!

A suitable atmosphere.—The asphyxiated baby's first need is for oxygen to revive the vital centres. Of carbon dioxide it already has a gross excess. The fatuity, therefore, of blowing carbon dioxide at its face must be obvious, and yet it is surprising how long it has taken for this practice to die out. Any alleged response was due more to the stimulus of the cold gas than to its composition, and it might as well be noted again that if the child was well enough to respond to such a stimulus it was well enough not to need it. Undoubtedly the portability of the very small carbon dioxide cylinders for a long time recommended their use.

To supply mixtures of 95 per cent oxygen and 5 per cent carbon dioxide is also pointless, at least during the first hour of life. Later on such a mixture may be given intermittently, when anoxia has been remedied, in the hope of encouraging alveolar expansion.

Now, pure oxygen is a pulmonary irritant if used over a long period of time but this is of no present concern when coping with an asphyxiated baby. The risks of inducing retrolental fibroplasia in premature infants do not arise until at least two or three days of excessive oxygen treatment.

In the emergency of frank asphyxia, the need for oxygen is so urgent that it should be given neat—even delivery through a glass funnel over the face is better than nothing. A polythene funnel is in fact better still as it can be moulded to a better fit round the child's face. Once breathing has become established the percentage of oxygen in the atmosphere to be breathed should be planned deliberately, ideally with the help of a gas oxymeter; percentages varying from 25 to 35, according to the maturity of the child and its general condition, should, if possible, be maintained in the incubator. Unfortunately, in most units the concentration of oxygen achieved depends more upon guesswork and the leaks in the apparatus than upon intelligent management, a matter to which cases of retrolental fibroplasia bear tragic testimony.

Aspiration of gastric contents.—As already mentioned, small quantities of gastric fluids, swallowed or indigenous, may be regurgitated and, in the very sick child, may either produce laryngeal spasm by being aspirated, giving rise to characteristic cyanotic attacks, or their inhalation may be even deeper. Gellis, White and Pfeffer found that the amount of fluid aspirated from the stomach was much greater after Cæsarean section (average 14 ml.), and where the mother had diabetes in addition the average amount was 20 ml., whereas after low forceps delivery the average was only 2 ml. These workers further observed that those babies whose stomachs were not aspirated at birth, and subsequently as necessary, developed respiratory embarrassment following Cæsarean section four times more commonly than those so treated. This is a very important observation and confirms our own practice. In fact, where resuscitative measures have to be taken with the child at Cæsarean section, gastric aspiration should be one of the routine procedures. Suction can be applied through a number four French rubber catheter passed down the œsophagus and aided by gentle manual pressure on the abdomen. The end of the catheter should be cut off square. This practically eliminates the risk of sucking mucous membrane into the lumen and damaging it.

The fluid aspirated contains the solid constituents of liquor amnii which has been swallowed in the natural course of events, but which remains in the stomach for want of the pressures supplied by the process of vaginal delivery. This is a matter which goes far towards explaining why Cæsarean section babies sometimes fail to do well.

With the vigorous baby, who is in no need of resuscitation, such

measures are not necessary, since it is well able to deal with its own secretions.

Drugs used in resuscitation.—There is not much choice here. Lobeline and nikethamide are the two in general use and are not without their dangers, as the margin between stimulation and convulsions is none too wide. In fact analeptic drugs are looked upon with increasing disfavour as they may do more harm than good.

Alpha-lobeline is said to act by lowering the threshold of the respiratory centre, though this is by no means certain. It must, in any case, reach the centre to do any good and is given intravenously into the cord in a dosage of 3·2 mg. ($\frac{1}{20}$ gr.), and milked towards the umbilicus in the hope that it will reach the general circulation and that the circulation will be adequate to carry it to its destination. Occasionally the immediate effect is gratifying, but it is very evanescent and may be followed by further respiratory depression. It is not so likely to provoke a convulsion as nikethamide.

Intramuscular injection of lobeline is useless; for one thing, any case which needs it has too poor a peripheral circulation to make use of it in time.

Intravenous injection into the umbilical cord can sometimes be difficult if the vein is empty and collapsed and accidental injection into an umbilical artery can be dangerous and produce necrosis over the buttock. Holmes (1961) recommends overcoming this difficulty by applying a sponge holder on the cord 10 cm. from the umbilicus, leaving a 15 cm. length of isolated umbilical vein remaining engorged proximal to the clamp and ligature at the point of separation of the baby. Drugs are now injected into the distended vein, the sponge holder is removed and a column of blood containing the drug is milked into the general circulation.

Nikethamide (Coramine) 0·5–1·0 ml. of a 25 per cent solution and like drugs unquestionably stimulate respiration, cardiac activity and the whole nervous system. The effect is often drastic and may do more harm than good, but its greatest use is in the narcotised apnœic baby. Again intramuscular injection is useless and the drug is most commonly given intravenously into the umbilical vein. Barrie *et al.* (1962) report that lingual administration proved as effective as intravenous injection in its effect upon respiration. A dose even as small as 0·125 ml. of the standard 25 per cent solution (30 mg.) produced forceful respiratory efforts within 30 seconds of being placed on the tongue. Larger doses have prolonged the effect: up to 10 minutes in the case of 125 mg. They recommend that this dose should not be exceeded.

Vanillic acid diethylamide has also been found by these workers to resemble the effects of nikethamide although its effect is slightly slower and shorter. It is effective both by intravenous and lingual

administration. Excessive dosage results in brief toxic effects consisting of flushing, restlessness and myoclonic twitching of the eyelids, but these pass off quickly. The smallest effective lingual dose is 1·5 mg. and the optimum is reckoned to be between 12·5 and 25 mg., or 5 mg. per Kg. of body weight. This drug is available as Vandid oral solution in glass dropper bottles containing 5 ml. solution of vanillic acid diethylamide 5 per cent (50 mg./ml.) in 25 per cent ethyl alcohol. The dose administered orally onto the tongue is thus twelve drops (25 mg.) for infants at term and 6 drops (12·5 mg.) for prematures. Needless to say the air passages should be first cleared by aspiration and if there is no response to this drug within two minutes, intubation should be carried out forthwith.

Adrenaline, often injected directly into the heart, is no more than a ritual performance, and I have never seen any good come of it, although I have often used it as a last resort, although external cardiac massage is more likely to succeed if anything can.

Where failure to breathe has been aggravated or provoked by the administration of morphine or its derivatives or of pethidine during the last few hours of labour, an antidote to the depressant effects on the baby of these drugs exists in N-allylnormorphine (nalorphine), marketed under the name Lethidrone. Given in dosage of 0·5 mg. into the umbilical vein, the effect is often dramatic, but this substance is useless against other sedatives such as the barbiturates.

Babies suffering from asphyxia at birth are intensely acidotic and, in fact, the worse their condition the lower the pH. Levels of pH 7·2 are common in early primary apnoea and as the child's condition worsens the pH may fall to 7·0. At a pH of about 6·8 the child's condition is frankly desperate and it is natural that the value of immediate infusion with sodium bicarbonate or with the buffer substance TRIS (Trishydroxyaminomethylamine) should be considered, but time is usually against one and nothing should be allowed to deflect those in attendance from the urgent necessity to oxygenate the baby, best of all by endotracheal intubation.

Methods of artificial respiration.—The old traditional methods of artificial respiration have now gone by the board, and rightly so, for three very good reasons. In the first place, they cannot be carried out without considerable exposure and handling, which is likely to be more vigorous as the child's condition appears more desperate, when in fact, bearing in mind its shocked condition, it really needs warmth and peace. Secondly, these methods, as a rule, rely on compression of the thoracic cage followed by natural recoil, in the hope that air will be drawn into the lungs. Since the baby is in a state of shock, and therefore toneless, there can hardly be much recoil. Thirdly, chest compression is supposed to drive air out of the alveoli which is then replaced by fresh air on recoil; although this may be

the case in adults whose alveoli were previously expanded, the principle cannot apply to the newborn whose alveoli are still collapsed so that there is no air to express in the first place.

These methods are, therefore, not only a waste of time but also harmful.

Mouth to mouth insufflation has been practised since antiquity. More recently a layer of gauze over the child's mouth has been added as a refinement for the benefit of the midwife in order to reduce her intake of vernix and meconium. The operator's mouth should include both the baby's nose and mouth. Any air insufflated finds its way, of course, not into the lungs but into the stomach, from which there can be little benefit and the risks of sepsis are considerable.

Intratracheal insufflation, already described, still holds pride of place among resuscitative techniques.

Bearing in mind the Queckenstedt phenomenon, any rise in intra-thoracic pressure is immediately matched by a rise in intracranial pressure via the great veins draining the skull cavity, which are without effective valves. Our pilot experiments on cats have shown a rise and fall in pressures within the skull which closely follow the pressure changes within the chest. It may follow, therefore, that anything which grossly increases thoracic pressure may have harmful effects on the brain. Now, where the skull bones are reasonably mature, and therefore firm, any rise in the intravenous pressure in the skull would be offset by the resistance of the skull to expansion. If this were not so, coughing and crying would be dangerous activities. With the very premature child, however, this protection is much less, and it may account for the high incidence of intracranial bleeding which occurs in the premature, however delivered. In the past this has been blamed on abnormal fragility of the blood vessels in prematurity, but I doubt whether this is really so and whether the mechanism has not hitherto been misunderstood.

Augmented respiration.—This is the principle underlying the author's method of artificial respiration. Fundamentally it involves synchronising the action of the respirator with any spontaneous respiratory efforts which the baby may be making. We have repeatedly demonstrated the mechanical load which a sick, shocked, narcotised or premature baby may have to shoulder in initially expanding its lungs, diverting the blood flow into the pulmonary vascular bed and overcoming the moist cohesion of its alveolar walls. Indeed, in such cases the respiratory effort required may be too much for it and it therefore fails to make that very important flying start to respiration, which we believe to be important.

In our earliest respirator experiments we soon found that mechanical devices which operated on a pre-set and arbitrary rhythm and without regard to the baby's breathing attempts were not only in-

effectual but often did more harm than good by actually working, from time to time, in direct opposition, or anti-phase, to the child's own respiration—if any, and often provoked what we termed "protest apnœa" (Donald and Young, 1952).

As a result of this I came to experiment with the principle of augmented respiration, in which a variety of respirators were produced all of which were triggered by a photoelectric mechanism that detected the onset of each spontaneous inspiratory attempt and immediately set the apparatus into an inspiratory phase to assist the baby's breathing. The baby thus automatically controlled its own respirator according to its needs. In the total absence of spontaneous respiration a pre-set rate of operation cut in, until the next inspiratory effort by the baby triggered the mechanism once more in step with the baby.

We are convinced that if there is any virtue in artificial respiration, and we believe there is and there appears to be a renewed interest in the subject, it must operate in accordance with this simple and rather obvious physiological principle.

The case for effective artificial respiration is further strengthened by the observations of Dawes *et al.* (1953) who found that artificial positive pressure ventilation immediately increases the rate of pulmonary arterial blood flow which is accompanied by (or indeed may be due to) a fall of nine-tenths of the pre-existing pulmonary vascular resistance. Jaykka (1957) also observed that the effects of artificial respiration and the erectile expansion of the lung capillaries are additive in effecting lung aeration.

Rocking methods.—Eve's rocking method is a very useful addition to treatment. By rocking the baby in its longitudinal axis the weight of the liver and abdominal viscera causes downward and upward displacements of the diaphragm, thereby encouraging the passage of air in and out of the lungs. There is, however, as Eve points out, the important advantage that circulation is first improved by increasing venous return, particularly from the head; this helps to remove carbon dioxide from the brain and vital centres; in other words "Restore the circulation and the brain restores itself".

Rocking can be done quite simply by holding the baby's body across one's chest and swaying from side to side through an arc of 40 to 70 degrees, performing about ten cycles a minute, the only disadvantage being that it is not easy to administer oxygen at the same time.

Phrenic nerve stimulation.—Cross some years ago developed a phrenic nerve stimulator on the lines of the Sarnoff apparatus. The electrical stimulus is applied at the appropriate point on either or both sides of the neck and delivered at about twenty-second intervals. The child is, therefore, forced to breathe in a series of hiccups. Since a baby's neck is so short it is often difficult for the

unpractised to stimulate the right point, and there is, in any case, some overflow to the sterno-mastoid and other muscles supplied by the upper part of the brachial plexus, but this aids rather than hinders chest expansion. Cross stated that spontaneous respiration is not inhibited.

Like other mechanical and electrical pieces of apparatus it has never caught on widely and in fact the store rooms of obstetric units are littered with discarded machines which no one can bring himself to throw out because of their admirable ingenuity and so they continue as dust-collecting, space-occupying nuisances. Our own department is no exception.

Administration of gastric oxygen.—Some years ago Yllpo drew attention to the fact that an oxygen bubble in the stomach of a baby disappeared, on radiological examination, within ten minutes.

This was followed up by the introduction of intragastric oxygen as a means of resuscitation by Akerren and Furstenberg (1950) and within a very few years the treatment was widely hailed and accepted throughout the whole world—as dramatically, in fact, as it has now been rejected by almost the same people who originally acclaimed it. After such a glorious innings it has now been thoroughly debunked from various quarters. Now it appears the disappearance of the oxygen from the lumen of the bowel is simply due to its utilisation by the intestinal wall and that even if it did get into the bloodstream it would be picked up by the hypoxic liver before it ever reached the heart and that even if it managed to by-pass the liver the Newcastle team (Cooper *et al.* 1960) reckoned that less oxygen could be absorbed from the entire alimentary tract into the mesenteric blood than would be necessary for bare cardiovascular survival let alone full resuscitation. Other experiments such as those of Coxon (1960) have shown that after collapsing the lungs of experimental animals by the injection of saline into the pleural cavities, the introduction of intra-gastric oxygen did not revive the animals or increase survival time, whereas lung ventilation succeeded. On all sides there is an increasing clamour against this line of treatment, pointing out that time may be dangerously lost by wasting it in this direction instead of getting on with pulmonary inflation. The really disturbing thing about this story is how far we are removed from being able to assess the value of any particular treatment and that the so-called scientific world in this respect is still subject to fashion and guesswork. There is no doubt, however, that the newborn baby very rapidly fills its intestinal tract with swallowed air and this would appear to depend on respiratory activity, including crying, so that these X-ray evidences furnish a good index of vigour at birth. It is now very much doubted that the phenomenon in any way assists the baby's oxygenation (Fig. 4).

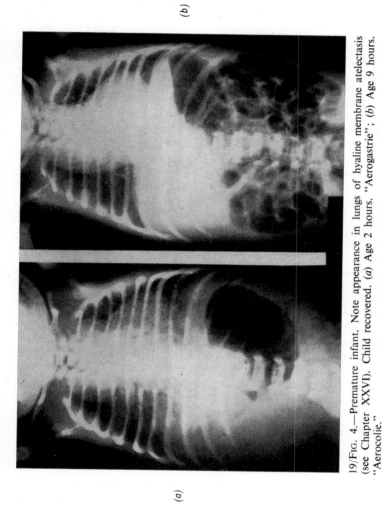

(b)

(a)

19/Fig. 4.—Premature infant. Note appearance in lungs of hyaline membrane atelectasis (see Chapter XXVI). Child recovered. (a) Age 2 hours. "Aerogastrie"; (b) Age 9 hours. "Aerocolie."

(By courtesy of Professor R. E. Steiner.)

Hypothermia.—Theoretically there would appear to be a case for this line of treatment in order to reduce the metabolic needs of the baby at birth and to play for time while some form of satisfactory oxygenation could be assured. This has led Westin and his team in Stockholm to introduce a system of rapid cooling with cold water. Using previable human fœtuses removed by abdominal hysterotomy for therapeutic reasons, often psychiatric, survival time has been impressively prolonged by perfusing with oxygenated blood in addition. This experimental approach to the problem is easier to carry out in Sweden than in most other countries because of different accepted indications for termination of pregnancy. Many of us have been too impressed with the difficulties of reviving a thoroughly chilled premature infant to feel inclined to adopt this line without more experimental evidence.

Cardiac massage.—This is clearly only applicable where a baby dies at the moment of birth or thereafter when the institution of this treatment can be immediate and before irrevocable brain damage is done. Open cardiac massage by thoracotomy, with all its entailed hazards, has been replaced by closed chest cardiac massage which is further facilitated by the softness of a baby's thoracic cage. Pressure is made downwards with two fingers just to the left of the sternum, towards the vertebral column, depressing the chest wall for about half to one inch, 80 to 100 times per minute. Needless to say pulmonary ventilation must be maintained at the same time and the single-handed operator will, therefore, have to employ mouth-to-mouth breathing as well (Gallagher and Neligan, 1962). If someone is present to maintain pulmonary ventilation by endotracheal oxygen so much the better, but it is important that both procedures should be combined. It is best to lay the baby on a hard surface such as a trolley top and although the heart may readily restart, inflation must be maintained until spontaneous respiration is satisfactorily re-established. A number of reports of success from this prompt line of treatment are now coming in, but clearly it is rather limited. In the case of stillbirths death has seldom occurred so recently before access can be obtained to institute cardiac massage and even if success could be won, it would only be rewarded by the tragedy of permanent cerebral damage. The neonatal babies who suffer from cardiac arrest usually do so for some gross reason which is already defying treatment. Nevertheless, if opportunities are not to be lost one must be mentally alert at the time of the crisis in order not to lose precious seconds.

Hyperbaric oxygen treatment.—Since a high pressure oxygen caisson was installed at the Western Infirmary, Glasgow, my pædiatric colleagues, Professor Hutchison and his team (1962), have been exploring this line of treatment in the case of asphyxiated babies.

At first only cases of respiratory distress syndrome could be treated in this manner because they had to be brought across the town from the Royal Maternity Hospital to the Western Infirmary and therefore acute respiratory emergencies at birth could not be treated by this means. It was soon found that this was a quick method of stuffing oxygen into a baby, but the treatment was unable to influence severe respiratory acidosis which complicates the respiratory distress syndrome. However, encouraged by the rapidity of oxygenation achieved, a small-sized caisson* was built and installed in the Maternity Hospital and since then it has been extensively used for correcting severe asphyxia at birth. It is now reserved for cases of primary apnœa mainly, and babies are only placed in the chamber if they have an Apgar score less than five and have failed to respond to the usual conservative methods within five minutes of birth. The pressure is rapidly built up to four atmospheres absolute (45 lb. per square inch). The baby may be in the caisson for fifteen to thirty minutes and if access to it is required decompression can be quite rapid (a matter of seconds) and because pure oxygen is used the problem of nitrogen bubbles within the circulation and central nervous system from decompression does not arise. It is clear that if the treatment is going to work it works rapidly and well and with a minimum of trauma to the baby. There have been no cases of oxygen poisoning nor oxygen convulsions. These babies are desperately in need of oxygen and the treatment is only a short-term one in any case. In a baby who is not showing any signs of spontaneous respiratory activity, such as this treatment is designed for, it is a little difficult to understand how the oxygen gets into it, but at this tremendous pressure there must be considerable absorption from any exposed mucous membranes and possibly through the skin.

It is always difficult to evaluate any new treatment of asphyxia neonatorum which may be due to so many different causes in babies of such differing weights and maturity as are likely to present one with the emergency. However, an attempt at a controlled trial of hyperbaric oxygen versus intubation and intermittent positive pressure with oxygen, as a method of resuscitation in babies, has been carried out jointly at the Queen Mother's Hospital and the Royal Maternity Hospital, Glasgow, selecting the patients by a system of cluster and random sampling (Hutchison et al., 1966). The trial was carried out over many months and covered a sufficiently large group of cases to be able to infer from its results that there was practically no significant difference between the two methods and whether the babies were mature or premature.

Nobody denies the value of endotracheal intubation and positive pressure assistance to the asphyxiated baby's breathing, but as

* Vickers Research Establishment.

Hutchison has pointed out, the availability of adequately trained personnel to carry out intubation safely in all maternity units at all hours of the day and night is simply not a fact; whereas unskilled people can put a baby, after airway clearance, into a simple pressure caisson and turn on the oxygen taps and it is suggested that this at least provides a safe and easily acceptable alternative. Experiments on asphyxiated animals at birth have very little relevance in assessing this sort of treatment. They are not strictly comparable to the case of the baby whose myocardial glycogen reserves may have been undergoing prolonged depletion before the moment of birth. Although Cross and his colleagues (1964) observed that in such a deliberate experiment of asphyxiating mature fœtal rabbits at birth beyond "the last gasp", 10 of 12 treated by intermittent positive pressure ventilation recovered whereas none of all the 17 which received hyperbaric oxygen survived. Gupta and Tizard (1967) have pointed out the difference between babies in primary apnoea and those terminal cases asphyxiated beyond the "last gasp", a matter which can only be decided retrospectively and they suggest that the efficacy of any new method of resuscitation should only be judged in the case of babies in terminal apnoea. Primary apnoea declares itself by babies whose heart rates accelerate before the start of resuscitation and who respond to treatment by gasping before an improvement in colour. The converse is not true necessarily, but the argument is that since endotracheal oxygenation is effective after the last gasp, all apnœic babies ought to be given the benefit of the doubt and intubated; but they admit that if a baby has even taken a partial gasp, exposure to hyperbaric oxygen might then be effective even through a limited alveolar bed. It is as well that terminal cases of apnoea are so relatively uncommon compared with the others or one might indeed find oneself constantly trying to salvage cases with a questionable long term prognosis.

Ideally every baby at its birth should have in attendance somebody capable of safe, atraumatic endotracheal intubation, whereupon the controversy would be quelled.

Prophylaxis.—One may well ask, in view of the frequent occurrence of the emergency of neonatal asphyxia, whether something cannot be done to reduce this hazard. Unfortunately, there is no specific prophylactic measure, for much of the whole art and science of obstetrics is challenged, and there is not a great deal of credit in delivering a baby barely alive as a result of its almost catastrophic entry into the world.

Good antenatal supervision should forestall many of the possible difficulties of labour, will prevent the greater part of eclampsia, and will play at least some part in mitigating the prematurity risk, to mention only a few examples.

In labour itself the early detection of fœtal distress is important, the choice of drugs and their timing should be judicious, episiotomy will often spare a baby the last lethal straw and skilful use of the obstetric forceps may make all the difference between intracranial hæmorrhage and survival. The use of pudendal block local anæsthesia, whenever possible, in forceps delivery makes an impressive difference to the incidence of neonatal asphyxia.

Late prognosis.—Obstetricians often lose sight of the infant they have delivered, and reports assessing the part which asphyxia at birth may have played in causing subsequent disability are not numerous.

Schreiber, in an analysis of 900 mental defectives, found that there was evidence of some birth asphyxia in 70 per cent. Although one of the editorials of the *British Medical Journal* (1952) rather played down the late damaging effects, one is inclined to the view that anoxia never did anyone any good, even a baby, and although it is no more than conjecture, it is more than likely that ten minutes' asphyxia will at least reduce a sixth form intelligence to that of the lower fourth. In Aberdeen, however, Fraser and Wilks (1959) have given a somewhat less depressing picture having followed up 100 children who had suffered delay in the onset of satisfactory respiration at birth. In 40 of the cases asphyxia had been severe. Nevertheless, neurological examination at the age of seven and a half years showed major abnormality in surprisingly few, but minor disorders of personality and perception as compared with the control group were noted. Likewise in Aberdeen Fairweather and Illsley (1960) investigating mentally handicapped children came to the conclusion that social and genetic factors were more responsible than obstetric complications for the development of the disabilities.

A study of school performance at the age of 11 has been undertaken in the case of 50,000 children whose birth records were known (Barker and Edwards, 1967). It was interesting to note that they found impaired performance mainly associated with only 5 of the obstetric complications studied, namely, prematurity, post-maturity, toxæmia, occipito-posterior position and delivery in an ambulance. This last-mentioned type of event was a little difficult to explain even on the basis of social grading of the mother.

Mention has already been made in Chapter I of "at risk registers" in order that the fate of children may be followed up by casting the observation net as wide as possible, but the value of this has been challenged by Richards and Roberts (1967) who maintain that such registers have led "to a situation in which an undefined population is being screened for undefined conditions by people who, for the most part, are untrained to detect the conditions for which they are looking," and rightly claiming that there is no alternative to sound

clinical examination of all infants in the neonatal period and appropriate screening thereafter, but this is a counsel of perfection.

The most severe cases which manage to survive may suffer cerebral diplegia. Cerebral palsy may not only be attributable to genetic factors, to maternal infection in early pregnancy or to toxæmia, but may be due to damage through anoxia or intracranial bleeding in the course of labour. Multiple pregnancy and prematurity and likewise kernicterus are also believed to be important causes. The significance of convulsions is particularly ominous and Craig (1960) noted that apart from the high mortality following them (42 per cent), in the survivors who are followed up for the next three years the incidence of mental or physical handicap was nearly three times (8 per cent) as compared with those who had had postnatal asphyxia without convulsions. The degree to which subsequent epilepsy may be caused by brain damage at birth has not yet been fully determined, but Earle *et al.* (1953) in necropsy studies of 157 cases of temporal lobe epileptiform seizures found that in 63 per cent there was evidence of compression or damage at birth to the temporal lobes believed to be caused by a temporary herniation, under pressure of the skull at birth, through the incisura of the tentorium cerebelli involving particularly one or both hippocampal gyri. In the intellectual field all gradations from mental backwardness to personality disorders and epilepsy may originate from life's first critical quarter of an hour, and it is as well to assume that in resuscitating the newborn one is fighting not only for the child's life but for its very wits.

In summary, resuscitation procedure is usually carried out in the following order

1. Clear the pharynx, mouth and nostrils by suction.

2. Lay child, head sloped downwards, in warm cot—until aspiration of stomach completed and then prop up to assist breathing.

3. Supply oxygen either by tent or face mask.

4. If child is limp, insert an airway to deal with sagging tongue.

5. If no improvement, rocking or a respirator may be employed.

6. If still no improvement after a few minutes', the trachea is intubated under direct vision and positive pressure lung inflation employed.

N.B.—If the child is born in marked white asphyxia, this is done earlier.

7. If respiratory depression can be attributed to morphine or pethidine given to the mother, inject 0·5 mg. N-allylnormorphine into umbilical vein.

8. Inject coramine 0·25–0·5 ml. intravenously into the cord.

9. External cardiac massage, combined with continuing pulmonary ventilation.

Fortunately, most cases revive before the whole of the above ritual has to be gone through, and those that do not are by now irretrievably dead.

Further Treatment—Cerebral Irritation

Once the immediate emergency of asphyxia in the labour ward has been overcome the baby may, nevertheless, continue in some jeopardy for the next 48 hours, particularly if fœtal shock was severe in the first place. It may demonstrate signs of cerebral irritation, of which the following are the more significant:

1. Liability to apnœic, grey or blue attacks.
2. Twitching and convulsions.
3. Hyperexcitability on switching on a light in the room or making a sharp noise.
4. High-pitched shrill cry.
5. Restlessness and wakefulness.
6. Grunting respirations.
7. Rapid, shallow or irregular respiration.
8. Blue lips.
9. Rolling eyes.
10. Neck rigidity.
11. Bulging anterior fontanelle.
12. Temperature instability.

The differential diagnosis is often a matter of great clinical difficulty. Atelectasis, especially with hyaline membrane, pneumonia, intraventricular hæmorrhage in premature babies and subdural hæmorrhage in the more mature, can be very difficult to distinguish without special tests, but radiology of the chest (Donald and Steiner, 1953) and spirometry may be of assistance. The treatment of cerebral irritation demands minimum handling, sufficient oxygen concentration in the atmosphere to maintain a good colour but no more than is strictly needed, warmth and repeated aspiration of pharynx and stomach by suction at the first sign of a blue attack. Because of the dangers of regurgitation it is necessary to withhold all fluid or feeding, for 48 hours often, except for the administration of sedatives, for example, phenobarbitone gr. $\frac{1}{8}$ (8 mg.) or chloral gr. 1–3 (60–200 mg.) in syrup, which may be repeatedly required to afford the child sorely needed rest.

REFERENCES

AKERREN, Y., and FURSTENBERG, N. (1950). *J. Obstet. Gynæc. Brit. Emp.*, **57**, 705.

APGAR, V. (1953). *Curr. Res. Anesth.*, **32**, 260–267.

BARCROFT, J. (1946). *Researches on Prenatal Life*. Oxford: Blackwell Scientific Publications.

BARKER, D. J. P., and EDWARDS, J. H. (1967). *Brit. med. J.*, **2**, 695.
BARRIE, H., COTTOM, D., and WILSON, B. D. R. (1962). *Lancet*, **2**, 742.
BARRIE, H. (1963). *Lancet*, **1**, 650.
BORN, G. V. R., DAWES, G. S., MOTT, J. C., and WIDDICOMBE, J. G. (1954). *Cold Spr. Harb. Symp. quant. Biol.*, **19**, 102.
CARTER, R. E. B. (1957). *Lancet*, **1**, 1292.
COOPER, F. A., SMITH, H., and PASK, E. A. (1960). *Anæsthesia*, **15**, 211.
CORNER, B. (1962). *Proc. roy. Soc. Med.*, **55**, 1005.
COXON, R. V. (1960). *Lancet*, **1**, 1315.
CRAIG, W. S. (1960). *Arch. Dis. Childh.*, **35**, 336.
CROSS, K. W., DAWES, G. S., HYMAN, A., and MOTT, JOAN C. (1964). *Lancet*, **2**, 560.
CROSS, K. W., KLAUS, M., TOOLEY, W. H., and WEISSER, K. (1960). *J. Physiol. (Lond.)*, **151**, 551.
CROSS, K. W., and ROBERTS, P. W. (1951). *Brit. med. J.*, **1**, 1043.
DAWES, G. S., MOTT, J. C., WIDDICOMBE, J. G., and WYATT, D. G. (1953). *J. Physiol. (Lond.)*, **121**, 141.
DAWKINS, M. J. R., MARTIN, J. D., and SPECTOR, W. E. (1961). *J. Obstet. Gynæc. Brit. Commonw.*, **68**, 604.
DONALD, I. (1954). *J. Obstet. Gynæc. Brit. Emp.*, **61**, 725.
DONALD, I. (1957). *Brit. J. Anæsth.*, **29**, 553.
DONALD, I. (1963). "Asphyxia neonatorum", in *The Obstetrician, Anæsthetist and Pediatrician*. Oxford: Pergamon Press.
DONALD, I., KERR, M. M., and MACDONALD, I. R., (1958). *Scot. med. J.* **3**, 151.
DONALD, I., and LORD, J. (1953). *Lancet*, **1**, 9.
DONALD, I., and STEINER, R. E. (1953). *Lancet*, **2**, 846.
DONALD, I., and YOUNG, I. M. (1952). *J. Physiol. (Lond.)*, **116**, 41P.
EARLE, K. M., BALDWIN, M., and PENFIELD, W. (1953). *Arch. Neurol. Psychiat. (Chic.)*, **69**, 27.
EVE, F. C., and FORSYTH, N. C. (1948). *Lancet*, **2**, 554.
FAIRWEATHER, D. V. I., and ILLSLEY, R. (1960). *Brit. J. prev. soc. Med.*, **14**, 149.
FLAGG, P. J. (1931). *Amer. J. Obstet. Gynec.*, **21**, 537.
FRASER, M. S., and WILKS, J. (1959). *J. Obstet. Gynæc. Brit. Emp.*, **66**, 748.
GALLAGHER, B., and NELIGAN, G. (1962). *Brit. med. J.*, **1**, 400.
GELLIS, S. S., WHITE, P., and PFEFFER, W. (1949). *New Engl. J. Med.*, **240**, 533.
GIBBERD, G. F., and BLAIKLEY, J. B. (1935). *Lancet*, **1**, 138.
GUPTA, J. M., and TIZARD, J. P. M. (1967). *Lancet*, **2**, 55.
HOLMES, J. M. (1961). *Brit. med. J.*, **1**, 1317.
HUTCHISON, J. H., KERR, MARGARET M., INALL, J. A., and SHANKS, R. A. (1966). *Lancet*, **1**, 935.
HUTCHISON, J. H., KERR, M. M., McPHAIL, M. F., DOUGLAS, T. A., SMITH, G., NORMAN, J. N., and BATES, F. A. (1962). *Lancet*, **2**, 465.
JAYKKA, S. (1957). *Acta paediat. (Uppsala)*, **46**, Suppl. 112.
JAYKKA, S. (1958). *Acta. paediat. (Uppsala)*, **47**, 484.
KARLBERG, P. (1960). *J. Pediat.*, **56**, 585.
LERMAN, S. I. (1967). *Lancet*, **2**, 265.

MacRae, D. J. (1962). *Lancet,* **2,** 701.

Mann, T. P., and Elliott, R. I. K. (1957). *Lancet,* **1,** 229.

Melchior, J. C., Svensmark, O., and Trolle, D. (1967). *Lancet,* **2,** 860.

Mott, J. C. (1961). *Brit. med. Bull.,* **17,** 146.

Potter, E. L., and Rosenbaum, W. (1943). *Amer . J. Obstet. Gynec.,* **45,** 822.

Richards, I. D. G., and Roberts, C. J. (1967). *Lancet,* **2,** 711.

Roberts, H. (1949). *J. Obstet. Gynæc. Brit. Emp.,* **56,** 961.

Roberts, H., Kane, K. M., Percival, N., Snow, P., and Please, N. W. (1957). *Lancet,* **1,** 128.

Schreiber, F. (1938). *J. Amer. med. Ass.,* **3,** 1263.

Shelley, H. J. (1961). *Brit. med. Bull.,* **17,** 137.

Stafford, A., and Weatherall, J. A. C. (1960). *J. Physiol. (Lond.),* **153,** 457.

Westin, B., Nyburg, R., Miller, J. A., and Wedenburg, E. (1962). *Acta. paediat. (Uppsala),* Suppl. 139.

Yllpo, A. (1935). *Acta paediat. (Uppsala),* **17,** Suppl. 1, 122.

CHAPTER XX

POSTPARTUM COLLAPSE

IN an emergency it is strange, but nevertheless true, that the more desperate the patient's condition the more difficult may accurate diagnosis become. If the delivery has been a difficult one, the attendant's powers of judgment may be undermined by temporary loss of morale, and reactions vary widely according to temperament from that of "Put her legs down, wrap her up, she will probably be all right presently," to gloomy speculations about the extent of hidden injuries inflicted, and only experience will counter the highly individual variations in outlook.

It is true, however, that in the absence of active bleeding, time and nature are on one's side, and it is generally wise to remember that if in doubt about what to do one should do nothing, apart from obvious routine resuscitative measures, until that doubt is clearly resolved.

Only a small minority of cases of collapse after delivery occur without hæmorrhage. Bleeding brooks no delay, both in stopping it and replacing quantitatively that which is lost; but from time to time it will appear that the deterioration in the patient's condition is out of all proportion to the amount of blood which she has lost, and it is the assessment of this factor, the factor of coincident or superimposed shock, which is the theme of this chapter, and an attempt is made to present the problem from the viewpoint of the doctor who finds himself confronted with such a worrying situation.

It is obvious that messy delivery, in which blood is allowed to run to waste on to sheets and bedding and into the bucket and which cannot, therefore, be even approximately measured, is going to deny the opportunity of relating the woman's condition to hæmorrhage alone, and the habit of tidy work is just as important as in other branches of surgery. As far as possible all blood lost should be carefully collected for measuring. Even an unsutured episiotomy can surreptitiously cost a patient a pint or two of blood and the slow but steady trickle may pass, for a time, unnoticed.

The importance of "blood accountancy" can, therefore, be stressed *ad infinitum* but never *ad nauseam*.

Where it can be reasonably certain that a patient has lost, for example, no more than 25–30 ounces and yet is collapsed, two groups of conditions must be quickly reviewed:

(*a*) Blood is being lost but not externally.

(*b*) Other shock-producing factors are operative.

650

Since the conditions in the first group demand the promptest treatment, a search in this direction should first be undertaken, and the most likely sites are within the body of the uterus itself, the peritoneal cavity and the retro-peritoneal spaces.

A uterus which is slowly filling with blood may often be fairly hard, and only the increase of its overall size may reveal what is happening; the impression of size on palpation is more important than actual height of fundus.

Quite large quantities of blood can lie in the peritoneal cavity without producing many physical signs locally, although general signs of shock are obvious; pain is often much less than would be expected, of abdominal rigidity there is of course none, tenderness may be very indefinite, and the most noticeable features may be bulging of the flanks, dullness to percussion and the patient's clear dislike of lying down flat and thereby allowing blood to run up under the diaphragm.

Many hæmorrhages into the retro-peritoneal tissue spaces and between the layers of the broad ligament are overlooked if not large, but they too add to the patient's shock over and above the amount of blood lost to circulation.

The following is a table classifying the various causes of post-partum collapse, bearing in mind always that shock and hæmorrhage are interlocked in a sort of synergism.

COLLAPSE

Hæmorrhage

Non-hæmorrhagic shock

Obstetric Accidents	Obstetric Shock ("Idiopathic")	Surgical Traumatic	Coincidental Accidents
1. Retained products		1. Ruptured uterus	1. Acute cardiac failure
2. Retained clot		2. Post-operative shock	2. Pulmonary collapse
3. Acute inversion		3. Retroperitoneal and broad ligament hæmatoma	3. Anæsthetic accidents, especially inhaled vomit
4. Pulmonary embolism, especially amniotic fluid embolism		4. Accidents to ovarian cysts	4. Reaction to drugs including local anæsthetics
5. Concealed ante-partum hæmor-rhage			5. Previous corticosteroid therapy
6. Eclampsia			6. Pneumothorax
			7. Ruptured aneurysm
			8. Subarachnoid hæmorrhage
			9. Coronary thrombosis
			10. *Status lymphaticus*

Published data on postpartum shock deal only with cases that end in death, and innumerable cases of profound shock occur in practice which never find their way into print because they recover and the reason for the shock cannot always be accurately attributed.

HÆMORRHAGE

In the hæmorrhage group, patients vary widely in their reaction to blood loss and the amount of collapse thereby suffered. The highly multiparous patient, besides being more liable to bleed on that account alone, stands hæmorrhage worse than the primigravid patient quite apart from the question of age; the stresses, moreover, of previous child-bearing and child-rearing may tell their tale. Antenatal health is therefore of very great importance. There is nothing like anæmia to beget anæmia, and the positive health measures of good antenatal care go a long way towards fortifying the patient against the vicissitudes of labour. A woman approaching labour with a hæmoglobin of 65 per cent (9·6 g.) or less faces it with some peril, and all antenatal conditions producing fatigue exaggerate the effects of labour itself. Where some complication of pregnancy has occurred such as antepartum hæmorrhage, be it due to placenta prævia or accidental placental separation, only a relatively small postpartum loss is necessary to tip the scales towards a state of collapse.

A lengthy, exhausting and dehydrating labour likewise magnifies the effects of postpartum bleeding.

It is, therefore, difficult to relate the degree of collapse absolutely to quantitative blood loss without taking such antecedent factors into account. At the end of the second stage of labour there is a physiological mechanism, akin to shock in miniature, which helps to protect the patient from hæmorrhage by reducing the blood pressure. Any shock factors which may develop or be already operative are superimposed upon this mechanism but with this important difference—their clinical manifestations are delayed, often by as many as ten minutes, so that by the time a further drop in blood pressure is recorded as the result, for example, of bleeding, one is already so many minutes out of date in assessing the general condition. To recognise this is to improve one's choice of the optimum moment for active intervention in ridding the patient of her placenta with the minimum of additional operative shock. This point is dealt with more fully in the chapter on postpartum hæmorrhage.

The general appearance of the patient, coupled with an exact knowledge of the amount of blood lost is, therefore, more objectively important even than the blood pressure at the moment or the state of the pulse.

NON-HÆMORRHAGIC SHOCK

This does not differ in its manifestations from shock encountered in other fields of medicine.

Sheehan (1948) has fully described his findings at autopsy in a large number of obstetrical disasters and made interesting observations.

Blood flow is greatly reduced, but not evenly throughout the body, since the processes of vasoconstriction spare the brain with its vital centres as far as possible. Blood flow through the skin is greatly reduced, hence the impression of pallor and coldness. Such circulation as persists in the skin is sluggish, and the damage done by a hot-water bottle, which a healthy person would regard as no more than very warm, can be very extensive because the heat is not carried away and dispersed and any toxic products from local overheating are not rapidly diluted in the circulation.

Muscle blood flow and all visceral blood flow is reduced, so that stagnation and pooling are general, except in the brain as aforesaid.

All renal filtration usually stops at systolic blood pressures of less than 80 mm. Hg, so that anuria results. The duration of uncorrected shock will determine in large measure the recovery of renal function.

The heart is operating under grave handicaps, the venous return is reduced and atrial filling is poor, so that cardiac output falls, and even acceleration of the heart cannot compensate for the deficiency because of a stroke output which may be as low as 20 ml.

These effects, namely vasoconstriction and tachycardia, are the result of sympathetic activity, and as Sheehan points out, are highly protective in cases of hæmorrhage by mitigating further blood loss and maintaining blood supply to the vital centres, but where shock without blood loss occurs, this mechanism may be harmful by embarrassing the heart's action through poor venous return and thus precipitating cardiac failure. To transfuse the patient liberally with blood under such circumstances, quite apart from increasing the general stagnant pooling of blood, will only increase the heart's difficulties, while the administration of adrenaline, by heightening sympathetic effects, will aggravate the process.

The need, therefore, to judge how much the patient's state is due to bleeding and how much to shock factors now becomes obvious and should discourage indiscriminate blood transfusion.

The latent period of delay in falling blood pressure has already been mentioned. There are two stages in the process. Initially, there is a fall in pulse pressure because the diastolic pressure is first increased due to vasoconstriction and the systolic pressure is for a time maintained; then, as the condition worsens, vasoconstriction

begins to fail, the heart meanwhile becoming more inefficient, and both systolic and diastolic pressures fall together. The awareness of pain is for some unknown reason dulled.

Other autonomic effects are to be found in dilatation of the stomach, the ascending colon and the proximal half of the transverse colon, corresponding to the predominant sympathetic nerve supply of the intestinal tract.

The liver is liable to suffer central necrosis in the lobules due to vasoconstriction and reduced blood pressure, a state of affairs made worse (Govan and McGillivray) if there is also pre-eclamptic toxæmia or if further vasoconstricting drugs are given, and these changes in the liver may have something to do with irreversibility in shock.

Postpartum Pituitary Necrosis

The anterior lobe of the pituitary is very susceptible to damage, and as a result of thrombosis in the vessels supplying it, suffers necrosis to greater or lesser degree. The immediate effects are less noticeable and serious than the remote. There is initially a tendency towards hypoglycæmia and lactation is never established. Later the signs of hypopituitarism are manifested (Simmonds' disease), a condition which used to be called superinvolution, and in which there is a degree of genital atrophy with amenorrhœa and usually sterility. The term Sheehan's syndrome is now used when referring to this type of hypopituitarism dating from hæmorrhage and shock at delivery. Murdoch (1962) analysed 57 cases admitted to Glasgow hospitals with this diagnosis since 1950. The commonest reasons for admission being lassitude, nausea and breathlessness of increasing severity. Of these patients, 10 were already dead at the time of review and it would appear that pryrexial illnesses are particularly dangerous in precipitating hypopituitary coma. Any disease associated with vomiting has likewise a bad effect. There may be some delay in the development of the full-blown Sheehan's syndrome and in any case in which there has been severe hæmorrhage or shock at delivery and in whom lactation does not subsequently occur, damage sustained by the anterior pituitary should be watched for in the course of the next year, declaring itself in amenorrhœa, intolerance to cold, lassitude and general debility. Microcytic anæmia often adds to the patient's wretched state and does not respond readily to iron therapy, but may be helped by the addition of testosterone.

The patients may be subjectively much improved by treating with thyroid extract and cortisone 25 mg. daily.

General listlessness, apathy and intolerance of cold will remain with the patient for the rest of her prematurely senile life, perhaps another thirty years, until, with increasing tendency to myxœdemat-

ous changes and a persistent anæmia, some intercurrent infection closes the tragic chapter. The fact that this disease is not more commonly seen is due to the number of candidates for it who die before it has a chance to reveal itself, and in the future the more prompt treatment of postpartum collapse, which is now more generally available, should lessen the incidence still further, for the duration of a state of shock is more damaging in the long run than the degree. Up to the present only the stimulus of another pregnancy, itself an unlikely event, will restore youthful health by bringing about a hypertrophy of such glandular tissue in the anterior pituitary as has escaped ischæmic necrosis.

Anuria

Another grave sequel of protracted shock is acute renal tubular necrosis, dealt with more fully elsewhere. It has already been stated that renal filtration ceases with systolic blood pressures below 80 mm. Hg, and, within the course of a very few hours of uncorrected shock, sufficient renal damage is sustained to stop the secretion of urine completely or reduce it to a few turbid ounces. Any case of severe shock ought, therefore, to be very carefully watched for several days for signs of urinary suppression.

The Factor of Prolonged Labour

Of Sheehan's 147 cases which he examined post-mortem, it was found that, leaving aside cases of uterine rupture, the fatal cases resulting from a strenuous delivery had in no instance laboured for less than two days, and it is clear that resistance to shock depends very much upon the condition in which the first as well as the second stage of labour leaves a patient. Fatigue, dehydration and acidosis are thus powerful contributory factors.

Turning now to the table previously given, some of the causes of collapse require some discussion.

OBSTETRIC ACCIDENTS

Retained Placenta without Bleeding

There is no creature more treacherous than a woman who retains her placenta after delivery of her child. Not only may she start a severe hæmorrhage at any unpredictable moment, and cannot therefore be left unattended, but as time goes on her general condition is very liable to deteriorate, though the mechanism of this phenomenon is not yet understood. Of Sheehan's 147 fatal cases, no fewer than 35 had retention of the placenta for over two hours, and even though manual removal might be very difficult, the shock thereof as a cause of death is very unlikely if undertaken within the

first two hours of the third stage. Where hæmorrhage has occurred it is, therefore, obviously desirable that the patient's condition should be restored sufficiently to allow manual removal of the placenta to be undertaken within that time interval, and, as is discussed in the chapter on postpartum hæmorrhage, this opportunity may be missed through neglect of very prompt restorative measures as soon as the primary blood loss occurs, so that by the time manual removal is decided upon the patient is sinking for the second time and cannot surface anything like so quickly. This is a thoroughly dangerous situation, in which the shock of the operation in an exsanguinated and hypotensive patient has to be weighed against the shock induced by longer retention of the placenta and the long time it may take for the blood transfusion to bring her to a safe level for operation.

If a placenta does not separate within two hours of delivery of the child, the chances of a safe and spontaneous separation are becoming too slender to count upon and there is, therefore, nothing to be gained by waiting. One knows of cases in which the placenta has been left in the uterus for several days without harm to the patient, but such sang-froid on the part of the attendant is little better than recklessness, and one wonders how thorough was the watch kept upon her throughout this time.

Authorities vary in the time limit they set; most of us take steps to deliver the placenta after one hour of waiting, and anything up to about four hours is probably safe though pointless, and two hours can be taken as a sensible maximum. At the end of the second stage the patient is naturally tired and in need of a good sleep, thus it is impossible to observe a protracted third stage and at the same time keep her both warm, dry and comfortable.

Retained Clot

To a lesser extent much of what has been said above applies here. Quite apart from the fact that clot will encourage further bleeding, such a patient often "perks up" very noticeably after the uterus has been emptied by a judicious squeeze which every midwife administers before turning her back on the patient. This sound and simple practice is often neglected at the end of a Cæsarean section while the patient is still anæsthetised and therefore in no state to object, and it is certain that it makes a great difference to the immediate postoperative condition on return to the ward.

Acute Inversion

This is dealt with fully elsewhere, but as a cause of collapse it must be very quickly excluded or treated, and should be one of the

first possibilities to cross the obstetrician's mind. Cord pulling is now more fashionable, but it is well to remember that about 15 per cent of cases of acute inversion occur spontaneously and for no apparent reason. In three-quarters of such cases the placenta is inserted at the fundus, the least common site of all, and there is no means of foreseeing this possibility.

The complete inversion of the third degree is the rarest variety, and it is where the inverted mass does not protrude into view that such a cause of collapse may be overlooked. Abdominal palpation should be made at once to determine the whereabouts and the shape of the uterine fundus, and where this is in doubt, for example in a case of gross obesity, a vaginal examination may have to be made.

Pulmonary Embolism

This rare complication of labour has been noted from time to time, and the embolus may consist of air, thrombus or liquor amnii with its ingredients of meconium, vernix caseosa, etc. (Steiner and Lushbaugh).

For an air embolus to enter the circulation, part at least of the placental site must be exposed which in the normal third stage is unlikely before its completion and delivery of the membranes. Nevertheless, it would appear to be a wise precaution to keep the patient's knees together and to wait for the uterus to harden before changing her position, for example from left lateral to dorsal.

An air embolus may be introduced in the course of intra-uterine manipulation which has been preceded by some placental separation. Attempts to hurry up blood transfusion by increasing the pressure of air within a transfusion bottle, usually by means of a Higginson's syringe, for example, may end in sudden catastrophe and I have had one such case in my own experience. I had just finished operating on her for a severe and hæmorrhagic vault laceration and left instructions for the remainder of the almost full bottle of blood which she was then receiving to be given. Leaving the department, I got no further than the hospital gate when I was recalled to find that the patient, who only a few minutes before had been making a good recovery, was now dead, yet only about half the bottle of blood had been given. In fact bloodclot had formed well up the filter inside the bottle and the pressure had been built up inside the bottle with a Higginson's syringe in order to complete the transfusion hurriedly and quite unnecessarily. A truly massive air embolus had been instantly fatal. Modern transfusion giving sets are far safer in this respect than the older patterns, but, even so, a watch must be kept to see that the bottle does not empty and that only blood and not air is being driven down the tubing. The effects of embolism are immediate

and shock will have to be treated at once. Intravenous morphia 15 mg. (gr. ¼) with oxygen therapy are the two most useful emergency measures. Transfusion and infusion are both contra-indicated if there is no blood loss to replace, inasmuch as they aggravate the pulmonary œdema which, in any case, is bound to develop. When cardiac arrest occurs because of an air embolus, cardiac massage is only likely to make matters even worse, because air will be driven into the pulmonary circulation. The correct treatment is aspiration of the air out of the right ventricle with a wide bore needle. Unfortunately there is seldom time for effective treatment which in any case is only likely to benefit the borderline case. A useful, immediate, first-aid procedure is to place the patient in the head-down, left lateral position in the hope of displacing the bolus of air towards the apex of the right ventricle. In the case of smaller volumes of air now in the right side of the heart it may be possible for pulmonary circulation to continue until the air bubble is gradually passed piecemeal and less dramatically into the pulmonary system.

Amniotic fluid embolism is more common than recognised and produces profound shock, dyspnœa, tachycardia, cyanosis and, if not immediately fatal, hyperpyrexia. The worst case of this sort which I have encountered was admitted in strong labour after artificial hind-water rupture to induce labour two days earlier. On admission she was obviously dyspnœic, grossly cyanosed, her temperature was 105° F., the fœtal heart was absent and her condition was indeed desperate. There had been no vomiting. As the cervix was almost fully dilated she was delivered with forceps without difficulty, but died without hæmorrhage in spite of oxygen and restorative measures 45 minutes later. Necropsy revealed massive amniotic fluid embolism but the site of entry of the liquor amnii into the circulation could not be demonstrated. Presumably the previous surgical induction, coupled with powerful uterine action, had established an entry track.

The emboli consist of particulate constituents of liquor amnii, namely epithelial squames, fat, lanugo hairs and meconium and can be demonstrated in the pulmonary arterioles and alveolar capillaries (Figs. 1 and 2).

Of all the causes of sudden disaster in labour, amniotic fluid embolism ranks high and, in fact, over a third of sudden deaths in a series reported from Liverpool (Tindall, 1965) would appear to have been due to this cause. The diagnosis can only definitely be established in the case of maternal death as a necropsy finding, and even so the evidences may have disappeared because of autolysis if there is much delay in carrying out the examination, as is often the case owing to inquest procedure; but the presumptive diagnosis is justified on clinical grounds when there is sudden collapse with tachycardia,

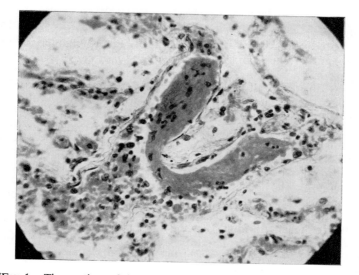

20/Fig. 1.—The section of lung capillary showing embolic mass of vernix material. The capillary is greatly distended and there is a leucocytic reaction in the vessel and in the capillaries of adjacent alveoli. (H. and E. × 500.)

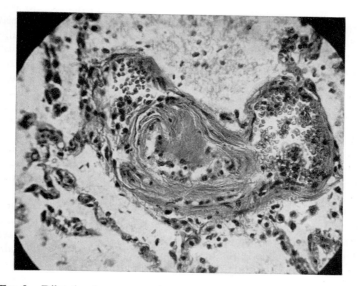

20/Fig. 2.—Dilated pulmonary vessel containing an embolic mass. The embolus consists of vernix material surrounded by bundles of squames. (H. and E. × 500.)

(Figs. 1 and 2 by courtesy of Dr. A. D. T. Govan.)

tachypnoea, cyanosis and hypotension. The two other conditions which produce an almost identical picture are acute pulmonary œdema due to mitral stenosis and the inhaled vomit syndrome presently to be described.

In by no means all cases, however, is death from amniotic fluid embolism immediate and clotting defects may develop within the course of the next hour or two due to intravascular microcoagulation involving particularly the pulmonary tree, thereby aggravating cyanosis. Blood coagulation failure from this variety of hypo-fibrinogenæmia may, in fact, be the first evidence that amniotic fluid embolism has occurred (see Chapter XIV). Although I have encountered serious hæmorrhage in such a case, this can be controlled by fibrinogen replacement. The lethal factor is the vascular obstruction to the pulmonary circulation. The very worst thing to do at this point is to prevent fibrinolysis by the use of antifibrinolytic agents and it is far preferable, almost paradoxically, to use heparin intravenously to prevent further vascular occlusion, using a loading dose of 5000 units intravenously immediately, followed by a drip administering 1,000 units per hour. No more fibrinogen should be given than is strictly necessary for the control of bleeding. The patient's danger is more immediate from her lungs than from her anæmic state. The diagnosis can to some extent be assisted by immediate X-ray, taken usually with a portable X-ray machine, because of the gravity of the patient's condition, but provided the patient does not die within the first few hours from the amniotic fluid embolus itself or, more likely, from injudicious treatment, resolution is rapid, presumably due to natural fibrinolysis of the widely scattered microthrombi (Fig. 3). If this variety of embolism, however, presents with pulmonary signs first, without signs of hæmorrhage, then heparin must be given courageously and without hesitation before the patient's lungs "solidify".

Figure 3 illustrates one of our own cases (Willocks *et al.*, 1966). The embolism occurred during the patient's third Cæsarean section and was associated with considerable blood loss. Pulmonary signs of cyanosis together with shock appeared during the operation which was carried out under endotracheal anæsthesia and not following it, as might have been expected, in the vomit aspiration syndrome. Ventilation was with difficulty adequately maintained with intermittent positive pressure using 100 per cent oxygen; at the same time attempts were made to maintain a degree of positive pressure during expiration to discourage increasing pulmonary œdema. Repeated tracheal aspiration was necessary to remove fluid from the lungs and aminophylline was administered. The base excess of –5 mEq/L. was quickly apparent and the pH of the blood rapidly fell to 7·28. This was corrected with 100 mEq. of sodium bicarbonate and low

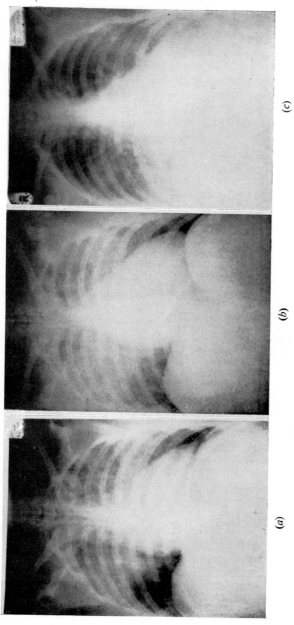

20/Fig. 3.—Amniotic fluid embolism

(a) Taken in operating theatre shortly after the occurrence.
(b) Five hours later. Patient's condition very critical.
(c) The following day nearly 24 hours after the onset.

Note the very rapid alteration in radiological appearances.

(a)

(b)

(c)

molecular weight dextran was given in the hope of increasing the pulmonary blood flow. Frusemide was also given intravenously (20 mg.) to reduce pulmonary œdema and digoxin 0·5 mg. together with intravenous hydrocortisone to maintain the circulation. It will be noted that fibrinogen was not given in spite of the hæmorrhage attending the operation. The blood loss was simply replaced. This case was much debated among us and we reckoned that the intermittent positive-pressure ventilation helped to reduce the pulmonary œdema, and at least we did not fall into the trap of aggravating the condition by giving the wrong treatment; the prompt correction of biochemical imbalance in the form of metabolic acidosis doubtless contributed to the recovery. These cases are sufficiently rare to leave one in considerable doubt as to how to cope with the emergency which is often completely unexpected and the above outline of treatment was unanimously agreed by all of us at the time.

Concealed Antepartum Hæmorrhage

The patient who has weathered this grave emergency to the point of delivery has little in reserve to withstand even minor third-stage difficulties. Attempts, therefore, to hurry delivery before recovery both of uterine tone and general condition are fraught with more than usual danger, and no less than 25 of Sheehan's cases died after delivery as a result of shock following concealed antepartum hæmorrhage. Precipitate labour following abruptio placentæ can lead to very profound shock, even in the absence of further hæmorrhage.

SURGICAL-TRAUMATIC

Ruptured Uterus (see Chapter XXII)

The fact that a woman has managed to deliver herself by no means rules out a diagnosis of uterine rupture, and where delivery has followed operative intervention, such a possibility is even more prominent.

I have known spontaneous rupture to occur both at the end of a straightforward delivery and during the apparently normal delivery of the second of twins.

It is a condition which carries a very high mortality, if neglected through failure to diagnose it, and even when treated still remains one of the worst hazards of childbearing. A previous Cæsarean section scar, particularly of the classical variety, should prime one's suspicions of uterine rupture in cases of collapse. Such scars may rupture rather insidiously. Internal version, difficult forceps operations, especially those involving rotation of the fœtal head, and, in fact, any major manipulative measure, all carry the obvious risks

of inflicting rupture which may only be appreciated after extraction of the child. The diagnosis is by no means easy, particularly in incomplete rupture, but where shock persists in spite of adequate blood transfusion to replace blood lost, this possibility should come readily to mind and the diagnosis promptly established by digital exploration of the uterus.

Operative Shock

Apart from any gross injury, the obstetric patient has no peculiar immunity from traumatic shock any more than the surgical case. It is nevertheless surprising how much sheer force the parturient woman will stand, provided that such force is not misapplied either in nature, timing or direction. However, the case is quite different if, for example, the cervix is not fully dilated and forcible delivery of the head, even though successful and without lacerating the cervix, is absolutely certain to produce some degree of shock, often very great. In such a case the lower segment of the uterus is pulled upon together with the attached ligaments with their rich supply of nerve fibres, and this fact, together with the light plane of anæsthesia usually employed, provides an adequate reason for shock; this complication is probably the commonest cause of all.

Antepartum hæmorrhage of any variety predisposes the patient to traumatic shock. Another all-too-frequent source of shock is the repeated use of Credé's method of attempting to deliver the placenta, and there are many obstetricians who have been so impressed by the damage thereby inflicted that they feel it is a manœuvre which should be abandoned; it has now disappeared from our own practice.

Innumerable such instances of misapplied force could be given; what makes matters so difficult is the uncertainty at the time whether or not some serious injury has been caused which calls for courageous surgery in a situation which is already grave.

Retroperitoneal and Broad Ligament Hæmatoma

These cases are usually due to incomplete uterine rupture, though occasionally there may be a traumatic rupture of the utero-ovarian venous system without tearing of the uterine wall. The source of the trouble is often not immediately obvious; the swelling may at first be very soft and boggy and only very careful examination may discover it.

Accidents to Ovarian Cysts

Torsion may occur in labour, and very occasionally a cyst finds itself in the path of the presenting part, and whether it ruptures or not shock is certain to occur.

COINCIDENTAL ACCIDENTS

The patient with a cardiac lesion may collapse and die within the first 24 hours. Here one is forewarned but not necessarily fore-armed, and even the most careful treatment (see Chapter IV) will not prevent every such disaster.

A case of eclampsia may suddenly show a most precipitate fall in blood pressure, a very serious sign and usually betokening a major vascular accident, often multiple. In some cases acute suprarenal failure is the likely mechanism.

Inhaled vomitus in anæsthesia is now becoming one of the more prominent hazards of midwifery as others are reduced or eliminated and in spite of the increased attention which is being given to this branch of anæsthetics. There is probably no obstetrician alive who has not, more than once, been frightened almost out of his wits by his anæsthetist.

The combination of inexperienced anæsthetist, Boyle's anæsthetic machine and Clauson's harness in a labour room without mechanical suction devices instantly available and without labour ward beds cap-able of immediate head-down tilt, has provided most obstetricians of my vintage with their full share of alarms. The calamitous effects of inhaled vomit are often even more lethal to the unborn baby.

Inhaled Vomit Syndrome

This is nowadays recognised much more readily as a clinical entity. There are two main varieties. The first, due to inhalation of solid material which blocks off a main branch of the bronchial tree, is an obvious and well-known matter. Lung collapse, pneumonia and lung abscess follow in the case inadequately treated by bronchoscopy. But this sort of accident is relatively uncommon in obstetric practice. More common and treacherous is the type of accident to which Mendelson (1946) drew attention. Here, liquid and highly irritant gastric contents are deeply inhaled and result in an asthmatic type of behaviour in a patient whose condition progressively deteriorates after apparent recovery from the anæsthetic. Clinically there is cyano-sis, tachycardia, wheezing from pulmonary œdema and deepening shock. It is by no means always obvious that vomit has in fact been aspirated and the differential diagnosis between amniotic fluid embolism, acute pulmonary œdema due to mitral stenosis and cardiac failure, and this syndrome may be difficult. More than half the deaths attributable to general anæsthesia are associated with inhaled acid vomit.

In reviewing seven cases Parker attributed the development of this "acid-aspiration" syndrome to progressive and generalised broncho-spasm, thereby explaining the interval which usually elapses between

the end of the anæsthetic and the onset of serious symptoms. Anoxia, cardiac failure and massive pulmonary œdema are the immediate causes of death, often within a dozen hours and sometimes a day or two later when pneumonia is usually superadded.

Treatment is a matter of urgency. The head should be turned to one side and the pharynx immediately emptied by mechanical suction. The patient should be tilted head downwards (and in how many labour wards is this possible?) and if there is any cyanosis a laryngoscope should be passed and any accessible solid foreign material removed. It will probably be necessary thereafter to proceed with the anæsthetic and operation, but if respiratory difficulties of any sort appear following the cessation of the anæsthetic, the likelihood of acid aspiration should be recognised. With the help of a bronchoscope, under renewed anæsthesia, the bronchial tree should be sucked clear as thoroughly as possible. Oxygen should be given and aminophylline (250 mg.) injected intravenously to relieve bronchial spasm. It is doubtful if the spontaneous breathing of 100 per cent oxygen is adequate when artificial ventilation with oxygen through an endotracheal tube is not only more efficient but reduces the tendency to pulmonary œdema (McCormick, 1966). Hydrocortisone, 200 to 300 mg., should be given intravenously followed by 100 mg. six-hourly intramuscularly, or maintained in an intravenous drip if one is being used, the dose being gradually tapered in the course of the ensuing four or five days. As hydrocortisone prevents the normal response to secondary bacterial invasion, broad spectrum antibiotics should be employed (McCormick). There has been debate whether lavage of the lungs with large volumes of bicarbonate or saline might be of use to neutralise the aspirated acid, but the general opinion is that this may only spread the trouble and in fact prove dangerous.

This is one of the big hazards of modern operative obstetrics and for this reason forceps deliveries are being increasingly performed under pudendal block local anæsthesia which is adequate for four out of five cases. Where, however, an inhalational anæsthetic has to be given, the stomach may have first to be emptied by stomach tube. Cases of prolonged labour also demonstrate gastric inertia and usually have treacherously full stomachs. Glucose drinks coaxed into them during the first stage of labour lie unabsorbed within the stomach to be regurgitated when anæsthesia is induced. Intravenous fluids are, therefore, not only more effective but very much safer from this point of view. Even the precaution of passing a stomach tube may not be enough to empty the stomach adequately, quite apart from its unpleasantness in a demoralised patient. Even though all fluids have been restricted since labour became fully established it is now our standard practice, as advocated by Taylor and Pryse-Davies (1956), to administer prophylactic antacid by mouth and for this purpose 14

ml. of magnesium trisilicate, B.P.C., are given shortly before anæsthesia is induced. This is sufficient to neutralise 140 ml. of gastric contents. Magnesium trisilicate is superior to half strength aluminium hydroxide which tends to be more viscous and therefore less beneficial if it should be aspirated. The aim should be to raise the pH of the gastric contents to above the critical level of 2·50, below which human lungs would appear to be particularly vulnerable quite apart from the mechanical dangers of aspiration.

Chloroform is now generally agreed to be a dangerous anæsthetic in spite of its traditional place in midwifery, and it is a pity that what it saves in producing a smooth induction it loses in the direction of ventricular fibrillation and liver damage, for there is no handier agent in domiciliary practice. It is the frequently repeated induction of anæsthesia which multiplies the risks particularly.

Previous corticosteroid therapy produces a hazard of increasing importance. It is now generally agreed that the adrenals may require as much as two years to recover fully from the suppressive effects of corticosteroids and during this period the patient may be incapable of mustering the normal physiological responses to stress, particularly of trauma and operation. Admittedly there is some compensation in the stimulus which pregnancy provides to the maternal adrenals and this may be enough for weathering a normal pregnancy and labour, but when pregnancy or delivery are complicated by vomiting, infection, blood loss, operation or any stressful complication, the patient faces the risk of sudden acute collapse and death unless additional supportive therapy equivalent to 200 mg. of cortisone acetate intramuscularly is supplied during each 24 hours, preferably for one day before the emergency, in so far as it can be foreseen, and for at least two or three days thereafter depending upon her general condition. In a real emergency it is wise to administer the corticosteroid in a glucose saline intravenous infusion, controlling the dosage by blood pressure readings. If the clinician is confronted with sudden collapse due to this cause of suprarenal inadequacy the intravenous route should certainly be chosen, as the rate of absorption from intramuscular injection is too slow and unpredictable. The need, therefore, to be aware of previous corticosteroid therapy is very real and in my own unit cardiac arrest occurred in a patient whose doctor at home had been treating her many months earlier with cortisone for "rheumatism" and of which we had no knowledge. Information of this sort is even more urgent than knowing the patient's blood group.

Another cause of sudden and unpredictable collapse is drug sensitivity. This may occur even in the case of local anæsthetic agents used, for example, in pudendal block. Fortunately lignocaine has a

very good record in this respect but accidental intravenous injection may produce some degree of collapse. There is probably no such thing as a drug to which some patient somewhere in the world is not sensitive and this possibility should be borne in mind in attempting a diagnosis of the cause.

Spontaneous pneumothorax is an uncommon complication but it becomes particularly dangerous if it goes on to tension pneumothorax, and we have indeed had such a case in a woman who smoked so heavily that she benefited the Chancellor of the Exchequer to the tune of 60 cigarettes a day. The state of her lungs can be imagined and she presumably managed to rupture a subpleural emphysematous bulla as a result of her coughing and chronic respiratory disease. Unfortunately, because of a complicating antepartum hæmorrhage, she had to have a general anæsthetic for vaginal examination, halothane in oxygen being chosen and positive-pressure ventilation being avoided. In the course of the ensuing labour epidural anæsthesia was given to avoid the need for respiratory depressant drugs and directly after the injection of the main epidural dose she collapsed with acute dyspnoea, bronchospasm and cyanosis. Naturally the immediate reaction was to blame the epidural anæsthetic but in fact it was fortunately noticed that there was tracheal deviation to the left. The patient was now *in extremis* but prompt relief of the intrapleural pressure, by the insertion of a needle in the seventh intercostal space, dramatically saved her life (Vance, 1958). This story serves to remind one of how quickly one has both to think and act in a case such as this where faulty observation, or the institution of routine antishock methods, would have been rewarded only by certain death of the patient.

Pulmonary collapse completes the list of commoner causes. The remainder are more in the nature of curiosities: anaphylactic phenomena, paroxysmal tachycardia, subarachnoid hæmorrhage, coronary thrombosis, ruptured heart valves and ruptured aneurysm, splenic, renal or mesenteric, to mention a few, and in doing so for the sake of completeness it must again be stressed that the commonest things most commonly occur and should be looked for first.

IDIOPATHIC OBSTETRIC SHOCK

The more carefully the case is considered and examined the less often will this diagnosis be made; in fact, there are many who deny that it exists. This is an overstatement. Every now and then a patient inexplicably collapses and dies, and at autopsy, usually by the coroner's pathologist, no causative lesion whatsoever can be discovered. Then, and then only, may the diagnosis of idiopathic obstetric shock be made, for there is no alternative.

One can only speculate on the mechanism by which it is produced and at the same time marvel that it does not occur more often when one considers that to some women, labour, even uncomplicated labour, is the greatest ordeal they have ever had to undergo. Stretching of the parts may be a factor in susceptible individuals, just as stretching of the anal orifice may produce surgical shock. Pain, bruising, dehydration and frank terror may all play their part, but it is very difficult to say how often such shock occurs without being certain of the thoroughness of postmortem examination in a large number of obstetric disasters. Sheehan found no such case in his 147 cases. In the *Report on Maternal Morbidity and Mortality in Scotland*, 1929–33, in 100 fatal cases quoted by Munro Kerr and Chassar Moir rapid labour was listed in two, and in seven cases the cause of death was undetermined, but it is not certain how far all other possible causes were excluded. The diagnosis of idiopathic shock, therefore, can only be made by a complete process of elimination which is impossible until after death and particularly in the case of amniotic fluid embolism postmortem autolysis very rapidly destroys the evidence.

PROPHYLAXIS AGAINST POSTPARTUM COLLAPSE

The first essential is to save blood loss at all times and in all places. There is no greater obstetrical commandment than this, and the second is never to overestimate a woman's powers of endurance.

Antenatal care should eliminate as far as possible and wherever possible the handicaps likely to operate during labour, particularly anæmia, and, where they cannot be eliminated, to mitigate their effects, for example by securing a week or two of maximum rest for the damaged heart.

In labour itself good supervision not only delays the onset of maternal distress, but also goes far towards preventing postpartum collapse by combating dehydration, discouraging ketosis by the timely use of an intravenous glucose drip and encouraging the maximum amount of rest and relaxation by the judicious use of sedatives.

THE FLYING SQUAD

Since Farquhar Murray established the first flying squad in Newcastle-on-Tyne in 1935 no fewer than 172 maternity hospitals in England and Wales have developed this service. About 3,000 such calls are dealt with annually (about 1 per cent of all domiciliary deliveries). This in itself might be regarded as a condemnation of domiciliary midwifery, but in the present state of maternity bed shortages in Great Britain the flying squad has a very vital rôle.

The original squad in Newcastle dealt with 353 cases in its first

twelve years of operation and Stabler (1947) gave an account of this pioneer work which is likely to be of historical importance as, apart from its other intrinsic interest, it covers the period before and after the institution of blood banks. Before 1940 intravenous saline was the main restorative, since stored blood was not yet available.

Twenty-seven cases of acute hæmorrhage or shock were transferred to hospital but nine of these died and Stabler blamed the journey. This was certainly true before the availability of adequate blood transfusion in the patient's home, but would not be the case nowadays. For this reason Stabler reckoned that the squad should be capable of, and equipped for, anything and everything on the spot. He therefore recommended not only staffing with an experienced obstetrician, assistants and anæsthetist, but six items of baggage as follows:

1. Large box for drugs, anæsthetics, syringes, bowls, instruments and intravenous giving sets.
2. Small box for gowns, drapes, dressings and gloves.
3. Small box sufficient for abdominal surgery.
4. Crate of dried plasma, saline and 3–4 pints of group O Rh-ve blood.
5. Bundle of blankets and hot-water bottles.
6. Oxygen cylinders and B.L.B. mask and fittings.

It is quite clear that many of the cases whose deaths are described should never, by present-day standards, have been booked for domiciliary delivery, for example, cases of previous Cæsarean section, diabetes, fibroids, previous postpartum hæmorrhage, cardiac disease and toxic goitre, and the existence of flying squads should not encourage this type of practice.

There are two ways of regarding the function of a flying squad. The area covered, the state of the roads and transport facilities will to some extent determine the choice although these are rapidly becoming more uniform, especially with the addition of helicopter ambulances for island communities.

The Stabler point of view envisages a squad capable and ready to perform Cæsarean hysterectomy, for example, on the kitchen table, on the ground that delay and transfer to hospital may be more dangerous than operating in primitive conditions. The other point of view, to which we subscribe, is that the function of the squad is to resuscitate the patient and to make her fit for the journey to hospital. With adequate transfusion this is nearly always possible.

The main difficulty about desperate surgery in desperate circumstances is the safety of anæsthesia and if the condition is not all that desperate the patient is far better off dealt with in hospital. On the other hand if her condition is truly desperate she is not in need of surgery but of resuscitation. The so-called minor anæsthetic can all

too easily end in major catastrophe. There is no such thing as a minor anaesthetic. In both 1960 and 1961, 188 Flying Squad calls were answered from our hospital (376 cases). Postpartum hæmorrhage, as might be expected, was the commonest reason, followed by retained placenta with or without bleeding. Antepartum hæmorrhage came third with abortion and eclampsia further down the list. The number of calls is higher than ever before, mainly because of increased use made of the service by doctors outside. The results of applying the principle of full resuscitation and then removal of the patient to hospital accompanied by the squad and in the case of third-stage complications coverage with ergometrine, and in all cases, where indicated, by continuing blood transfusion would appear to justify this policy. There were no maternal deaths over many years and full aftercare of the patient is made possible. In our part of the world there is a shortage of anæsthetists and unless full and competent anæsthetic facilities can be provided, including mechanical suction and head-down tilting facilities, we feel that more lives are likely to be lost from anæsthetic accidents than will be saved by being operated on in the home. With our practice in a very crowded area, the distances are short and the ambulance service first-class. A different state of affairs exists, for example, in Lanarkshire where calls have to be answered from as far away as 20 miles. Liang (1963) has given a full account of the Flying Squad service of the Bellshill Maternity Hospital in this county. This squad is equipped with an ambulance with major resuscitating facilities, including the ability to tip the head down on a stretcher (Leslie, 1963). Even so it is felt by this squad that manual removal of the retained placenta is the only operative treatment that a Flying Squad team should perform in the home, or possibly the rapid extraction of a baby in a case of prolapse of the cord when the state of the cervix is suitable. Certainly our own policy is to remove the placenta, if possible, by the Brandt-Andrews technique or simple expression if it is already separated, rather than admit the patient unnecessarily to hospital, but we are not alone in our policy of regarding the Squad as primarily a resuscitation team. Fraser and Tatford (1961) describe a similar set-up from St. James's Hospital in South London, where it is agreed this type of practice is suited to the urban type of service. Again in this service, if signs of placental separation are present the placenta is delivered by maternal effort, by simple fundal pressure, or by the Brandt-Andrews technique. If signs of separation are doubtful the patient is catheterised and if the placenta does not separate, an intravenous drip is set up and the patient is removed to hospital. She is not removed until her blood pressure has been restored to 100 mm. systolic and is always kept in hospital under observation for 48 hours, and with this practice we

If an endotracheal tube is already in place and an anaesthetist present, ideal pulmonary ventilation can be properly maintained. Various double-ended airways are also often available amongst first-aid equipment.

The single handed operator is at an enormous disadvantage without any equipment or help and the best he can do is to adopt an alternating pattern of activity of about two or three breaths of exhaled air for every dozen or less compressions of the heart. Help should, of course, be sent for but as Milstein has remarked "should not be waited for."

External cardiac massage by the closed method described above is not as efficient as internal cardiac massage following thoracotomy, but the difference is not all that great. Both types of cardiac massage produce a cardiac output of about one-sixth of what might be expected with a normally functioning heart. Nevertheless life can be effectively maintained for half an hour or so by the efficient use of it, while preparations to restart the heart are undertaken. Unfortunately, and this applies particularly to obstetrics, external cardiac massage is even less effective than internal when there has been massive hæmorrhage, because the heart fills very poorly; hence the need to avail oneself of every possible drop of blood by raising the legs vertically. This unfortunately requires another pair of hands which one may not be able to spare. Obviously if there has been massive hæmorrhage little will be gained by massaging an empty heart and massive transfusion will be required to fill it. Some favour intra-arterial transfusion, or, if the chest is already open, direct infusion into the cavity of the left ventricle via the apex. Normally there is no time for such refinements.

Air embolism as already discussed may produce a type of cardiac arrest which will not respond to cardiac massage; in fact the situation may be aggravated unless the air can be evacuated from the right side of the heart at once.

At the earliest possible moment the trachea should be intubated so that effective positive pressure ventilation can be maintained regardless of cardiac massage, although it is preferable for the anæsthetist to regulate his ventilation of the lungs usually by manual bag squeezing, so as not to coincide with the acts of sternal compression.

Internal Cardiac Massage

If external cardiac massage is to have any hope of success it must be capable of producing a palpable carotid or femoral pulse; in fact quite reasonable perfusion pressures can be achieved by this method, but, particularly after hæmorrhage, this objective may not be achieved.

It should be possible to make up one's mind within the first minute or two whether external massage is being effective and if in any doubt to proceed at once to internal massage by thoracotomy. The first time I ever carried this out I made the mistake of remaining on the right hand side of the patient with the result that I had poor control of the extent of my incision or its depth and, in my haste, cut the underlying lung because of failure to wait the fraction of a second necessary for the lung to fall away from the parietal pleura with the opening of the cavity and I also accidentally incised part of the ventricular muscle wall of the heart, so that a few valuable seconds were lost in suturing, as well as yet more blood.

The incision should extend from the left edge of the sternum along the fourth, fifth or sixth intercostal space, right back, if possible, to the posterior axillary line, or as far as the hardness of the operating table will allow. Too small an incision makes the insertion of one or both hands very difficult. The time for care in making the incision is in opening the parietal pleura, as already suggested. If possible the internal mammary artery should be avoided at the anterior end of the incision but at the moment this hardly matters since it will not be bleeding anyway and can be ligated later before closing the chest. Asepsis though desirable is immaterial in such an emergency.

Having made the incision, extending as far back as possible, the ribs are retracted using both hands at first in order to insert one hand into the chest cavity, usually the left hand, if one is standing, as one should, on the left hand side of the patient. The use of a rib retractor will prevent a great deal of wrist discomfort and chafing. The hand should be passed right behind the heart and then a compression towards the deep surface of the sternum carried out. The other hand can supply counterpressure over the front of the sternum.

The heart may start beating on its own after the first few compressions, but if it does not there should be no hesitation in slitting open the pericardium, making first a small incision to allow the entry of air as in opening the peritoneal cavity in ordinary abdominal surgery and then extending the incision from the apex to the base of the heart anterior to the phrenic nerve which should be avoided. The incision can be enlarged towards the right at its lower end. Now it is possible to work with both hands, and very efficiently too, and the palms and thenar eminences should be used in preference to the points of the fingers which may damage the myocardium.

What is particularly discouraging is when the heart appears not to fill adequately between each compression and this is very likely to be experienced where massive hæmorrhage has been one of the precipitating causes of the cardiac arrest. It is a mistake however which I have made in the past of waiting for cardiac filling as felt by the hands, which may reduce the massage rate to less than 50 a minute,

and one should proceed at a rate of 80 whether the heart is filling or not, while awaiting the proper restoration of blood volume. If bleeding now begins to appear from the incision one has reason for congratulation, as there must be some sort of a circulation establish-ed. The bleeding points can now be secured.

The patient after half an hour begins to lose heat to a dangerous extent and it will not be easy to restore the heart beat below a temperature of 30 to 31° C. Warm Ringer's solution poured into the chest may help to raise the heart temperature but this should be done with caution.

Once efficient cardiac massage, either internal or external, has been established the immediate emergency is over and some thought can be given to the cause of the cardiac arrest, its type and the method of restoring the heart beat. It is now important to distinguish between the two main types, namely cardiac asystole and ventricular fibrilla-tion. An electrocardiograph machine will by now have been attached to the patient. The trace in the case of asystole simply shows a straight line whereas ventricular fibrillation shows a random and irregular electrical wave pattern. If the pericardium is already open the differential diagnosis can be made by looking at the heart. Coarse fibrillation is a more welcome sign than very feeble fibrillation which may escape notice. The former is said to feel like a "bag of worms".

In asystole the heart is soft, relaxed and motionless and as hypoxia is one of the commonest causes the coronary veins may look almost black. Ventricular fibrillation is revealed as an irregular twitching or unco-ordinated writhing.

The damaging effects of hypoxia on the heart must be realised and the need to counter it by adequate pulmonary ventilation at the same time must be met before one can hope to restart the heart. Hypoxia will, of course, be aggravated by hæmorrhage resulting in an in-adequate circulating blood volume, by hypercapnia and anæsthetic drugs and the effects of a high level of serum potassium are particu-larly damaging. The conducting mechanism within the heart is sharply reduced by hypoxia. Hyperkalæmia can in fact be associated with either asystole or ventricular fibrillation, and potassium is released from all the tissues of the body under the influence of anoxia and can be still further raised by the transfusion of stored blood. A high potassium level causes a loss of conductivity within the heart whereas calcium ions increase the contractility and prolong systole and shorten diastole. The ratio of potassium to calcium ions is therefore important and must presently be corrected by the injection of calcium gluconate. In addition to this if, as is likely, a large transfusion is being given, the calcium ions will be necessary to combat the citrate effect of stored blood and it is our own practice after the first two units of blood to give 1 g. usually as 10 millilitres

of a 10 per cent solution of calcium gluconate for every two units of blood given after the first couple.

Quite apart from the damaging hydrodynamic effects of hypovolæmia, hæmorrhage causes a release of large quantities of adrenaline into the circulation, one of the effects of which is to stimulate the liberation of potassium from the liver, so that hyperkalæmia may itself be an immediate precipitating cause of cardiac arrest. The avoidance therefore of hæmorrhagic hypotension by prompt correction of blood volume deficiencies is an important prophylactic measure. To some extent intravenous digoxin may help to counter the effects of potassium intoxication of the heart which is now suffering from diminished myocardial contractility.

The importance of distinguishing between asystole and ventricular fibrillation at this stage lies in the fact that there are certain differences in treatment, although asystole can turn to ventricular fibrillation and vice versa. If cardiac massage restores the heart beat the point is academic and this may suffice in cases suffering from an overdosage of the cocaine class of drugs, but if the heart beat does not recover following massage and the diagnosis of ventricular fibrillation is made, electrical defibrillation is most clearly called for. This procedure is bound to fail unless full oxygenation of the myocardium can first be obtained by cardiac massage and forced pulmonary ventilation. It is easier to defibrillate a heart which is in coarse ventricular fibrillation than in feeble, but massage may help to coarsen the variety of fibrillation in the first place. If not, the injection of adrenaline may help. Defibrillation can be carried out either externally or by direct application of electrodes to the front and back of the heart, preferably covered with lint made wet with Ringer's solution in order to distribute the area of electrical shock. All assistants should stand well clear because voltages of some hundreds are used. Defibrillation may be followed by asystole and one should wait for at least a quarter of a minute in the hope of a spontaneous contraction starting up. Failing this the heart must again be massaged. Most defibrillators work with alternating current. My own personal experience of high voltage (2,000 volt) direct current defibrillation on each occasion has been while I was under an anæsthetic. I understand the jump on the table is impressive but I am glad not to have witnessed it. Most units now have electrical defibrillators to hand, but in their absence one may have to resort to the use of procaine which diminishes myocardial irritability and helps to control fibrillation. It is not, however, an effective alternative to electrical defibrillation, although adrenaline may improve its efficacy. If procaine hydrochloride has to be used the dose is from 50 to 200 mg. If, however, it merely produces reduced tone in the myocardium and the defibrillation fails, 5 to 10 ml. of 1 in 10,000

adrenaline should be given intravenously to restore a more vigorous type of fibrillation before making another attempt (Milstein).

Treatment of asystole.—As before, the first treatment is cardiac massage and forced pulmonary ventilation with 100 per cent oxygen. Five to ten millilitres of a 1 per cent solution of calcium chloride should be given at once, either intravenously or directly into an exposed heart chamber. A 10 per cent solution of this dosage has been recommended but is caustic and may cause necrosis if it misses its target. Adrenaline, 5 to 10 ml. of a 1 in 10,000 solution, may also be effective in starting up a heart in asystole but may precipitate ventricular fibrillation which, however, can be electrically reversed. Again it must reach the coronary circulation to be effective locally and therefore active cardiac massage must be maintained in order to obtain an effect.

The direct intracardiac injection of drugs like calcium chloride or adrenaline in the case with the closed chest who has been maintained with external cardiac massage, is best made by inserting a long needle about 10 cm. vertically through the fourth left space close to the sternum. If the heart is exposed the injection should be made into the left ventricle entering via the apex and taking care to aspirate blood to ensure that the point of the needle is within the ventricular cavity.

There is still hope as long as the myocardium shows signs of responding to massage, drugs or electrical defibrillation, even though repeated attempts to restart the heart may have to be made. Indeed coarse fibrillation is a far more encouraging sign than complete asystole or very fine and feeble fibrillation. Once the heart has been started the chest should not be closed for at least half an hour because of its liability to stop again and mechanical respiration through an endotracheal tube should be maintained for hours, although if spontaneous respiration does not reappear within 12 hours the outlook is very gloomy.

Acidosis in cardiac arrest.—The damaging effects of hyperkalæmia have already been mentioned and these can be to some extent countered by improving the potassium/calcium ionic ratio by the intravenous injection of calcium gluconate, but it must not be forgotten that very severe metabolic acidosis comes on in a matter of minutes of cardiac arrest even though cardiac massage is promptly instituted. Our own rule-of-thumb method is to give 200 mEq of sodium bicarbonate, i.e. 200 ml. of 8·4 per cent solution, as an immediate measure once other more pressing matters have been attended to, but Gilston (1965) has recommended the following formula:

$$\text{Dose of sodium bicarbonate in mEq} = \text{weight of the patient in kg.} \times \text{the duration of cardiac arrest in minutes} \times \tfrac{1}{10}$$

The immediate availability of micro-Astrup biochemical control of the blood chemistry is a great help.

Further care.—After half-an-hour's observation to see that cardiac activity is maintained, the pericardium may be closed. This should only be partial and designed to prevent the apex of the heart from herniating outwards, and water-tight closure may embarrass the heart's action or may cause tamponade from hæmopericardium. Milstein recommends the use of interrupted sutures at intervals of 2 cm. along the lowest 5 to 6 cm. of the percardial incision, the upper two-thirds being left open. The mammary artery must be secured preferably by under-running sutures as its ends retract easily and after dealing with any other bleeding points a spray of polybactrin may be squirted into the wound, or some other antibiotic powder, and the ribs should be approximated with a few pericostal sutures of strong catgut. The intercostal muscles are then sutured with continuous catgut as much as possible and a separate suture layer for the pectoral muscles. The incision must be made air tight to enable the patient to breathe and a drainage tube of wide bore should be inserted into the pleural space in the lateral chest wall well below the original incision and sutured to the skin. The free end is connected to an underwater seal. A mechanical suction pump applied to the drainage bottle may assist pulmonary expansion and pleural cavity drainage.

At the earliest safe opportunity the patient should be moved into an intensive care unit for follow up treatment, which may include hypothermia for suspected brain damage and supervision for anuria, assisted respiration and biochemical control.

SUMMARY OF IMMEDIATE EMERGENCY STEPS

1. Don't waste time—it only wastes life.
2. Head down and tilted back.
3. Two or three precordial punches.
4. Clear airway and inflate lungs for three or four breaths.
5. External cardiac massage—if necessary on hard floor.
6. If ineffective, perform thoracotomy without wasting time on asepsis.
7. Internal cardiac massage.
8. Continue pulmonary ventilation.
9. Transfuse as necessary.
10. If internal cardiac massage ineffective open pericardium and massage heart.

Total permissible elapsed time to date—3 minutes.

From now on, treatment can be more planned and deliberate with the help of assistants.

There is no longer any such thing in maternity hospitals as acceptable sudden death. A harrowing three-hour ritual lies ahead before the diagnosis of maternal death is likely to be acknowledged and all hope finally abandoned.

REFERENCES

1. *British Medical Journal* (1957). Editorial, **1**, 453.
2. FRASER, A. C., and TATFORD E. P. W. (1961). *Lancet*, **2**, 126.
3. GOVAN, A. D. T., and McGILLIVRAY, I. (1950). *J. Obstet. Gynæc. Brit. Emp.*, **57**, 233.
4. HAGBERG, C. J. (1956). *S. Afr. med. J.*, **30**, 1140.
5. LESLIE, D. W. (1963). *J. Obstet. Gynæc. Brit. Commonw.*, **70**, 291.
6. LIANG, D. Y. S. (1963). *J. Obstet. Gynæc. Brit. Commonw.*, **70**, 83.
7. McCORMICK, P. W. (1966). *Proc. roy. Soc. Med.*, **59**, 66.
8. MENDELSON, C. L. (1946). *Amer. J. Obstet. Gynec.*, **52**, 191.
9. MILSTEIN, B. B. (1963). *Cardiac Arrest and Resuscitation*. London: Lloyd Luke (Medical Books).
10. MURDOCH, R. (1962). *Lancet*, **1**, 1327.
11. PARKER, R. B. (1954). *Brit. med. J.*, **2**, 65.
12. SCOTT, W. A. (1947). *Brit. med. J.*, **2**, 647.
13. SHEEHAN, H. L. (1948). *Lancet*, **1**, 1.
14. SHEEHAN, H. L., and MURDOCH, R. (1938). *J. Obstet. Gynæc. Brit. Emp.*, **45**, 456.
15. STABLER, F. (1947). *Brit. med. J.*, **2**, 878.
16. STEINER, P. E., and LUSHBAUGH, C. C. (1941). *J. Amer. med. Ass.*, **117** 1245 and 1340.
17. TAYLOR, G., and PRYSE-DAVIES, J. (1966). *Lancet*, **1**, 288.
18. TINDALL, V. R. (1965). *Proc. roy. Soc. Med.*, **59**, 63.
19. VANCE, J. P. (1968). *Anaesthesia*, **23**, 94.
20. WILLOCKS, J., MONE, J. G., and THOMSON, W. J. (1966). *Brit. med. J.*, **2**, 1181.

CHAPTER XXI

POSTPARTUM HÆMORRHAGE

"If you can fill the unforgiving minute with sixty seconds worth of distance run."—KIPLING.

THIS is indeed the unforgiving stage of labour, and in it there lurks more unheralded treachery than in both the other stages of labour combined. The normal case can, within a minute, become abnormal and successful delivery can turn swiftly to disaster. The obstetrician's judgment must be sure and swift, and errors of commission carry with them penalties as great, or greater, than those of omission. Increasing experience serves only to sharpen one's alertness during this stage, and there is no room for complacency in any case, however normal, until the placenta has been delivered for at least half an hour, with the uterus well retracted and with minimal bleeding.

It is far more important to understand the physiology of this stage of labour than to know the mechanisms of the second stage and the only safe management is one based upon this knowledge.

PHYSIOLOGY OF THE THIRD STAGE

An excellent opportunity is afforded at Cæsarean section to observe the process of placental separation and uterine retraction, for both the inside and the outside of the uterus can be watched at the same time. The shrinkage of the uterus which occurs after the delivery of the baby is not a rapid phenomenon as in the case of skeletal muscle contraction, but occurs almost surreptitiously. It is after a few minutes that the pallor of the uterus and the wrinkling of its surface bear witness to the immense degree of retraction which has been taking place. As seen at operation this shrinkage would appear to be a gradual and progressive phenomenon, and this fact alone should stress the importance of never hurrying the third stage.

Intermittent contractions are of course superimposed, but as a rule they are not usually noticeable to the hand palpating through the abdominal wall for at least ten minutes; it would appear that the contractile activity of the uterus is, for a short while, somewhat in abeyance after the effort of delivering the fœtus, although retraction continues progressively. In twin delivery the uterus appears to take a similar rest after the delivery of the first child.

The method of placental separation can also be witnessed profitably at Cæsarean section. The commonest mechanism is that

682

associated with the name of Schultze, in which the central portion separates first, followed by a concentrically enlarging area so that the placenta bulges into view with the centre of the fœtal surface presenting. For a long time it was thought that this mechanism was caused by the collection of blood behind the centre of the placenta which spread towards its margin, thus completing separation, but this retroplacental hæmatoma is now regarded as a result of separation rather than a cause.

The other method is that described by Matthews Duncan in which the placenta as a whole is sheared off the uterine wall and presents with its inferior margin first. It is very much less common and is probably more often associated with difficulties in spontaneous delivery of the placenta. The membranes, moreover, are more easily torn instead of being peeled off progressively as in Schultze's method.

The reason for placental separation is almost certainly the mechanical effect of shearing, for the area of the placental site is reduced to a diameter of 4 inches or less, to which the bulk of the placenta cannot readily accommodate itself. In normal cases there is not much resistance in the decidua at the plane of cleavage. The membranes, however, are often very adherent and, having no appreciable bulk, are not sheared off the uterine wall by the reduction in area to which they are attached. This phenomenon, too, can be demonstrated at Cæsarean section. The placental mass progressively peels off the membranes, but it is not uncommon for the latter to delay for a time the spontaneous delivery of the placenta. It is at this stage that fundus fiddling becomes particularly dangerous as, thereby, retroplacental blood may be forced to track towards the outside world between the membranes and the uterine wall. Once this track has been formed, blood can trickle away continually while the placental mass, by its retention *in utero,* discourages uterine retraction. Further bleeding can now go on to the point of exsanguination. A failed attempt at Credé's expression often demonstrates this, but in more serious degree.

The presence of blood clot, or placenta, or both within the uterine body may stimulate contractions, but inevitably interferes with retraction, and only the latter will safeguard the patient against postpartum hæmorrhage.

The greater part of the uterine musculature is composed of the intermediate criss-cross layer of muscle fibres which are arranged trellis fashion, and through the interstices of which the maternal blood vessels supplying the placental site run a tortuous course. Closing the gaps in this trellis by retraction shuts off the supply of blood to the placental site, and for this reason these fibres are known as "the living ligatures of the uterus".

More often than not the placenta is separated from its attachment to the uterine wall with the contraction which completes the delivery of the baby's body, provided this is not hurried, and only the adherence of the membranes, the temporary cessation of further uterine contractions and the rest from bearing down efforts which the patient takes, delay the immediate delivery of the placenta.

A marked change overtakes the patient as a whole immediately following the birth of her child. Whereas she was hot, she now feels cold and starts to shiver, and often the maternal blood pressure undergoes a temporary fall following the exertions of the second stage. This may contribute some protection against the risks of postpartum hæmorrhage. There does not, hitherto, appear to have been much study of the immediate behaviour of the blood pressure in the first few minutes following delivery, but the hypotension is only transitory. There is some rise in blood pressure during the uterine contractions of the second stage.

It is popular nowadays to refer to a fourth stage of labour and its dangers, but this seems to be unnecessary, for the patient who bleeds half an hour after the delivery of her placenta is, in fact, a case of third-stage hæmorrhage, inasmuch as it is due to inadequate retraction of the uterus which is part of the essential mechanism of the third stage.

MANAGEMENT OF THE THIRD STAGE

More tuition is concentrated upon this matter in the training of undergraduates and midwives than on any other part of the subject, yet faulty management remains one of the commonest sources of trouble. It is customary to conduct this stage with the patient in the dorsal position, mainly for two reasons: firstly, the abdomen can be more easily examined, and secondly, the exact amount of blood lost can be collected in a dish, the edge of which is kept pressed against the perineum. A very suitable dish for the purpose and one which we use in preference to the usual kidney dish has been designed and described by Murdoch (1958). The importance of blood accountancy is dealt with fully in the chapter on postpartum collapse; suffice it to mention here that it is impossible to relate a patient's general state to the factor of hæmorrhage without knowing exactly the extent of the loss involved. Blood allowed to run over the sheets or into a bucket is blood left out of the reckoning and the amount is usually a great deal more than appearances would suggest.

On the vexed subject of early or late clamping of the cord and its influence on the amount of blood "transfused" from placenta to baby, the strength of uterine contraction at the very end of the second stage, or the very beginning of the third stage, is what really determines the quantity rather than the time interval before clamping.

In the healthy baby the transfusion is partly completed by the end of one minute and fully at three minutes. Oxytocic drugs accelerate the process so that one minute suffices to complete it.[7] Respiration does not appear to affect placental transfusion.

In this country many patients complete the second stage of labour in the left lateral position, it being believed, perhaps wrongly, that the perineum can be more easily saved from "damage". The great disadvantage, however, is the need to turn the patient over on to her back in the third stage, and this is always one of the more anxious moments. Many times I have witnessed a brisk gush of blood accompanying the shift of position, and it occurs at a time when one is relatively more disorganised. For those, therefore, who conduct normal delivery in the left lateral position, certain precautions should be taken in turning the patient on to her back, the most important of which is to ensure that the fundus of the uterus is hard and well contracted before starting and the knees should be kept together while moving. This will keep the labia in apposition and discourages the possibility, admittedly remote, of air embolism through the placental site should placental separation have occurred already.

During the ensuing period of waiting the patient is cold and acutely conscious of the wetness round her buttocks, and it is difficult to keep her warm because of the need to keep the abdomen uncovered for examination and inspection. The only safe coverings for the thighs at this time are sterile drapes which are not always available although they certainly should be. While waiting for the signs of placental separation to appear, the time can profitably be passed by allowing the patient to handle her child and, wherever feasible, to put it to the breast. This has a remarkable effect on uterine activity.

Signs of placental separation.—There are only two of really convincing value. The first of these, namely feeling the placenta by vaginal examination, is commonly frowned upon, although I have no hesitation in surreptitiously making such an examination after a forceps delivery because already enough intravaginal interference has occurred to make further cautious vaginal examination of no moment. The other convincing sign is that of lengthening of the cord, and when observed there is never any doubt about it, for it is never less than several inches and often as many as six or more. This invaluable sign is all too often missed and usually unnecessarily so. In separating the baby from its mother the very first step should be to apply a clamp to the cord as close as possible to the vulva after gently lifting up any slack which may be in the vagina. The other clamp can then be applied towards the fœtal end of the cord, as usual, and the cord severed.

Now, for some reason which I have never been able to fathom, tutors in midwifery persist in the ridiculous ritual of making the clumsy-fingered student tie bits of twisted string neatly, and about half an inch apart, at the chosen point of cord division. A little piece of wool is then applied to collect the small drop of blood which appears on cutting the cord with scissors, as if such finesse mattered at all in the face of the general messiness of labour! What matters, of course, is that during all this misguided activity cord lengthening passes unobserved, whereas a clamp applied at the vulva as afore-said will leave one in no doubt. A very senior midwife once told me that it would not be safe to teach the method of applying the proximal clamp close to the vulva for fear of the adventitious structures which might be included by the flustered pupil. Horrid thought!

The other signs of separation are less conclusive. The fundus of the uterus becomes globular, like a cricket ball, instead of pyriform and somewhat flattened. This is because the placenta has left the upper uterine segment which is now empty and well retracted. Un-fortunately, especially in well-covered patients, mistakes in inter-pretation are made every hour of every day. The uterus is said to become more mobile, as is indeed the case when the bulk of the placenta is sitting in the vaginal vault, but the elicitation of this sign savours of fundus fiddling. The level of the fundus rises after ex-pulsion of the placenta from the upper segment, but this is also true of the uterus which is filled with blood and is too unreliable a sign. A bulge is sometimes visible above the symphysis pubis, but this too may be misinterpreted and may be due to the presence of urine in the bladder. Lastly, a test of placental separation fre-quently employed must be mentioned only to condemn it in un-equivocal terms: it consists in drawing the uterus upwards by manipulation through the abdominal wall and observing if any length of cord is dragged into the vagina from its previous position over the fourchette and perineum. This is hardly good asepsis. Such a test is both unreliable and meddlesome.

Very often, as if to satisfy curiosity, the fundus is seized and pushed downwards to see if this effects delivery of the placenta and, times without number, this hit-or-miss type of diagnosis is the signal for a train of events which starts with a trickle of blood and a protest from the patient and ends in near disaster. Many books still refer to the small gush of blood as being one of the signs of placental separation. This is bad teaching and true only in so far that bleeding could not occur at all unless there was some degree of separation. Unfortunately, this sign gives no indication of whether or not the separation is complete. It does, however, indicate that blood collect-ing behind the placenta has now found a vent to the outside world

and that the former restrictions on handling of the fundus now no longer apply.

"Controlling the fundus."—A hand is gently laid upon the abdominal wall over the fundus to observe it, but in some institutions the fear is so great that the fundus will be kneaded, pummelled, pushed about and generally fiddled with that this practice is forbidden and reliance is placed upon visual observation of its contour, looking tangentially across the abdominal wall. Anyone, however, who cannot be taught to keep his hand on the fundus absolutely still should be strongly advised not to take up midwifery. It is commonly thought that the hand in this position can control the fundus from rising and from filling up with blood. This of course is nonsense, because an atonic uterus will fill up with blood wherever one's hand is placed. One might well ask, then, what is the purpose in applying the hand to the abdominal wall at all. It is undoubtedly valuable and superior to visual observation: firstly, the state of uterine activity can be observed as the uterus hardens and softens with the return of uterine contractions; secondly, the subsidiary signs of placental separation can be observed, and thirdly, and perhaps this is the most important reason, the fundus does not get lost. Without a hand constantly aware of the exact position of the fundus one may, in the presence of a sudden brisk hæmorrhage, be in doubt at first as to whether the fundus is under the costal margin or inverted into the vagina, and some valuable seconds may be lost in the search.

Throughout the period of waiting the right hand is kept immersed in a bowl of antiseptic, not so much in order that a manual removal of the placenta may be immediately undertaken as to keep the hand sterile for the subsequent examination of the perineum. "With the patient's welfare in mind, an impatient obstetrician is far better off doing gynæcology."[18]

Since the third stage is always a time of anxiety which no obstetrician ever wholly outlives, there is a very natural tendency to wish to get it over, and in cases in which oxytocic drugs have not been given at the end of the second stage it is a valuable rule to regard a minimum period of twenty minutes as essential for the safe delivery of the placenta, even though one may be reasonably satisfied that the signs of placental separation have already occurred. Now this may seem an extreme view, and one might argue that it is pointless to wait after the placenta has left the upper uterine segment. Mistakes, however, are so often made that it is a pity to grudge the few extra precautionary minutes. In almost all cases this patience will be rewarded by the uterus completing its physiological functions fully, and there are only three admissible reasons for ignoring this simple practice, firstly, hæmorrhage, which of course demands treatment in its own

right; secondly, in cases in which the patient is already under an anæsthetic and there may be very good reasons for terminating the operation; and thirdly, after the intravenous use of oxytocic drugs. As a student I attended for a fortnight a hospital where this twenty-minute rule was in force, and although the rule was not always intelligently applied, inasmuch as attempts were often made to secure the delivery of the placenta whether signs of separation had occurred or not, nevertheless these injudicious attempts were made with impunity, because sufficient time had been allowed for the uterus to assume full control of the situation. Only if the patient voluntarily expels her own placenta should the third stage be shortened in the normal case.

Delivery of the placenta.—After the lapse of a measured twenty minutes and with the evidences of separation present, it is infinitely preferable to get the patient to expel her own placenta than to resort to pressure upon the fundus. The routine use of the uterus as a piston to drive out the placenta is usually unnecessary and probably damaging to the uterine supports, and to many patients, in retrospect, this is accounted the most unpleasant part of labour. The patient's co-operation should in all cases be sought and encouraged.

Cord traction.—This has been traditionally denounced as a dangerous practice. To be honest, we all do it from time to time. It is, of course, particularly humiliating if the cord breaks off and it makes a surprising amount of mess too. There is little harm in the practice provided the placenta is wholly out of the upper uterine segment, in which case there is less need for it. Counter control through the abdominal wall should always be applied on the body of the uterus with the other hand, otherwise the cervix, and perhaps more, may easily appear at the vulva. The position is altogether different when the placenta is still within the upper segment, and inversion of the uterus is only as uncommon as it is thanks to the fact that fundal insertion of the placenta is unusual, and to the fact that most people respect the rules! To exert cord traction with the fundus of the uterus anything but firmly contracted is certainly asking for trouble.

The use of one hand, with the palmar surfaces of the fingers applied to the anterior surface of the uterus at the level of the junction of upper and lower segments, thus drawing the uterus upwards, is an important part of the cord traction manœuvre. This method of delivering the placenta is now usually known as the Brandt-Andrews method of delivery, after the two men who described and practised it independently.[2, 1] It is also known as "controlled cord traction". The important feature of the manœuvre is not the pulling on the cord, as has been witnessed in apes at delivery, but the dragging upwards at the same time of the uterus towards the umbilicus. The direction in which the cord is pulled is also important. This should

be somewhat downwards and backwards. The attendant stands on the patient's right and with the flat of the left hand facing towards the patient's head the uterus is pushed upwards and backwards while the right hand draws the cord downwards and backwards. This has the effect of straightening out the genital canal in line with the pull on the placenta. To those formerly used to delivering the placenta by pushing on the fundus as a piston, the temptation to pull on the cord and at the same time press downwards on the fundus is very natural, but this defeats the whole object of the exercise because it curls the uterus over in anteversion, re-forming the right angled bend of the genital canal and making the traction on the cord totally ineffective unless the placenta is already in the vagina. Another common mistake is to pull the cord too far forwards and upwards.

Cords vary enormously in their tensile strength and with firm and steadily increasing tension a tearing sensation may easily be felt. Clearly the cord is now going to break and it may be necessary to desist and wait for further descent of the placenta spontaneously. The patient can greatly reduce the amount of tractive effort necessary on the cord by bearing down herself at the same time.

These attempts can be repeated every two or three minutes only synchronously with complete hardening of the uterus of course, but if delivery of the placenta is not achieved within twenty minutes by this technique one should be ready to recognise the need for manual removal of the placenta.

Controlled cord traction, following the use of intravenous ergometrine given with the delivery of the anterior shoulder, is recommended as a routine procedure in normal cases by Spencer (1962), who considered the method safe and a desirable alternative to Credé's expression. In a thousand of her cases the umbilical cord broke in twenty-six but no harm came of this. She believes that if the placenta is still attached to the uterine wall, controlled cord traction will not succeed and this is certainly true wherever there is morbid adherence of the placenta, but in such cases nothing short of manual removal is likely to succeed. It is claimed for the method that the third stage is appreciably shortened and the total amount of blood lost much reduced even in normal cases. The manual removal rate is not increased as a result of using this technique. Amongst many other authors on the management of the third stage nowadays Kimbell further describes the use of amyl nitrite inhalation, one capsule broken under the nose, and repeating the procedure if the first attempt fails. This is designed to relax the cervix, or an hour-glass constriction, if present, but he goes on to say that further failure calls for manual removal of the placenta forthwith.

There is one possible disadvantage of controlled cord traction as

a routine method of shortening the third stage and that is, in my experience, the somewhat increased tendency of the uterus to relax and fill with blood about ten minutes or so later, but this has to be offset against the frequent occurrence of slow filling of the uterus with blood before delivery of the placenta in cases of unhurried spontaneous third stage.

The practice in my own unit is to give an intramuscular injection of Syntometrine (1 ml. containing 0·5 mg. ergometrine and 5 units of synthetic oxytocin) at the end of the second stage and not to use other routine methods of accelerating the third stage. Where labour is completely normal and there is no bleeding we teach our students to wait and to watch for signs of spontaneous placental separation, to keep a hand on the fundus only when it cannot be clearly seen through the abdominal wall in order to avoid losing it and, after the lapse of adequate time for full spontaneous placental separation, to get the patient to deliver the placenta by her own expulsive efforts. We are discouraging the use of the fundus as a piston and prefer the controlled cord traction technique to aid the patient's expulsive efforts, if necessary, but only if the placenta has unquestionably separated. This is undoubtedly the right approach for pupil midwives and undergraduate students. Any third-stage difficulty calls for more qualified intervention, as is described later.

Retained membranes.—The weight of the placenta after delivery should always be supported so that it does not wholly drag upon the membranes and tear them. Suspending the placenta by the cord and twisting the membranes into a rope is quite good practice but, above all, the complete delivery of the membranes depends upon gentleness, patience and care. The fundus of the uterus should be massaged vigorously during the procedure, and this helps to loosen the membranes from the uterine wall by ensuring full uterine retraction. Should a portion of chorion break away and not be delivered, it is no very serious matter and certainly does not justify exploring the uterine cavity.

Retention of placental tissue.—The placenta should be examined as soon as possible, and if it is found that a cotyledon or a succenturiate lobe is missing, the only safe thing to do is to anæsthetise the patient and explore the uterine cavity with the gloved finger forthwith. To yield to the temptation of hoping that all will be well and that the administration of ergometrine will suffice is to take a serious risk. One may be tempted to adopt this foolish, optimistic attitude either because the patient has had a perfectly normal delivery and one is, therefore, reluctant to take radical measures once everything is apparently over, or because the patient has had a dangerous delivery and one is reluctant to add to her trials by yet further operative procedures. It can only be answered that, in the first instance, the

patient is easily well enough to stand it, and in the second, she may be too ill to withstand the far more serious risk of the inevitable secondary postpartum hæmorrhage. It is customary to examine the placenta for missing cotyledons by cupping it, concave, in the palms of two hands, but this method easily conceals any missing gaps and it is better to examine the placenta convex over the backs of both hands to reproduce its attitude *in utero*. In nearly all cases of secondary hæmorrhage from whom quite sizeable amounts of placental tissue have subsequently been removed on uterine exploration, reference to the notes indicates that there was no sign of any missing cotyledons, which shows the inadequacy of the traditional method. The possibility of a retained succenturiate lobe will be indicated by the appearance of torn vessels running up to the edge of the rent in the membranes.

In exploring the uterus one may be dismayed by the impression of roughness of the placental site to the examining finger, but careful examination will reveal whether or not placental tissue is still within the uterine cavity.

Leaving the patient.—The patient should not be left unattended as long as the placenta is still within the genital tract, nor should she be left until a full hour after delivery is completed. The so-called fourth stage has already been referred to and is a period commonly marred by hæmorrhage. Apart from retained placental tissue, already mentioned, the chief cause of bleeding is the gradual collection of a large clot of blood within the uterine cavity. Nothing begets hæmorrhage so much as hæmorrhage, and the presence of a clot *in utero* interferes with uterine retraction and encourages atony.

Before leaving the patient, therefore, the fundus should be examined, firm contraction secured by kneading, and the body of the uterus should then be squeezed to make quite sure that the uterus is empty. The amount of blood appearing at the vulva which is permissible should be no more than sufficient to soil a pad in the course of an hour or two. Any bleeding in excess of this amount demands treatment.

Ergometrine in the Third Stage of Labour

This life-saving drug has made all the difference to the safety of labour. Formerly its use was taboo until after the delivery of the placenta because, it was preached, a constriction ring with hour-glass retention of the placenta would occur. This theory, in common with so much traditional teaching, is not true, and the use of ergometrine as a prophylaxis against hæmorrhage before placental separation has everything to recommend it, provided that the uterus

is not subjected to handling. Anything is better than the loss of blood—even a constriction ring, should it occur.

It is now known that the incidence of hour-glass contraction is not increased by the use of oxytocic drugs at the beginning of the third stage, and that in those cases in which this complication occurred a history of abortive attempts at Credé's expression could nearly always be elicited. It can be argued that the use of pituitary extract might be more physiological, but there is nothing that pituitary extract can do which ergometrine will not do better and a good deal more safely. In the past, accidents from pituitary preparations were not uncommon and were occasionally associated with profound shock. Modern commercial preparations of oxytocin are better purified and safer than before, nevertheless there seems to be no good reason for preferring even these to ergometrine, which is known to be both safe and reliable. The combination of both in one preparation such as Syntometrine (Sandoz) appears to be ideal.

In many hospitals throughout the country an intramuscular injection of 0·5 mg. of ergometrine has become routine as soon as the head is delivered or alternatively at the very beginning of the third stage. The injection can be simply given by the midwife, and within a few minutes the uterus demonstrates a very healthy tone. Workers in these institutions are usually emphatic about the benefits, and although the actual incidence of postpartum hæmorrhage is only to some extent lowered, the significant fact is that the size of the hæmorrhage, when it does occur, is very much less. In other words, there may be almost as many blood losses of over 20 ounces, but there are many fewer cases of blood losses of over 40 or 50 ounces, and it is this second factor which matters most.

It might be as well to ask if there are any drawbacks. There is certainly one serious risk, namely the case of the undiagnosed twin. To give ergometrine while the second twin has still to be delivered is certainly a serious matter, made even worse should the lie not be longitudinal, and the child must be very expeditiously delivered if it is to survive the uterine spasm which occurs as a result of ergometrine. Unfortunately, medical assistance may not be at hand, and this risk more than any other makes one hesitate to recommend its general application throughout domiciliary practice.

If ergometrine is given intravenously as a prophylactic measure against hæmorrhage, the timing of the injection is important if the best results are to be obtained. Its administration should coincide with the crowning of the head or with the delivery of the anterior shoulder. Thereafter, the delivery of the body should await the contractile response of the uterus. By this means satisfactory separation of the placenta is encouraged.

An effect which is almost as rapid can be obtained by the intra-

muscular injection of ergometrine coupled with hyaluronidase and Kimbell in comparing 1,700 cases, so treated at the moment of crowning, with 700 untreated controls, found that the incidence of hæmorrhage was nine times as high in the latter and that the manual removal rate was not increased as a result of ergometrine so given. He too inclines to the view that retention of the placenta may be encouraged if the drug is given too late, for example, after the delivery of the child's body.

With the help of tocographic studies Embrey and his colleagues at Oxford have explored the advantages of using a combination of oxytocin for its speed of action and ergometrine for its duration of effect (Syntometrine). They confirmed tocographically that hyaluronidase accelerated the action of intramuscular ergometrine by about two minutes. Having found that the full effect after intramuscular injection of ergometrine alone was as slow as seven minutes this, in their opinion, was a rather disappointing improvement, and the addition of oxytocin was found to speed up the response of the uterus.[6, 7] The observations of the Oxford workers have been abundantly confirmed by others using Syntometrine in Worcester, Manchester and by ourselves and it would appear that intramuscular Syntometrine makes as good a substitute as can be obtained for intravenous ergometrine under circumstances in which such an intravenous injection cannot be given. There remains the one debateable point, having given Syntometrine whether to adopt a highly active policy and secure delivery of the placenta forthwith by fundal pressure, or controlled cord traction, or to wait for signs of placental separation. Our own view at the moment is that after giving Syntometrine, and provided there is no bleeding, there is nothing to be lost by waiting a few minutes and allowing time for the placenta to descend at least some distance down the genital canal, peeling off the membranes behind it.

The oxytocic response of intravenous ergometrine is fully established within forty-one seconds (average time) as against nearly five minutes with intramuscular ergometrine plus hyaluronidase and seven minutes with ergometrine alone intramuscularly, but Syntometrine is effective within two and a half minutes.[8]

Definition of postpartum hæmorrhage.—The definition of postpartum hæmorrhage is arbitrary. Blood losses of over 20 ounces are almost universally accepted as indicating postpartum hæmorrhage, whether it comes from the placental site or from laceration of the genital tract. This standard is not wholly satisfactory, for the danger of postpartum hæmorrhage depends more upon the rate at which blood is lost than upon its actual amount, and the patient's ability to withstand hæmorrhage has also to be taken into account. However, for statistical purposes, it serves well enough. The usual time

limit set for the application of this definition is up to 24 hours after delivery. Thereafter bleeding is designated "secondary postpartum hæmorrhage" (see later).

CAUSES OF POSTPARTUM HÆMORRHAGE

Apart from lacerations, uterine inversion and clotting defects (which are dealt with elsewhere), there is only one cardinal cause of postpartum hæmorrhage, namely anything which interferes with retraction of the uterus as a whole and of the placental site in particular. In the majority of instances this is because the uterus is, for various reasons, atonic. Less commonly mechanical factors may play a part, such as the presence of fibroids or a partial pathological adherence of the placenta to the uterine wall preventing emptying, however good the uterine tone. Inversion is dealt with elsewhere, but it must be remembered that it may be accompanied by severe hæmorrhage. It will be seen, therefore, that the majority of cases are due to imperfect retraction as a result of uterine atony, and the remarks just made about the routine use of ergometrine apply in this direction. It is therefore necessary to seek for the factors which predispose to uterine atony. The retention of the placenta may be the cause of imperfect retraction because of morbid adherence, but is far more commonly the effect, since morbid adherence is rather unusual and certainly not as common as operators describe in recounting their experiences in manual removal.

Factors which predispose to uterine atony in the third stage.— High degrees of multiparity probably constitute the commonest cause, and this fact has never been wholly satisfactorily explained, for the grand multipara usually goes through the first and second stages of labour exhibiting the very reverse of sluggish uterine action. It may well be that, in her case, uterine contractions occur with a vigour out of all proportion to the ability of the uterus to retract, a fact which comes fully to light only in the third stage. After the first four or five deliveries each successive labour carries a somewhat greater risk of postpartum hæmorrhage, and since these women, often as a result of rapidly repeated childbirth, overwork, poverty, malnutrition and chronic iron deficiency anæmia, are in a poorer condition to withstand even a moderate postpartum hæmorrhage, it will be seen that the effects are far more serious.

The next most important predisposing factor is that of multiple pregnancy. In cases of twins (and hydramnios too) the uterus, because of over-distension, may be lacking in retractile power; but even more important is the fact that in twins the double placenta is a relatively large structure, which is less readily delivered, and the area of the placental site is greatly increased so that bleeding, when

it does occur, is doubly profuse. Added to all this there is the possibility that some of the large placental site area has overlapped on to the lower uterine segment where retractile power is poor.

Placenta prævia itself, besides causing inevitable antepartum hæmorrhage, is often a cause of postpartum hæmorrhage the effects of which are aggravated by the antecedent bleeding, and it is a strange paradox that one of the commonest causes of death in A.P.H. should be P.P.H. The same obtains in cases of accidental hæmorrhage, and the most terrible hæmorrhage I have ever witnessed followed delivery of a woman with abruptio placentæ.

Uterine exhaustion following a prolonged, inert labour is often classed as one of the principal causes of postpartum hæmorrhage, though this has not been my experience. It is certain that when hæmorrhage does occur its effects are more pronounced because the patient is already dehydrated as a result of her labour. It is the loss of available circulating fluid rather than the number of available red cells which accounts for the immediate evidences of shock in postpartum hæmorrhage. With regard to prolonged labour it must be remembered that many of these cases have been fairly heavily narcotised and the uterine atony in the third stage is often due to drugs and anæsthetics.

Precipitate labour is quite often followed by postpartum hæmorrhage which is not necessarily due to grand multiparity. It is probable that in these cases the placenta is detached at the end of a precipitate second stage, and the uterus, which in any case requires a few minutes to achieve retraction, is unable immediately to follow up its sudden emptying with suitably maintained shrinkage.

Anæsthetics produce atony more as a result of the depth of general narcosis achieved than because of individual drug propensities, and for this reason chloroform and ether are reputedly dangerous in high dosage. Nevertheless, certain drugs seem to affect the uterus less adversely than others, notably cyclopropane, which I always welcome during Cæsarean section, not only for this reason, but because of the high oxygenation rate with which it is given. Relaxant drugs of the curare class do not interfere with uterine contraction, nor do the lighter anæsthetics like nitrous oxide or Trilene. General debilitating diseases predispose the patient to some extent to postpartum hæmorrhage, but their chief contribution lies in magnifying its effect.

Most people are agreed that a patient with a previous history of retained placenta runs an appreciably greater risk of the same misfortune in subsequent deliveries. It would seem only prudent, therefore, to deliver such a case in an institution. Dewhurst and Dutton (1957) in a review of 132 labours in which there had been a previous history of abnormal third stage found that in 23 per cent this stage

was again abnormal and that even one or more intervening labours without trouble did not eliminate the dangers of recurrent mishaps in the third stage of the next labour. A woman, therefore, who has once had third-stage trouble, be it hæmorrhage, placental retention or manual removal, should be suspected of being capable of a repeat performance.

They recommend in such cases the routine prophylactic use of intravenous ergometrine at the delivery of the anterior shoulder. Yet even this precaution did not prevent serious hæmorrhage in all cases —a sobering thought. The availability of suitable cross-matched blood for transfusion is clearly essential in the patient with a bad third-stage history and hospital confinement indicated absolutely.

Fibroids undoubtedly increase the likelihood of third-stage bleeding, not only because they may mechanically interfere with uterine retraction, but also because when they impinge upon the inner surface of the uterus the decidual reaction in this region is sometimes less complete. Should the placenta happen to be sited here, some degree of morbid adhesion may be encountered. This is a matter which cannot be foreseen in a case complicated by fibroids, but it is as well to bear the risk in mind. Fortunately, bleeding usually ceases once the uterus is empty, even though fibroids may be present in marked size or number. Should bleeding continue after the uterus has been proved empty by exploration, it may be necessary, in rare instances, to resort to hysterectomy.

Lastly, as already stated, one of the most common if not the most trivial cause of postpartum hæmorrhage is the presence of clots in the uterus. Their very presence seems to paralyse the uterus from further retractile activity and they are all too often overlooked. Their effect can hardly be wholly mechanical, because it is such a simple matter to squeeze them out.

Estimates of blood actually lost at delivery vary from guesswork to near mendacity, according to temperament, but the amount is nearly always greater than reckoned. Using a hæmodilution technique (Perdometer) in which we have collected all blood, swabs, soiled towels and gloves in a sort of washing machine with a known volume of hæmolysing detergent, it is possible, after correcting for the patient's known hæmoglobin level, to calculate the blood loss accurately.

For years it has always bothered me that hæmoglobin levels in patients 3 days after Cæsarean section were so often a couple of grams or more per cent lower than the estimated blood loss would account for until this investigation produced the likely explanation. In a study of over 500 cases[21] it was found that the average blood loss at Cæsarean section was nearly one litre (!) and at forceps delivery just over 400 ml. Spontaneous vaginal delivery, as might be expected,

cost the patient least blood of all (less than 300 ml. in 83 per cent of cases to which episiotomy added a further 130 ml.). It is quite clear therefore that one can safely double a colleague's estimate of blood actually lost, and in some cases treble it, without fear of exaggeration.

PROPHYLAXIS

The first important step is to spot the losers, or rather the blood losers, and arrange for their delivery in an institution which is capable of supplying immediate anæsthesia, resident skilled, obstetric cover and full laboratory services, including those necessary for massive transfusion. General practitioner obstetric units do not normally fulfil these requirements. Patients in the following categories should have blood cross-matched on admission to the labour suite:

History of postpartum hæmorrhage.
Antepartum hæmorrhage.
Previous Cæsarean section.
Hæmoglobin under 10g./100 ml.
Intra-uterine death.
Fœtal distress.

In general, whenever there is a possibility of Cæsarean section or excessive hæmorrhage, blood should be cross-matched.[22] In the first chapter of this book the indications for hospital booking are fully given. Many of them are concerned with the risk of hæmorrhage and, of these, all cases of grand multiparity, multiple pregnancy, antepartum hæmorrhage of any variety and a past history of third-stage troubles constitute the most important groups. The incidence of postpartum hæmorrhage is also higher in women under the age of twenty years, whatever their parity, and in those over the age of forty.

Vigilance during the third stage there must always be, but it would be well to consider more specific measures. Of these the most important is to be ready with ergometrine. Valuable minutes may easily be lost in procuring a syringe and opening an ampoule, and the syringe should always be charged with 0·5 mg. of ergometrine or Syntometrine some time during the second stage and kept in readiness in some standard position. In domiciliary practice the mantelpiece is suggested. The drug will in any case not be wasted, for it can be given before leaving the house should its use not have been previously necessary.

Antenatal supervision, in so far as anæmia is routinely diagnosed and corrected during pregnancy, is also an important measure to insure the patient against the possible effects of hæmorrhage.

The chances of postpartum hæmorrhage can be reduced by good

management. Even one's management of the second stage of labour is of importance. Only an irresponsible person would deliver a woman with forceps in the complete absence of uterine contractions, and anyone sufficiently ignorant to commit this crime could be expected to be incompetent to cope with the inevitable hæmorrhage rewarding his folly. Even in normal delivery, however, it is important to deliver the baby's trunk slowly in order to allow a little time for uterine retraction to follow up the egress of the baby's body. This rule applies particularly after the intravenous use of ergometrine if the full benefits of this treatment are to be enjoyed.

Once bleeding starts, even though the amount is not initially serious, it is far better to act too soon than too late. A common and treacherous situation is one in which very small gushes repeatedly occur, none of them, by themselves, at all alarming, but whose effect is cumulative. It is important here not only to measure very accurately how much the loss is adding up to, but to be quite clear about what is happening inside the uterus. At a time when one of these little gushes is taking place, it will usually be found that the uterus is hard. The gush then stops and, for a time, it is thought that all is well, yet when it recurs the uterus is again found to be firm and well contracted. What is happening of course is that during the periods of arrested external bleeding the uterus is relaxing and filling itself with blood and the gush which occurs with the observed hardness of the uterus represents blood actually lost a minute or so earlier. Once this sequence of events is established, it becomes less and less likely that the placenta will be spontaneously delivered, and although the case may be nowhere near classification as one of postpartum hæmorrhage, it is far better to take note of the warning before it is too late.

One is often reluctant to intervene because, for the time being, the patient's general condition seems so satisfactory but, as explained in the chapter on postpartum collapse, the signs of a rising pulse and a falling blood pressure are usually ten minutes out of date, so that intervention, when it comes as a result of these indications, comes too late.

One's only defence, therefore, is to start thinking alertly when the 10-ounce mark is reached and to be prepared to act when the loss reaches 15 ounces. If one waits until the statutory 20 ounces has been lost, intervention will only have to be undertaken under conditions far less favourable. Beware therefore of inertia not only in the uterus but in the attendant!

The patient's own blood is more precious than any that a blood bank can provide and a surer defence against puerperal sepsis than all the antibiotics in the world. It would be better to carry out manual removal of the placenta with imperfectly sterilised hands,

while the patient still remains in possession of most of her own circulating blood volume, than to carry out the same operation with the most rigid asepsis in a patient already dangerously exsanguinated.

Treatment of Postpartum Hæmorrhage

The uterus must be emptied of its contents whether they be blood clots, placenta, or both. This is the first principle of treatment, and the order in which the various measures are employed differs in some respects, depending upon whether the placenta has already been delivered and upon the briskness or persistence of the hæmorrhage.

Bleeding after Delivery of the Placenta

The fundus of the uterus should at once be sought and kneaded by brisk massage through the abdominal wall until the uterus hardens with a contraction. Then, and not before, it is firmly squeezed to expel the blood clots which are almost certainly present within its cavity. This alone may suffice.

In carrying out this simple measure it is important to avoid pressing the uterus down into the pelvic cavity, which is not only useless but may be harmful, because venous drainage is to some extent obstructed and hæmorrhage is, therefore, likely to be increased. While squeezing with one hand, the other hand should steady the uterine body from below, being placed on the abdominal wall just above the symphysis pubis. Quickness of movement is more useful than sheer brute force, from which the patient cannot protect herself by contraction of her very lax abdominal wall.

At the earliest opportunity the placenta should be examined to make sure that it is complete and that there is no evidence, in the form of torn vessels at the edge of the chorionic rent, to suggest that a succenturiate lobe has been left behind. If either a cotyledon or a lobe is missing, exploration of the uterine cavity will, of course, be necessary.

Ergometrine should be injected as soon as possible, and the choice of the intravenous or the intramuscular route will depend on the urgency of the hæmorrhage. For this reason a sterile syringe already loaded with ergometrine and kept in a standard position in readiness for the injection will often prove a great standby. The intravenous route is to be preferred where seconds rather than minutes count and an almost certain effect is assured within forty seconds. The intravenous dose favoured is 0·25 mg. of ergometrine. This is twice the dose recommended by Chassar Moir, but the margin of safety is wide. It is not necessary to exceed this dose intravenously, as some patients may exhibit side-effects, such as

dizziness, vomiting and weakness of the limbs. Intramuscular injection of ergometrine will usually produce its effect within seven minutes and often less, the standard dose in this instance being 0·5 mg. Syntometrine, already described, is even better, and acts more quickly.

If the uterus refuses to harden up with the initial rubbing, and this is rather uncommon, no time should be lost in injecting one of these drugs. Massage of the uterus will now be effective.

A uterus which keeps softening and losing successive little trickles of blood, especially after twin delivery, may be kept in a better state of activity by maintaining an oxytocin drip infusion for an hour or two.

If bleeding still continues a laceration of the cervix or vagina should be suspected, as discussed later, but one should not forget as a possible cause of prolonged trickling after a complete delivery of the placenta and with no evidence of a tear of cervix or vagina and where there is no clotting defect that the cause may, in fact, be due to a minor degree of uterine inversion. Bimanual compression of the uterus is very seldom called for in such cases and hot intra-uterine douches even less frequently.

The uterus can often be compressed very efficiently through the abdominal wall, without resorting to vaginal manipulations, by raising it with the right hand out of the pelvis and passing the left hand behind the fundus. This hand now presses the uterus forward over the right hand and, moreover, the lower part of the uterus can be compressed against the sacral promontory.

Bleeding before Delivery of the Placenta

One's immediate reactions will depend upon whether or not the patient is under an anæsthetic, because if she is already anæsthetised, for example for forceps delivery, manual removal of the placenta can be undertaken more readily. In these cases intravenous ergometrine should already have been injected as soon as the anterior shoulder was born (see chapter on Forceps) and one is now working at a considerable advantage.

When a patient is not under a general anæsthetic, decisions are usually harder to make. It is true that manual removal of the placenta can be undertaken without a general anæsthetic; in fact 1 have done so myself with the help of self-administered Trilene, but except in grave emergency or when the placenta is obviously loose in the lower uterine segment and controlled cord traction has just failed to deliver it, such a practice is not to be recommended. I was once rash enough to give a talk to the Mother's Union of our Church on "what to do about a woman upstairs unexpectedly having a baby", but the meeting soon degenerated into a series of personal obstetrical reminiscences

by the various members of my audience. One of these included a description in graphic terms of having one's placenta removed without anæsthesia, which electrified the audience. It made the evening!

The first thing to do, of course, is to massage the fundus of the uterus vigorously until it hardens, and, whether or not this is success-ful in temporarily arresting the bleeding, no time should be lost in in-jecting ergometrine intravenously or intramuscularly, according to the rapidity of the blood loss. This is far better treatment within the first minute than resorting to possibly fruitless and damaging attempts at Credé's expression of the placenta in the unanæsthetised patient.

The importance of not fiddling with the fundus during the con-duct of the third stage has already been dealt with at length, and one's actions now are in strange contrast to this previous inactivity. Once blood has started to appear at the vulva the arguments for keeping hands off the fundus of the uterus no longer apply, and so-called fiddling, to the extent of purposive massage, is now called for. Rubbing up a contraction in any case produces no more than a temporary respite from bleeding. This is bound to recur until the placenta has been safely delivered.

Credé's Method of Expression of the Placenta

This is a subject on which strong views are held by some author-ities in opposing directions. That it is resorted to more often than necessary there can be no doubt, and it is equally certain that it can produce or aggravate shock. Consequently many obstetricians think that there is no justification whatsoever for its use. Controlled cord traction or the Brandt-Andrews technique may make Credé's ex-pression unnecessary in many cases and should be tried first. On the other hand, by its judicious use it is possible to save many a patient from the need for manual removal of the placenta, and most of us now take a middle view, permitting one attempt at Credé's expression before the patient has received an anæsthetic, a further attempt once anæsthesia has been induced, to be immediately followed by manual removal of the placenta should this second attempt fail. (If possible, the bladder should be emptied first by catheterisation provided time allows.)

Unless one is possessed of a very powerful masculine hand it will usually be found that two hands are required. A common method is to pass the fingers behind the body of the uterus and to squeeze the front wall with the opposed thumbs. Alternatively, in a thin woman, it may be possible to squeeze the uterus between the palms of the two hands. The upper part of the uterus should be

squeezed first, and in doing so the uterus should not be driven down into the depths of the pelvis, which is both shocking and ineffectual.

On no account should Credé's expression ever be attempted unless the uterus has first been made to contract either by brisk massage or by the injection of ergometrine. If the uterus cannot be made to harden up, then Credé's method of expression is absolutely contraindicated, for not only will it fail but acute inversion of the uterus is likely to result.

If a large clot has already collected in the uterus, it is necessary to maintain the pressure in order to secure the delivery of the placenta. This is a method which calls more for knack than for force. Much of the latter is often grossly misapplied by the novice. As soon as the placenta has been expelled, it is necessary to rub the uterus again to maintain a good state of contraction until bleeding ceases. The effect can be reinforced by the injection of more ergometrine.

The amount of ergometrine given in the repeated injections should not exceed 1·0 mg. If, as often happens, the attempt fails, and one is simply rewarded by further bleeding, it may be necessary to give a further injection of ergometrine while anæsthesia is being induced.

Stock should at all times be taken of the patient's general condition. Fortunately, where shock is profound, bleeding will usually greatly diminish, if not stop altogether, and this temporary respite should be made use of to set up an intravenous infusion. If crossmatched blood is already available, so much the better, but usually there will be some delay in obtaining it and, in the meantime, normal saline may be given. The patient's most urgent need is for an adequate circulating blood volume. The decision when to proceed to deliver the placenta under anæsthesia will depend upon the state of the patient's blood pressure. If the systolic pressure is less than 100 mm. Hg there are considerable risks in proceeding further until the state of shock and exsanguination has been to some extent corrected, and in the chapter on postpartum collapse details are given of how to choose the best moment for operative intervention.

Until the patient's condition warrants an anæsthetic, ergometrine, blood transfusion and oxygen are one's main standby. During this anxious period, the blood pressure must be repeatedly observed, and no time must be lost, as soon as the systolic pressure exceeds 100 mm. Hg, in proceeding to the removal of the placenta. If there is delay now, the patient will assuredly bleed again, and shock this time will be less easily corrected.

In making the second attempt at Credé's expression under an anæsthetic all preparations should be at hand for proceeding to manual removal should the attempt fail and, if possible, an intravenous drip should already be in action. These circumstances demand the presence of another practitioner, and in domiciliary

practice one would be well advised not to proceed further single-handed.

In most large population centres there are, nowadays, "flying squads" who will come readily to one's aid. While waiting for the arrival of help the bladder should be catheterised, the patient should be given morphia and, if available, oxygen. She should be kept warm, for shock is greatly aggravated by cold, and one has to rely on the ergometrine already given to protect the patient from further bleeding.

Every obstetrician should carry in his bag some fluid suitable for intravenous use. Even saline is better than nothing. Where no fluid suitable for intravenous use is to hand, ordinary tap water, run slowly into the rectum, will help to restore the patient from a state of complete pulselessness. Dextran is not without drawbacks. In the first place it must not be given until a specimen of the patient's blood has been taken for grouping and cross-matching as its presence in the patient's circulating blood may interfere with the test. Secondly, it may interfere with the mechanism of blood coagulation.[19]

It is far better to rely upon these measures than to resort to further traumatic attempts at Credé's expression, pending the arrival of help. Before the days of "flying squads" one had only the choice of transferring the patient to hospital, in a condition already precarious, or of coping with the situation on the spot with the help of a partner. The more desperate the patient's condition the more likely was the second of these alternatives to be the safer procedure, unless transport to a nearby hospital was readily available. The advantages of transferring the patient to hospital, however, are that really massive transfusion becomes possible and expert anæsthesia is available. Local circumstances, therefore, must decide the choice.

The institution of the "flying squad", with its ready supply of Rh-negative Group O blood, has simplified the dilemma and has been responsible for the saving of many lives. We always keep a fresh stock of four units of Rh-negative, Group O blood, screened for Anti-A hæmolysins at the ready for immediate transfusion to any recipient in urgent need, and have on occasion used all of it too.

Let us now assume that the patient's general condition is fit for anæsthesia, that an attempt at Credé's expression or, preferably, controlled cord traction has already failed, the placenta still remaining *in utero*, and that all preparations are to hand.

The patient is anæsthetised with some quick-acting anæsthetic, of which thiopentone is one of the most useful, and during the induction the obstetrician dons sterile gloves. It is a regrettable fact that the shortage of skilled anæsthetists may, in many instances, deny otherwise up-to-date maternity units the immediately available service they should have. Rather than wait for expert anæsthetic

help, manual removal of the placenta under a sort of "hypoanæs-thesia", using a combination of pethidine (Demerol) 50 mg. intra-venously, pudendal block and trichloroethylene has proved a useful expedient[5] which, however, is to be deplored since it might encourage Regional Board Staffing Committees to view full anæsthetic cover with less urgency. After drenching the vulva with antiseptic solution a catheter must be passed, for, if there is time for anæsthesia there is also time for catheterisation. The abdomen must be covered with a sterile towel. Through the towel the second attempt at Credé's expression may be made, again having assured oneself that the uterus is well contracted. If this attempt fails or if it cannot be undertaken because the uterus cannot be made to contract satis-factorily, one is now ready to proceed in a matter of seconds to manual removal of the placenta. The above precautions of asepsis are always worth while before attempting expression, in order to obviate delays if manual removal is necessary.

MANUAL REMOVAL OF THE PLACENTA

To quote Bruce Mayes, "The really difficult part about manual removal is the decision to undertake it." Under the procedure out-lined above, this decision will have already been taken and there will now be no hesitation.

The vulva has already been cleansed with antiseptic lotion and the bladder has been emptied. The cord should be cut off short at the vulva. One hand in the shape of a cone is insinuated into the vagina. Time should not be wasted removing perineal sutures. If necessary they can be replaced later. The cord is followed until the placenta is found.

The other hand is just as important as the hand inside the uterus. There is a very natural tendency to forget about the existence of this second hand whose function is to steady the fundus of the uterus and prevent it from being pushed up towards the costal margin. During manual removal of the placenta the uterus is very inclined to relax, with the result that the internal hand has to be introduced almost to the entire length of the forearm if this precaution is not taken.

Using the external hand correctly, it should not be necessary to introduce the other hand farther than two or three inches above the level of the wrist, the fundus being guided on to the fingers inside by external manipulation. If, through faulty technique, the fundus of the uterus is allowed to drift into the upper abdomen, the placental sinuses are opened up and hæmorrhage becomes profuse. The risk of perforation of the uterine wall is also considerably increased.

Finding the placenta is not usually difficult and can be facilitated by keeping the cord taut while inserting the hand. It now has to be

remembered that no retreat is permissible until the placenta has been completely detached.

Having reached the insertion of the cord in the placenta the periphery is sought. Some now proceed to separation by working from above downwards, but in actual fact it is easier to work by starting from the already detached portion. This is usually the inferior margin, and a plane of cleavage is here already demonstrated.

As far as possible the fingers should be kept together, working in the manner of an egg slice removing an egg from a frying-pan, at all times remembering the functions of the external hand pressing through the abdominal wall.

If a fold of the membranes can be kept in front of the advancing fingers, so much the better. Frenzied clawing with the individual fingers is to be deprecated, because the placenta will be torn to ribbons and much of it will be left behind. In few operations is there a greater need for patient determination.

Working from the detached margin upwards, the placenta will have been completely detached by the time the upper margin is reached, but it should not be removed from the uterus until one's fingers have reached above this margin.

Having now satisfied oneself that the whole placental mass is free within the uterine cavity, it is best delivered by traction on the cord, retaining the hand inside the uterus for a final exploration of its cavity.

Carried out deliberately and carefully, this operation can sometimes be remarkably bloodless but, in any case, bleeding must not undermine resolve. A failed attempt at manual removal is nothing short of disastrous.

The operation is not usually difficult, but there are certain points which are worth discussing. Occasionally there may be difficulty in reaching the placenta because of the presence of an hour-glass contraction ring. This is dealt with later. The other main difficulty is when an area of morbid adherence of the placenta is encountered. There is no doubt that this is far more often diagnosed than is actually the case, and I have now noted that right-handed operators tend to attribute morbid adhesion in the region of the right cornu of the uterus, whereas left-handed operators seem to diagnose this trouble in the left cornu, and it is suggested that this finding is occasionally more subjective than objective. When, however, this pathological condition is encountered, the difficulty may be very great, and it is almost impossible to remove the placenta without leaving shreds of tissue behind. Under these circumstances one has to be content with the best that one can do.

Having successfully completed manual removal of the placenta, most cases will usually stop bleeding. Occasionally, when there is

gross uterine atony, hæmorrhage continues unabated. Intravenous ergometrine is more likely to be successful than any other measure, but sometimes one may have to resort to bimanual compression of the uterus forthwith.

Bimanual Compression of the Uterus

The clenched fist is placed in the anterior fornix and the body of the uterus is compressed against it by a hand placed behind the uterus through the abdominal wall. Considerable hæmostatic pressure can be applied in this way, but it cannot be maintained for more than two or three minutes because of fatigue. During this time, however, the uterus usually contracts and arrests hæmorrhage.

There is one great pitfall about this procedure, namely that the case most urgently in need of it often has a uterus so atonic that it cannot be felt and therefore cannot be convincingly compressed. When the uterus is too soft to be palpable, one may even doubt whether the clenched fist is in the anterior fornix. In such cases it may be necessary to resort to a hot intra-uterine douche.

Intra-uterine douche.—A hot intra-uterine douche is a very certain method of stimulating an atonic uterus to contract. It is not without its obvious dangers, and should only be used when other measures fail to control the bleeding. It is customary to put some antiseptic lotion in the douche, but it is the heat which matters rather than the constituents. To be effective, therefore, the temperature should be not less than 118° F. in the douche can. Temperatures greater than this carry with them the risk of producing a sloughing of the vagina, especially in a patient who is severely shocked, under an anæsthetic, and in whom the blood circulation rate is very slow.

All air should be driven out of the piping before the douche nozzle is inserted into the uterus, because of the risk of air embolism. The can should be held not more than 2 feet above the level of the uterus, because greater pressures may force fluid along the Fallopian tubes. The risk of sepsis is, of course, increased by using an intra-uterine douche, but the dangers of present hæmorrhage are far more pressing.

Uterine tamponade.—This is a desperate measure and is very seldom employed in this country, although it is more popular in the United States. Enormous quantities of sterile roll gauze have to be used, each length being knotted together.

The gauze is best introduced by a hand passed well into the uterus with the other hand steadying the fundus from outside through the abdominal wall. It is most important to pack the upper portion of the uterus thoroughly, and a common mistake is to introduce some half-hearted packing only into the lower part of the uterus, leaving a large cavity above, which of course just fills with blood.

The packing is most likely to exert its effect by stimulating the uterus to contract rather than by direct pressure upon the placental sinuses. If, however, the uterus relaxes above the pack instead of contracting, as it may well do, matters are made very much worse.

It is impossible to pack the uterus properly without an anæsthetic, and the operation is both dangerous and useless unless done with great thoroughness.

I have only used this method of controlling hæmorrhage once, and that was in a case who had been delivered by a colleague by classical Cæsarean section for placenta prævia. A large portion of the placenta was found to be accreta and the placenta could only be removed piecemeal. Much of it was left behind, and hæmorrhage during the operation was torrential. I first saw the patient some hours after operation, and she was then receiving her eleventh pint of blood. Her bed had been changed twice because of soiling with blood, she had air hunger and was pulseless. Her blood pressure was less than 50 mm. Hg systolic. She was far too ill for hysterectomy and was moreover still bleeding. In this case I explored the uterus, removed a large quantity of retained blood clot and as much remaining placental tissue as I could, and packed the uterus firmly with gauze. The effect was dramatic and the patient rallied, leaving the hospital a fortnight later none the worse for her experience and with her uterus still *in situ*. The pack was removed under morphine premedication 24 hours later.

It is in cases of placenta prævia which continue to bleed postpartum that packing is likely to be more useful than at any other time. This is because the placental site is situated in a non-retractile portion of the uterus and, rarely, packing alone may control the hæmorrhage.

On the whole it is not an operation to be lightly considered, and the case well enough to stand it in safety is likely not to need it, and other measures should suffice. Oxidised cellulose gauze has been used by some obstetricians, but Titus reports that he found its use unsatisfactory, because he had to remove large portions of partially dissolved material piecemeal at a later date.

ATTENTION TO THE PATIENT'S GENERAL CONDITION

So long as the patient is actively losing blood no general resuscitative measure can ever hope to keep pace with the deterioration so caused. Therefore, the first step must always be to arrest acute hæmorrhage. Many cases, however, will subside into a condition of uncorrected shock unless prompt resuscitative measures are taken. Of these, blood transfusion is by far the most important, and no time should be lost in setting one up, as already mentioned. Pending

the arrival of cross-matched blood, plasma or even normal saline may be given, but the sooner the patient receives whole blood the better, for this is what she is losing.

It is very easy to waste time by busying oneself with minor and less effectual measures to restore the patient's general condition when one's whole concentration should be directed towards the intravenous drip.

If the veins are collapsed it may be difficult to make the drip run at more than a drop every second or two. Nikethamide 0·25 ml. injected into the drip tubing sometimes encourages it to speed up and

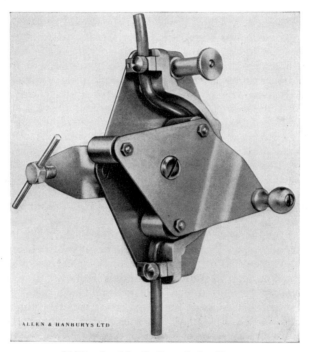

21/Fig. 1.—Martin Transfusion Pump.

(By courtesy of Allan & Hanburys, Ltd.)

warming of the limb occasionally helps. Rapid transfusion can be given under positive pressure with one of the rotary roller-type pumps now on the market (Fig. 1) and no maternity unit should be without some such device. On no account should positive pressure within the blood bottle be generated by means of a Higginson syringe attached to the vent tube, a common but terribly dangerous practice.

I have seen a patient killed within a few seconds by a massive air embolus which forced its way into the delivery pipe.

Most patients are undertransfused rather than overtransfused since the blood loss is usually greater than reckoned and the effective blood contents of the standard bottle amount only to 400 ml. since the remainder is made up of citrate.

Pulse and blood-pressure records may not reveal the full degree of exsanguination and the adequacy of blood replacement because a circulating blood volume as low as 70 per cent of normal may fail to cause variations in pulse rate or blood-pressure level.[12] Usually, therefore, the amount of blood transfused depends upon guesswork, but the measurement of central venous pressures provides the readiest guide in an emergency. The method is not only simpler but more useful than estimating blood volumes by dye or isotope dilution techniques.

To measure central venous pressure a plastic catheter of previously estimated length is passed into the superior vena cava through a No. 14 gauge needle, either via a jugular vein or from an arm vein, which we prefer. It is connected both to drip infusion and to a water manometer by a three-way tap and the column of water height is measured above the manubriosternal junction which is 5 cm. above the level of the superior vena cava with the patient in the dorsal position. Using the manubriosternal junction as a reference point the normal range of central venous pressures is from 5 to 12 centimetres of water. Transfusion should be maintained until this range is achieved and pulmonary congestion due to overtransfusion will not occur unless the upper limit is exceeded.

The foot of the bed is raised, morphia is given to allay restlessness and the patient is wrapped up in dry, warm bedding. The blood pressure and pulse are recorded every quarter of an hour and a watch is kept for renewed bleeding. In extreme degrees of hypotension Methedrine intravenously, will raise in half a minute a blood pressure of, for example, 70/60 to over 100/70 mm. Hg, and the effect is not so transitory as might be expected.[11] The dose is up to 20 mg. and it may be added to the drip. This treatment is a useful ancillary measure, but is no substitute for blood transfusion. One should aim, so far as possible, at replacing quantitatively the measured amount of blood lost. Where there is difficulty in maintaining a reasonable blood pressure Aramine is a useful addition to the drip, or hydrocortisone (see Chapter XX).

The longer a patient remains in uncorrected exsanguination and shock, the longer will it take for the above resuscitative measures to succeed, and if they are instituted with the minimum delay, one is usually rewarded by a remarkable recovery in the patient within three hours.

NOTES ON TRANSFUSION

The following notes are extracted from an admirable pamphlet on the subject issued by the Ministry of Health, in association with the Department of Health for Scotland, for the National Blood Transfusion Service, 1958.

Banked blood should not be used unless there is a clear line of demarcation between the sedimented cells and the supernatant plasma, which should be straw coloured and free from visible signs of hæmolysis. The latter may be indicated by a reddish-purple discoloration in the supernatant plasma spreading upwards. The blood should have been stored at 4° C. and should not be time-expired. At no time should the blood have been allowed to freeze, as frozen and thawed blood may be lethal and blood which has been out of a refrigerator for more than 30 minutes should not be used.

Packed cells, made by discarding the plasma and adding the cells of one or more other bottles should only be prepared from blood less than a fortnight old and should be used within twelve hours of preparation.

Plasma is supplied with 400 ml. of pyrogen-free distilled water in which it is dissolved after 5 minutes shaking. Failure to dissolve within 10 minutes indicates rejection. Reconstituted plasma should be used within 3 hours.

In a previously healthy patient in urgent need of blood following hæmorrhage a transfusion rate of 100 ml./minute until the systolic blood pressure reaches 100 mm. Hg is well tolerated, but the rate should thereafter be cut back according to the state of the blood pressure.

In correcting chronic anæmia and in patients suffering chronic debilitating disorders, especially cases of cardiac disease, the rate of administration should not exceed 20–40 drops/minute for fear of embarrassing the heart. Signs of overload are jugular vein filling and moist sounds from pulmonary œdema at the lung bases.

The clinician administering the blood is responsible for ensuring that grouping and compatibility testing have been adequately carried out—preferably under proper laboratory conditions and only in the gravest emergency should Group O Rh-negative blood be used blindly since even this may contain anti-A or anti-B antibodies and uncommon immunization against even Rh-ve antigens is possible.

Samples of the patients' serum for testing should always be taken before any dextran-like substance has been infused. 5–10 ml. is collected with a dry sterile syringe and placed in a dry sterile tube after removing the needle (to avoid the damage caused by squirting).

Full compatibility testing and grouping takes a few hours but

laboratories can carry out modified compatibility tests within about half an hour in emergencies, which are preferable to the crude pre-war methods we used to employ of mixing a drop of the blood to be given on the back of a saucer with a drop of the patient's serum, obtained from the lumen of a broken-off capillary pipette end, and watching for signs of agglutination. Proper testing therefore means a 24-hour laboratory technician service.

Blood should not be warmed after removal from the refrigerator except in cases of exchange transfusion in babies.

Venepuncture is far preferable to cut down and cannulation, and a number of ingenious needle mechanisms are now available for introducing polythene catheters into veins.

In setting up the transfusion bottle and giving set, a clip should be closed on the tubing just proximal to the needle. After the air vent to the bottle has been opened the afferent tubing should be hung down and the clip near the end opened over a dish until blood runs out. The clip is then closed and the distal end, lifted in a U until it is at the same level as the bottom of the drip chamber. The clip can then be slowly opened until all air has been expelled from the tube. This avoids flooding the drip chamber.

The patient should be carefully watched for the first 30 minutes to stabilize the drip rate and to observe any unfavourable reactions.

All urine should be kept, measured and tested for albumin. The samples should not be discarded for 24 hours in case of any hæmoglobinuria or subsequent signs of transfusion reaction develop.

Treatment of Transfusion Reactions

In the event of a severe transfusion reaction occurring due to the giving of incompatible blood, the following treatment is suggested in order to lessen the risk of anuria:

500 ml. 10 per cent Rheomacrodex in dextrose (or approx. 1 g./Kg.) to be given as soon and as quickly as possible, followed by a further similar quantity given over the next hour.

The decision that incompatible blood has been given may be made on the basis of:

1. The severity of reaction, or
2. A comparison of the group shown on the bottle with that given in the patient's case notes, or
3. Subsequent verification in the laboratory that either the patient's alleged group or that of the bottle was erroneous.

It would not necessarily be justifiable to delay treatment until laboratory confirmation was obtained.[22]

Complications of Blood Transfusion

1. *Febrile Reaction.* Grade 1. Temperature to 100° F. Grade 2. Temperature above 100° F., with sensation of chill but no shivering. Grade 3. Rigor.

2. *Circulatory Overload and Pulmonary Œdema.*

3. *Hæmolytic Reaction.* This follows the giving of incompatible blood or blood already partly hæmolysed by freezing, heating, infection or prolonged storage.

The symptoms are often of rapid onset and include fever, dyspnœa, headache, constricting sensation of chest and intense lumbar pain.

Hæmoglobinuria and jaundice develop subsequently, the former in a few hours and the latter within a few days.

Death, when it occurs, is usually due to acute cardiac failure or suppression of urine.

4. *Air Embolism* is another dangerous complication usually due to connecting a Higginson's syringe to the transfusion bottle to speed up the drip, but it can also occur from faulty apparatus, even after puncturing the tubing to inject substances into the blood being given. This last hazard is reduced if the puncture is made at the distal end of the tube nearest the needle.

Air embolism should be promptly treated by clamping off the source and turning the patient on to her left side for two hours and giving oxygen.

5. *Allergic Reactions* such as urticaria, rashes and angioneurotic œdema.

6. Transfusion of already infected blood may produce symptoms at first indistinguishable from those of a hæmolytic reaction, except that there is extreme hypotension with warm extremities. There may also be vomiting, diarrhœa and abdominal pain. Antibiotics and vasopressor agents will be required.

7. *Homologous Serum Jaundice* may follow transfusion with blood or plasma, although all dried plasma in this country is prepared from pools from not more than 10 donors nowadays. The condition is clinically indistinguishable from infective hepatitis but the incubation period is from 40–150 days.

RISKS OF POSTPARTUM HÆMORRHAGE, IMMEDIATE AND REMOTE

Postpartum hæmorrhage in 1945 accounted for 9·4 per cent of all maternal deaths (Registrar-General) and even now accounts for 20–30 deaths a year in England and Wales. It is doubtful, however, whether figures from this source give a true picture, and many

patients who do not die as a result of their hæmorrhages remain handicapped for many years to come with indifferent health and chronic anæmia.

If the patient escapes immediate death from hæmorrhage, she still remains very liable to develop puerperal sepsis, for nothing so predisposes the patient to infection as the loss of blood. The saving of blood at all times and in all places is far more important than the most rigid aseptic technique, and no chemotherapy, however advanced, can guarantee the mastery of infection in the case of the seriously anæmic patient.

Gibberd once quoted a mortality for manual removal of the placenta of between 5 and 15 per cent, but it is usually the severity of the hæmorrhage indicating the manual removal which is lethal, rather than the operation itself. Nowadays, when manual removal is much more readily undertaken, the mortality has shrunk to low proportions.

The operation of manual removal is, however, easily fatal if undertaken in a patient whose blood pressure at the time is below 80 mm. Hg systolic, and, if possible, it is preferable to secure a blood pressure of over 100 before undertaking it.

The choice of anæsthetic makes an appreciable difference, nitrous oxide being particularly dangerous because of anoxia in a patient already anæmic.

If the systolic blood pressure remains below 80 mm. Hg for more than a very few hours, the patient is liable to develop anuria due to tubular nephrosis. All renal filtration ceases when the blood pressure reaches these low levels, and these cases should be watched carefully for signs of oliguria during the next few days.

After a severe postpartum hæmorrhage it is common for a patient to be unable to establish lactation, and chronic sub-involution may undermine her gynæcological health for years to come.

Anterior pituitary necrosis (Sheehan's syndrome), though fortunately uncommon, is a very serious risk in a patient who remains shocked and acutely anæmic for any length of time. This is discussed more fully in the chapter on postpartum collapse.

A chronic iron deficiency anæmia may remain as a permanent sequel to postpartum hæmorrhage unless steps are taken to correct it during the puerperium. The hæmoglobin should, as a matter of routine, be estimated 48 hours after delivery, and it will often be found that the patient has lost far more blood than was thought likely at the time. Blood transfusion, especially of packed cells, greatly expedites convalescence, but in less severe cases intramuscular iron therapy very often suffices, and it should be one's aim to restore a normal blood picture to the patient within the first six postnatal weeks.

EXTRA-PLACENTAL BLEEDING

If a patient continues to bleed although it is known that the uterus is empty and, by its hardness on palpation, it appears to be well retracted, the source of the hæmorrhage must be sought in the cervix, vaginal vault, vaginal walls or perineum.

An episiotomy usually bleeds far worse than a second-degree tear, and efficient suture will deal effectively with it. The worst hæmorrhage from the vulva usually occurs from tears in the neighbourhood of the clitoris. This can be controlled by underrunning a mattress suture.

More commonly the continued loss of bright blood usually indicates a laceration of the cervix. As a source of postpartum bleeding this is not common following normal delivery, but after forceps delivery or breech extraction it is a relatively frequent complication. One is often tempted to extemporise in the hope that the bleeding will cease spontaneously, which admittedly often occurs, but it is not wise to procrastinate for more than a minute or two. During this time the necessary instruments should be mustered for obtaining a proper view of the whole extent of the cervical perimeter. These instruments are: (1) A large Sim's speculum. (2) Three pairs of sponge forceps. They are far more satisfactory than vulsella, which tend to tear the cervix. (3) A liberal supply of gauze swabs. (4) A good light.

The cervix is often œdematous and bruised, and its lips may be very much distorted at the end of delivery, so that it is not always an easy matter to identify a laceration and the bleeding point at its base. Digital palpation from inside is not satisfactory, and it is far better to obtain a proper view by dragging each successive portion of the cervix well into sight, with the help of the speculum and the sponge forceps. One obtains a hold of any accessible portion of the cervix with the sponge forceps, and then, with the help of a second pair, works round the margin of the cervix towards the lateral edges. By pulling the speculum laterally and the sponge forceps medially a good view of the lateral fornices can be obtained.

Arterial bleeding from the cervix will be seen coming usually from the depth of the cleft caused by the laceration. As a temporary measure this bleeding region can be grasped with the third pair of sponge forceps while sutures are prepared.

The main indication for suture of a cervical laceration is to control hæmorrhage. It is very doubtful whether it is worth sewing up a laceration which is not causing bleeding because, for some reason, these lacerations never heal well however carefully sutured, and the cosmetic effect at postnatal examination is almost invariably disappointing.

It is often easier to put the first suture in, not at the base of the

laceration, but at the corners of its most distal margin. A finger can then be passed inside the cervix deep to the tear, and by gentle traction on the first suture the remaining sutures can be inserted very accurately (Fig. 2).

Occasionally, and this applies particularly to vault lacerations, as well as cervical, it may be possible to control hæmorrhage by applying sponge-holding forceps to the rent edges but impossible to

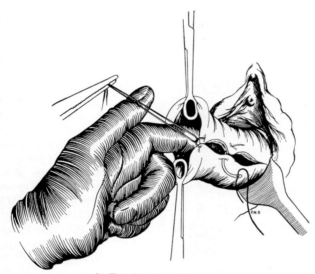

21/FIG. 2.—Cervical suture.

replace them with hæmostatic sutures because of cutting out, or inaccessibility combined with a parlous state of the patient. In such cases the safest course may be to leave the clamps in place for 24–48 hours, strapping them together. To prevent the patient dislodging them with her thighs one foot should be bandaged to the knee of the opposite leg (Fig. 3).

HOUR-GLASS CONSTRICTION RING (CONTRACTION RING)

The incidence of this troublesome complication to some extent varies with the amount of meddlesome interference which is undertaken during this stage of labour. The old fear that the use of oxytocic drugs before the delivery of the placenta would evoke it has not been borne out by experience since the routine use of these drugs in this manner was introduced. In almost all cases in which constriction ring occurs after the use of an oxytocic drug, some evidence can be found that the body of the uterus has been irritated by

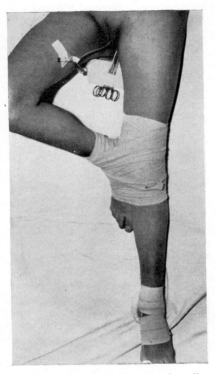

21/Fig. 3.—Method of preventing dis-
lodgement of hæmostatic clamps.

attempts at Credé's expression or by general mishandling. Intra-uterine manipulations during the second stage of labour to some extent make the uterus irritable and such a ring may develop during the third stage. Its occurrence is considered by many to be far more likely to be provoked in cases who have been given pituitary extract injections than in those who have received ergometrine; nevertheless, injudicious interference is more often to be blamed than either of these drugs.

The diagnosis can only be made, of course, by inserting, or attempting to insert, a hand into the uterus, and in the course of manual removal of a placenta the development of such a ring may be noticed. Fortunately, its onset is fairly gradual, and it is often possible to complete the removal before the ring has closed down too tightly.

In extent, a contraction ring varies from a complete constriction, making the upper portions of the uterus totally inaccessible, to minor degrees of ridging. In the former instance, if the hand is introduced in order to remove the placenta, the cord will be found to disappear through the vault of a smooth dome which represents the part of the uterine cavity below the ring. The placenta is thus completely out of reach. These cases, because of the very tightness of the ring, are incapable of bleeding for the time being. This ring cannot be penetrated, and as the patient is not bleeding, time can safely be allowed for it to wear off. The patient should be given morphia 15 mg. (gr. $\frac{1}{4}$), and within four hours it will be found that the ring has relaxed and the placenta can now be removed. During this period the patient should, of course, be kept under careful observation and the appearance of bleeding during this period will indicate, firstly, that the ring is relaxing, and secondly, that the placenta is endeavouring to separate and intervention should thereupon be undertaken.

The less extreme varieties of ring will allow the passage of two or more fingers, and in such cases the constriction will often yield to passive dilatation. Deep general anæsthesia encourages relaxation of the ring and in many cases amyl nitrite works like a charm. This drug is made up in small capsules of 3 or 5 minims and is highly volatile. The capsules are surrounded by little cotton bags to prevent the scatter of glass splinters. They are broken and immediately placed underneath the anæsthetic mask. However quickly one does this, much of the vapour will escape, and it is usually advisable to use two capsules. Often within a few seconds a ring which has appeared impassable seems to vanish, and the examining hand finds itself within the main cavity of the uterus without further difficulty. As soon as the placenta has been removed it matters not at all whether a ring reforms.

RETENTION OF THE PLACENTA WITHOUT BLEEDING

This is by no means uncommon and, because of the concern which it is likely to cause, it is hard to remember that as long as the patient is not bleeding she is in no immediate danger. A scrupulous vigilance of the third stage must be maintained throughout the period of waiting, and it is particularly important to satisfy oneself that the uterus is not slowly and silently filling with blood behind the placenta. This will be indicated not only by a rise in the level of the fundus, which may be very gradual, but by a very definite impression of an increase in size of the uterus as a whole. These signs point to the fact that bleeding is occurring and supply the indications to interfere.

In other cases the uterus seems merely to be inert and no signs of placental separation appear. One soon begins to wonder how long it is profitable to continue the wearisome observation of the third stage. While waiting, however, it is as well to remember that the apparent uterine inertia may be due to a full bladder, and a catheter should always be passed. It is common to find that somewhere between 6 and 10 ounces of clear pale urine have surreptitiously collected in the bladder since the delivery of the child. One was originally assured by catheterisation that the bladder was empty at the end of the second stage and this apparent diuresis in the third stage may come as a surprise. Much of this urine has probably been dammed back within the dilated ureters and renal pelves by the mechanical pressure of the child's head during the second stage.

After passing a catheter the uterus often appears to wake up and the signs of placental separation then follow.

If the placenta does not separate within an hour it is rather unlikely to do so spontaneously for a long time and most obstetricians are prepared to intervene before two hours have elapsed.

There are certain good reasons for discouraging an unduly prolonged retention of the placenta. Firstly, so long as the placenta remains undelivered, the patient is liable to start bleeding at any time. Secondly, supervision cannot be relaxed throughout this period. Thirdly, the patient cannot be left undisturbed in her own warm bed where she would be only too glad to have a sleep after the exertions of her recent labour. Fourthly, there is the occasional risk that the patient may develop a variety of postpartum collapse due to retention of the placenta alone. Finally, the longer the placenta is left in the uterus the greater are the chances of puerperal sepsis.

Every now and then an enthusiast for conservative methods decides to leave a placenta *in situ* for an indefinite period, in the hope that it will safely autolyse and ultimately be discharged, just like in cattle, and we have all heard of cases in which the placenta has been left in for several days without apparent ill effects. If the attendant prescribing this treatment were prepared to remain with the patient throughout this time and not to relax vigilance, we would have more respect for his attitude, but in many of these cases the placenta is removed by his house surgeon as soon as his back is turned.

If, after catheterisation and waiting, the placenta is still retained, preparations should be made for its removal, if necessary under anæsthesia. Although this may sound pessimistic, it is far better to be prepared for every eventuality before starting to rub up a contraction and squeezing the uterus, because, if anything goes wrong and bleeding starts, delays in completing delivery of the placenta may now be serious.

If the patient has not already received some ergometrine, 0·5 mg. should be injected intramuscularly. This alone may do the trick, but in any case it is far better than pushing on the fundus of the uterus to see what happens, a mistake that is often rewarded by the onset of bleeding which one may not be able to arrest immediately.

An anæsthetist should now be summoned, sterile drapes should be at hand and preparations made for the possibility of having to proceed to manual removal of the placenta if simpler measures fail.

Causes of retention of the placenta.—There are four main causes of retention of the placenta:

1. *Inertia.* This can often be countered by the injection of ergometrine which is preferable to uterine massage.

2. *Adherence of the membranes to the uterine wall.* This is a common cause, and one in which treatment by Credé's expression is most likely to succeed, or as an alternative, cord traction (see earlier).

3. *The presence of a constriction ring.* This has already been dealt with.

4. *The placenta may be totally morbidly adherent (placenta accreta).*

This last condition will not be diagnosed until an attempt at manual removal has to be made. In a study of 14 cases of placenta accreta in Glasgow, Millar (1959) noted the greatly increased incidence of placenta prævia as an ætiological factor, a point which my own experience confirms. The cause is thought to be primarily the result of a defective decidual reaction, probably hormonal in origin, rather than the result of previous trauma such as manual removal and curettage which themselves are required because of it. The association with uterine inversion is also recognised.

Treatment for this rare and ugly condition (which, be it remembered, may be encountered by those undertaking manual removal of the placenta in domiciliary conditions) consists of "grubbing out" the placenta as best one can and controlling the hæmorrhage as far as possible by bimanual compression, blood transfusion and even by uterine packing. Finally, severe degrees of placenta accreta may require hysterectomy.

Operative procedure.—Once the decision has been taken to terminate the third stage and all preparations, as outlined above, are to hand, the procedure is in the first place to ensure a well-contracted uterus, if necessary by massage, and then to employ the Brandt-Andrews manœuvre and failing that, not more than one attempt at Credé's expression. This is done initially without an anæsthetic and after catheterisation of the bladder. If this fails, anæsthesia is induced and Credé's expression is again attempted, which, if unsuccessful, must be immediately followed by manual removal of the placenta.

There is often some difference of opinion about the repair of a perineal laceration or an episiotomy during the waiting period of an abnormally prolonged third stage, but one should have no hesitation in proceeding with it, for not only will it save time, but it will also save blood. The patient is bound to continue to lose a certain quantity of blood from any sizeable laceration and even more so from an episiotomy. Not only is this more humane to the patient, but does not in any way interfere with the completion of the third stage.

SECONDARY POSTPARTUM HÆMORRHAGE

This is bleeding which occurs after an interval of 24 hours or more following the birth of the child and is most often due to the fact that something abnormal is retained within the uterus, usually a portion of placenta, occasionally a large blood clot or a submucous fibroid. In a series of 97 cases from Sheffield,[3] labelled as secondary postpartum hæmorrhage, there was no satisfactory cause for the bleeding found in over half those requiring surgical exploration and in less than a third of them was the retention of retained placental tissue

confirmed histologically. In others, only organising clot, fragments of decidua and uterine muscle were found, yet the results of evacuation of the uterus were good whether placental tissue was found or not. Unfortunately in no less than 3 cases the uterus was perforated by instrumentation for which laparotomy and suture was indicated.

Œstrogens for suppressing lactation are a fairly common cause and bleeding follows usually within a fortnight of their withdrawal.

Retained chorion seldom causes secondary postpartum hæmorrhage, and chorion epithelioma, an unlikely possibility, does not cause bleeding before at least three or four weeks after delivery.

Most secondary postpartum hæmorrhages reveal themselves within the first week or nine days of the puerperium, but sometimes much later, and often supply advance warning in the form of increased red lochial loss and a low-grade puerperal pyrexia. The condition is potentially very dangerous, and one cannot afford to ignore even a small secondary postpartum hæmorrhage because it is almost certain that a very much larger and possibly fatal hæmorrhage will follow. I have seen some very alarming hæmorrhages of this type.

It is, therefore, essential to explore the uterine cavity without undue delay and to be certain that a supply of cross-matched blood is available, because the operation may be by no means bloodless.

If a portion of placenta has been retained for any length of time it tends to become organised and rather densely adherent to the uterine wall, so that its removal is not only difficult but its presence within the uterus may escape detection. I well remember one such case in which the uterus was explored twice and no placental tissue found, yet the patient continued to have alarming hæmorrhages and had to be repeatedly transfused. At hysterectomy, which was undertaken eventually as an emergency measure, a large portion of placenta was found densely adherent to the uterine wall in the region of the fundus.

REFERENCES

1. ANDREWS, C. J. (1940). *Sth. Med. Surg.*, **102**, 605.
2. BRANDT, M. L. (1933). *Amer. J. Obstet. Gynec.*, **25**, 662.
3. DEWHURST, C. J. (1966). *J. Obstet. Gynaec. Brit. Cwlth.*, **73**, 53.
4. DEWHURST, C. J., and DUTTON, W. A. W. (1957). *Lancet*, **2**, 764.
5. DICKINS, AILEEN M., and MICHAEL, C. A. (1966). *J. Obstet. Gynaec. Brit. Cwlth.*, **73**, 460.
6. EMBREY, M. P. (1961). *Brit. med. J.*, **1**, 1737.
7. EMBREY, M. P., BARBOR, D. T. C., and SCUDAMORE, J. H. (1963). *Brit. med. J.*, **1**, 1387.
8. EMBREY, M. P., and GARRETT, W. J. (1958). *Brit. med. J.*, **2**, 138.
9. KIMBELL, N. (1954). *Brit. med. J.*, **2**, 130.

10. KIMBELL, N. (1958). *Brit. med. J.*, **1**, 203.
11. LLOYD, HILDA N. (1947). *Proc. roy. Soc. Med.*, **40**, 372.
12. MACGREGOR, W. G., and TOVEY, A. D. (1957). *Brit. med. J.*, **2**, 855.
13. MILLAR, W. G. (1959). *J. Obstet. Gynaec. Brit. Emp.*, **66**, 353.
14. Ministry of Health (1958). *Notes on Transfusion* issued for the National Blood Transfusion Service. London: H.M. Staty Office.
15. MOIR, J. C. (1944). *J. Obstet. Gynaec. Brit. Emp.*, **51**, 247.
16. MOIR, J. C. (1947). *Brit. med. J.*, **2**, 309.
17. MURDOCH, R. (1958). *Lancet*, **2**, 731.
18. ROBERTSON, S. (1967). Ob-Gyn. Collected Letters. *Internat. Correspondence Soc. of Ob-Gyn.*, **8**, 103.
19. SCOTT, J. S. (1955). *Brit. med. J.*, **2**, 290.
20. SPENCER, P. M. (1962). *Brit. med. J.*, **1**, 1728.
21. WALLACE, G. (1967). *J. Obstet. Gynaec. Brit. Cwlth.*, **74**, 64.
22. WILLOUGHBY, M. L. N. (1964). Personal Communication.
23. YAO, ALICE C., HIRVENSALO, M., and LIND, J. (1968). *Lancet*, **2**, 380.

CHAPTER XXII

MATERNAL INJURIES

LACERATIONS of the cervix are not included in this chapter, having been dealt with in the chapter on postpartum hæmorrhage, but acute inversion will be considered here, for it is in a sense an obstetrical injury.

UTERINE RUPTURE

There are two types of uterine rupture, complete and incomplete, distinguished by whether or not the serous coat of the uterus is involved. In the former the uterine contents, including fœtus and occasionally placenta, may be discharged into the peritoneal cavity, and for this reason it would appear to be the more dangerous of the two varieties. This, however, is not necessarily the case, and the terms complete and incomplete are unfortunate in that they give such an impression. The uterus, once empty, is able to retract, so that the amount of blood in the peritoneal cavity is often mercifully limited. On the other hand, most incomplete ruptures start in the lower segment, where retraction is deficient, so that bleeding can continue briskly both *per vaginam*, between the layers of the broad ligament, and retro-peritoneally.

Incomplete rupture with resulting broad ligament hæmatoma is commoner than recognised, but fortunately only a proportion of the cases develop to an alarming extent.

When the cervix tears in labour, the lateral rent easily extends into the lower segment, where large veins may be torn and may bleed furiously. In milder cases there may be no more than a troublesome puerperal pyrexia to show for it.

Not all cases of lower segment rupture are incomplete, and in obstructed labour or in difficult and traumatic instrumental deliveries a rent, usually oblique, may occur through all the layers, including the visceral peritoneum. As a general rule, rupture occurring during labour occurs in the lower segment, whereas in pregnancy it is usually in the upper segment, and in this case the onset is often fairly silent and insidious, particularly when a previous classical Cæsarean scar gives way.

Ruptures often extend to involve both the cervix and the vaginal vault as well, an accident which not only increases bleeding but often makes any conservative surgical procedure impracticable.

Causes of uterine rupture.—The incidence of uterine rupture is about 1 in 2,500 cases and is not becoming so very much rarer now-

adays because of an extended ætiology. Between the years 1950 and 1964 there were 143 reported cases in Dublin of which forty-three followed previous Cæsarean section. The incidence of scar rupture was 1·4 per cent following lower segment section and 6·4 per cent after the classical operation.

The remainder were traumatic, including 13 due to oxytocin infusion of which eight were in grand multiparæ.

The maternal mortality from traumatic rupture was as high as fifteen per cent.[10]

During pregnancy the commonest cause is a previous Cæsarean section scar, chiefly the classical variety. Any history of genital tract infection during the puerperium following such an operation raises serious doubts about the integrity of the scar, and if, as is not un-likely, the placenta in the present pregnancy happens to be sited over the scar, the burrowing action of the villi into what is often an imperfect decidua and the increased vascularity of the area weakens the uterine wall.

Myomectomy scars in the uterus are often quoted as causes of rupture, especially when the uterine cavity has been opened at the previous operation, but this disaster is very rare. Personally I have never met it, and Bonney, a great protagonist of myomectomy, never encountered it in his very large series. The difference here lies in the fact that the uterus after myomectomy is not undergoing in-volution with the rhythmical contractions which follow Cæsarean section, and the tissues, because they are at rest, heal better.

Direct trauma to the uterus is another recognised cause but is extremely uncommon, and it is surprising how much violence the pregnant uterus will withstand.

The uterine wall may be weakened by previous wounds, for example, after manual removal of a morbidly adherent placenta or curettage, with or without perforation, for retained products of conception following abortion. The later in a previous pregnancy that abortion followed by curettage has occurred the greater the risk of perforation at that time, often undiagnosed, and of uterine rupture in a subsequent pregnancy. One of the worst such cases I have personally encountered was that of a woman admitted so ill that it was difficult to make a diagnosis at all—as is often the case in really desperate emergencies. She was in acute pain and very shocked. The uterus, corresponding in size to thirty-four week's gestation, was not hard enough to encourage a diagnosis of abruptio placentæ. The fœtal heart was absent and the urine was normal. In spite of transfusion her condition rapidly deteriorated. A provisional diagnosis of hæmoperitoneum was made though its source was not expected to be uterine in view of her past obstetrical history which was negative, apart from a previous abortion at six months followed by curettage.

Laparotomy revealed an enormous quantity of free blood in the peritoneal cavity coming from a small hole in the fundus uteri through which a portion of placenta was presenting. She collapsed on the table in the course of Cæsarean hysterectomy and was pulseless for over an hour, but following massive transfusion of eight pints of blood she made an uninterrupted recovery.

Concealed antepartum hæmorrhage is very occasionally associated with uterine rupture, which adds to the great gravity of the condition, but this too is fortunately a rare complication.

Nowadays no gynæcologist worthy of the name performs the operation of ventrifixation, especially in any woman likely to become pregnant again, for in this case the uterus can only enlarge by the mechanism of sacculation, if abortion does not first occur.

Lastly, pregnancy in a rudimentary horn or an angular pregnancy may result in uterine rupture. Notwithstanding all this, however, there are a number of cases in whom no cause whatsoever can be found, particularly in grand multiparity.

After labour has started, additional causes come into the field, and it is now particularly that a uterus, weakened by rapid and repeated childbearing, may be unequal to the strain.

The use of oxytocic drugs in labour is dangerous from the point of view of rupture, and for this reason alone they are only employed with full precautions and supervision before the end of the second stage.

Grand multiparity is a contra-indication to their use because of this hazard. The response of the uterus may be unpredictably violent and in a case of my own, a para 9, the first few ml. of a dilute oxytocin infusion proved lethal. In spite of supervision and the immediate shutting off of the drip, the uterus "stood on its head" and burst. Cæsarean hysterectomy was a matter of minutes but she died ultimately of uncontrollable renal failure.

Version in labour, especially internal version, is a very common cause, and the more advanced the labour the greater does this risk become. Even the gentlest handling provides no guarantee against it. I have myself caused a very extensive rupture of the uterine wall, extending from the round ligament to the cervix and vaginal vault, in performing an internal version in a case of transverse lie with hyperextension of the fœtus, although I was surprised at the time by the very great ease and lack of force with which the operation was completed.

Any instrumental delivery, especially if the cervix is not fully dilated, may cause rupture of the uterus, except in cases of low forceps extraction, but with careful application this accident should not occur in experienced hands. Cranioclasm, however, may result in tearing of the uterus, and vaginal walls as well, if great care is not taken in extracting the exposed portions of bone.

Forceful stretching of the cervix which, after all, is no more than a variety of *accouchement forcé*, may cause a tear of the cervix which extends upwards into the lower segment to an uncontrollable degree and is a practice now generally condemned.

The uterus may be ruptured during the course of manual removal of the placenta, but this risk is lessened by keeping the fingers of the hand close together and by avoiding any temptation to claw at the placenta. The steadying influence of the outside hand on the abdominal wall also helps to reduce this risk, which is in any case surprisingly small.

By far the majority of cases of uterine rupture occur either as a result of a previous Cæsarean section scar giving way or of obstructed labour. The latter comes into a class of its own. The risk of rupture of a uterus bearing a scar is apparently increased by each pregnancy thereafter, by each succeeding vaginal delivery, by high parity, twins, large fœtus and hydramnios.[3]

Labour may be obstructed as a result of disproportion, malpresentation, pelvic tumours and strictures of the cervix which are the result of previous cauterisation, amputation, trachelorrhaphy or, very rarely, some congenital defect. In these cases either the uterus or the cervix must tear, and occasionally an annular separation of the cervix may occur (Fig. 1). In disproportion causing obstructed labour the uterine rupture is sometimes favoured by ischæmia, due to the pressure of the presenting part. The tear in the uterus then spreads from this area.

Threatened rupture and prophylaxis.—Occasionally a uterine scar that is about to give way may give some advance warning in the form of pain and tenderness localised to the region of the scar.

In obstructed labour with an intact uterus, the lower uterine segment becomes progressively thinned while the upper segment, as a result of retraction, becomes thicker, so that the junction between the two (Bandl's ring) can often be both seen and felt through the abdominal wall. This visible ridge rises progressively in level and is usually oblique. At the same time the intervals between the contractions shorten, until the condition of tonic contraction or tetanic spasm of the uterus is fully developed. Rupture is now imminent. The combination of a Bandl's ring rising appreciably within 20 minutes or so, together with the threat of tonic contraction, indicates the immediate need for delivering the patient by the simplest and therefore safest possible method before rupture actually occurs. Under these circumstances internal version is nothing less than disastrous and, in the case of a shoulder presentation, decapitation is not only simpler but more expeditious. If the child is still alive, Cæsarean section is the only reasonable treatment, but when, as is

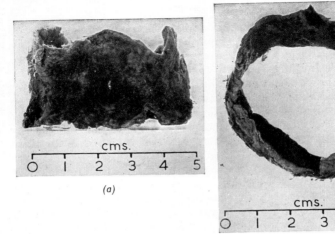

(a)

(b)

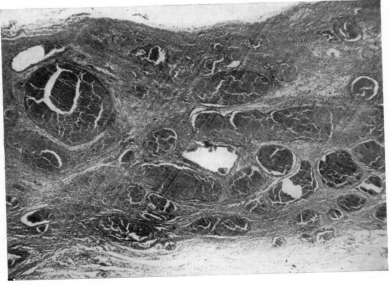

(c)

22/Fig. 1.—(*See opposite.*)

726

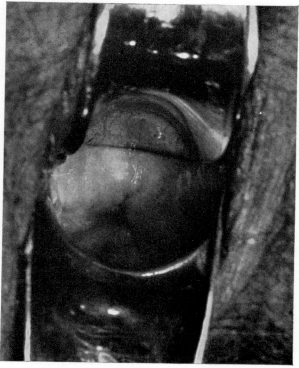

(d)

22/Fig. 1.

(a) and (b). Annular detachment of cervix.

(c) Photomicrograph of section of detached cervix showing intense engorgement of the blood vessels, advanced necrosis of all tissues and areas of hæmorrhage.

(d) Remaining stump of cervix three months after delivery.

(By courtesy of Dr. J. P. Erskine and the R.C.O.G. Museum).

usually the case, the fœtus is already dead, craniotomy in a cephalic presentation and other destructive operations as appropriate still have a place. Few obstetricians in civilised communities nowadays have much experience in these operations, because with proper supervision the situation does not arise.

Consequences of rupture.—As a rule, rupture in labour is far more dramatic than that occurring in pregnancy and is more dangerous because shock is greater and infection is almost inevitable. Hæmorrhage and shock are the two most immediate risks and may be rapidly fatal.

Prolapse of the bowel is also likely to occur and is also assuredly fatal unless dealt with. Hypofibrinogenæmia may complicate uterine rupture and add defective coagulation to a situation already sufficiently disastrous. It is suggested that amniotic fluid may be forced into the circulation through vessels exposed by incomplete lower segment rupture, commonly in multiparous patients with precipitate delivery.[6] The resulting microcoagulation throughout the vascular tree, especially pulmonary, defibrinates the blood and, besides hæmorrhage, the patient suffers collapse with cyanosis and respiratory distress. Finally, sepsis may carry off a patient who manages to survive the other catastrophies. Many cases of incomplete rupture, however, settle down spontaneously, and the hæmatoma in the broad ligament is ultimately absorbed.

The outlook for the next pregnancy is seriously prejudiced, and to allow a woman subsequently to deliver herself *per vaginam* is very questionable, however carefully and skilfully the rent has been sutured and however successful the antibiotics have been in controlling infection. It is usually wisest to perform elective Cæsarean section in the next pregnancy about ten days before term, and in those cases where it is decided to take the risk of vaginal delivery, the forceps should be ready at full dilatation. This eliminates the increased dangers of the second stage.

Symptoms of uterine rupture.—Classically the patient experiences a severe bursting pain, although in a few cases of insidious rupture she may complain of no more than severe discomfort. Fainting is common, and usually there is some external bleeding, although this is variable. Silent rupture is more likely with a lower segment scar and may be accompanied by no more than a rise in pulse rate. This sign is highly significant in a woman who is now labouring following a previous lower segment Cæsarean section.

Diagnosis of uterine rupture.—In the acute case the diagnosis is not usually difficult because labour comes to an abrupt stop to the accompaniment of great pain and ensuing shock.

Where, however, the onset is insidious, these signs are very much less marked. Nevertheless, contractions cease. The patient is not always shocked at first, and occasionally her condition may remain reasonably good for up to half an hour.

A characteristic sign is the loss of the presenting part from its former position within the pelvis. Indeed, as the fœtus is extruded into the abdominal cavity, the fœtal parts become easily palpable through the abdominal wall, especially if the patient is thin. The child usually dies, the fœtal heart ceasing shortly after rupture.

In cases of complete rupture the now empty and retracted uterus forms a firm swelling to one side of the fœtus, while in cases of incomplete rupture the bulge of a retro-peritoneal hæmatoma in the

broad ligament can often be felt to one side of the uterus and it may extend into the pelvis down one side of the vagina, bulging into its lumen.

Occasionally rupture occurs at the very end of the second stage of labour, so that vaginal delivery of the fœtus is successfully completed. There now follows a very characteristic sign, namely shortening of the cord. This is practically pathognomonic of uterine rupture, with extrusion of the placenta into the abdominal cavity, and I have seen such a case in which this was the first and only obvious clue, since the patient's condition remained, for the time being, very good. The diagnosis was finally confirmed when an attempt was made to remove the placenta manually. On this occasion I well remember the firm, rounded, slippery swelling of the posterior wall of the uterus in front of my hand and the coils of intestine at the back of my fingers as I followed the cord into the peritoneum. The actual rent in the uterus was not noticeable to the examining hand at first.

Sometimes the diagnosis of uterine rupture will only be made after the completion of the third stage, and I recall another case in which collapse occurred during the third stage with the placenta still *in situ* and with only a moderate degree of external bleeding. I removed the placenta manually from the posterior wall of the uterus and did not observe the rupture of a previous classical Cæsarean scar in the anterior wall. In the hours which followed, the patient's condition seemed to be far more anæmic than warranted, considering the six pints of blood which had already been transfused. Her blood pressure was satisfactory, but, on removing the hot blankets, her flanks were noted to be bulging with blood from an extensive hæmoperitoneum. She made an uninterrupted recovery following hysterectomy.

After delivery any case exhibiting a severe degree of shock which is unexpected or unexplained calls for exploration of the uterus forthwith, since many cases of maternal death occur from unsuspected uterine rupture and lacerations of the genital tract.

In Feeney and Barry's series of 45 cases of uterine rupture and perforation there were seven maternal deaths of which six were regarded as avoidable. Three of these deaths were due to failure, within hospital, to diagnose the condition in time.

All cases of previous Cæsarean section who have just completed a subsequent vaginal delivery should be examined to assess the state of the old scar in the uterus. This can be done immediately after delivery without an anæsthetic by passing two fingers through the cervix and exploring the lower part of the uterine cavity. Pushing the uterus downwards over the fingers by pressing on the fundus facilitates the examination.

When bleeding continues in spite of a well-retracted uterus, for

example after a forceps delivery or breech extraction, it is as well to remember that a laceration of the cervix, if present, may have extended far up into the uterus, and it is necessary to identify the apex. Sometimes, however, the cervix is intact and the bleeding may be coming from a rupture of the vaginal vault. This may not be easy to determine unless the cervix is first grasped with ring forceps and retracted to one side so that the vault can be inspected.

The differential diagnosis is concerned with the other causes of acute abdominal catastrophe, chief among which, in obstetrics, is concealed antepartum hæmorrhage, in which pain, shock, absence of uterine contractions and the disappearance of the fœtal heart sounds likewise occur. Usually, too, there is vaginal bleeding. The uterus, however, in this case is regular in outline, and no swelling either of broad ligament hæmatoma or extruded fœtal parts can be felt to the side of it. The history of the case may be of some help; nevertheless, it is easy to be mistaken.

Shoulder presentation with the head in the iliac fossa may feel remarkably like a uterus pushed to one side by a fœtus extruded through a uterine rent, but in this case rhythmical contraction and relaxation of the uterus will be observed.

After delivery the differential diagnosis is concerned with the other causes of postpartum collapse which have been dealt with in the chapter on that subject, but it behoves one especially to bear in mind the possibility of acute inversion. If in doubt, a vaginal examination should be made, because this is a condition which does not lightly forgive procrastination.

Treatment.—In full-blown complete uterine rupture, laparotomy should be undertaken as soon as possible after a blood transfusion has been started. Having opened the abdomen, three courses of action can be considered, namely hysterectomy, repair of the rupture, and repair and sterilisation of the patient. Of these, hysterectomy is undoubtedly the safest course, for a uterus which has once ruptured may well do so again, and removal of the dangerous and infected organ gives the best prospects for a smooth convalescence. However, especially in a young woman, there may be strong reasons for taking the risk of preserving the uterus and the nature of the rent itself will largely influence the decision.

Undoubtedly the advent of the antibiotics has made the repair and conservation of the uterus a less hazardous procedure, and I have delivered a young woman of two normal babies by the vaginal route, following a previous uterine rupture in which the bowel prolapsed into the vagina. Needless to say, the case caused considerable anxiety, but she was particularly anxious to increase her family and continually threatens to repeat the procedure yet again. It is not desired to give the impression that this line of treatment is favoured,

but the patient in question, though well aware of the risks, was insistent. In the majority of cases there can be no doubt that, in a subsequent pregnancy, the safest course is to perform elective Cæsarean section just before term.

The third alternative treatment, namely repair and sterilisation, has rather less to recommend it than the other two, because it takes every bit as long as hysterectomy to perform. The only advantage is that the patient is left with the questionable blessing of continued menstruation.

In repairing a uterine rupture it is customary to freshen up the edges of the wound by dissection, but too much time should not be wasted on this. The uterus should be repaired with interrupted sutures in layers, starting with one traction suture at the upper end of the rent and then working from the bottom upwards. In this way it is possible to examine the lowest and therefore the most difficult parts of the repair with the finger passed inside the uterus through the rent before it is finally closed. Great care must be taken not to include the ureter in any of the stitches, especially when the rupture extends to the sides of the lower segment. Prophylactic chemotherapy is of course obligatory.

In the lesser degrees of incomplete rupture in which the patient's condition remains satisfactory and the parametrial hæmatoma does not continue to enlarge, it is often possible to adopt a more conservative line, and these cases can be treated by plugging. The hæmatoma should be cleared out *per vaginam* and the space firmly packed with gauze impregnated with sulphonamide and penicillin. It is important at the same time to exert counter-pressure by means of a pad and abdominal binder, as otherwise blood may collect beyond the pack and behind the peritoneum. Uterine retraction should be maintained with ergot, and full anti-shock treatment should be continued, as appropriate. The pack is removed after 48 hours, the patient being well morphinised and several hours being spent over its gentle withdrawal. In less severe cases, in which the patient's general condition warrants it, morphine, blood transfusion and cat-like observation may suffice.

INVERSION OF THE UTERUS

This is one of the most serious complications in all midwifery. Fortunately it is very rare, although it is impossible to obtain reliable figures of incidence. Reports in the literature estimate it variously as between 1 in 17,000 and 1 in 200,000 deliveries. Most well-run obstetrical services supply reports of their work, and in these inversion is naturally extremely rare. It is in parts of the world where obstetrics is less enlightened that inversion is more common, and it is from these very regions that reports are not as a rule available.

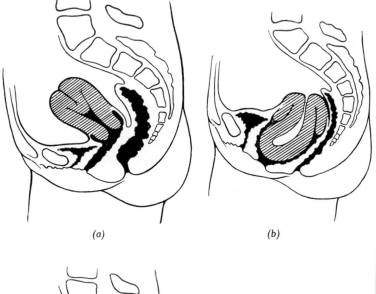

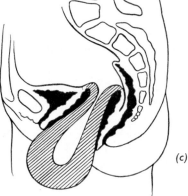

22/Fig. 2.—Stages of Inversion

(a) 1st stage inversion.
(b) 2nd stage inversion.
(c) 3rd stage inversion.

There are three degrees of uterine inversion (Fig. 2). The first degree, which is likely to be missed, is that in which the fundus, in turning itself inside out, does not, however, herniate through the level of the internal os. In the second degree the fundus passes through the cervix and lies within the vagina, and in the third degree, which is very uncommon, the entire uterus is turned inside out and hangs outside the vulva, taking much of the vagina with it (Fig. 3). In other words, in all but the third and rarest degree the inverted uterus does not present to external view and consequently the diagnosis may not be as obvious as would appear.

Causes of inversion.—In about four-fifths of the cases some error of management is responsible, although the existence of spontaneous inversion cannot be denied. A fundal insertion of the placenta would appear to be a necessary prerequisite, and has been established in 75 per cent of spontaneous inversions.[2] A second prerequisite at the time of inversion is atony of the uterus. In other words, the hard and well-retracted uterus cannot be inverted.

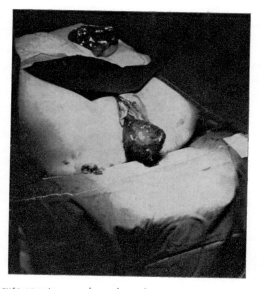

22/Fig. 3.—Acute spontaneous inversion of uterus. Photograph taken within a few minutes of its occurrence with a Polaroid camera, while anæsthetist and colleague made preparations for reducing it. (In my haste the photograph was badly torn). Cardiac arrest occurred a few minutes later during anæsthesia. Thoracotomy was repeated four times in course of the next 36 hours because of recurrent cardiac arrest. Patient ultimately died without regaining consciousness.

The association of fundal placental insertion and uterine atony allows a number of more immediate causes to operate. Firstly, pulling on the cord under these circumstances will clearly provoke inversion, and the strongest argument against this practice is that one cannot be certain at the time that the placenta is not inserted at the fundus, although it is the least common position for it to occupy. It takes very little traction to pull such a uterus inside out, and I have demonstrated it to students at Cæsarean section, an experiment not to be recommended, because in this case the drop in the patient's blood pressure was quite remarkable and I had some difficulty in re-

placing the inversion as the remainder of the uterus began to retract behind it.

Again, pressure upon the fundus of the soft uterus in order to expel blood clot or placenta may easily provoke inversion. Thirdly, a short cord may start a spontaneous inversion during the second stage of labour, although more commonly the placenta itself becomes detached. Sometimes, although the cord is not unduly short, it may be wound several times around the baby's neck, and this will produce the same effect.

Precipitate delivery, especially in the erect position, is more likely to provoke inversion than when the patient is lying down.

It has been postulated that occasionally there may be a localised area of uterine atony in the region of the placental site and that a sharp rise in intra-abdominal pressure, for example from violent bearing-down efforts or severe coughing, may initiate the process. In fact, inversion may be due to traction from within via the cord or pressure from without. In the former case, some degree of abnormal adhesion of the placenta is probably necessary to invert the uterus.

Fibroids at the fundus are possible causes of inversion, but more commonly they only produce the chronic variety in cases wherein a submucous fibroid develops a pedicle and becomes a fibroid polyp. This is a state of affairs which is not met in obstetrics, although it is fairly common in gynæcology.

The rôle of Credé's expression of the placenta in producing inversion must be mentioned. Properly performed with a firm retracted uterus, the danger is practically non-existent, but any such attempt without first ensuring a uterine contraction is, of course, asking for trouble.

There is no specific prophylaxis against inversion except the avoidance of pulling on the cord or pressing on the fundus of the uterus while it is soft. The patient should not be instructed to change her position, for example from the left lateral to the dorsal position, in the third stage without first ensuring that the uterus is firm, because the rise in abdominal pressure which the effort of movement entails might, in rare instances, initiate inversion.

Risks of inversion.—The immediate effect upon the patient is one of shock, often extremely profound, which comes on even faster than that associated with acute uterine rupture. It should be one of the first diagnostic possibilities to be considered in any patient developing postpartum collapse. Hæmorrhage is variable but may be quite severe, especially when the placenta is already detached. The patient who weathers these two risks is still exposed to the likelihood of puerperal sepsis, which the various therapeutic measures adopted to reduce the inversion are likely to aggravate. As in all conditions producing severe shock, anuria and Sheehan's syndrome are possible

sequelæ. The untreated case is likely to die, but in a few instances spontaneous reduction occurs. In those in which it does not, the inverted uterus becomes infected and proceeds to slough.

Diagnosis.—The patient is usually too shocked to register much in the way of symptoms which, if recorded, consist mainly of severe lower abdominal pain with a strong bearing-down sensation.

The first step in arriving at a diagnosis is to find the whereabouts of the uterine fundus and to note any cupping, dimpling or irregularity of its upper surface. In severe cases the body of the uterus cannot be found at all on abdominal palpation, since it has turned itself inside out into the vagina. Abdominal palpation alone is not enough, and Spain (1946) described two cases in which, although the patients were thin, the abdominal signs of cupping of the fundus could not be demonstrated although they were deliberately looked for. One of the patients died ten days later. In both, the diagnosis was only made on vaginal examination. Any possibility, therefore, that the uterus may be inverted demands vaginal examination. The differential diagnosis is concerned with other causes of postpartum collapse dealt with in another chapter.

Treatment.—The best person to treat uterine inversion is the attendant present at the time of its occurrence. If it can be reduced within a few seconds of its development, the very factors which produce shock will be removed. The treatment is immediate replacement without attempting to remove the placenta from the inverted fundus. As a general rule it is preferable to reduce the inversion with the placenta still attached and to deal with its delivery later. In many of these cases the placenta is morbidly adherent and, in any event, removal exposes the maternal sinuses, which are intensely engorged, to infection. Moreover, bleeding is likely to be very severe and will aggravate the already developing shock. There is another very real risk in removing the placenta from the inverted uterus, namely that the uterine wall can be easily torn and perforated.

There are only two indications for removing the placenta before replacement of the uterus. The first is the necessity to reduce the bulk of the inverted mass in order to get it through a narrowing cervical ring, and secondly, when all but a portion of the placenta is already separated. If immediate replacement is not feasible, shock supervenes so quickly that further attempts are no longer safe until the shock is first treated. Within a very few minutes even vaginal examination, unless very gentle, can precipitate or aggravate shock.

Unfortunately, in a number of cases acute inversion occurs in the absence of skilled assistants, so that when first seen the patient is already too shocked for replacement there and then. In these circumstances, or where it is not possible to replace the inversion straightway, the first thing to be done is to convert a third-degree

inversion into one of the second degree and to raise the foot of the bed to maintain the inverted mass within the vagina instead of hanging outside. This reduces shock to some extent and, to a lesser extent, the inevitability of infection. Attempts at replacement in the presence of shock may easily prove fatal and should only be made either before shock has come on or after it has been treated.

Having replaced the inverted mass into the vagina, the patient should be given morphia 15–20 mg. ($\frac{1}{4}$–$\frac{1}{3}$ gr.) and a plasma or saline drip should be set up pending the arrival of cross-matched blood for transfusion.

In domiciliary practice the patient should be treated adequately for shock before submitting her to an ambulance journey into hospital, and the assistance of a "flying squad", if available, is invaluable. While awaiting help the patient should be kept warm, and on no account should ergot or pitocin be given, as these will only aggravate matters and make reduction or replacement virtually impossible for the time being. The vulva is meanwhile kept covered with a sterile pad.

Replacement of the inversion.—The longer this is deferred the more difficult is it likely to be because of the tightening of the cervical ring. A fairly deep anæsthetic should be given, and following the usual antiseptic ritual, an attempt may be made by manual and digital pressure to reduce the inverted mass. If possible an attempt should be made to reduce that part of the uterus which has inverted last, in other words, the part nearest the cervix, rather than dimpling the inverted fundus and trying to push extra thicknesses of uterine wall through the cervical ring. While carrying out this manipulation the other hand should be placed over the abdomen to supply counter support, otherwise the still inverted uterus may be pushed high up into the abdomen with the vagina on the stretch. This increases shock. If this manœuvre is successful in replacing the uterus, the hand should be kept within its cavity until ergometrine has been given and taken effect. This will reduce the likelihood of a recurrence. Titus, in his book *Management of Obstetrical Difficulties*, recommended packing the uterus to prevent the inversion recurring, but opinion in this country is much less inclined to favour packing of the uterus at any time.

O'Sullivan in 1945 published a simple and very effective method of dealing with inversion by applying intravaginal hydraulic pressure. He himself told me that he came on this method of treatment purely by accident. He was about to reduce an inversion by the traditional methods and, preparatory to doing so, gave the patient a warm antiseptic vaginal douche, in the course of which his forearm blocked the vulval outlet. To his astonishment the inversion disappeared and the uterus returned to its normal position. He has

since used this method in at least two dozen further cases deliberately. He passes a douche nozzle towards the posterior fornix and, with the douche can raised no more than 3 feet above the level of the vagina, he runs in a copious warm antiseptic solution. An assistant gathers the labia around his forearm so as to block the vulva, and in practically every case the treatment is dramatically successful. This method would appear to be a real advance and is certainly less likely to cause further shock to a patient than manipulation and taxis. I once had a case in which acute inversion of the third degree had occurred four hours previously in domiciliary practice. The mass was pushed into the vagina and covered with a sterile pad and the patient admitted to hospital. Profound shock supervened following vaginal examination which transfusion could not correct. Under deep anæsthesia replacement was undertaken but I found the cervical ring so tight that in spite of combining O'Sullivan's hydraulic method and direct manipulation I could at first prevail nothing. The whole mass felt like a doughy pudding. Presently the ring appeared to move upwards towards the fundus and the last half of the inversion suddenly and miraculously disappeared under the hydraulic pressure of the douche. The patient's recovery was immediate and dramatic.

If all the above methods fail, it is usually because the cervical ring has become too tight and its forcible dilatation will only make matters worse. In long-standing cases Aveling's repositor may be tried, coupled with repeated hot douches but, as a rule, provided the patient's condition can stand the surgical procedure, it is better to resort to operation, of which there are several types. Of these the best known is that of Spinelli in which, using the vaginal approach, the bladder is dissected upwards and pushed out of the way. The ring and the lower part of the inverted uterus, i.e. that part of it nearest the cervix, is divided anteriorly, and the inversion is then replaced, following which the incision is closed with interrupted sutures. An alternative method is that of Küstner, in which the cervical ring is divided posteriorly.

Operation by the abdominal route is another alternative, and an attempt may be made to drag back the inversion from above by the use of Allis forceps. The recently delivered uterus, however, is very liable to tear, in which case reposition may be more easily achieved by incising the ring posteriorly from above according to the method of Haultain. Full anti-shock treatment must be maintained until the patient is out of immediate danger. Bacteriological cultures should be taken from the cervix at the time of replacement, so that appropriate antibiotic treatment may be started with the minimum of delay and as early as possible in a puerperium which is almost bound to be stormy.

PERINEAL AND VAGINAL TEARS

The adoption of the erect posture has endowed humanity with certain well-known penalties. One of these is the fact that the pelvic floor literally lives up to its name at the bottom of the pelvic cavity and is subjected to stresses which in no way apply to quadrupeds. As a result the shape of the birth canal becomes that of a right-angled pipe, the far wall of which is formed by the muscles of the pelvic floor. As the perineum constitutes the common point of insertion for most of these, it comes in for the brunt of the burden in vaginal delivery.

The casual view that the perineum was ordained by nature to tear in childbirth cannot be upheld, for it is a structure of considerable functional importance. A damaged perineum means an ineffective pelvic floor, and the condensations of pelvic fascia, which maintain the pelvic viscera in their normal anatomical positions, cannot afford indefinitely to do without the active muscular support of the levatores ani. Thus, after a latent period of many years, the supports of the uterus, bladder and bladder-neck yield, often in the process of menopausal atrophy, and the patient all too often becomes the victim of prolapse, stress incontinence or both. In this respect a stretched perineum may be almost as bad as a torn perineum, for both lose some of their functional capacity. Furthermore, a torn perineum is a wound in a none too sterile part of the body at a time when unnecessary infection cannot be countenanced, and it is only the great vascularity of the part and its local resistance to infection which prevent it from becoming a dangerous portal of entry for sepsis.

TYPES OF PERINEAL TEAR

There are three main degrees of perineal laceration; the first degree involves the hymen, or what is left of it, and fourchette, together with a small distance of vaginal and perineal skin, but the perineal body itself is undamaged. In second-degree laceration the perineal body is ruptured, together with a variable length of posterior vaginal wall. In severe forms the external anal sphincter may be damaged, but provided the lumen of the anal canal is not opened, the case should properly be included in the second degree. The third degree laceration is obviously the most serious because the anal canal is opened up, in fact, the tear may extend to include the rectum. The patient is incontinent of fæces and the whole wound is inevitably infected from the bowel. This type of injury is a major obstetrical disaster, and unless effectively dealt with may wreck the patient's whole future and make a social outcast of her.

There are a few minor subdivisions of less importance, such as the

so-called central tear of the perineum in which an anterior bridge remains intact, the baby being delivered as the term would suggest. The existence of the anterior bridge of unruptured tissue is of no importance and in any case it must be divided before repairing the tear.

Labial lacerations are seldom of any structural significance and do not often call for any reparative procedure. They are, however, very tender, and can be quite a nuisance during the puerperium when they are particularly liable to produce reflex retention of urine.

The causes of perineal tearing are not necessarily the fault of the medical attendant, although the extent thereof may to some extent be a measure of clumsiness. In the past much harm has been done by sister tutors of midwifery who have regarded the torn perineum as a matter for disciplinary admonition of the midwife, with the result that a policy of saving the perineum at all costs tends to be adopted. This is highly undesirable, because an overstretched and devitalised perineum ends up far worse off than a perineum which has been torn and properly sutured. If the perineum is kept on the stretch for a long time by the baby's head, it transmits great pressure to the back of the symphysis pubis and to the region of the bladder neck, so that its supports become permanently weakened, and stress incontinence, even without prolapse, may result. In the reports of most well-run maternity units the episiotomy rate exceeds the perineal tear rate.

Very rapid delivery, on the other hand, is not only unnecessarily damaging to the perineum but is bad for the baby's head. The head may be crowned without causing damage, but the perineum may be needlessly torn in the course of delivering the face. If possible this should be achieved between uterine contractions. The delivery of the posterior shoulder frequently causes damage which the patient has hitherto escaped, and in training students and midwives more emphasis should be placed on skilful handling at this stage than in the delivery of the head itself, because the majority of lacerations caused by the posterior shoulder are unnecessary and largely due to clumsiness.

The narrower the subpubic arch, the more acute the subpubic angle, and the more android in type the pelvis, the farther back will the head have to pass to emerge from under the symphysis pubis. This will certainly increase the extent of perineal damage.

Face-to-pubis delivery, because of the larger fœtal diameters concerned, does more damage than delivery with the occiput anterior, and the worst degrees of tear, frequently involving the rectum, are those caused by the unwitting forceps extraction of a head in the unreduced persistent occipito-posterior position.

Breech delivery has a high perineal tear rate, because there is less

opportunity for the perineum to stretch adequately, and in primi-gravidæ it is most undesirable that the perineum should hold up the delivery of an aftercoming head, so that episiotomy is more or less standard practice.

Prevention of perineal tears.—It is not intended to give the impression that the perineum should just be allowed to rip, in fact, a conscientious attempt should be made to limit the extent of tearing. Timely episiotomy (under local infiltration anæsthesia) will often forestall a ragged tear. It is certainly impossible to guard the perineum with the fingers, as is so frequently taught, for the force so applied is misdirected and misapplied. Much can be done by allowing completion of the delivery of the head only between pains and by care with delivery of the posterior shoulder. It seems probable that the use of the left lateral position in normal labour is less likely to favour tears than the dorsal position, although the latter has so many other advantages that its use is becoming increasingly general in this country.

Method of repair.—This should be done soon after delivery, and the practice of accumulating the night's tears in hospital until they can all be liquidated the following morning is to be deplored. For one thing, freshly damaged tissues can be more satisfactorily sutured, for another, less time is allowed for the introduction of sepsis, and lastly, the patient deserves to be tidied up after labour and left in peace without the anticipation of stitching in hours to come. There is much to be said for proceeding with the repair while awaiting delivery of the placenta, especially if the tear is not extensive. The only argument against getting to work straightway is in the case of the extensive tear when a good view must be obtained, and it may be very inconvenient to deal with the arrival of the placenta before at least the vaginal skin is properly sewn up.

A good light is essential to work by and a relatively bloodless field is a great help, otherwise the apex of the rent in the vagina will be missed. It is a good plan to cut a vulval pad in two and to push the half pad up into the vaginal vault to absorb any trickle of blood from above. Very adequate anæsthesia can be obtained by the injection of 1 per cent lignocaine infiltrated directly round the region of the tear. Twenty millilitres should be perfectly adequate for the purpose.

The apex of the vaginal tear is now identified, and the vagina is first sutured with continuous catgut so as to produce a good blood-tight joint. This prevents the seepage of lochia into the depths of the perineal wound, which will assuredly occur if the posterior vaginal wall is not properly closed. Failure to observe this precaution results in many repairs breaking down. The perineal body is then stitched, usually with about three or four interrupted No. 1 catgut sutures.

While inserting them, the index finger of one hand should press the rectum backwards out of harm's way. These stitches should not be tied tightly; this is a common mistake and discourages rather than facilitates healing. There remains now only the perineal skin. My own preference is for interrupted fine catgut sutures inserted with the knot buried inwards. Some prefer a running subcuticular stitch, but any continuous suture in the event of sepsis tends to prevent drainage. Interrupted nylon or silkworm gut is still very popular in units still accustomed to barbarity and the use of black silk has a touch of black magic about it. Apart from being a natural tissue irritant it involves the patient in the miserable puerperal ritual of stitch removal.

I have never had any trouble from burying under the skin the knots of interrupted fine catgut and the patient is always very comfortable.

The old-fashioned method was to take silkworm gut on large harpoon needles and go through all layers, taking up enormous bites of tissue. This is a very unsatisfactory method, and while the end result may look all very well from the outside, it often leaves no more than a "dashboard" perineum with relatively little substance deep to the skin. My students have attributed to me the remark that women do not micturate on barbed wire fences. I cannot remember making it but at least they got the message. It might be feared that the delivery of the placenta would break down one's repair, but this is not so, for the placenta is very soft, and any suturing which could not withstand its passage has not been properly done. The possibility of having to undertake manual removal of the placenta may also discourage one from embarking on perineal suture during the third stage, but this should not deter one. The deep sutures need not be tied until after the arrival of the placenta.

It is a common mistake to sew up too tightly, with the result that the patient is considerably embarrassed subsequently by dyspareunia. The tissues of the vulva and vagina shrink during the process of involution, and it should be a rule to ensure that three fingers can be easily inserted simultaneously into the vagina at the end of the operation.

THIRD-DEGREE TEAR

There is no place for local anæsthesia in repairing a third-degree tear. The job has to be done very thoroughly in a proper theatre and a general anæsthetic should be given. The first step is to repair the anus and rectum. Interrupted catgut sutures are used, starting from above and working downwards. They should be inserted in such a way that the knots come to lie within the rectal lumen (Fig. 4). An alternative

and more fussy method is to insert Lembert sutures which necessitate the tying of knots on the perineal aspect and no advantage is to be gained thereby.

Having repaired the anal canal, the torn ends of the anal sphincter must be found. One side nearly always retracts out of view and must be deliberately sought, whereupon two or three fine mattress sutures are used to produce satisfactory end-to-end apposition of the sphincter. If the tear has been very deep, it may be found to have

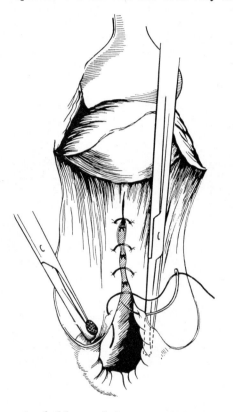

22/Fig. 4.—Repair of rectum in third-degree tear.

extended beyond the upper apex of the perineum, in which case the vaginal and rectal rents will correspond, so that it is difficult to repair the rectum as a separate layer. This step is essential nevertheless, and in order to achieve it the rectum should be dissected upwards from the vagina for a distance of about half an inch. This is a common region for a residual rectovaginal fistula, not only from failure to observe this precaution, but because there is no appreciable thickness of tissue which can be brought between.

The third-degree tear has now been converted into one of the second degree and the steps of the operation are continued as described above.

The after-treatment is important, and the patient should be kept on a low residue diet for the next week. Liquid paraffin by mouth is commonly recommended from the second day onwards, but paraffin is extraordinary stuff for finding out leaks and will seep through any available crevices in the surgical repair, thus encouraging non-union, and the patient may be left with a fistula. It is necessary to leave the bowels strictly alone for at least five or six days; thereupon a gentle instillation of a few ounces of olive oil with a soft rubber catheter twice a day should suffice to soften down any fæcal masses, so that when the patient has a bowel action at about the end of a week it is a soft atraumatic one.

In spite of the most careful technique, it not infrequently happens that the repair of a third-degree tear breaks down. There are two reasons for this: either the repair was imperfectly carried out or it breaks down because of sepsis. The patient is now left with a very real disability in the form of some degree of rectal incontinence and will not be comfortable until the trouble is dealt with. Nevertheless, it is not safe to attempt further repair until all signs of local sepsis have cleared up. Usually one prefers to wait for about four months for involution to complete itself, in the hope thereby of operating upon more satisfactory tissues, but in favourable circumstances secondary suture may be undertaken earlier. Every failed attempt prejudices the outlook for subsequent operations.

It is worth noting here, in passing, that patients with unhealed third-degree tears very seldom develop prolapse, in spite of the perineal damage. This is because of the constant effort which the patient unconsciously makes, with what is left of her pelvic floor, to maintain some degree of rectal continence.

A patient who has had a successfully repaired third-degree tear must be carefully managed in any subsequent delivery. If there has been much previous difficulty in curing her, there is much to be said for elective Cæsarean section but, if vaginal delivery is decided upon, a generous episiotomy is obligatory. On no account should the scar of the previous repair be subjected to the stresses of labour.

VAULT RUPTURE

This is more common than is usually recognised, and is one of the causes of continued trickling of blood after the completion of the third stage. The lateral margin of the cervix is often involved as well, and if large vessels at the base of the broad ligament are opened up, hæmorrhage can be very profuse. In lesser degrees quite a large

paravaginal hæmatoma may form and give rise to a pyrexial puerperium. Attempts to repair a rent in the vaginal vault are fraught with the danger of damaging a ureter, and on the whole these injuries are safest left to themselves to heal. However, if any appreciable degree of bleeding continues, the rent and the space in the cellular tissue beyond it should be packed with gauze, and to prevent the development of a parametrial hæmatoma, a firm abdominal pad and binder should be applied to exert counter-pressure. The bleeding point is often on the torn vaginal edge and careful suturing deals with it. Nevertheless, if the rent is a large one, it is worth partially suturing, at the same time inserting a drain into the hæmatoma cavity. These measures will nearly always suffice, but where the hæmorrhage is really torrential and cannot be controlled by packing from below, it may be necessary to resort to laparotomy and in very rare instances to hysterectomy, or as an alternative, ligation of the anterior division of the internal iliac artery on the affected side.

EPISIOTOMY

The importance of this little operation is out of all proportion to its simplicity. Nevertheless, it is frequently abused. As an alternative injury to a second-degree tear its value is somewhat debatable, and to inflict a cut for no other reason than to prevent a tear is of dubious advantage, because the former may be more extensive than is actually necessary. Both, if properly sutured, heal equally well.

An episiotomy is infinitely preferable to an overstretched and devitalised perineum, with its parallel weakening of the supports of the bladder neck. Timely episiotomy can prevent a great deal of damage in this respect and is regarded as an important factor in the prevention of subsequent prolapse. An episiotomy, moreover, will save what might otherwise have been a perineal tear extending to the third degree, because it deflects the direction of tearing to one side of the anus.

The chief virtue of episiotomy lies in the saving of unnecessary wear and tear upon the fœtal skull. This is particularly important in cases of prematurity.

A second stage prolonged because of rigidity of the perineum can often be completed satisfactorily without the need for forceps, and the patient may be saved a great deal of unnecessary misery. Lastly, the uterus may be spared some exhaustion, and this will reduce the likelihood of postpartum hæmorrhage.

In forceps deliveries, episiotomy is becoming increasingly general, because delivery can be completed with less traumatic force to mother and baby, since it relieves the fœtal head of the undesirable rôle of acting as a battering ram on the maternal pelvic floor.

Flew's episiotomy rate in primigravidæ was over 50 per cent, yet combined with the forceps operation, the rate was only 12 per cent, suggesting in other words that episiotomy dispensed with the need for forceps in many cases.

To withhold episiotomy when indicated would be wanton; nevertheless, it constitutes a mutilation, although mild, and if ruthlessly abused without good reason, it will leave a number of women exposed to the likelihood of further perineal troubles in subsequent deliveries, often necessitating repeated episiotomy. This is a minor objection, but it has to be remembered that occasionally a painful and unsatisfactory scar may give rise to dyspareunia. It is as well to repeat episiotomy, when indicated, on the same side as before. It heals just as well and causes less ultimate scarring and possible dyspareunia.

Indications

There are many indications, and the following is a list of most of them:

1. All cases of fœtal distress in the second stage demand episiotomy to spare the child further delay, damage and asphyxia in labour.

2. All cases of prematurity for reasons given above.

3. All cases of primigravid breech delivery. It is too late to start thinking about an episiotomy when one runs into trouble with the after-coming head or with extended arms.

4. All cases of face-to-pubis forceps delivery.

5. After previous colpoperineorraphy and after any operation for the cure of stress incontinence in which a vaginal delivery has been decided upon.

The above are absolute indications. To these many would add all cases of forceps delivery in primigravidæ.

There follows a list of relative indications:

1. When the subpubic arch is narrow, and the head, because of its consequent posterior displacement, has difficulty in emerging.

2. Failure to advance because of perineal rigidity.

3. When the presenting part has been on the pelvic floor for more than half an hour.

4. Most cases of face presentation, excluding anencephaly.

5. When the perineal skin starts to split and a sizeable tear appears to be a certainty.

A very ragged vaginal tear is an unsatisfactory thing to sew up and this can often be avoided by episiotomy. If an episiotomy is inadequate for the demands made upon it, it will split further, but very seldom indeed into the rectum, whereas tearing of the perineum may easily extend uncontrollably.

Technique

The usual practice is to direct the cut to one side of the midline. A so-called midline episiotomy or perineotomy has little to recommend it, as any extension of the wound will be directed towards the rectum. The time to perform the episiotomy is when the perineum is unquestionably bulging. The length of incision required is then easier to determine, and to do it earlier may result in an unnecessary amount of blood loss which normally the pressure of the presenting part tends to control. On the other hand, to perform episiotomy too late, when the damage from stretching is already done, is also a mistake.

It is sometimes taught that an anæsthetic is not necessary on the argument that the patient is feeling such excruciating pain at this

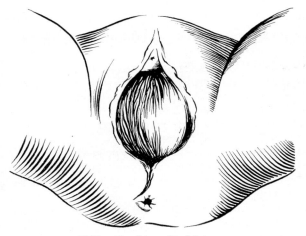

22/Fig. 5.—Line of episiotomy.

stage of labour that she is unlikely to notice any addition to it. This is nothing less than horrifying brutality, and it is inexcusable not to infiltrate the area of the incision with a few millilitres of lignocaine, a simple procedure taking a few seconds.

The best instrument to use is a strong pair of curved scissors, and the incision should start anteriorly from the midpoint of the fourchette (Fig. 5). It is a common mistake to make an oblique cut starting too far from the midline, for not only may this defeat satisfactory suture but a more vascular area is opened up and bleeding may be excessive. The best procedure is to cut directly backwards for the first part of the incision and then to use the curve of the scissors to direct the incision laterally in the shape of the letter "J"

so that it runs to one side of the anal margin. By keeping 1 inch away from the latter one can be certain of avoiding damage to the anal sphincter. Personally, I prefer to map out the incision with an unmounted scalpel blade held in the left hand using the scissors only for cutting the vaginal wall.

A finger should be inserted into the vagina as a guard and the whole depth of tissue should be convincingly divided, if possible in one determined cut rather than in a series of nibbles. If brisk bleeding occurs, it is probable that the episiotomy has been done too early, but in any case a powerful bleeding point ought to be picked up with a hæmostat, for a patient can lose a surprising quantity of blood from an episiotomy wound in quite a short space of time.

The repair of an episiotomy follows exactly the same lines as for a second-degree tear, but the inner side of the wound tends to retract more than the lateral margin and care must be taken to secure satisfactory alignment.

The practice of performing bilateral episiotomy has now been almost universally abandoned because, although it provides an enormous exposure and the anal canal tends to hinge backwards out of the way like a trap-door, there is a strong likelihood of sloughing, since the blood supply has been interrupted from both sides. For this reason it is better to do a wide single episiotomy than two small bilateral cuts.

There are very few dangers in episiotomy, the chief being blood loss which can always be controlled. Sepsis occurs occasionally and the wound breaks down, but secondary suture as soon as the sepsis has been cleared up is a perfectly satisfactory procedure.

On rare occasions Bartholin's duct is damaged, and some time later a Bartholin's cyst develops. This should never occur if the incision has been started correctly in the midline and only results from recklessly wide lateral cuts.

If deepening shock occurs, as occasionally it may, following episiotomy repair, it is worth including a large paravaginal hæmatoma among the diagnostic possibilities. Vaginal examination will at once reveal the characteristic lateral bulge. In such a case the repair must be undone, the clot evacuated and proper hæmostatic suturing undertaken. Only rarely should packing be necessary.

INJURIES TO THE URINARY SYSTEM

It is not surprising that the urinary tract occasionally suffers some degree of wear or tear considering its unfortunate anatomical proximity to the field of obstetrical battle. All manner of urinary disabilities therefore, ranging from the mild to the severe may be encountered.

STRESS INCONTINENCE

During early and late pregnancy some degree of this is common enough to be almost physiological, but the stresses of labour may so weaken the fascial supports of the bladder neck that a permanent disability results, if not forthwith, at least in years to come, particularly at about the time of menopausal involution.

The bladder neck in difficult labour becomes the nut between the crackers, being compressed and devitalized between the back of the symphysis pubis and the advancing fœtal head.

Sometimes the anterior vaginal wall is pushed down in front of the presenting part, and it is important to press it up and out of the way during the second stage. Often a perineal tear is carefully avoided at the cost of diminished urinary control, and it is far preferable to perform episiotomy than to leave the head a long time on the perineum. The expeditious use of the low forceps operation, or Ventouse, will also cut short prolonged stress upon the bladder neck supports, but forceps applied before full dilatation of the cervix is a potent cause of stress incontinence.

After delivery, postnatal exercises are of great value in forestalling the development of this miserable condition, and it is important that they should be continued after return home when urinary control is inadequate or cystocele threatens. Physiotherapy, here, can perform a very useful function.

If the condition persists at the time of postnatal examination, the temporary support afforded by a suitable pessary until involution is complete may render subsequent operation unnecessary.

If, however, stress incontinence is still troublesome six months after delivery, operative repair by colporrhaphy should be performed regardless of the patient's age or the prospects of further childbearing. The need for this, however, is usually the result of the patient's failure to co-operate in her postnatal exercises and physiotherapy. Stress incontinence is a preventable condition.

Having successfully cured the case surgically, labour must, in later instances, be conducted with due regard to the operative result. Episiotomy at the very least is emphatically indicated, and in occasional instances Cæsarean section may be advisable.

URETERIC FISTULA

This is fortunately a very rare complication of vaginal delivery and only the most extreme forms of misdirected trauma are likely to inflict it.

VESICO-VAGINAL FISTULA

This is uncommon in enlightened obstetrics, but was a common result of neglected disproportion, particularly in cases of flat pelvis.

It may arise either as the result of pressure necrosis of the bladder neck, in which case the fistula develops about a week after delivery when the slough separates, or it may be directly caused by laceration with instruments, or, in the operation of cranioclasm, by the jagged ends of skull bones. After symphysiotomy, too, the bladder, no longer fully supported by the pubic framework, may suffer damage.

Howsoever caused, the invariable symptom is total urinary incontinence regardless of posture or activity.

The diagnosis is not difficult. The larger fistulæ can either be seen, or felt with the finger but the instillation of methylene blue into the bladder may help to reveal very small lesions.

The fistula is usually situated on the anterior vaginal wall, but occasionally it may open into the anterior fornix or even into the cervix or uterus. At lower segment Cæsarean section failure to displace the bladder downwards and out of harm's way before incising the uterus, or careless suturing later, may damage the bladder wall and cause a vesico-uterine fistula. Damage to the bladder at the time of the operation is usually demonstrated by bloodstained urine which is easily tested for by pinching the catheter before withdrawing it and then emptying the urine within over a white towel or swab.

Treatment should be immediate and never deferred even until next day if there is to be any hope of obtaining spontaneous closure. A catheter should be passed into the bladder and anchored with sutures; continuous gentle suction drainage should be maintained for two, or preferably three weeks, keeping the bladder absolutely empty and at rest. I have seen very unpleasant fistulæ close spontaneously without more elaborate treatment, but success depends entirely upon instituting drainage before the fistulous track has a chance to epithelialise.

If this treatment fails to close the fistula, operative repair must be undertaken, and there is no need to prolong the patient's wretchedness by waiting for more than three months, since it can safely be assumed that if it has not closed before then nothing short of surgical repair will succeed in effecting a cure.

OBSTETRICAL PALSIES

Although the literature has paid rather scant attention to this subject, palsies as a result of pregnancy and labour are by no means rare, and they constitute a fairly important source of postnatal disability. The commonest form is the appearance of foot drop, usually unilateral, shortly after delivery or during the first day or so.

The muscles most frequently affected are the dorsiflexors of the foot and toes, though occasionally the glutei, hamstrings, quadriceps and adductors of the thigh may be severally involved.

The lesion is of the lower motor neurone type with flaccidity and wasting. Sensory loss or disturbance is less prominent but is often present. Strenuous vaginal delivery, usually terminating in a forceps operation, is an accepted predisposing condition, but the complication can occur after easy, rapid and normal delivery with a roomy pelvis.

The old explanation that the lesion was caused by direct pressure, either by the fœtal head or the forceps blades upon the lumbosacral cord or sacral plexus, is not accepted nowadays, because it does not explain the onset of symptoms many hours after labour, nor the appearance of damage of femoral nerve distribution, and if direct intrapelvic pressure could so operate, one would expect vesical and rectal injury even more often.

Backward rotation of the sacrum in labour has also been thought to result in stretching of the lumbosacral cord and may account for some cases of postnatal sciatica, but the most likely explanation lies in the theory of intervertebral disc protrusion. O'Connell (1944), in giving details of four cases, discussed the likelihood of this factor very clearly, and he considered that the prolapsed disc theory can account for all cases, excluding of course those of peroneal palsy due to misuse of lithotomy poles and stirrups. This explanation is not accepted for all cases however; Chalmers (1949) traced 142 cases in the literature and added another four of which only one was attributed to disc protrusion, the other three being due to compression (two cases) and sacral rotation (one case) and he concluded that different mechanisms could produce the condition. Now, as is well known, the joints of the pelvis increase their mobility in pregnancy, and in pathological degree this may give rise to symptoms of pelvic arthropathy. The effect is believed to be due to "relaxin" or progesterone and can be reproduced in experimental animals. Since it is unlikely that an endocrine effect would select only the pelvic joints, it is reasonable to assume that the vertebral column, too, takes part in the general loosening-up process. In pregnancy, furthermore, lordosis of the lumbar spine may be exaggerated, so that the intervertebral discs become vulnerable to the stress of labour and may herniate. The type of neurological lesion and whether or not it is bilateral will then depend only upon the extent and direction of the disc protrusion. The disc most commonly involved is that between the fifth lumbar and first sacral vertebral body.

On this basis treatment is formulated. Firstly, rest in bed is necessary, sometimes for six weeks in cases which do not readily clear up and where pain persists. A hard board should be placed under the mattress and over the bed-springs to prevent sagging of the back while the patient is relaxed in sleep. Secondly, splinting is applied to prevent damage by unopposed overstretching of the para-

lysed muscles. Massage and electrical stimulation to the muscles are started fairly early, and active exercise is encouraged with the return of function.

The prognosis is usually favourable and many cases clear up within a few weeks, though it may be necessary to prescribe a spring to raise the front of the shoe in the early stages of ambulation. In severe and resistant cases, in which disability or pain and backache persist, operation upon the prolapsed disc may be required. Nevin (1951) has suggested that cases who develop disc lesions in pregnancy should be delivered by Cæsarean section unless a straightforward and easy labour can be confidently anticipated.

REFERENCES

1. CHALMERS, J. A. (1949). *J. Obstet. Gynæc. Brit. Emp.*, **56**, 205.
2. DAS, P. (1940). *J. Obstet. Gynæc. Brit. Emp.*, **47**, 525.
3. FEENEY, K., and BARRY, A. (1956). *Brit. med. J.*, **1**, 65.
4. FLEW, J. D. S. (1944). *Brit. med. J.*, **2**, 620.
5. HIGGINS, L. G. (1957). *Lancet*, **1**, 618.
6. JOSEY, W. E. (1966). *Amer. J. Obstet. Gynec.*, **94**, 29.
7. MOIR, J. C. (1964). *Munro Kerr's Operative Obstetrics*, 7th edit. London: Baillière, Tindall & Cox.
8. NEVIN, S. (1951). In *Medical Disorders in Pregnancy*, edited by S. G. Clayton and S. Oram. London: J. & A. Churchill.
9. O'CONNELL, J. E. A. (1944). *Surg. Gynec. Obstet.*, **79**, 374.
10. O'DRISCOLL, K. (1966). *Proc. roy. Soc. Med.*, **59**, 65.
11. O'SULLIVAN, J. V. (1945). *Brit. med. J.*, **2**, 282.
12. SPAIN, A. W. (1946). *J. Obstet. Gynæc. Brit. Emp.*, **53**, 219.

CHAPTER XXIII

CÆSAREAN SECTION

CÆSAREAN section is now performed with increasing impunity, thanks largely to antibiotics, improved anæsthesia and the availability of blood transfusion. It is natural, therefore, that the indications for this operation are being continually extended; nevertheless, there is no excuse for resorting to it because one lacks the obstetrical skill of a previous generation, and it would be a great mistake to regard it as a means of finding a happy issue out of all our obstetrical afflictions. "Cæsarean Section—a lethal operation?" was chosen, in fact, as the title of Sir Andrew Claye's William Hunter Memorial Lecture in Glasgow in 1960, in which he reviewed disasters precipitated by ill-chosen indications, unsatisfactory operating conditions, indifferent or inexperienced technique and bad timing.

In these days of small families the baby's right to survival is increasingly recognised, and consequently many of the indications for the operation are now solely concerned with the interests of the infant.

Indications.—The following is a list of indications more or less in order of importance, which singly, or in combination, may sway the obstetrician's decision in favour of abdominal delivery (vaginal by-pass):

1. Fœtal distress in the first stage of labour. This indication accounts largely for the rising incidence of Cæsarean section in hospital practice. Often the vigorous condition of the baby at birth, in spite of being coated with thick meconium, causes one to wonder how genuine was the distress. The growing use of fœtal blood sampling by the Saling method as described in the chapter on prolonged labour may help however to reduce the incidence of unnecessary Cæsarean section for this indication.

2. More than minor degrees of disproportion.

3. Where previous Cæsarean section has been carried out following a failed trial of labour for disproportion.

4. Certain cases of uterine inertia, especially with the membranes ruptured for a long time. In these cases the fœtal prognosis worsens as labour becomes more and more prolonged.

5. The bad obstetric history. This subject is dealt with more fully elsewhere.

6. Severe degrees of placenta prævia or any case of severe re-

vealed antepartum hæmorrhage, when the patient is not in labour and primigravid and the baby still alive.

7. Failed surgical induction. As discussed in the chapter on induced labour, the indications for embarking on induction must be sufficient to make one ready to proceed even farther in order to secure a patient's delivery, should induction fail.

8. Certain cases of fulminating pre-eclamptic toxæmia, in which surgical induction will not terminate the pregnancy quickly enough.

9. Certain classes of malpresentation, usually in association with other abnormalities.

10. Prolapse of the cord with the child still alive and the patient still short of full dilatation of the cervix.

11. A previous repair operation in which symptoms of urinary or rectal incontinence have, with difficulty, been cured. This of course applies also to a history of repair of vesico-vaginal fistula.

12. The presence of an established constriction ring in the course of labour with the child still alive and labour prolonged.

13. Many cases of diabetes mellitus.

14. Ovarian tumours complicating pregnancy at term if they cannot be pushed from in front of the presenting part.

15. Cases of fibroids which occupy the pelvis and persist in their threat to obstruct the advance of the presenting part.

16. Elderly primigravidæ, in association with other abnormalities. Cæsarean section is no guarantee of live birth of the child but, especially after a prolonged period of infertility, subsidiary indications for Cæsarean section will, in this case, carry more weight.

17. Certain cases of cardiac disease, in which a perfectly straightforward labour cannot be confidently anticipated as a result of associated abnormalities, major or minor. The use of Cæsarean section to provide a means of carrying out sterilisation at the same time is not a valid indication.

18. Cases of carcinoma of the cervix discovered late in pregnancy.

19. Structural abnormalities of the vagina which cannot be expected to stretch adequately or safely to allow the passage of the fœtal head. These abnormalities may be either congenital or the result of previous plastic operations on the vagina.

20. History of two previous Cæsarean sections.

The case for the lower segment operation.—For nearly all practical purposes there is only one type of Cæsarean section today, namely the lower segment operation. Its almost universal adoption has contributed a great deal to the safety of Cæsarean section. Although the approach is still transperitoneal, there are many reasons for preferring it to the older, classical upper segment operation. For one thing, it is usually possible to perform the operation with relatively much less blood loss. For another, it takes

very little longer to perform; but one of its chief virtues lies in the reduced chances of infection of the general peritoneal cavity because of the low position of the operation area which can be excluded by gauze packing. The scar in the uterus lies deep in the pelvis and behind the bladder during the puerperium and the spread of infection tends thereby to be limited. Its greatest advantage, however, lies in the fact that the uterine scar is placed in an area of the uterus which is at rest during the puerperium; this allows far more satisfactory healing. The classical scar in the upper segment is undermined by the rhythmical uterine contractions which follow delivery and loosen the sutures, often causing them to cut out so that only the serous coat of the uterus holds that organ more or less together Any uterine infection still further interferes with sound healing, and the chances of uterine rupture in a subsequent pregnancy are too high to be countenanced. The classical scar, moreover, is very liable to ooze blood at the end of the operation. This not only encourages infection, but invites the formation of bowel adhesions which rarely complicate the lower segment operation. In the course of the latter, coils of intestine should not even come within view, and this fact must contribute, to some extent, to the diminished incidence of postoperative ileus.

Lower Segment Section and Placenta Prævia

There is still a tendency in some quarters to prefer the classical operation for cases of placenta prævia, and for some years the author held this mistaken view, largely out of fear that he might run into uncontrollable bleeding in incising the lower segment. It was not until he started doing the lower segment operation for placenta prævia that he came to believe what others had already told him. It is true that the front of the lower segment may be very vascular, but with a good technique this should not be troublesome, and certainly the upper segment is, as a rule, more likely to bleed whether the placenta is situated beneath the incision or not.

Another objection advanced is that one may encounter the placenta prævia anteriorly. This should not deter one, for it is only the matter of a second to brush it aside or, if necessary, to rip straight through it. Perhaps the most serious objection is that with an anteriorly placed placenta the uterine wall in the lower segment may be more friable and, therefore, uncontrollable tears may occur, making suture difficult and threatening satisfactory union. There is the further danger that the fœtus may bleed from the placenta if the latter has to be incised instead of being pushed aside. Butler and Martin (1954) reported 5 cases of neonatal anæmia as a result of this and Neligan and Russell (1954) likewise encountered the placenta on incising the lower segment in 20 out of 45 cases of placenta prævia.

It is recommended, therefore, that the umbilical cord should be clamped as soon as possible if the placenta has been damaged in order to reduce the fœtal blood loss, and a careful watch, by repeated hæmoglobin estimations, should be maintained in any baby in which this complication is thought possible. Blood transfusion should be given if the baby's hæmoglobin level falls to 90 per cent.

It is unlikely that the scar in the lower segment will again be the site of placenta prævia in future pregnancies. This is an important consideration, because it is very often those cases in which the placenta, in a subsequent pregnancy, is situated over the previous uterine scar that the uterus is most liable to rupture.

Classical Cæsarean Section

Unfortunately, this cannot be dismissed without some discussion, for it is still too commonly practised. As already hinted, the indications for it must be very few indeed. The following are the only indications which would appear to be valid:

1. The mother is already dead, and one is performing post-mortem Cæsarean section in the hopes of securing a live child.

2. When the patient is already so moribund from antepartum hæmorrhage due to placenta prævia that every second in delivery may count.

3. When hysterectomy is contemplated at the same time.

4. When some relevant structural abnormality of the uterus exists which makes approach to the lower segment technically impossible.

5. Occasionally in cases of transverse lie no proper lower uterine segment can be identified.

6. In cases of gross kyphosis in which the distance between sternum and pubis is so reduced that the belly is pendulous and the lie transverse. I have only once encountered such a case and it was as much as I could do to avoid placing the incision in the uterine fundus.

Extra-peritoneal Cæsarean Section

This operation might have had a great future but for the discovery of the antibiotics. In the lower segment operation both the peritoneal cavity and the pelvic cellular tissues are exposed to infection, whereas only the latter are involved in the extra-peritoneal approach. Nevertheless, this is no great matter, since the pelvic peritoneum is, in any case, more capable of dealing with infection than the pelvic cellular tissue. Extra-peritoneal Cæsarean section is undoubtedly more difficult technically and is more time-consuming, and the very circumstances which might therefore call for its performance would, in themselves, tend to contra-indicate it for this

reason alone. Whatever method is used, it is a common accident to open the peritoneal cavity and thereby destroy the whole virtue of the procedure and the bladder is even more liable to injury. In an attempt to circumvent the technical difficulties, various surgeons have devised exclusion types of operation in which the peritoneal cavity is first opened and then, after exposing the outer side of the lower uterine segment, the remainder of the peritoneal cavity is excluded by suturing the visceral and parietal peritoneum together above the operation site. I myself devised such an operation and performed it in three cases, tearing a large hole in the bladder in one and in no instance being satisfied with the exposure obtained. Although convalescence proceeded uneventfully in all three, there was nothing remarkable about it.

The extra-peritoneal Cæsarean section as occasionally practised nowadays may be one of two types: firstly, the *Waters' operation*, in which the approach to the lower segment is made centrally by literally skinning the peritoneum off the dome of the bladder and then dislocating the bladder downwards. The area of approach is by no means avascular, and since the peritoneum over the bladder dome is densely adherent, very sharp dissection is called for, during which either bladder or peritoneum are easily opened.

The other type of extra-peritoneal operation is the *Latzko operation*, in which the lower segment is approached by the para-vesical route, the bladder and utero-vesical pouch of peritoneum being together displaced to one side. I have no experience of this operation, but I should imagine that it is technically far from easy, and that in approaching initially from one side fairly severe venous bleeding might be expected. Injuries to bladder or peritoneum would be liable to occur as before.

Porro Cæsarean Section

American authorities are inclined to use this term to cover cases of Cæsarean sub-total hysterectomy, but this use of the name Porro is incorrect. As performed in 1877 by Porro, it involved amputation of the uterus at the internal os together with the adnexa and the fixation of the cervical stump in the lower end of the abdominal wound. Nowadays, of course, the cervical stump is dealt with as in routine sub-total hysterectomy.

History

The operation of Cæsarean section dates of course from antiquity, and was usually employed in the hope of obtaining a living child when the mother was dead or so near to death that maternal survival

was not a practical consideration. While the mother was still alive, even so-called primitive peoples employed, as a rule, some form of narcosis, usually alcoholic. The introduction of anæsthetics, however, in the last century brought the operation into more serious consideration.

In 1870 the death-rate from Cæsarean section was still in the region of 75 per cent. In 1878 Murdoch Cameron in Glasgow achieved the feat of performing a series of eight Cæsarean sections without a maternal death. One of the cases lived to the ripe age of 75. She had an illegitimate pregnancy and a true conjugate of $1\frac{1}{2}$ inches —not a good combination in the Scotland of those Victorian days. A meeting of the senior obstetricians of the city debated her fate and Cæsarean section was finally agreed, one of the disputants insisting that a minority view be minuted since he regarded the case as borderline!

Quite apart from shock and sepsis, the main reason for maternal death was hæmorrhage, because it was the practice, up to that date, to return the uterus to the abdomen unsutured. The success of uterine wound suture revived interest in the classical type of operation during the last thirty years of the nineteenth century.

All these operations were of the classical variety, and the Porro operation at once produced an enormous improvement in mortality figures for, by suturing the cervical stump into the lower end of the abdominal wound, there was no opportunity for continued intraperitoneal bleeding. Moreover, the main focus of sepsis, namely the body of the uterus, was removed by amputation, and drainage of what was left was of course complete.

The history of lower segment Cæsarean section is older than one would expect, for in 1805 Osiander performed an operation of this type, and in 1821 a disastrous attempt at extra-peritoneal Cæsarean section was made by Ritgen, in which the patient died although the child was born alive.

At the beginning of this century Frank developed a type of exclusion operation in which he sutured the upper edge of the parietal peritoneum to the visceral peritoneum and incised the uterus transversely through the lower segment, and by 1910 Sellheim was doing an operation which was not very dissimilar from the lower segment operation of today. The operation, however, appears to have taken a long time to come into vogue, and it was Munro Kerr who did most of all in this country to popularise it.

It is strange to think that the general adoption of the lower segment operation has taken place only in the last quarter of a century. The maternal mortality figures speak for themselves, and the improvement cannot be attributed to antibiotics or to blood banks, neither of which made their appearance until shortly before

the war, and to this operation alone must go the major credit for the increased safety of Cæsarean section.

Incidence of Cæsarean Section

This varies very widely in different centres. Hospital statistics give no true picture of how commonly the operation is in fact performed amongst the population as a whole, because the more abnormal cases gravitate there. The figure varies between 1 per cent and 8 per cent according to the nature of the hospital and also according to geographical conditions; for instance, in areas where contracted pelvis, due to rickets, is still relatively common, the incidence of Cæsarean section is higher. Our own figure was 7·1 per cent for 1964–5.

Safety of Cæsarean Section

The operative mortality had fallen from the level of 75 per cent during the middle of the last century to less than 10 per cent at the beginning of this one, although the classical operation was almost universally performed during this period.

The reasons for which the operation is performed have very often more to do with the death-rate than the operation itself, and cardiac disease, diabetes mellitus, placenta prævia and concealed accidental hæmorrhage are noteworthy examples.

At present the overall maternal mortality in England and Wales in cases delivered by Cæsarean section is 3·5 per thousand and in spite of recent improvements in facilities and techniques the figure remains between 8 and 10 times as high as after delivery by the vaginal route.

The risk of pulmonary embolism, as with all pelvic abdominal operations, still remains with us, but this is very largely a preventable condition. It is not wholly fair to compare the operative mortality of Cæsarean section with the mortality of vaginal delivery. Such a comparison, to be valid, should take into account the indications.

Preparation of the Patient

Of all measures, undoubtedly the most important is to exclude any anæmia or to treat it if present. Where blood loss prior to operation has been acute, it should be replaced quantitatively as far as possible before operating. Where chronic anæmia exists, the blood condition ought to be restored at least to a hæmoglobin level of 80 per cent pre-operatively. Needless to say, the patient's blood group must be known, and preferably some serum should have been taken already for cross-matching and a supply of a compatible blood

should be assured. It would be sheer pessimism to anticipate the need for routine blood transfusion in all one's cases but, when needed, circumstances may brook no delay. The patient who is anæmic is ill-equipped to withstand further hæmorrhage at operation, and the effects of bleeding will be magnified. But this is not all, for anæmia not only aggravates the effects of shock but also predisposes the patient to puerperal thrombosis; also resistance to infection may be so lowered by anæmia that the patient's chances of recovery may be prejudiced. It is now our practice in all cases to have a saline drip set up and running slowly before starting the operation. Any intravenous injection or blood transfusion can then be given without delay if necessary.

Another wise precaution is to take a straight X-ray of the abdomen where time permits, in order to exclude the presence of a fœtal abnormality in so far as this is possible. There are two main absolute indications for Cæsarean section even when fœtal abnormality is radiologically demonstrable. These are, cases of central placenta prævia, and secondly, gross pelvic contraction. In most other cases, however, where a fœtal abnormality exists, every attempt should be made to secure vaginal delivery.

In all cases in which the possibility of infection is suspected, it is a wise plan to take a specimen from the vault of the vagina for bacterial culture before operating. The report on the culture will then be available so much the earlier, so that appropriate chemotherapy can be readily instituted. Where there has been no opportunity to take this pre-operative specimen, a swab should be taken from the uterine cavity at operation.

The advisability of operating under what is now referred to as a "chemotherapeutic umbrella" in suspect cases is a debatable matter. Undoubtedly the practice is abused, and antibiotics are given to all sorts of cases quite empirically, with the result that accurate diagnosis of a puerperal infection may be prejudiced and the patient's recovery, far from being accelerated, may actually be delayed. The "umbrella", however, is certainly indicated in cardiac cases in whom the risk of heart valve vegetations is too serious to countenance.

The stomach should be empty. Unfortunately, especially in those cases who have been some time in labour and have throughout this period been encouraged to drink as much as possible, the stomach is likely to contain large quantities of fluid, and this fact provides one of the greatest risks in the induction of anæsthesia. It is safer to pass a stomach tube and to administer by mouth 14 ml. of magnesium trisilicate mixture (B.P.C.) to neutralize any remaining gastric acid.

The abdominal wall and vulva of the patient are shaved and some suitable antiseptic paint is applied. A pre-operative soap and water

enema is given, provided there is no antepartum bleeding, and a catheter is passed before the patient leaves the ward. The catheter is left *in situ* throughout the operation unspigoted and draining, so that the bladder at all times is unquestionably empty. Premedication is usually restricted to atropine 0·6 mg. (gr. $\frac{1}{100}$) to dry up secretions, and narcotic drugs are not usually given at the same time because of the possible effect they may have upon the baby's readiness to breathe.

ANÆSTHESIA

The greatest danger period is during the induction of anæsthesia, when vomiting from a full stomach is particularly liable to occur and may result in dangerous degrees of aspiration. Maternal asphyxia is even more dangerous to the baby than it is to the mother herself, and because of the very slow and sluggish circulation of the uterus it may be anything up to a quarter of an hour before the uterus becomes well oxygenated again following acute asphyxia. During this period the baby, even if it does not die, is liable to undertake premature inspiratory movements.

The fairly general improvement in anæsthetic standards is progressively eliminating the once common preference of many obstetricians for spinal and local anæsthesia, often administered by the obstetrician himself.

Epidural anæsthesia, introduced by the lumbar route has largely replaced spinal anæsthesia, especially in cases of prolonged incoordinate labour where it might have been instituted earlier on.

The advantages which apply to both epidural and spinal anæsthesia are that hæmorrhage is reduced because uterine tone is not affected. The effect, moreover, on liver and kidneys is negligible, while during the post-operative period there is very little vomiting or intestinal ileus. The child suffers no effects whatsoever from the anæsthetic. Nevertheless, there are certain grave disadvantages. A severe fall in blood pressure may occur in the course of the operation and may be very hard to correct. It is not a safe form of anæsthetic in patients who are severely shocked or suffering from hypotension from any cause. Cases with heart disease are liable to collapse and severe degrees of anæmia make this type of anæsthetic unsuitable. Highly excitable patients are not likely to co-operate well, and in them the technique may be almost impossible to carry out. The later complications of spinal anæsthesia also have to be borne in mind, namely meningitis, paraplegia, incontinence and diplopia, and on the whole the risks are too great to justify its use for Cæsarean section.

Local anæsthesia still has a useful place in situations where general anæsthetic service is inadequate. Shock is reduced to a

minimum and pulmonary complications are very rare. Again, the liver and kidneys suffer no toxic damage and cardiac muscle is not in any way affected. Uterine tone is good throughout, and this also diminishes hæmorrhage. Cases of heart disease are regarded as usually suitable.

Unfortunately, there are certain drawbacks to local anæsthesia which prevent its more general adoption. It takes time to secure adequate anæsthesia and often one fails to achieve it completely so that the patient, already frightened, finds that she has to suffer also a certain amount of pain. It is usually impossible by local infiltration methods to make extraction of the head, especially when deep in the pelvis, a painless procedure, and very often the local anæsthetic has to be reinforced at this time with some short-acting general anæsthetic such as thiopentone. Remembering the patient has usually had no narcotic premedication, there can be no doubt that the experience, even if it is not particularly painful, must be psychologically traumatic. The surgeon is often handicapped by the fear of hurting the patient, and this will tend to limit his exposure. The peritoneal cavity will, for the same reason, be less efficiently packed off and the removal of all traces of blood and liquor at the end of the operation is likely to be less thorough. On the whole the Cæsarean section carried out under local anæsthesia is often an unpleasant experience for both surgeon and patient, and general anæsthesia is more widely preferred.

Of the inhalation anæsthetics, chloroform has to be mentioned, although its use is dying out. It has the one great advantage that induction is usually smooth, but this feature is more than cancelled by its great dangers, not the least of which is the liability to produce uterine atony and therefore postpartum hæmorrhage. In this respect, because chloroform is such a powerful uterine relaxant, it is the worst anæsthetic to use.

Ether is much safer, of course, but the dangers of uterine atony are almost as great. Both ether and chloroform are liable to interfere with the baby's respiratory centre and they are definitely contraindicated in prematurity and in cases of established fœtal distress. Induction of anæsthesia involving the use of ether takes very much longer, and during this time the patient is in considerable danger of vomiting and induction asphyxia. Following ether the post-operative course is likely to be much less pleasant for the patient because of air swallowing, vomiting and ileus.

Halothane, though satisfactory from this point of view, relaxes the uterus dangerously in a manner which ergometrine will not counter, although oxytocin may be more effective. It is therefore not recommended.

Trichloroethylene anæsthesia, although very safe, unfortunately is

not usually adequate by itself for the performance of the operation, and there is no inhalation anæsthetic which is entirely satisfactory. I prefer cyclopropane, because induction is smooth and quick, the patient remains well oxygenated and the uterus loses very little retractile power. Nitrous oxide is fraught with more perils than is generally realised, mainly because of the high risk of vomiting.

The introduction of the relaxant drugs of the curare class has made possible the use of very much smaller quantities of inhalation anæsthetic agents with, therefore, a great increase in their safety. The short-acting relaxants are particularly useful and they do not interfere with uterine tone.

Intravenous barbiturates may expose the child to the risk of apnœa as a result of barbiturate depression. A dose not exceeding 250 mg. of thiopentone may be given at the beginning of induction provided the trachea can be intubated forthwith, otherwise this drug cannot be considered as safe in Cæsarean section. The majority of our anæsthetics now consist of brief thiopentone induction followed immediately by a short-acting muscle relaxant and immediate tracheal intubation. Any anæsthetist worthy of the name is skilful at passing endotracheal tubes. Those who are not should be discouraged from undertaking obstetric anæsthesia. Anæsthesia is thereafter maintained with nitrous oxide and oxygen and sufficient relaxant to facilitate exposure and wound suture. The patient should regain some measure of consciousness and certainly her cough reflex within a few minutes of the end of the operation.

The choice of the best anæsthetic is a thorny subject on which very few obstetricians agree and still fewer anæsthetists. It shows that no ideal method yet exists. One thing, however, is certain: this type of anæsthesia is not for the occasional anæsthetist, for there are too many pitfalls and dangers, not merely to one life but to two.

Technique of Lower Segment Cæsarean Section

The position of the patient during the operation should be level, and the use of the Trendelenburg position is not only unnecessary but may be harmful. Under certain circumstances it may be necessary to tip the patient in the head downwards position, especially if the anæsthetist gets into difficulties with induction vomiting, and very occasionally the use of the Trendelenburg position may facilitate delivery of the head when it is deep in the pelvis. For these reasons it is important to ensure that the patient's legs are well and firmly tied on to the table, or, better still, to use iliac crest supports, because should the Trendelenburg position be needed, the circumstances which call for it will not afford time for fixing the legs and the patient may be in danger of sliding off the table. Shoulder rests

are very dangerous things, and brachial palsies seem to be particularly easily produced in pregnant women at term, especially after the use of relaxants which abolish all muscle protection in the brachial plexus. If one of the arms has to be abducted for the purpose of giving an intravenous injection during the operation, the likelihood of the risk is greatly magnified. The new corrugated mattresses prevent this risk entirely.

The catheter is left *in situ* and drains into some loose wool between the patient's legs. The fœtal heart should be checked.

After painting and towelling the patient, the operator should examine the abdomen and satisfy himself about the position of the child. In the case of a transverse lie it is better, if possible, to correct this before starting the operation than to rely upon internal version through the incision in the lower segment. In vertex presentation it is worth noting on which side the occiput lies, because, in delivering the head, the occiput should be rotated so that it presents through the uterine wound first.

Incision

It is a common mistake to make this unnecessarily long, and it should not be extended below the level of the top of the symphysis pubis, for this will not only produce troublesome bleeding but does nothing to increase the exposure. Five inches is perfectly adequate, and it should seldom be necessary to carry the upper level above that of the umbilicus. A midline incision is still commonly employed. A paramedian incision has only theoretical advantages which are not borne out in practice and the incidence of scar hernia is not reduced thereby. Moreover, it is unsightly.

The aponeurosis is sought in the region of the linea alba and is incised vertically, practically down to the symphysis pubis. Every half-inch gained in this downward direction will produce noticeably more room. It is not necessary to cut through the pyramidalis muscles, but one can guide the blade of the knife between the outer border of this muscle and the inner border of the corresponding rectus muscle.

We now mostly use a transverse incision of the Pfannenstiel type about two fingersbreadth above the symphysis pubis. The rectus sheath is then divided transversely and peeled off the underlying rectus abdominis muscles, cutting with blunt pointed scissors to free it deep to the linea alba in the midline and sparing, as far as possible, vessels and nerves laterally. It is desirable to leave the pyramidalis muscles attached to the lower aponeurotic flap and to dissect bluntly behind them as far down as the top of the symphysis pubis. The more practice one has at making this incision the fewer

the number of bleeding points that have to be picked up as a rule. The rectus muscles are separated in a vertical direction.

This incision, because it has a better blood supply than the vertical varieties, heals better (Willocks and Gebbie, 1963) and, as in thyroidectomy scars in the neck, the skin edges lie more naturally together and a more cosmetic scar results. A further advantage of this incision is that the fundus of the uterus can be more easily palpated during the first few post-operative hours.

The peritoneum is now picked up and incised in the upper third of the incision. It is important not to open the peritoneum any lower than this because, during labour and also in late pregnancy, the bladder may be a lot higher than expected and may be accidentally opened. Should this mistake be made, the bladder should at once be repaired in two layers with fine catgut. In enlarging the incision in the peritoneum the upper edge of the bladder should be both felt and looked for. Often a little ooze of blood from the margins of this incision will give warning that one is getting close to the edge of the bladder. Occasionally, because the bladder is so high, it may be felt that an inadequate exposure is being obtained. In these circumstances the incision in the peritoneum can be skirted to one side or the other round the bladder margin. A Doyen's retractor is now inserted, although I now often dispense even with this in order to reduce trauma to the abdominal parietes which may discourage mobility and deep breathing during the recovery phase.

It is better to use a small Doyen retractor than a wide one. Paradoxically a better exposure is obtained thereby, because the assistant can swing a small Doyen retractor to either side of the wound in order to improve the surgeon's access to any particular corner of it. The anterior surface of the uterus is now in view, and it should be noted whether or not there is a serious degree of dextro-rotation which is by no means uncommon, and brings the very vascular left lateral border of the uterus too closely into the field of operation. If large veins present themselves to view on the surface of the uterus, one should suspect such uterine rotation and confirm it by passing a hand in and feeling for the round ligaments and correcting it. It is not always possible to centralise the uterus satisfactorily, but it is as well to be aware of this anatomical variation so that eventually the incision may be started farther on the right side and consequently nearer the uterine midline.

The remainder of the peritoneal cavity is now packed off with roll gauze six inches wide. The left side should be well packed first, because this will help to correct dextro-rotation of the uterus, and the pack should extend well down in front of the broad ligament so that spill will not occur. The packing is now continued beneath the margins of the upper part of the incision in the abdominal wall and

then well down in front of the right broad ligament. Packing is an important step in the operation, and one's aim should be to prevent any blood or liquor from reaching the general peritoneal cavity. Dry gauze is more efficient than gauze wrung out in warm saline, as it is more absorbent.

Identification of the Lower Segment

This is not difficult. The level at which the serous coat of the anterior wall of the uterus ceases to be intimately applied to the uterine wall and can be slid over the underlying muscle (because of its very loose attachment to it) marks the upper margin of the lower segment. In labour this limit is considerably raised, and often a slight groove marks the junction with the upper segment. In the absence of labour contractions, in prematurity, in cases of transverse lie and in cases of placenta prævia the length of the lower segment is much reduced in comparison, and it is very easy to incise the uterus far too high, perhaps even into the upper segment, which is most undesirable.

The upper edge of the bladder is applied to the front of the lower segment, and is seldom less than 2 inches below this demarcation line, which can usually be seen as a definite ridge. The peritoneum of the uterovesical fold is now picked up in the midline with forceps and a stay suture is inserted, the ends of which are cut 1 inch long. This is a useful identification mark in suturing the visceral peritoneum later. The peritoneum is now cut with scissors in the midline above the marker suture and the closed scissors are inserted beneath it both to the left and to the right to open up the space of areolar tissue behind it and to satisfy oneself that there is no danger of injuring the bladder (Fig. 1).

The visceral peritoneum is incised transversely in a curved direction convexity downwards, almost as far laterally as the round ligaments on each side, taking care not to injure the uterine veins. A layer of thin cellular tissue will be found deep to this incision, and it should be picked up with forceps and incised likewise. There may be some venous bleeding at this stage, but for the time being it should be ignored. The lower flap of peritoneum, together with the bladder, is now sponged down behind the symphysis pubis in order to expose a reasonable area of lower segment and to enable the uterine incision to be made as low as possible.

Incision of Uterus

The Doyen retractor is now adjusted so as to include the bladder behind its lip and to keep it out of harm's way during the next stages. Occasionally some large veins may be seen coursing over the uterus, and they should be avoided in making the initial incision. A suitable point is selected roughly in the midline and as low down as

CÆSAREAN SECTION

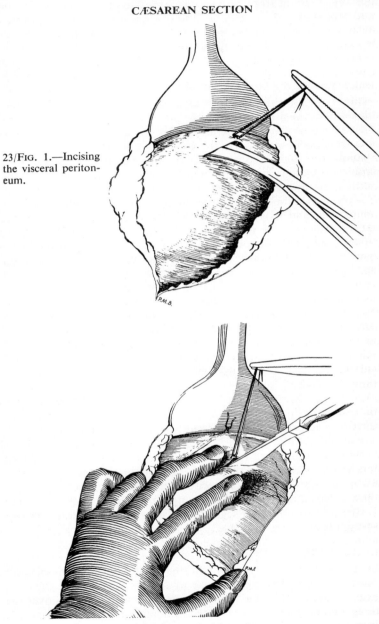

23/Fig. 1.—Incising the visceral peritoneum.

23/Fig. 2.—First incision of uterus.

possible and a stay suture is here inserted whose ends are left long and held in a clamp. Traction on this suture elevates the uterine wall away from the underlying fœtal head and a small transverse incision is made just above it, not more than half an inch wide (Fig. 2). By restricting the size of the initial incision and by carefully selecting its site it should be possible to proceed without undue hæmorrhage, which in any case can usually be controlled temporarily by pressing with the second and third fingers of the left hand on either side of it. Bonney's isthmo-compressor has been devised to circumvent troublesome bleeding, but this should not be needed if the initial incision is kept very small. The incision is deepened, and between strokes with the knife its depth is palpated with a finger of the left hand. In this way it is often possible to complete the incision without opening the amniotic sac.

Very occasionally one's view may be obscured by fairly brisk venous bleeding from a varicocele of the utero-vesical fold or from large veins in the bed of the bladder, but an assistant working a suction apparatus should be able to keep the field sufficiently clear at least to complete the initial incision by touch if not completely by sight.

As soon as the thickness of the uterine wall has been penetrated, first one finger and then two of the left hand are inserted through it and between the membranes and the lower segment itself. These fingers raise up the uterine wall and protect the underlying fœtus and the incision is extended laterally in each direction with curved scissors, concavity directed upwards (Fig. 3). It is best always to enlarge the incision to the right before the left, because of the prevalence of some degree of dextrorotation of the uterus which exposes the vessels on the left side to greater risk of injury. Having thus enlarged the incision by 2 inches in both directions, the index fingers of both hands are now inserted into its lateral angles and it is stretched upen sufficiently to allow the head to be delivered (Fig. 4).

By using the hook of the finger to extend the incision, one is far less likely to damage the great vessels at the sides of the uterus. It is a common mistake not to extend the incision sufficiently far, a mistake which is aggravated by now using the scissors.

By adopting the above precautions one should seldom encounter severe hæmorrhage from the lateral angles of an incision which has gone too far outwards. Only on rare occasions is it necessary to deal with large, abnormal vessels on the surface of the uterus by preliminary ligation. Some surgeons having made an initial opening in the uterus rely entirely upon digital traction to extend it, but by using scissors in the first place as described, the direction of extension is somewhat determined in advance and laceration of the lower uterine flap, especially downwards, is largely

CÆSAREAN SECTION

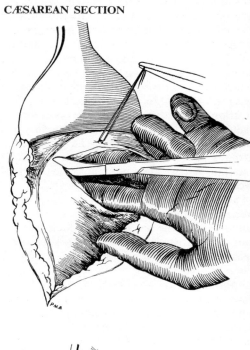

23/Figs. 3 and 4.—Enlarging uterine incision.

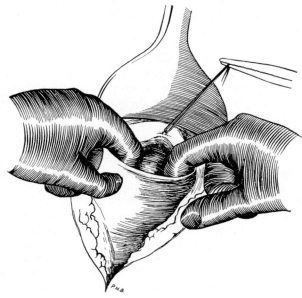

prevented. Uncontrolled tears of the lower segment have to be very carefully identified afterwards and sutured.

In this country the transverse uterine incision, as described above, is generally preferred, but across the Atlantic a vertical incision is still popular, so it might be as well to review the arguments in favour of each. The case for the vertical incision is firstly that hæmorrhage is likely to be less from the edges of the wound which, being midline, is less vascular. Secondly, in sewing up a vertical incision there is no disparity between the thicknesses of the two edges of the incision, whereas in the transverse incision the upper edge is much thicker than the lower and it is therefore not possible to make such a tidy scar. Thirdly, if the wound becomes infected, it is said by some that thrombosis is less likely to involve the veins at the side of the uterus and encourage embolism, and moreover the lowest end of the vertical incision is lower than the transverse and this may facilitate drainage.

It might appear from the mechanics of labour that a transverse scar in subsequent delivery might prove weaker than a vertical one. This has not been borne out by the experiences of uterine rupture.

The case for the transverse scar, on the other hand, is if anything stronger. A great proportion of the muscle fibres low down in the lower segment are arranged in a circular fashion so that a transverse scar is more suitable anatomically. It is also easier to control the extent of a transverse incision, whereas a vertical one may accidentally be extended too far downwards behind the bladder, and it is often difficult to make a large enough opening without encroaching in an upward direction on the upper uterine segment, thereby defeating the whole purpose of the lower segment operation. In any case, from the point of view of infection, the transverse incision, being lower than the highest part of the vertical incision, is less dangerous. Lastly, the bladder is less likely to be damaged with the transverse incision if the technique described above is carefully followed.

Delivery of the Head

Having opened the uterus, the Doyen retractor is removed in order to make room for the surgeon's hand, which is carefully insinuated so that the fingers can be passed below the head (Fig. 5). Either hand may be used for this manœuvre, and in the case of a deeply engaged vertex I find it easier to use my left hand in the first place in order to secure disengagement, as I stand on the patient's right. One may be dismayed at first to find that there is not apparently enough room to pass the hand down between symphysis and baby's head, but it is always possible to worm the half hand between them, especially on the side on which the baby's face lies. No force

CÆSAREAN SECTION

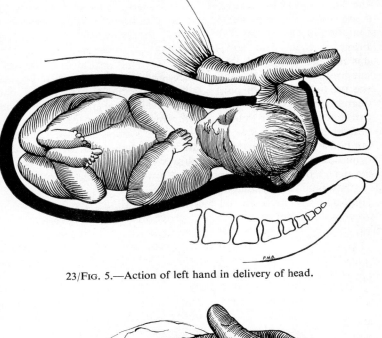

23/Fig. 5.—Action of left hand in delivery of head.

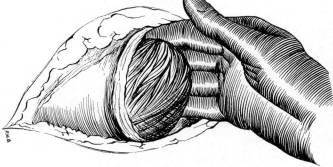

23/Fig. 6.—Right-hand delivery of head.

should be used and gentle persistence will succeed. It may help if the baby's anterior shoulder is pushed upwards by the other hand. A common mistake is to try to lever the head out of the pelvis before the fingers have been passed right round the corner below the baby's head. The difficulty in disengaging it is as much due to vacuum as to tightness of fit, so that it sometimes pays to spread the fingers slightly

to facilitate the release of this negative pressure. This is the crucial stage of the operation, and occasionally in difficult cases the use of the Trendelenburg position, already referred to, may help.

As soon as some air manages to get below the head it will be found that the vertex can be quite easily raised to the level of the pelvic brim. It should not be lifted beyond this point. The right hand, if it has not hitherto been used, should now be inserted in place of the left hand so as to act as a scoop in directing the head out through the uterine incision (Fig. 6). It is important to encourage as much degree of flexion of the head as possible, to bring smaller diameters through the incision and, remembering on which side the occiput lies, slight rotation should be imparted to the head to encourage the lambda to present through the wound first, instead of delivering it broadside on and thereby involving the large occipito-frontal diameter. The head is then allowed to be born very slowly.

Difficulties in Delivering the Head

Firstly, there may be some difficulty in reaching below the head with the fingers, and rough handling may provoke accidental tears of the lower segment. Secondly, the head may be found to be so tightly wedged that nothing will move it. This impression is usually false, and more often than not is due to a faulty technique, since if the head has managed to get that far, retreat must surely be possible. As a last resort some recommend thrusting the hand into the vagina and pushing the head up from below, with all its attendant risks of sepsis. An alternative measure is to incise the uterus vertically in the midline so that the original incision becomes an inverted T. This will of course involve the upper segment, but the child can now be delivered by the breech and the head extracted from the depths of the pelvis by traction.

As already mentioned, the head should not be pushed up above the level of the pelvic brim, for it may easily bob out of reach, in which event the uterine incision tends to shrink, and it can be quite difficult to steer the vertex through it.

Alternative Methods of Delivering the Head

Many surgeons use a pair of obstetric forceps as a routine. It is felt, however, that more damage is likely to be done by cold steel than by the soft hand, and the use of the forceps is either unnecessary, dangerous, or both. The blades are applied with the concavity of the pelvic curve directed towards the patient's feet. It is clearly undesirable to apply them over the antero-posterior diameters of the head which is likely to occur unless the head is first rotated. Now, if the head occupies the pelvis with a loose enough fit to make this rotation

possible, it is surely loose enough to allow the passage of a hand. The correct procedure is to rotate the head so that the mouth faces upwards, and then, having applied forceps, to deliver the face first. This at least is a more certain and scientific way of doing it than merely putting on the forceps and hoping that the occiput will emerge first. If there is difficulty in extracting the head from the pelvis with the hand, the brute force which a metal instrument can bring to bear is contra-indicated.

Another commonly practised method, which has nothing whatever to recommend it, is to use a single blade of the obstetric forceps as a lever and vectis. This clumsy, unwarranted and dangerous procedure carries the following risks: firstly, the point of the blade may be accidentally passed through the cervix so that the posterior lip of the cervix and the posterior fornix are levered up with the head and are likely to be lacerated. If the damage is recognised, the necessary repair may tax the surgeon's skill to the uttermost. The leverage which is possible with this instrument compresses the bladder against the symphysis pubis and may damage it. Lastly, the head may swivel on the blade and be very difficult to control. In the past, I have had considerable experience of this method and cannot condemn it too roundly.

Another method of delivering the head is to use Willett's forceps or the Solomon's modification thereof, but simplicity is its only merit. It is true that the head can be delightfully and easily steered out of the uterine incision with the help of this instrument, and when one considers how very little force is needed, one realises that the strength exhibited by some surgeons during the delivery of the head by hand must surely be unwarranted and misapplied. The Willett's forceps have two great disadvantages: for one thing an area of scalp may be avulsed, particularly in premature infants, and I myself once removed a whole thickness area of scalp about the size of a penny using only the lightest traction. The child fortunately made a satisfactory recovery but bears the scar to this day. The other disadvantage is that the small spikes of the forceps make puncture holes in the scalp which very easily become septic during the neonatal period. These two risks together make the use of this instrument undesirable.

Delivery of the Child's Body and the Prevention of Postpartum Hæmorrhage

As soon as the head is delivered the anæsthetist gives an intravenous injection of 0·25 mg. ergometrine. This is an important step and enormously reduces the amount of blood lost. Ampoules usually hold 0·5 mg. of ergometrine, and the second half of this dose can be kept in reserve should further intravenous injection be necessary.

Given intravenously, the effect is both certain and rapid, and the intramuscular route cannot compare with it in efficacy.

There are many who adopt the fatuous procedure of injecting ergometrine directly into the uterine muscle. Now this is only an intramuscular injection and, as in the case of all such injections, the drug must first find its way into the circulation before it can exert its full effect upon the uterus, with the result that there may be anything up to a few minutes delay before any effect is apparent. Moreover, of all the muscles to choose, the uterine muscle is probably the least suitable, because any spontaneous retraction which it may have undergone after delivery of the head will restrict circulation and, to some extent, delay absorption. It may be thought that the local effect of the drug at the site of injection in the uterus will quickly spread over the whole surface of that organ, but this is unlikely.

Within a few seconds of injecting ergometrine intravenously the uterus contracts well and should be allowed to assist the expulsion of the child's body so that by the time it is completely delivered the uterus has already shrunk considerably. It is then reassuringly firm and placental separation has usually started.

While the intravenous injection is being given immediately after delivery of the head, the child's mouth, pharynx and nostrils are cleared of mucus and blood, etc., with a mechanical suction apparatus. Frequently the baby will now take its first breath. In delivering the shoulders it is usually best to raise the head and allow the posterior shoulder to appear first. There is no need whatever to hurry, and rough handling is only likely to tear the lower segment. The rest of the child's body is now slowly and gently extracted or expelled by the uterine contraction.

The Third Stage

If the above steps have been carefully followed, there should be very little bleeding, and one can profitably wait a minute or two to allow the placenta to separate spontaneously. There is still some debate about how soon the cord should be clamped and divided. Certainly the traditional practice of hurriedly holding the child by the heels high above the uterus while separating it has nothing to recommend it, because fœtal blood will syphon back into the placenta from this position. If the need for resuscitation is all that urgent this unnatural type of "venesection" is unlikely to improve matters.

Alternatively the baby may be held below the level of its placenta until pulsation stops, although this is a clumsy manœuvre without proven value. Our own practice is to allow the baby to lie on the mother's thighs on its side, at the same level therefore as the placenta, while pharynx and nostrils are aspirated by mechanical suction.

Usually the baby will cry by this time and make further resuscitation assaults unnecessary, although it is hard to stop nurses from annoying it thereafter with oxygen funnels.

If pulsation in the cord ceases, or is slowed in cases of fœtal asphyxia, the cord is clamped and divided as no further placental transfusion is likely in such instances.

Gunther (1957) showed, by weighing, that babies acquired about 80 ml. of blood from the placenta after normal vaginal delivery if cord clamping was delayed. Uterine activity squeezes the placenta and is partly responsible for this physiological type of transfusion.

After dividing the umbilical cord, the stay suture originally placed in the lower flap of the uterine wall is picked up and the Doyen's retractor is replaced. The uterine incision can now be carefully inspected and the lateral corners can be marked by applying Littlewood clamps.

Occasionally one or two vessels on the edge of the incision may be bleeding rather briskly, and these can be controlled by applying Green-Armytage clamps to the wound edge, but they are seldom necessary and can be rather a nuisance by flopping about and getting in the way.

By now the placenta will probably have separated, and firm pressure on the fundus through the abdominal wall will deliver it. Some surgeons make a habit of inserting the right hand and removing the placenta manually. This, however, is only very rarely necessary and is likely to provoke more bleeding than allowing the placenta to separate unaided. Cord traction should be "controlled" as described in the previous chapter. I once unwittingly inverted the uterus through the lower segment incision by pulling on the cord, and the effect on the patient's blood pressure was striking. In any case, the cord should not be pulled upon unless the fundus is well contracted and hard. The membranes are often very adherent to the uterine wall and should be delivered very carefully and gently to prevent tearing and leaving large shreds behind. It is often surprising how relatively bloodless the third stage can be by the careful adoption of these procedures.

Drainage of Lochia

If a patient was already in labour at the time of operation, one may not be concerned about uterine drainage, since the cervix will already be partially open, but in elective Cæsarean section the closed cervix may prevent discharge of blood. It is most unusual for the cervix not to open sufficiently by the end of the operation to allow blood to drain, but a portion of chorion may, for a time, overlie the internal os and prevent drainage. It is a wise practice to pass the finger down to the internal os from inside the uterus and to satisfy

oneself that drainage is possible. In the very rare instances in which the internal os is tightly closed, a Hegar's dilator may be passed through it from above and removed from the vagina at the end of the operation.

Constriction Ring

About 90 per cent of these occur at the junction of the upper and lower uterine segments and, on the rare occasions when present, may prevent delivery of the shoulders. Steady traction will usually succeed in delivering the body of the child, but occasionally it may be necessary to incise the ring vertically. Much more commonly a constriction ring may cause retention of the placenta, in which case the placenta will have to be removed manually.

Suture of the Uterine Wound

The lower flap stay suture now demonstrates its usefulness and prevents a very common and dangerous mistake which I have seen committed twice by surgeons far senior to myself. The posterior wall of the lower segment often bulges into the wound after the delivery of the placenta and the lower flap, if not marked by a stay suture, is liable to drop down into the depths of the pelvis, out of sight in a pool of blood, with the result that one can easily suture the upper edge of the incision to the posterior uterine wall. The mistake is almost certain to be recognised later, but it will mean undoing the stitches.

Blood may well up into the operative field fairly copiously at this stage, and it is necessary to waste as little time as possible in inserting the first layer of sutures. To preserve one's landmarks in the face of this bleeding it is a good plan to mark the centre of the upper edge of the wound with an Allis clamp and to cross this clamp and the stay suture, already mentioned, across the palmar surface of the index finger of the left hand, thus approximating the edges of the incision in the midline. The index finger is now pointing into the left corner of the incision and, using the Reverdin needle with the right hand, it is possible to start the suture line with great accuracy, beginning at the left corner, and thus being certain that no gaps are being left by checking the suture line from inside the uterus with the finger (Fig. 7). The whole thickness of the uterine wall, excepting the decidua, is included in a continuous suture of chromicised catgut, and the fact that one is often sewing a thin edge to a fat one should make no difference. On the whole it is undesirable to penetrate the decidual layer as there is the hypothetical possibility that a track may thus be formed for infection to ooze outside the uterus. Accurate suture, excluding the decidua but no more, is reckoned to improve

the healing result and the strength of the scar in subsequent labours (Poidevin).

Having inserted the first continuous suture, the situation, so far as hæmorrhage is concerned, should be well under control and the field of operation can now be mopped out. A second continuous chromicised catgut suture is now inserted to reinforce the first and

CÆSAREAN SECTION

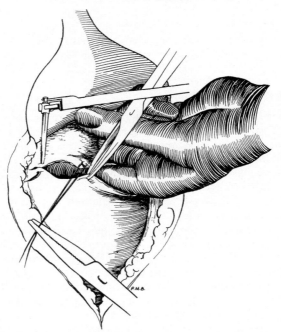

23/Fig. 7.—Closing uterine incision.

should include the layer of pelvic fascia which was originally displaced in exposing the lower uterine segment. This will usually complete hæmostasis of the uterine wound, but, if necessary, isolated bleeding points can be underrun with interrupted mattress or "over and over" sutures.

Hæmatomata may occasionally occur, especially at the lateral corners of the incision, as a result of puncturing veins with the needle. These should be controlled from spreading by mattress sutures. All blood is now mopped out of the field and the 1-inch-long stay suture originally placed in the lower flap of the uterovesical peritoneum will be seen in the depths of the pelvis and is picked up.

The visceral peritoneum is now closed with a continuous catgut suture which will automatically replace the bladder over the wound in the uterus. The resulting scar in the peritoneum of the uterovesical fold will be no more than 1–2 inches long.

All traces of blood are now removed and the roll gauze packing is withdrawn. If the packing has been properly inserted, there should be hardly any visible trace of blood or liquor in the peritoneal cavity.

Closure of the Abdominal Wall

This is closed in layers in the usual manner. Deep tension sutures in the case of vertical incisions produce an unsightly scar. It is better to reinforce the rectus sheath continuous suture line with three further interrupted catgut sutures. The skin is closed with Michel clips, or better still with subcuticular stitching. I have not used dressings, apart from a Nobecutaine "varnish" spray for many years. One is not infrequently confronted with the case that already has a ventral hernia from previous Cæsarean sections which have employed vertical instead of Pfannenstiel incision and it is tempting to use the occasion of repeat section to repair it. It is far preferable, however, not to attempt formal repair of a hernia amounting to more than simple divarication of the rectus abdominis muscles at the same time as Cæsarean section because of the increased shock which is likely and the danger of post-operative distension. The use of the Pfannenstiel incision is still preferable to the vertical even where the latter has been used before, unless it is intended to excise a very unsightly scar. Dressings simply prevent ready inspection of the wound and are uncomfortable to remove. The idea that gauze, no matter how many layers, with its coarse mesh can keep out bacteria is simply Crimean nonsense. The best dressing of all is Nature's coagulum.

I seldom forbid anything in my unit except unthinking traditionalism and stupidity. The application of a many-tailed bandage, or a "cuirass" of adhesive strapping is one of them. Their only function is to restrict deep breathing during recovery and thus to encourage thromboembolism.

Before leaving the theatre the surgeon should satisfy himself that the uterus is well retracted and any clots which may have collected within its cavity should be squeezed out while the patient is still under an anæsthetic and in no condition to protest. Failure to take this simple precaution may result in a brisk loss of blood when the patient arrives back in the ward.

The catheter is pinched between the finger and thumb and withdrawn, and then any urine within it is released and inspected for the presence of blood. The absence of any naked eye appearance of blood in the urine is a fairly reliable reassurance that the bladder has not been damaged. If bladder damage is suspected or there is more

than a faint degree of hæmaturia, the patient should be put on continuous catheter drainage for at least a week.

After Care

If no blood appears at the vulva at the end of the operation even after squeezing the uterus, it is probable that the cervix is too tightly closed to allow its escape or it may be covered by a sheet of chorion. Nearly always, however, the cervix will open sufficiently within the next hour, but if no blood appears by then, ergometrine 0·5 mg. should be injected intramuscularly. If, after a further hour, blood still fails to appear, it may be necessary to dilate the cervix from below with a pair of artery forceps, for the retention *in utero* of lochial discharges is almost certain to produce a stormy convalescence.

For the first few days it is very difficult to be certain that the patient is emptying her bladder completely, unless she has a Pfannenstiel incision which will often permit palpation of a distended bladder and a consequently raised uterine fundus. Retention is unlikely with early ambulation and allowing the patient out of bed to micturate. Our patients, provided their general condition is satisfactory, are encouraged to get out of bed as soon as they want to pass water and certainly within the first 24 hours. The use of bed pans is steadily diminishing.

It is during the early post-operative phase that the services of the physiotherapist are particularly useful. Deep breathing should be firmly encouraged from the first. This, by improving the venous return from the extremities to the heart, does more than anything else to stave off thrombosis in the deep vessels of the calf, etc., and is more important than early ambulation in preventing pulmonary embolism. I have heard of a hospital on the Continent in which the incidence of pulmonary embolism was, for a time, unduly high, so a notice was put up in one of its surgical wards which read, "Breathe hard, cough hard, spit hard", which well illustrates the principle. Leg and ankle movements, if necessary with the encouragement of a physiotherapist in attendance, should be persisted in from the very first. To turn an unwilling patient, however, out of bed and sit her in a chair is simply a travesty of the principle of early ambulation. Huddled in a chair and with her legs dependent, nothing could be more calculated to discourage a healthy venous return from the legs and she would be far better off doing her exercises and deep breathing in bed.

The Cæsarean section patient has not had her pelvic floor and pelvic ligaments stretched in the process of vaginal delivery, so that the hypothetical risk of prolapse as a result of getting up too soon does not apply. On the second post-operative day there is nearly always a certain amount of gaseous distension of the bowel and the

patient may be much troubled by flatulence. As soon as good peristaltic movements can be auscultated, an enema should be given, following which the intestinal tract will rapidly deflate. It is a mistake to give the enema before reasonable peristalsis has returned to the gut because, in that case, the enema is likely to be retained. As a general rule the enema can be given towards the end of the first 48 hours. A Dulcolax or a glycerine suppository may be used instead and we are now giving fewer enemata.

Whether or not the patient lost a large quantity of blood at the time of the operation, the hæmoglobin level should always be estimated on the third day, for these patients are often found to be more anæmic than expected. Appropriate treatment will greatly hasten full convalescence. The quantity of blood lost at Cæsarean section is always more than most surgeons will admit to, as though their surgical skill is being questioned. The average loss as measured by Wallace using the Perdometer technique was found in fact to be not far short of a litre, and far higher than in most forceps deliveries. Surgeons should recognise that Cæsarean section is a "bloody operation" and should be more ready to acknowledge the benefits which transfusion may contribute to speedy post-operative recovery.

Breast feeding can be started on the second day and managed as in normal cases. If convalescence is uneventful the patient can be discharged home safely within ten or twelve days. Earlier dismissal is not a mark of slicker surgery and if embolism is going to occur (as occasionally it will in spite of all precautions) the patient has a better chance of surviving it in hospital.

COMPLICATIONS OF CÆSAREAN SECTION

The first and most important of these is, of course, primary hæmorrhage and, as already stated, blood of a suitable group should always be available and unhesitatingly given as indicated. Shock is not usually a common complication unless associated with hæmorrhage. It is recognised and treated on the usual lines.

Sepsis, frequently mild, occasionally severe, still remains one of the commonest complications. Many of the cases who have been in labour for some while at the time of the operation are infected and a swab taken at this point will reveal the responsible organism far earlier and make possible the prompt institution of appropriate chemotherapy. Operating under an antibiotic umbrella has the serious drawback that the causal organism may be partially suppressed for the time being and therefore not recognised later. Troublesome resistant strains may be bred. This is particularly true of *Staph. pyogenes*, which is one of the commonest and most serious of the infecting organisms complicating Cæsarean section. In

spite of modern technique, about a quarter of the cases have to be classified as puerperally morbid. Unfortunately, when serious infection does occur, the peritoneal cavity is inevitably involved and the patient will be more dangerously ill than if she had received the same infection in the course of vaginal delivery.

When Cæsarean section has perforce to be undertaken in the presence of already recognisable sepsis, it is as well to anticipate peritonitis and ileus and to pass a naso-duodenal tube at the end of the operation and maintain "suck-and-drip" therapy from the very beginning of the post-operative phase until the bowel regains peristaltic activity. The suction must be continuous and not intermittent and should be limited to about 10 cm. water negative pressure to prevent blocking the tube by forcibly sucking gastro-intestinal mucous membrane into its openings. This can be achieved by a very simple device (Fig. 8) which, when connected in series between pump and collecting bottle, safely and effectively limits suction.

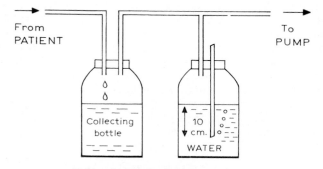

23/Fig. 8.—Limited suction drainage.

The purpose of continuous suction is to remove swallowed air at once and before it has a chance to distend the gastro-intestinal tract for want of peristalsis to pass it on. Intermittent suction fails in this respect and it is the unseen gas which is removed rather than the brown fluid which matters. We now believe that distension causes ileus rather than vice versa.

During the period of continuous aspiration the patient is losing electrolytes, particularly chlorides, and twice daily biochemical electrolyte balance studies should be undertaken in order to control the drip infusion therapy which is mandatory at the same time. It is the biochemical imbalance of paralytic ileus which is the final killer in peritonitis. Antibiotics may trample down her infection but will not of themselves restore her biochemistry.

It is indeed impressive to watch the convalescence of such a case, whose death from peritonitis would have seemed a certainty a few

years ago. With a flat, undistended abdomen, a clean moist tongue, well hydrated, free from vomiting and passing urine of normal specific gravity she soon masters her infection and emerges from the valley of the shadow of death. I recall the hideous post-operative distension of bygone years, the metallic tinkle on auscultation of otherwise silent intestines, the acute mental awareness of the patient, her rising and weakening pulse and her copious brown vomits, often too large for the standard bedside bowl. How readily prevented and treated today when maternal deaths from peritonitis are almost culpable!

Chest complications are also much commoner after abdominal delivery and account for a number of cases of puerperal pyrexia. The formation of a retrovesical hæmatoma is fairly common after the lower segment operation, and although the condition usually resolves without much trouble, it probably causes many of the apparently inexplicable post-operative temperatures. The importance, therefore, of hæmostasis in producing a smooth puerperium cannot be overstressed.

Some degree of hæmaturia may occur for the first day or two after operation and may suggest some damage to the bladder. Most commonly it results from the pressure of an unsuitable Doyen retractor and the ministrations of a rough assistant manipulating it. If there is any doubt, however, about the integrity of the bladder, continuous catheter drainage should be instituted.

All temperatures, even though not notifiable, call for full investigation, and in every case a high vaginal or cervical swab should be taken for culture together with a midstream specimen of urine. It is both lazy and foolish to wait until the next day in the hope that the temperature will have subsided, and it should be an absolute rule never to start empirical chemotherapy before unadulterated specimens have been taken. A high post-operative pulse and a niggling temperature frequently signify the onset of venous thrombosis or the development of a hæmatoma which may not be fully apparent for some days. Pulmonary embolism, unfortunately, still remains one of the great risks, although it is very largely a preventable accident. This subject is dealt with more fully in the next chapter.

REPEAT CÆSAREAN SECTION

It used to be said "once a Cæsarean always a Cæsarean" partly because the operation was done mainly for disproportion, and for this condition the old saying is largely true provided the original diagnosis was genuine. Subsequent babies tend to be larger for the same period of gestation, and if a patient was previously incapable of delivering herself with an intact uterus it would hardly appear

reasonable to expect a uterus with a scar in it to perform better. Many primigravid trials of labour, however, fail because of uterine inertia or because of the complicating factor of a persistent occipito-posterior position, and the need for the previous section may have been more due to these than to actual bony disproportion. Under favourable circumstances, therefore, a repeat Cæsarean section may not be necessary. Nevertheless, a previous Cæsarean section casts "a shadow over any future pregnancy" (Jackson, 1961). Today a more up-to-date version of the old saying would be, "Twice a Cæsarean, always a Cæsarean".

The main fear, of course, in subsequent pregnancy and labour after Cæsarean section is that the scar will rupture. Holland in 1921 reported an incidence of over 4 per cent of scar rupture after previous Cæsarean section, but this referred to the classical operation.

Rupture of the lower segment scar is rare. It may appear treacherously thin at operation, yet is still unruptured for all that, and it is by no means true to judge that rupture would have occurred just from appearances alone. Poidevin (1959) found that on opening all uteri which have previously been subjected to lower segment Cæsarean section a larger or smaller depressed scar will always be seen. The deformity usually takes the form of a wedge depression but provided it is not more than 5 mm. deep the scar can be relied upon not to give way. But when the deformity is deep or irregular the scar should be suspect. These deformities of the uterine wall can only be demonstrated by radiohysterography between pregnancies. Usually, however, one is presented with the problem in a patient already pregnant and has to fall back on the usual gamble on probabilities.

Three factors are mainly responsible for subsequent scar rupture. Firstly, infection of the scar during recovery from the previous section. A history of genital tract infection should always make one suspicious of the scar's integrity. Secondly, implantation of the placenta over the site of the old scar is a common way in which it becomes undermined. This implantation is far less likely to occur over a lower segment scar than over one in the upper segment. Thirdly, lack of immobility of the healing tissues interferes with sound healing, and this is one of the great reasons why the classical scar so often comes to grief. After delivery the lower segment remains at rest, but the upper segment is undergoing constant and rhythmic activity in the form of "after pains" during the early days of the puerperium, with the result that the stitches tend to cut out or work loose and only the serous coat, which heals very rapidly indeed, may be left intact.

Repeat Cæsarean section, then, is chiefly indicated in cases of established disproportion and more commonly after a classical

CHAPTER XXIV

PUERPERAL MANAGEMENT AND COMPLICATIONS

THE puerperium, that period of recovery and involution from pregnancy and childbirth, usually regarded as lasting for six weeks, is rapidly losing medical interest and importance, perhaps dangerously so, because of our modern preoccupation with antenatal care. The lying-in period in maternity hospitals is getting progressively shorter under a variety of stimuli, not the least of them being a shortage of maternity hospital beds, and, one by one, standard nursing procedures which were hitherto regarded as more or less sacrosanct are being thrown overboard. The days of the peasant woman who produced her baby in the fields and then continued with her work now do not seem quite so far away.

Neither the patients themselves nor the doctors who look after them will interest themselves much in a lying-in period of fourteen days, as has been deemed desirable. Consultants themselves are much to blame for the neglect of this period in a woman's life since so many of them tend to spend only a very small fraction of their time visiting their lying-in wards as compared with the trouble they take over their antenatal cases. The present decline in breast feeding has tended further to rob this period of medical interest and the problems of the baby are coming more and more into the sphere of activity of the pædiatrician. It is small wonder, therefore, that patients, once safely delivered, feel that it is all over "bar the shouting" and are anxious to get home.

This tendency to shorten the lying-in period in hospital has received further impetus from the acknowledged risk of the baby acquiring a hospital staphylococcal infection the longer it stays in hospital, but, above all, the medical profession are to blame for this trend by their intellectual neglect of lying-in care now that maternal puerperal sepsis has ceased to be the problem of bygone times.

When I was a student patients lay in bed for over a week until they felt thoroughly weakened by the experience and then were got up and given some hurried lessons in baby bathing and sent home on the tenth day, debilitated by bed rest, and still frightened strangers to their babies whom they had had little opportunity to get to know and were told to report again for postnatal examination in six weeks'

time. To them the intervening period must have seemed like a very rough sea somehow to be crossed. The institution of Health Visiting on arrival at home provided opportunities for helping a woman at this difficult period in her life and many hospitals, including my own, ran a splendid "after-sales service" in the form of mothercraft advice, largely thanks to the initiative of a devoted nursing staff.

Nowadays the increasing practice of early ambulation and rooming-in at least ensure that when a patient does leave hospital after an abbreviated lying-in period she receives less of a psychological and physical jolt.

At present, in Glasgow, the puerpera hardly expects to stay in hospital more than six days and, however many more hospital beds are provided, it is unlikely that the working-class women of this city will come to accept a longer period in hospital as desirable. At the extreme end of the scale we have what is popularly known as the Bradford Experiment (Theobald, 1959) in which, in order to secure a greater number of hospital deliveries and the safety thereby provided, a large number of women who are safely delivered and fit are discharged home on the second day. Now it should be pointed out first of all that it was not the primary objective of this so-called experiment simply to increase the number of hospital deliveries on the "sausage machine" principle, but it came about because of an urgent need to increase the number of antenatal beds which could only be got at the expense of the lying-in wards and in so far as this objective is considered the results were highly rewarding. Furthermore a very satisfactory liaison was established with the general practitioners, the local authorities and the domiciliary midwives, which, alone, could make such a scheme satisfactory and workable. Hellman *et al.* (1962) have also described the results of this very early discharge principle in action, usually about the third or fourth day, in Brooklyn, and it is clear that unless the baby, as well as the mothers, are carefully followed up as they would have been had a longer period been spent in hospital, important findings such as neonatal jaundice might escape notice. One cannot help feeling, however, that this is a sorry doctrine of expediency rather like "bowing down and worshipping the devil" and may readily encourage Planning Authorities to curtail their maternity hospital building programmes in the interests of economy and to overwork their hospital staffs at no extra cost to the exchequer. Such a trend could only end in disaster and a rising rate of hospital sepsis the inevitable result. At a time when there is so much talk about personal relations in obstetrics nothing could be more calculated to undermine the happy and fruitful relationship established between most patients and those in hospital who look after them than this sordid and mechanistic view of delivery and its aftermath.

It would not come amiss at this point to consider the Registrars, Housemen and midwives whom such an abuse can easily expose to overwork. They shoulder the heat and burden of the day, and the night as well, and they deserve to be treated as human beings every bit as much as their patients. We have now established under the auspices of the Ministry of Overseas Development and the University of Glasgow an explant of the Queen Mother's Hospital in Nairobi and here, in a rapidly emerging country, in spite of obvious and very great pressures we have shown that it is possible in the teaching and training unit at the Kenyatta National Hospital to maintain the same standards and ideals which we preach at home.

Two reasons are often given for the 48-hour dismissal scheme, or even lesser periods. The first is so-called pressure on beds. There is only one honest answer to that problem and that is to provide more beds. If this can be achieved in Glasgow it can be achieved anywhere else and the administrators must be suitably stimulated. The second reason commonly given, particularly from general practice, is that patients dislike hospitals in the same way that many children dislike boarding school. The answer to the second problem is to have better and nicer hospitals. Alas, many British maternity units are structurally quite nasty places, outdated, dingy and depressing, with a rigid discipline, indifferent food and general dreariness, but within the years since the second world war nearly all of them have had a face lift. What matters more than paint and flowers is the attitude of the staff, particularly the nursing staff.

The decision to allow small children to visit their mothers and the new baby brother or sister was a difficult one to reach. I had always preached in the past that small children were walking test tubes of infection, but this is probably untrue and anyway the patient will be returning to such a milieu with her new baby within a very few days. The children are only supposed to visit their own new baby and not the others. This matter is discussed more fully in Chapter 1.

The mothers are thus looked after and relieved of the household responsibilities from which they certainly deserve a rest in the early days of the puerperium, without any of the usual heartache, and it is as well to consider how much better off such a mother is than one sent home very often to conditions which no amount of general practitioner of Health Visitor supervision can ameliorate; in fact as Garrey and his colleagues from the Royal Maternity Hospital, Rottenrow, on the other side of the town, have pointed out, there is often a background of social deprivation and the care or supervision possible at home simply cannot equal that which a modern hospital can provide. There are still far too many homes in the poorer cities without bathrooms, or even indoor sanitation, and the more multiparous the patient, the more does she appreciate the benefit from a

period of tender, loving care in a hospital which manages to eschew the traditional types of discipline.

A woman emerging from the months of pregnancy and the hazards of delivery, however normal, deserves a period of tranquillity in which to establish a satisfactory psychological "rapport" with the most important member of the house in a relationship which is most adequately expressed in breast feeding. It is probably better, therefore, that changes in environment such as being sent home should occur either immediately after delivery, as in the case of the Bradford experiment, or after the tenth day. Nothing is to be gained by the present practice of letting patients home at the end of the first week, or somewhat earlier at a time when lactation is neither safely established nor satisfactorily suppressed.

The simplification of lying-in care has already been mentioned. Over the years in our unit to a large extent we have abolished juggings, swabbings, enemas, catheterisations, removable perineal sutures and in Cæsarean section dressings, adhesive strapping, manytailed bandages and as much as we can condemn as nursing mumbo-jumbo. A similar attitude applies to the newborn. On the other hand we attach considerable importance to good feeding, fresh air and adequate periods of rest both at night and in the afternoon, free of visitations from doctors, students or relatives. Physiotherapists have a particularly important role in training the patient in deep breathing, perineal exercises and leg exercises designed to improve circulation. Women should be encouraged to take an interest in regaining their figures, advised on their diet and brainwashed in a positive attitude towards good health. Unfortunately this cannot be achieved in six lying-in days and to practice gynæcology even in this day and age is to force on one the realisation of how commonly a patient's disabilities date from childbirth, such as backache, discharge, poor urinary control, dyspareunia, varicose veins, swollen ankles, obesity and a host of psychosomatic ailments, surely an indictment of postnatal care. The following is our present schedule of lying-in care.

Schedule of Lying-in Care

(a) *Mothers*

1. They are allowed out of bed to go to the lavatory within the first twenty-four hours.
2. They are given a bath on the second day.
3. They wash their own breasts and those who are not yet ambulant are supplied with a basin for the purpose.
4. If the nipples are badly crusted on arrival in the lying-in ward the nurses assist the mothers to bathe the crusts off and, in severe cases, apply olive oil.

5. The mothers apply their own nipple dressings consisting of a mixture of lanoline, gentian violet and tinct. benzoini co. or Massé cream on small squares of lint.

6. Where the breasts are hard, but not obviously engorged, manual expression is carried out, with the assistance of the nurses since the patients are often unpractised in the art. Breast expression is not carried out in more than the mildest cases of engorgement, instead reliance is placed upon the use of stilbœstrol (5–10 mg.).

7. Nurses assist the mothers in the early stages in fixing the baby on the breast.

8. Bedpans and vulval toilet are practically non-existent, except for patients confined to bed for medical reasons.

9. Since the method of suturing the perineum is by using catgut throughout the Crimean ritual of suture removal on the sixth day is dispensed with.

10. Uncomplicated cases of Cæsarean section are treated more or less in the same manner.

11. The use of bidets with running water sprays has made a wonderful difference to perineal comfort and healing.

(b) Babies

1. The baby is bathed when it is a few hours old in order to remove vernix, meconium and blood. We have considered abolishing this procedure on the ground that vernix is probably a very good skin dressing, but some of these babies are in a very offensive condition after birth and it is feared that the mothers might take it upon themselves to scour the offending material off the babies to their consequent detriment. The first bathing is done, of course, by the nursing staff, but thereafter the baby receives no further bathing until the day before discharge when the mother undertakes it herself. Phisohex cream removes vernix effectively.

2. At the same time as this initial bathing the cord is cut short and tied and spirit is applied, without a dressing, again by the nursing staff.

3. The cord thereafter is treated by the mother three times a day by the application of spirit.

4. Twice a day the mother powders the baby with hexachlorophane. This takes the place of standard baby powder in our unit.

5. The baby is "topped and tailed" once a day by the mother.

6. The mother does all the nappy changing on her bed and obtains the nappies from a wheeled trolley. At each changing of the nappies the mother cleans up the baby's bottom herself.

7. The baby goes to the breast at the age of six hours and thereafter four hourly, for three minutes on each side.

8. The baby stays as much as possible with the mother, including the nights, and if it cries during the night the mother is free to feed it herself, provided that not more than one interruption occurs to her sleep. The baby who is restless and won't settle down and is likely to disturb the mother's sleep and that of the other patients is taken outside, but the babies are moved out of the lying-in ward as little as possible. Allowing the babies into bed with the mothers as at the Coombe Hospital in Dublin has been considered, but we feel that the occasional accident, even though rare, cannot be chanced, nor could it be defended in the eyes of the public.

9. Bottle-fed babies are fed by nurses only at night, if they require it.

EXAMINATION OF THE NEWBORN BABY

General.—Firstly, check the identity of the baby and that its name tapes are correctly positioned.

In a warm room and in a good light the baby is now examined from head to toe. Caput, any cephalhæmatoma and moulding should be noted as this information may be useful in subsequent labours. Cleft palate must be looked for in a good light or it will be missed. Make sure that the arms are fully movable and that there is neither dislocation nor paralysis. Count the fingers.

Always take the first temperature per rectum in order to exclude imperforate anus, unless meconium has been passed already.

There should be full movement of the feet. A calcaneo-valgus deformity is usually self-correcting within the next few months, but equino-varus is much more sinister and should be brought to the notice of an orthopædic specialist.

The spine should be examined with the fingers to exclude spina bifida. If there has been hydramnios, a stomach tube should be passed as soon as possible after birth to exclude œsophageal atresia. In any event the first feed at 6 hours should be one of boiled water, before milk is given or the baby put to the breast, in case there is a tracheo-œsophageal fistula, the effects of boiled water being so much less disastrous.

Look behind the ears for accessory auricles.

The baby's mouth is easily opened by pressing on the lower jaw.

Look behind the anus for any sinus.

The cord clamp or ligature should be secure.

The antero-posterior diameter of the chest should be about the same as the transverse diameter and the heart should be examined for coarse murmurs. The liver is normally about $2\frac{1}{2}$ cm. below the

right costal margin and the spleen too may be palpable without signifying anything pathological.

Even at birth the testicles are usually in the scrotum. It is futile to try and pull back the prepuce. This cannot be done at this age. The only medical indication for circumcision is ballooning of the prepuce when the child attempts to micturate.

The central nervous system can be readily examined by observing the Moro reflex (startle reflex). It can be evoked by banging the side of the cot or making a loud noise, or even putting a cold hand on the baby's skin, or allowing the head to drop unexpectedly a few inches from one hand to the other. The baby responds by throwing out its arms and then immediately adducting them. The fingers are usually thrown open as well. Absence of this reflex suggests cerebral damage or depression. Sucking reflex is present at birth and the rooting reflex can be demonstrated by touching the corner of the baby's mouth with a teat or the mother's nipple when the baby will immediately search in order to get a hold with its lips. The grasp reflex is demonstrated by stroking the back of the fingers whereupon they extend and the baby will then close them over the examiner's finger.

An attempt at walking with giant strides is made if the baby is held upwards with hands round the thorax as though encouraging it to walk.

Congenital dislocation of the hip.—This must be sought for in all babies before they leave the obstetrician's care. Failure to carry out this simple examination in the neonatal period may mean that the missed case will not be diagnosed until it fails to walk a year or two later and may then be permanently crippled. It is possible that this failure to examine properly within the first few days of birth may expose the doctor to an action for damages, because the condition is so easily curable if picked up within the first week or two of life. The incidence of congenital dislocation of hip is by no means negligible at about 1·5 per 1,000 and the diagnosis depends upon demonstrating instability in the hip joint. The test for what is commonly referred to as Ortolani's sign only takes a few seconds. To carry it out, the baby is placed on its back with the legs pointing towards the examiner, with the knees fully flexed and the hips flexed to a right angle. The thighs of the baby are grasped in both hands with the middle finger of each placed over the greater trocanter on the outside and with the thumb placed on the inner side. The thighs are then abducted and the middle fingers of the examining hands press forward on the greater trocanters (Fig. 1 a, b, c and d). In congenital dislocation of the hip the femoral head suddenly slips forward into the acetabulum with a distinctly palpable "clunk". If pressure is now applied with the thumbs outwards and backwards on the inner side of the thigh, the femoral head again slips out over the posterior lip of the acetabulum.

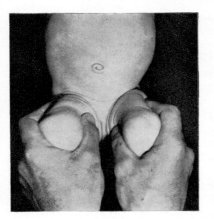

(a)

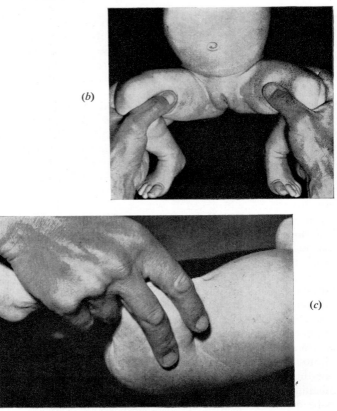

(b)

(c)

24/Fig. 1

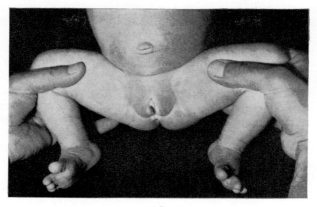

(d)

24/FIG. 1 (*see opposite*).—Ortolani's sign. (*a*) Grasping a child's knees and thighs. (*b*) Abducting the hips and pressing forward with the middle fingers of the examining hands. (*c*) Lateral view of the above manoeuvre. (*d*) The heads of the femora have slipped into the acetabulum with the characteristic "clunk".

If the femoral head slips back into the acetabulum again when the pressure is released it is merely unstable, rather than dislocated. Further confirmation in doubtful cases can be obtained by using one hand to grasp the pelvis firmly between a thumb on the pubis and fingers placed behind the sacrum and the other hand can repeat the test on one hip joint at a time.

This test is important because the treatment in early neonatal life is so simple and efficient, and consists simply in maintaining the hips in full abduction and at least 90° flexion with malleable metal splints, which can produce permanent cure by the age of three or four months if applied at once. On the other hand failure to nip in the bud this disabling condition will expose the child to a whole series of difficult operations in later life, with a high failure rate and a strong chance of osteo-arthritis developing at an early age, to say nothing of the likely permanent crippling which it will suffer.

Hydrocephalus and spina bifida.—The quicker these cases can be brought to a pædiatric surgeon the less terrible may be the disability in the event of the child's survival, which is nowadays quite likely. It is now reckoned that if operation can be undertaken within the first 24 hours of life, 75 per cent of cases of spina bifida will survive, one-third of them with minimal disability. Even those cases of open meningomyelocele are not beyond salvage. The essential thing here is to prevent drying of the exposed neural canal. A sterile swab soaked in saline should be immediately applied and the child

transferred to a pædiatric centre without even an hour's delay if there is to be much hope of salvaging neurological function below the waist, including sphincters. With early closure and proper management of hydrocephalus, practically all cases of pure meningocele and 20 per cent of those with meningomyelocele, may be spared lower limb paralysis and in only 20 per cent of the latter is paralysis likely to be complete or severe. Associated lower limb deformities may also need correction. Effective surgical treatment of hydrocephalus gives a fair chance that the child will be educationally normal and the condition tends to be self-limiting after the first few years of life. The important thing is to preserve the brain tissue between the ventricles and the inner skull. Sometimes, however, this tissue amounts to no more than a rind.

Neonatal hypoglycæmia.—Normally the blood sugar drops to about 50 mg. per 100 ml. within the first few hours in babies born at term. It falls even lower in premature babies and adult levels are only slowly regained during the first month, with premature babies again taking longer. The respiratory distress syndrome and exposure to cold greatly increase the tendency to hypoglycæmia.[39] Other ætiological factors, besides prematurity, are dysmaturity or the small for dates baby, diabetes, hypoxia, intracranial hæmorrhage and infection. The condition may be asymptomatic or symptomatic and when clinical signs appear they most often do so between the ages of 2 to 3 days when the blood sugar may be found to be lower than 20 mg. per cent. Unless treated promptly the brain may suffer irreversible damage or the child may die. The symptoms and signs consist of apnœic attacks, reluctance to feed, jittery movements and a depressed Moro reflex. Convulsions and coma may supervene. The differential diagnosis is that of tetany, meningitis and intracranial hæmorrhage. Diagnosis and therapy can be combined by the immediate injection of 1 to 3 g. of glucose intravenously—the child's immediate recovery confirming the diagnosis. Asymptomatic hypoglycæmia is thought unlikely to damage the brain,[39] but cerebral damage and mental retardation are more likely if clinical signs are manifested.

Since February, 1965, it was decided in Glasgow to perform a "Dextrostix" test on every infant admitted to the special care nursery at the Queen Mother's Hospital, and repeated six hours later in all those in whom feeding had not yet started. The test was also applied to all infants who had apnœic attacks or demonstrated other abnormal behaviour. The "Dextrostix" enzyme strip was found very suitable for screening for possible hypoglycæmia and certainly did not fail in any case where the true blood sugar was confirmed as being below 20 mg. per 100 ml. In the first 1,000 consecutive cases so tested no less than 31 cases of hypoglycæmia were picked up.[10] Ten of these cases were asymptomatic and only six were associated with

other severe disorders, the remaining 15 being cases of what were called ideopathic symptomatic hypoglycæmia. Of these so-called ideopathic cases, five were dysmature and one premature, most of them had twitchings or convulsions and in about half of them there was cyanosis, apnœa or lethargy. Troublesome vomiting was reported as an almost invariable symptom. This tended to undo the benefits of oral glucose and the most satisfactory treatment has been found to be the intravenous injection of 5 to 10 ml. of 50 per cent glucose, followed by a scalp vein 10 per cent glucose drip at the rate of 60 ml./Kg. per 24 hours. The crisis is rapidly mastered on this treatment and oral feeding with the addition of glucose 2·5 to 5 g. added to the feeds is established as soon as possible.

In the asymptomatic cases of hypoglycæmia 8 out of 10 cases had had some degree of asphyxia at birth and it is suggested that all babies at risk to hypoglycæmia should have "Dextrostix" screening, six-hourly by heel prick during the first 48 hours, whether or not feeding has been started, in order to reduce the later complications of mental retardation. It is thus the practice in our hospital not to wait for signs and symptoms to appear.

Cold injury.—The very great dangers of chilling of the newborn were pointed out from Brighton,[33] although by no means the coldest part of the United Kingdom. The danger would appear to be particularly great in the case of coalfire heated rooms when, in the small hours of the morning, the fire dies out and the parents continue asleep and unaware of their baby's peril. The hazard is not by any means confined to the homes of the poor. During the two winters from 1961 to 1963, no less than 110 hypothermic babies were admitted to the three major admitting units in Glasgow.[1] The criterion of severe hypothermia was a rectal temperature of 90° F. or lower, with the thermometer left *in situ* for not less than a minute. The seriousness of such a condition, whether the baby is premature or not, is revealed by the fact that in this series over 40 per cent died. Birth asphyxia and prematurity increase the hazards of this condition and the drowsy, anorexic baby with red cheeks should put the physician on guard. Apart from red skin, the baby feels very cold to the touch and there may be œdema and sclerema and the limbs may even be frostbitten. The diagnosis is immediately confirmed by the use of a low reading thermometer. It is noteworthy that of the 110 babies described in this series the diagnosis of severe hypothermia was made in only seven before admission.

Very careful rewarming over a prolonged period of up to two or three days in a properly equipped pædiatric unit provides the best chance of recovery.

It is amazing, in fact, what babies will stand in the way not only of asphyxia, but of exposure to cold, and Mann (1963) described the

case of a baby which was buried alive in a garden and survived after being dug up by the family dog.

INBORN ERRORS OF METABOLISM

So far about 80 of these have been recognised and they are commonly due to a primary enzyme abnormality which is genetically determined. Two of the most important are phenylketonuria and galactosæmia.

Phenylketonuria.—This is an autosomal recessive trait in babies who are homozygous with a deficiency in the enzyme phenylalanine hydroxylase. Normally phenylalanine, which is an aminoacid derived from milk, is converted by this enzyme into tyrosine in the liver. In the absence of this change phenylalanine collects in the blood and results in later mental retardation, possibly because of tyrosine deprivation. It appears in the urine as phenylpyruvic acid which can be detected by adding 5 to 10 per cent aqueous ferric chloride drops that produce a green colour. This is the basis of the Phenistix test paper which is applied to the wet nappies, provided the child is already ingesting milk and is old enough (i.e. a few days old) to demonstrate the rising level of unconverted phenylalanine. Unfortunately this simple test may miss some cases or may wrongly diagnose others.[38] This is an important matter in both directions because the missed case may later present as one of mental retardation whereas the wrongly diagnosed case, not properly confirmed biochemically, may be subjected for a long time to an unnatural diet, which has to be low in phenylalanine content causing unnecessary distress to the child and to those looking after it. Therefore the Guthrie test is more favoured.[22] The Guthrie test depends upon a method of bacterial inhibition assay.

The growth of a certain strain of *Bacillus subtilis* is inhibited by beta-2-thienylalanine but this inhibition can be specifically prevented by the presence of phenylalanine and phenylpyruvic acid. A drop of blood is collected by heel prick from the baby, at the age of about a week, onto a piece of rather thick type filter paper. This is autoclaved in order to fix the blood pigments and a small disc of the blood-impregnated filter paper is placed on the surface of a medium containing spores of this bacillus and inhibitory beta-2-thienylalanine. In the presence of phenylalanine, growth of the bacillus will not be inhibited and the diameter of the growth halo is more or less in direct proportion to the amount of phenylalanine in the original blood drop.[40] The same test method can be used to detect maple syrup urine disease or histidinæmia by substituting 2-beta-leucine or 8-azaserine for the inhibitory agent beta-2-thienylalanine. Phenylketonuria, commonly referred to as P.K.U., is believed to have an

Bacteriology

The denizens of the past, namely the hæmolytic streptococci, Groups A, B, C and G, have become much less important numerically, particularly the first-mentioned, and the anærobic streptococcus now heads the list. In the Calman and Gibson series already mentioned, the organisms responsible were listed as follows in 141 cases of genital infection:

Anærobic streptococcus, 34 per cent.
Staph. pyogenes, 23 per cent.
Non-hæmolytic streptococci, 19 per cent.
Strep. viridans, 11 per cent.
E. coli, 8 per cent.

There were no cases due to the Group A hæmolytic streptococcus in this series, although Gibson subsequently had a crop of them. The "also-rans" include the *Cl. welchii*, the *Strep. fæcalis*, pneumococci and gonococci.

The most ugly feature, however, in the changing bacteriology of our time is the rapid emergence of antibiotic-resistant bacteria, the chief offender at present being the staphylococcus, although other species are beginning to follow suit. This is a man-made problem entirely and is due to the injudicious use of powerful antibiotics. To quote an American witticism, "Fewer bugs are nowadays sensitive to pencillin and there are fewer patients that aren't!" Staphylococcal infection in hospital which is penicillin-resistant (as is likely) is almost certainly a cross-infection, whereas 95 per cent of staphylococci in the world outside are sensitive.

The situation is likely to deteriorate steadily in spite of teaching and propaganda in medical schools, and junior medical officers in hospitals are as remiss as general practitioners in prescribing the wrong antibiotic in inappropriate dosage to the patient who could have recovered without it anyway.

The pathogenicity of staphylococci is initially determined by finding out whether or not they can produce the enzyme coagulase which is responsible for the formation of protective fibrin round the infecting bacteria. The term "staphylococcus pyogenes" refers to coagulase-positive staphylococci.

In tracking down the source of staphylococcal epidemic, phage-typing is undertaken. Bacteriophages, of which over 20 are used in the classification of staphylococci, are in fact viruses which cause lysis of bacteria. By the use of different phages it is possible to identify characteristic lysis patterns and thus to track down the common source of infection. Phage-type 80/81 is a particularly troublesome strain in causing staphylococcal epidemics in maternity

hospitals and the most recent epidemic in Glasgow was due to this cause.

Streptococcal typing first of all depends upon demonstrating the capacity to hæmolyse blood. Where this is complete, the colonies show clear zones surrounding them on blood agar plates. This is called beta-hæmolysis. A less complete type of hæmolysis (alpha-hæmolysis) applies to the *Streptococcus viridans*. Only some of the beta-hæmolytic streptococci, however, are virulent and these have to be further grouped and typed. Lancefield grouping, of which Group A is by far the most important and virulent, is undertaken by using precipitation tests with anti-sera prepared against the different carbohydrate surface antigens which each streptococcal groups possesses. There are thus 13 Lancefield groups of hæmolytic streptococci from A to O, missing out I and J. Although B, C and G may be pathogenic, Group A is the important one. In each Lancefield group the streptococci can be further typed which again is important in tracking down the source of an infection.

The two most important anaerobic organisms in obstetrics are the anaerobic streptococcus and *Cl. welchii*. Growth of these is inhibited in the presence of oxygen. Culture must therefore be undertaken in truly anærobic conditions and in requesting a bacteriological report in cases of suspected genital tract infection it is important to ask for anærobic as well as ærobic culture.

If an infection cannot be stamped out at once with the initial loading dose, the less susceptible mutants, which are liable to appear at random at any time, may survive and with continuing inadequate dosage resistant strains will develop by selective breeding. This is called multiple step resistance and inadequate dosage is largely to blame. Certain species of organism, however, can develop high resistance to streptomycin in a single step, for example, *Mycobacterium tuberculosis* in which mutants with natural high resistance already exist in considerable numbers. This is why it is necessary to treat tuberculous infection with not less than two antibiotics because, statistically, one is much less likely to encounter organisms with double resistance.

Staphylococci are less dependent than most organisms upon random mutation to produce penicillin resistant strains and the resistant population is thus very easily produced even with large doses of penicillin. Such staphylococci produce the enzyme penicillinase which destroys the penicillin molecule. The importance of the newer types of penicillin lies in their ability to avoid destruction by penicillinase, for example, methicillin (Celbenin), cloxacillin (Orbenin), or cephaloridine (Ceporin). The following table lists the usual antibiotic sensitivities of some of the commonly encountered pathogens in obstetric practice:

TABLE XVI

ANTIBIOTIC SENSITIVITIES OF THE COMMON PATHOGENS

	Penicillin	Erythromycin	Fusidic Acid	{Methicillin {Cloxacillin	Ampicillin	Cephaloridine	Chloramphenicol	Tetracyclines	Nitrofurantoin	Neomycin	Streptomycin	Kanamycin	Polymyxins
Staph. pyogenes	v	v	+	+	v	+	v	v			v	v	v
Str. pyogenes	+	+			+	+	+	+			h	h	
Str. fæcalis	vh	+			+	v	+	+	+		h	h	
Hæmophilus	h	+			+	v	+	+			+	+	+
Coliforms	h				+	+	+	+	+	+	+	+	+
Proteus	h				v	+	+	h	+	+	+	+	
Pseudomonas							h	h			+	+	+
Cl. welchii	+				+	+	+	+					
Neisseria gonorrhœæ	v	+	+		+	+	+	+			+		

+ : sensitive

h sensitive to high concentrations

v variably sensitive

(With acknowledgments to W.H.O. Technical Report No. 210)

The sensitivity of a given organism to various antibiotics is determined by exposing the organism to concentrations of the antibiotic such as would be found in the tissues in the treated patient and observing whether or not growth is effectively inhibited. This can be done either by using standard dilutions, commonly made up in broth to which the organism is added, or quite a number of antibiotics can be tested out at the same time on a single culture plate impregnated with a series of discs which will produce zones of growth inhibition of bacterial growth depending on the degree of sensitivity. A large number of sensitivity results may be produced at one time but it is essential to use pure cultures of the organism, which means that other bacteria in the case of mixed flora must first be got rid of by obtaining pure cultures. This alone takes about 36 hours, so that a full sensitivity report, unless one is dealing with a single organism, cannot be obtained in under a couple of days. As a result antibiotic therapy cannot be truly definitive, except in clear-cut and obvious cases at the very start of an infection, the severity of which, however, may demand immediate action. The initial choice of antibiotic must therefore be a wise one depending upon the likely type of infection and the efficacy of the antibiotic used, bearing in mind the danger of breeding resistance or encouraging the growth of

other organisms so that the last state of the patient is worse than the first, and there should be no delay in delivering the specimen at the earliest possible moment to the bacteriologist in order to facilitate his task of obtaining pure cultures for sensitivity testing.

Penicillin is destroyed by gastric acid and therefore can only be given by mouth if in an acid resistant form such as phenoxymethyl penicillin (Penicillin V). Otherwise it must be given by injection. The penicillinase resistant penicillins such as methicillin and cloxacillin have already been mentioned. The latter is reasonably acid resistant and can be given by mouth one hour before meals in 500 mg. doses, six hourly. Cloxacillin can also be given by intramuscular injection, 250 mg., four to six hourly. The broad spectrum penicillin, ampicillin (Penbritin), is particularly useful because it resists gastric acid, can be efficient given by mouth, and concentrates highly in the urine. Unfortunately its resistance to penicillinase is less marked.

Streptomycin although having a broad spectrum has the double drawback of being useless by mouth and relatively toxic, particularly towards the eighth cranial nerve. I once had a case of bilateral wrist drop which was attributed to this drug. It should not be used for the treatment of coliform infections, for example, when other safer drugs are available. Kanamycin is also ototoxic and, like streptomycin, may accumulate in the bloodstream if there is renal impairment. The ability of any antibiotic to be excreted in the urine must be taken into account in both the choice and dosage of drug. Kanamycin has to be given by injection whereas neomycin must be given orally. Neomycin is also useful topically and for "sterilising" the gut from which it is not absorbed. It has therefore a limited place in obstetrics quite apart from its discouraging toxicity which contra-indicates parenteral administration.

The tetracyclines should never be used in pregnancy because of the evil effects of discoloration which they produce on a baby's teeth. They may also interfere with foetal bone growth. Their use should be restricted entirely to women who are puerperæ and who are not breast feeding their babies. There is thus seldom an indication to use tetracyclines in obstetrics. The damage to the foetus is not related to the dose nor the duration of administration.

Chloramphenicol would be one of the most useful of all antibiotics because of its wide range of activity and ease of administration, usually by the oral route, were it not for the very real danger of agranulocytosis which practically contra-indicates its use in obstetrics where other antibiotics can be used instead.

Nitrofurantoin (Furadantin) is mainly useful against organisms infecting the urinary tract including E. coli, Proteus and Str. fæcalis. It is given in tablet form four times a day after meals, commonly 100 mg. each dose.

The erythromycin group (Macrolides) is mainly useful in reserve against penicillin resistant staphylococci. Most other Gram-positive organisms are sensitive as well. Because of low solubility the drugs are usually given my mouth in enteric coated capsules, 1–2 g. daily, in divided doses. If given parenterally a larger volume has to be administered in order to dissolve the drug than when given intravenously.

There is more to the choice of an antibiotic than a knowledge of sensitivity which may have to be awaited over the course of a couple of days. If the art of prescribing is not to degenerate into mere witchcraft, it is as well to take some note of how these drugs are believed to act.

Sulphonamides compete with para-aminobenzoic acid which is structurally similar and which certain bacteria require in the course of folic acid metabolism. In other words they produce a metabolic pathway block. If, however, the bacteria do not require para-aminobenzoic acid they demonstrate sulphonamide resistance and even in the case of sensitive organisms the presence of pus will supply the metabolites which would otherwise have been blocked; therefore sulphonamides become ineffective where there is frank suppuration.

The penicillins on the other hand interfere with the formation of tough bacterial cell envelopes which alone protect them from lysis due to osmotic pressure. The polymyxins, however, alter the function of the cell membrane so that important substances leak out of the cell causing its death.

The tetracyclines and chloramphenicol interfere with protein synthesis, thus discouraging growth.

It will now be seen that there are two types of effect. Either the antibiotic kills the cell by its effect upon the cell membrane or the envelope, as in the case of the penicillins and polymyxins, or the metabolism necessary for the survival of the cell is interfered with as in the case of the sulphonamides and tetracyclines. The bactericidal drugs, as their name implies, can kill the bacteria outright, whereas the bacteriostatic merely inhibit their development and growth, preferably until such time as the host has had time to build up his own defences, but withdrawal of the drug too soon will allow the original bacterial population to go ahead unchecked. The following drugs are bactericidal:

    Penicillins
    Streptomycin
    Polymyxins
    Erythromycin in high concentration
 and Fusidic acid

The following drugs are bacteriostatic:

Sulphonamides
Tetracyclines
Chloramphenicol
Erythromycin in low concentrations

Bearing these points in mind and taking account of the likely infecting organism from the clinical condition of the patient, an intelligent choice of antibiotic drug can be made while still awaiting confirmatory sensitivity reports. Therefore, if possible in the early stages of an infection a bactericidal drug, which will kill the organism outright, is preferable to a bacteriostatic drug which will merely hold the infection in abeyance during the course of treatment. It is infinitely preferable to start with a narrow spectrum antibiotic rather than to shoot one's bolt with a broad spectrum drug which may presently confront one with resistant organisms of a most intractable kind, unless the patient's condition is so serious as to warrant the risk.

Pseudomonas infections are a particularly ugly reward for using broad spectrum antibiotics ill-advisedly. A less serious secondary infection following antibiotic therapy is infection with *Candida albicans*, which, if it becomes established in the intestinal tract can be very troublesome for a long time. I, myself, have personal experience of this very unpleasant complication of antibiotic therapy.

In many respects it is better to use combined therapy with more than one antibiotic rather than one very broad spectrum drug and as a general guide the bactericidal drugs are usually synergistic and do not antagonise each other, for example, penicillin and streptomycin, whereas antagonism is usual between bactericidal and bacteriostatic drugs.

When confronted with an acute infection one's immediate choice, if appropriate, is penicillin because of its low toxicity and its potent bactericidal effect. Unfortunately some patients are allergic to the penicillins and this extends as a rule to the newer drugs of this class. One must bear in mind the ease with which resistant strains can be easily selected out with the chosen drug especially in hospital practice and for this reason drugs like streptomycin and erythromycin should not be used alone. The presence of pus will render the sulphonamides useless and in considering the treatment of urinary infections one wants to choose a drug which is excreted in high concentration and active form in the urine, but must at the same time ensure that there is no renal excretory impairment, otherwise dangerously high blood concentrations of the drug may develop. This danger is particularly true of streptomycin and kanamycin. The general condition of the patient and whether vomiting is persistent

or not may determine the route of dosage, for example intravenous or oral.

As a general rule one should not use a steam roller where a sledge hammer will do. On the other hand the intention is to give the bacteria a proper clout, not just a gentle stroke. Underdosage therefore is dangerous.

In our unit in Glasgow no antibiotic may be prescribed without the specific sanction of the consultant in charge of the case and never before the necessary swabs have been taken for culture. In New Zealand, antibiotic prescribing seemed to go "hay-wire". In 1955, for example, the antibiotics bill, in a population of only 2 million, exceeded £400,000 and this figure excludes penicillin and strepto-mycin; nor does it include those drugs used in hospitals. (*Lancet* Editorial, August 11th, 1956.)

The public, too, is as much to blame as the less-thinking members of our profession, in automatically linking antibiotic therapy with an elevation of temperature, whatever its cause—a sort of shilling-in-the-slot medicine, and general practitioners are often subjected to a lot of moral pressure in this respect. My waste-paper baskets are filled nearly every day with attractively coloured brochures from manufacturers who proclaim for their products ever-increasing potency, allegedly fewer reactions and lower toxicity, and, worst of all, a yet broader spectrum. This last feature presumably attracts by suggesting that proper bacteriological investigation can be dispensed with and that the mental discomfort of choosing the specific remedy can be eliminated.

It is certain that as a result of such expensive folly the bacteriology of infective processes will have to be evaluated anew within the next 25 years, and urgently, too!

MORBID ANATOMY

The nature and extent of the pathology in puerperal sepsis de-pends upon certain factors. Firstly, the patient's general resistance to infection is of paramount importance because it influences both the efficacy and the speed of operation of the general defence mechanisms of the body. It depends upon the state of the blood, the absence of anæmia, particularly recently acquired anæmia as a result of exsanguination, and the state of general health which it is one of the objects of good antenatal care to promote. Next comes the initial state of the tissues locally at the beginning of the puerper-ium, the effects of trauma being obviously adverse. Thirdly, the nature of the pathology depends on the one hand upon the organism responsible and its virulence, and on the other the nature of the inflammatory response and its ability to localise the infection at its site.

It matters less whether a patient has pelvic peritonitis or parametritis than whether her infection is due to the anærobic streptococcus or the *E. coli*, and the gross manifestations of the disease, upon which the clinical signs are based, are profoundly influenced by the type of organism responsible and the characteristic type of response. For example, in the case of the hæmolytic streptococcus, the local response is not gross; abscesses, if present at all, tend to be small and the barrier erected to the spread of the infection is often ineffective. The clinical signs of inflammation are the result of the struggle between attack and defence, and since, in this instance, the defence is more mobile than static, the body as a whole is readily overrun with the infection and septicæmia may quickly develop. The rise in pulse rate is often far more characteristic than the rise in temperature, and where the inflammatory response is minimal, as in the most serious cases, the temperature may be sub-normal. The small vessels draining the uterus contain infected thrombi which liberate the bacteria into the blood stream in showers. Likewise the infection may sail through the wall of the uterus, hardly bothering it enough to interfere with involution, and may infect the peritoneal cavity which, too, may put up a very half-hearted protest. This is the picture in the cases coming to a fatal issue. A more efficient inflammatory response locally will save the patient's life, often with the formation of an abscess.

The above is in marked contrast to infections due to *E. coli*, in which the local response is far more vigorous and large abscesses are readily formed.

The *Staph. pyogenes*, characteristically, causes the formation of multiple small abscesses. Although a satisfactory response to infection more readily occurs, septicæmia and metastatic infection are common. The *Strep. viridans* is important because of its property of causing vegetations to grow on heart valves previously deformed either as a result of rheumatic disease or through congenital anomaly.

The anærobic streptococcus, now numerically so important, is associated with a history of trauma, particularly lacerations of the cervix opening up the tissues of the parametrium and the presence of retained products of conception. The inflammatory response is considerable, resulting in offensive lochia and often a type of induration of the pelvic cellular tissues which has been likened to plaster of Paris. The veins draining the pelvic organs become the seat of gross thrombophlebitis, from which little chunks of infected clot are liable to break away, producing pyæmic abscesses in the lungs. These cases run a prolonged course with intermittent fever and rigors.

The *Cl. welchii* is often present in a healthy vagina, but it becomes invasive in the presence of traumatised and devitalised tissue. A dead

fœtus retained *in utero* also provides such a culture medium, and for this reason surgical induction of labour should not be practised in cases of intra-uterine death. The two outstanding features in infection from this organism are hæmolysis and the formation of gas which, in fatal cases, not only produces marked tissue emphysema, but also what is known as the "foamy liver".

INVESTIGATION

Any case of pyrexia in the puerperium should be regarded as due to a genital tract infection until the contrary is proved, because of the great risks at stake. It is a wise rule, therefore, to take vaginal and cervical swabs, as well as a clean specimen of urine, for culture forthwith and not to await developments. This rule should be followed even though the physical signs unequivocally suggest an extra-genital infection. The temperature and the bacteriology are far more important nowadays than physical signs in the abdomen and pelvis. Until recently a high vaginal swab was considered adequate, but we no longer think so. It is true that in the case of an infection of the uterine cavity with the hæmolytic streptococcus, culture from the vagina is just as likely to demonstrate an overwhelming predominance in the growth of this organism as a swab taken from the cervical canal, but high vaginal swabs can be misleading in less outspoken cases, in that they may, in the absence of an overriding intra-uterine infection, yield cultures of normal vaginal inhabitants which are not necessarily pathogenic.

What is almost as important as the collection of the bacteriological specimen is its method of despatch. The late afternoon on a Friday is about the worst possible moment because it may not reach the laboratory in time for proper culture to be set up, so that all manner of irrelevant bacteria may falsify the picture. Even urine is a first-class culture medium and it is increasingly the practice now to send specimens to the laboratory as soon as they are obtained without even waiting for the end of a round or a clinic. If working, however, at a distance from a bacteriological department it is worth preparing a Gram-stained film on the spot. In the case of urine some of the specimen should be examined forthwith after spinning down and looking for pus cells and bacteria in a wet specimen under a cover slip. There are still antisocial individuals who have not the common decency to cover a wet specimen with a cover slip and simply soil the objective lens of the microscope, much as day trippers soil the countryside with their litter. The mentality is roughly the same.

Large numbers of vaginal squames and very few pus cells in a urine specimen will almost certainly indicate a badly taken and contaminated specimen (Fig. 2).

If sending specimens by post, sometimes a transport medium such

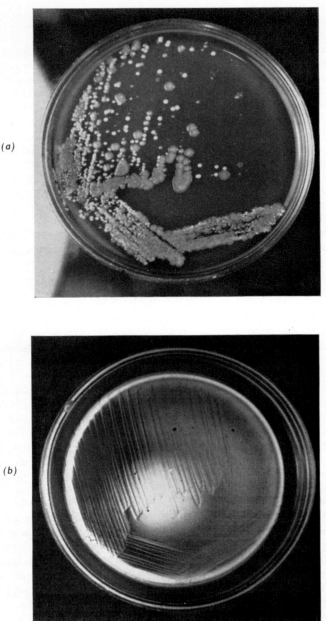

(a)

(b)

24/Fig. 2.—Culture plates showing the heavy contamination of a casually taken MSU; (a) compared with a catheter specimen, (b) taken 2 hours later from the same patient.

as Stuart's may be used, in which case the best plan is to dip the swab with which the specimen was taken into the little bottle of medium and break off the stick inside the bottle before applying the screw cap.

In setting up one's own cultures it is best to use blood agar plates both ærobically and anærobically for pus, and for urine a Mac-Conkey medium is likely to be best for coliforms and enterococci (Fig. 2).

The next best thing to immediate delivery to the bacteriologist is refrigeration until the specimen can be collected. The report from a badly handled or mishandled specimen is worse than no report at all.

It goes without saying that these specimens should be taken before any chemotherapy or antibiotics are prescribed. Among the many evils of prophylactic chemotherapy is the partial suppression of relevant bacteriological evidence without suppression of the disease process. As soon as the specimens have been taken, antibiotics may now be given empirically at first while awaiting the bacteriologist's report and later corrected or modified in accordance with these findings. Anærobic culture is just as important as ærobic and should never be omitted. Whenever there is a spiking temperature, or rigors, blood culture should be undertaken as well. Even in the absence of concrete bacteriological evidence, any case exhibiting a temperature which has defied the usual treatments for more than 10 days should be regarded as possibly due to the anærobic streptococcus.

Lastly, and I say lastly advisedly, a proper clinical examination of the patient must be carried out. The reason for putting matters in this order is that the possibility of a genital infection is so often discounted by the absence of local physical signs but, as has been said before, these signs depend upon the nature and the extent of the inflammatory response and, if present, represent a willingness on the part of the tissues to resist the infection. This examination will not only include the urine, a sample of which should always be examined on the spot with a microscope before waiting for the pathologist to announce the presence or absence of pus cells, but the breasts should be scrutinised, the chest gone over and the legs searched for signs of puerperal thrombosis. The perineum should be inspected for infection of any wounds sustained, in which case the removal of some of the sutures may be necessary and a rectal examination will detect a pelvic inflammatory collection. A point to remember is that puerperal pyelitis, apart from pyrexia, is usually symptomatically silent with neither loin pain nor tenderness.

GENERAL TREATMENT

The patient is nursed in isolation and all the usual details of general nursing care apply as in any acute febrile illness. An adequate fluid

intake must be maintained and sufficient rest must be ensured by the administration of analgesics or sedatives. Any serious degree of anæmia must be combated by blood transfusion in order to give the patient a fighting chance to resist her infection. All the antibiotics in the world will avail little if the patient is exsanguinated.

Local treatments, intra-uterine glycerine (except for certain saprophytic types of case) and the application of local heat have all gone by the board, and the specific treatment of today is now concentrated in the judicious use of the appropriate antibiotic, hence the importance of the bacteriologist.

The general hazards of antibiotics.—The ills which may affect the patient treated with sulphonamides or the antibiotics have been categorised under five main headings (Kekwick, 1956): 1. Allergic and anaphylactic reactions. 2. Gastro-intestinal disorders. 3. Renal lesions. 4. Neurological disorders. 5. Blood dyscrasias.

The first group, due to hypersensitivity, comprises angioneurotic œdema, asthma, sweating, collapse and sudden death. Emergency treatment consists in the immediate subcutaneous injection of 0·1 ml. of a 1 in 1,000 solution of adrenaline hydrochloride, repeated and repeated as necessary, keeping the syringe needle *in situ* until a total of 1 ml. has been given. The more chronic types of allergic response, mainly urticarial, can be treated by antihistamines given orally.

The tetracycline group are particularly liable to cause diarrhœa and gastro-intestinal upsets, often due to a resistant staphylococcal enteritis and occasionally to infection with *Candida albicans*.

The dangers of crystalluria and anuria from sulphonamides are well known, but, with the main exception of penicillin, the antibiotics also are occasionally capable of causing albuminuria and lower nephron nephrosis.

The chief neurotoxic effects are vertigo and deafness due to damage to the vestibular and auditory divisions respectively of the eighth nerve.

Of the blood dyscrasias, leucopenia and agranulocytosis are the commonest and expose the patient to the risk of fulminating streptococcal infection without the natural powers of resistance. Penicillin, which is guiltless in this matter, may be urgently necessary to combat such an infection in a patient half-killed by other antibiotics. The production of white cells may, in fortunate instances, be stimulated by intramuscular injection of nucleotide (B.P.C.) 40 ml. per day, and the oral administration of pyridoxine hydrochloride 50 mg. t.i.d. and folic acid 20 mg. daily.

Bone marrow aplasia occasionally occurs, especially after sulphonamides and chloramphenicol, and may necessitate repeated transfusion with whole fresh blood.

PROPHYLAXIS

It goes almost without saying that good midwifery comes foremost. Throughout the chapters of this book reference is constantly made to the adverse effect in respect of maternal morbidity which follows so many of the complications described. Many of these cannot be prevented, but the skill exhibited in meeting them with the maximum regard for the maternal tissues is reflected in straightforward puerperal convalescence. The saving of blood at all times and in all places is not only one of the first objectives of sound obstetric practice, it is vital to the patient's speedy recovery, and no amount of prophylactic chemotherapy can justify or mitigate a disregard for this principle. Notwithstanding all the care in the world, however, puerperal sepsis will continue to occur sporadically, but epidemics surely demonstrate serious loopholes in technique.

Although the sting has been removed from the hæmolytic streptococcus, epidemic staphylococcal infection has to some extent taken its place. The investigation of a high rate of staphylococcal infection in infants (which, as stated before, gives a good indication of surgical cleanliness or the lack of it) occurring in a large institution in London in 1949, as described by Barber, Hayhoe and Whitehead, is a model of bacteriological detective work, and many similar reports have followed since then. The findings of these workers are worth quoting. Firstly, infections encountered were predominantly penicillin resistant, from which the inference can be drawn that they were due to hospital cross-infection, since resistant strains of staphylococci in the population at large are in a distinct minority. The investigation was continued throughout the better part of the year, and it was found that between 60 and 70 per cent of the nursing and medical staff were at some time nasal carriers of *Staph. pyogenes* and that the strains were penicillin resistant in over 80 per cent. The heaviest growths were obtained from the members of the permanent staff, and the proportion of nurses and pupil midwives carrying these resistant strains rose with the duration of their stay at the hospital, rising from about 20 per cent on their first enrolment on the staff to 66 per cent after three months there. A control series was taken from a London store, from which 62 of the employees were examined, and although half of them were carriers of *Staph. pyogenes*, there were no penicillin resistant cases among them. There was also noted a seasonal variation in the incidence of infection among the babies, which reached its peak in February at 22 per cent and fell to 8 per cent in August, but in most of the other months was fairly constant between 11 and 14 per cent. It would appear, therefore, that there is inevitably a reservoir of infection in the noses of a high percentage of workers in hospital from which bedding, hands, clothes, instruments and utensils may become

infected. Hospitals, too, breed their own varieties of pathogenic coliforms, particularly in gynæcological wards, which put up the risks of catheterization for example. Every time a bed is made the air becomes filled with dust, impregnated with organisms from the bedding, so that it is remarkable that the infection rate is not higher than it is.

From the above, the lessons to be drawn are obvious. Clearly the institution so investigated is no isolated instance. Every hospital in the land is seeking to curtail staphylococcal cross-infection. Since it is not practicable to send two-thirds of the staff of hospitals off duty, one has to fall back upon the rigid observance of a first-class aseptic and antiseptic technique. The following steps are therefore recommended:

1. **Mask wearing.**—Colebrook's recommendations have lost none of their force, yet how seldom does one meet a proper technique. The masks should be supplied sterile and, once put on, should not

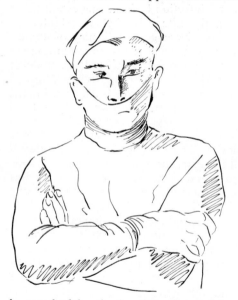

24/Fig. 3.—Bad mask wearing. A travesty of aseptic technique. Note also the left hand! The axilla, even after gowning, is not a sterile area.

be touched by the hands and certainly not pulled down under the chin. A very deplorable practice must be mentioned here in order to condemn it, namely the wearing of the mask over the mouth *but under the nose!* (Fig.3).

Unfortunately there are many who are guilty of this serious breach of technique and, worn in this fashion, a mask is worse than useless, as it just rubs staphylococci off the lower end of the nasal septum and scatters them at large.

2. **Gowns.**—Freshly laundered gowns or coats should be kept at the entrance to each lying-in ward and donned on entry. Clothes are dirty things, and it is only prudent to avoid, by a change of outer clothing, the carrying of infection from one ward to another. This practice is far from usual, unfortunately.

3. **Gloves.**—Dry sterile gloves should be used for all vaginal examinations and operative work, after a conscientious scrub-up. Putting on non-sterile gloves and then rinsing them in antiseptics or rubbing them over with antiseptic cream is not satisfactory, and the attitude should be that what is good enough for general surgeons (who would not dream of operating without dry sterile gloves) should be *almost* good enough for obstetricians!

4. **Isolation facilities.**—These must be adequate, and the accommodation for septic cases should be provided, preferably in another building or at least in another part of the block, and the staff concerned should not do duty in both clean and unclean wards. Barrier nursing constitutes no more than a dangerous pretence at taking adequate precautions. Maternity departments in general hospitals should be in buildings separated from the general wards. Unfortunately, in many hospitals of the older type this is not feasible.

5. **Infection among personnel.**—Members of the staff suffering from sore throats, colds, boils, whitlows, paronychia and other such ailments, even though mild, should be swabbed and immediately suspended from duty, and whenever infection occurs that is anything more than sporadic, a search should be made for the source.

6. **Septic babies.**—These should be sent, together with their mothers, to the isolation ward. They are a potent source of epidemic infection.

7. **Antiseptics.**—These, though indispensable, should be regarded as a subsidiary line of defence. Creams should be coloured with some dye to indicate the areas of application. Our present preference is for Phisohex. Chlorhexidine ("Hibitane") is a magnificent antiseptic but it is expensive. Savlon is cheaper and very satisfactory.

8. **Control of dust.**—Dust is an important source of cross-infection, always worse after bedmaking. The oiling of blankets and floors has been tried out. The first has certain laundering difficulties and the second has a depressing effect upon the appearance of the floor. Colebrooke has found that staphylococci can remain viable in blankets for many weeks. Boiling blankets shrinks them and autoclaving turns them into felt. Soaking them in antiseptics or oils has the further disadvantages of being likely to induce sensitivity reactions in some patients. The ultimate answer is to provide Terylene blankets in hospitals. These can be safely sterilised.

All dry-sweeping and the use of brooms should be replaced by vacuum cleaning.

9. **Bed-pans.**—These should be sterilised with steam as soon as used. On no account should cloth bed-pan covers ever be used. Disposable bed-pan linings have now replaced the traditional bed-pan with us, thus eliminating yet another source of cross-infection.

10. **Disposal of vulval pads.**—These should be placed at once in a bin with a fly-proof, automatically closing lid and should be collected twice a day and burnt. Strong paper container bags are very useful for lining the bins. Disposal lifts are ideal. They are safer than chutes which have been found to "funnel" bacteria from one floor to another.

The Problem of Neonatal Sepsis

During the 1950s this problem in maternity units had become so acute as to question, once more, the desirability of institutional confinement in completely normal cases. Within twelve months no less than four maternity departments in the West of Scotland, for example, had epidemic outbreaks necessitating the temporary closure of two of them, including the whole of our own maternity hospital. The trouble is endemic in all units and those who say they have none are usually those with the poorest facilities for bacteriological investigation, the lowest standards of observation and the least clinical honesty.

We now recognise that no septic lesion in a newborn baby is trivial, however superficial or minor it may appear to be. Even a small septic skin spot may apparently heal rapidly in hospital yet provide a latent focus of infection which, some weeks later, breaks out as a fixation abscess, for example in lung, or osteomyelitis, meningitis or septicæmia. The connection of this major illness with the earlier transient lesion is often missed and the maternity unit remains blissfully ignorant of its part in the subsequent disaster.

In an allegedly "clean" maternity department Barber and Burston reported that 65 per cent of all babies went home with penicillin-resistant strains of staphylococci, and Hutchinson and Bowman in Newcastle-on-Tyne found that colonisation of the infant nose and umbilical stump by *Staph. pyogenes* occurred in exactly two-thirds of all babies in one or other site within 24 hours of birth. Cross-infection appeared to be from infant to infant. They too found that some of the hospital strains of staphylococci carried home persisted and spread within the family for up to six months. It would appear that babies in hospital cannot avoid being colonised with staphylococci. What really matters is what sort of staphylococci. The umbilical stump is now increasingly recognised as a primary site of multiplication of these organisms and source of spread. Open exposure of the umbilicus to the air is favoured in most units as a means of accelerating

mummification of the umbilical stump and the usual modern practice is either to clamp or ligate the stump very close to the umbilicus and remove the distal tissue. Occlusive dressings, though favoured in certain units like St. Thomas's Hospital (Huntingford *et al.* 1961), are distrusted by most of us on the grounds that it is hard to believe that bacteria cannot penetrate them, that they encourage moisture and interfere with inspection. We prefer in our unit to powder the umbilical stump with hexachlorophane powder (Gillespie *et al.* 1958) as a method of achieving dry antisepsis.

The anterior nares of the babies also become quickly infected with staphylococci and so great is the problem that Williams (1958) observed that 15 per cent of babies developed at least some staphylococcal lesion, even though trivial. In an interesting experiment involving the positioning of babies in nurseries in relation to an index baby carrying a recognisable strain of staphylococcus, Wolinsky *et al.* (1960) found that the spread of infection was predominantly by organisms carried by the nurses and not by the index babies and even after one sole exposure over 50 per cent of the babies could acquire the strain from the appropriate nurses as determined by umbilical and nasal cultures. From this work it is clear that a baby is in more peril from being handled by a nurse than by lying in a cot next to an infected baby. The magnitude of the problem has been particularly well recognised in Australia where as many as 41 per cent of babies have been found to have developed clinical evidence of staphylococcal infection and 100 per cent of them at five days old carried staphylococci. Plueckhahn (1961) blamed the busy life which the babies suffered at the hands of the nursing staff, ranging from full bathing to weighing, eye toilet four-hourly, cot making and being changed, to the accompaniment of much coming and going of the staff and dirty linen being sorted within the same atmosphere. As a result of these disturbing figures the nursing management of these babies was drastically overhauled and produced a most astonishing decrease in minor staphylococcal disease from 41 per cent in 1956 to 4·7 per cent in 1960, achieved by restricting these routine nursing procedures, by employing rooming-in and dry-washing the babies with Phisohex. The institution of these more up-to-date techniques was also rewarded by a reduction in subsequent admissions of babies to hospital for staphylococcal disease and a considerable fall in the incidence of breast abscess in the mothers. Since babies must acquire staphylococci they are more likely to acquire epidemic varieties of virulent and antibiotic-resistant strains in hospital than if born at home and certainly Elias-Jones *et al.* (1961) found this rate to be more than double in the case of the former. Nevertheless, as Williams (1961) has pointed out in a survey of North-West London, there was also an appreciable

incidence of nasal carriage of *Staph. aureus* in babies born at home; in fact little different from those born in hospital and one cannot assume that domiciliary delivery protects the baby altogether from what has now become a modern widespread problem. The possibilities of competitive colonisation by harmless staphylococci as an alternative to high-powered methods of protection from exposure has yet to be worked out.

Unfortunately not only the staphylococcus but now the *E. coli* is providing new problems in cross-infection. The latter is now identifiable by serotyping and it would appear that many of these infections are transmitted from the mother's own bowel. Often, however, hospital strains of *E. coli* are the source of trouble.

The epidemic strains of staphylococcus are all penicillin resistant and already resistant to many or most of the commonly used antibiotics. This situation is likely to get worse with the present indiscriminate misuse of all and every drug unless some potent antibiotic, e.g. erythromycin, is kept strictly up one's sleeve and used only to save life in certain segregated instances.

Staphylococci of phage-type 80/81 are common offenders—as in our own epidemic in Glasgow, and also in Australia, New Zealand, Canada and the United States. Phage-typing, however, gives little indication of virulence but serves to track down a possible source of infection.

What then can one do in the face of so widespread a problem? The most rigid enforcement of the rules of surgical asepsis must come first. Domiciliary delivery might get over the difficulty but would expose the patient and her child to too many other hazards, except in cases "carefully selected" for their expected normality. Early dismissal from hospital is a compromise solution but is hardly fair on the type of patient most in need of rest and attention. The increased use of rooming-in and entrusting the mother with as much as possible of the handling of her baby certainly cuts down cross-infection between babies and constitutes yet another reason for early ambulation in the fit puerperal mother.

Additional Steps to Control or Curtail Infection among Babies

1. Any case of neonatal sepsis, however minor, must be isolated.

2. Overcrowding in the nurseries is dangerous and should be avoided.

3. Baby bathing is a fatuous, unnecessary and sentimental ritual which is largely overdone and provides opportunities for the spread of infection. The babies should be cleaned in their cots, sterile wool should be used and their towels should be separate.

4. Masks should always be worn by the staff whenever handling babies.

5. The number of nurses handling any individual baby throughout its stay in hospital should be limited as far as possible.

6. There should be no communal changing tables.

7. In addition to wearing gowns, the hands should be properly washed and dried on paper towels. Hospital hand towels are dangerous and should be abolished.

8. All feeding utensils should be boiled after use.

9. The cot bedding should be of Terylene. An alternative, although less efficient, method is to enclose the blankets in small cotton bags.

10. The babies should be removed from the lying-in wards while floor sweeping or bed making is in progress. The commonest type of neonatal infection is the "sticky eye". The use of prophylactic eye-drops, once so important in the prevention of gonococcal ophthalmia, has now been abandoned in many institutions. It does nothing to cut down the incidence of sticky eye and, in fact, it may provoke its increase. It is, nevertheless, important to take swabs at once from any eye showing conjunctival infection, after which eye-drops such as albucid or penicillin may be started straightaway pending the bacteriologist's report and the baby, and its mother with it, must be isolated.

BREAST INFECTIONS

There can be no doubt about the advantages of breast feeding for both mother and child and yet, except in the more intelligent strata of the community, breast feeding is unquestionably on the decline. Newson and Newson (1962) have disposed of the popularly held belief that it was the desire of the mother to get back to gainful employment which made her anxious to give up breast feeding at the earliest possible moment. They showed in their survey in Nottingham, an area of high level of employment of women, than even by the time the baby was twelve months old fewer than 2 per cent of the mothers were back at their full-time work and less than 8 per cent had even part-time jobs; they observed that over and over again the physical reasons at first given for failure to breast feed were cover for underlying attitudes of mind ranging from a vague sense of inconvenience to a deep-seated revulsion. Fifty-five per cent of those interviewed admitted that they had not wanted to breast feed and would not have continued anyway, 28 per cent said they would have liked to breast feed and the remainder were in the "don't know" class. Only about 1 in 10 of the mothers had continued to feed for as long as six months. So much for the success of medical and nursing propaganda. The position in Glasgow is exceptionally discouraging. Many of the older multiparæ do their best to discourage the young primigravida and take the line that it is an awful nuisance and a terrible tie. This attitude is most marked amongst

those living in the worst and most overcrowded housing conditions, where lack of peace and privacy militate against breast feeding, but one often feels that family doctors find it easier and less trouble to put a baby on the bottle than to encourage the falterer with all the determination which it sometimes requires. It is no use trying to encourage a favourable attitude towards breast feeding in the few hectic days which the Glasgow working-class woman is prepared to stay in hospital after delivery. The brainwashing can only succeed, if at all, in the course of antenatal care. We ascertain, earlier in pregnancy, the patient's wishes in regard to breast feeding and prepare accordingly. Breast milk is every baby's birthright. Failure to breast feed is a source of very real disappointment to many women, and in the large majority of cases is due to neglect on the part of the patient's nurses and doctors.

The psychological aspects and importance of breast feeding are incalculable but, on the more phsyical plane, human breast milk is the ideal diet for the neonate which no substitute, however ingenious its composition, can wholly replace. The statement so often made to mothers who are having difficulties with lactation, that their milk is disagreeing with the baby is in every instance a flagrant travesty of the truth, and it would be far more accurate to diagnose that the nurse was disagreeing with the mother. The following is a brief summary of the advantages of breast feeding:

1. Human breast milk, by having a relatively higher content of lactalbumen as compared with cow's milk, which has relatively more caseinogen, is more easily digested.

2. It is safe.

3. The chances of gastro-enteritis are much reduced.

4. It is far simpler than the conscientious preparing of feeds.

5. It is cheap.

6. Overfeeding at the breast is practically impossible after the first fortnight.

7. Uterine involution is unquestionably assisted. Suckling provides powerful sensory stimuli in the highly innervated nipple. These reach the innervation of the posterior pituitary and stimulate the production of oxytocic hormone. This not only provokes the milk-ejection reflex by its action on the myo-epithelial elements surrounding the mammary alveoli but acts, of course, directly upon the uterus as well.

8. Subsequent breast carcinoma is less common after a series of successful periods of lactation.

Feeding bottles are hardly necessary for the woman who succeeds in breast feeding her child, because she will manage to lactate until the child is old enough to drink directly from a cup at about eight or nine months, which is about the correct time for weaning, although

from the age of six months or from the time when the child has reached a weight of 15 pounds, whichever is the sooner, additional food in the form of groats, Farex or simple broths will have been given.

Maternity hospitals, in their reports, are often showing figures of over 90 per cent "successful breast feeding" at the end of the lying-in period, but this means practically nothing, because it will be found that only a minority have managed to keep it up by three months' time, and, as Waller said, "At the end of the first fortnight the term *wholly breast fed* cannot be construed as *securely breast fed*". What, then, has gone wrong since the patient's discharge from hospital? In fact the seeds of failure were sown during the patient's stay in hospital and, paradoxically, it is often the patients who, during this period, seemed to have a super-abundance of milk that dry up so often shortly after their return home. The cause of the trouble nearly always lies in an uncorrected over-distension of the breasts occurring during the first puerperal week. A rise of milk pressure within the breast alveoli discourages secretion by flattening the alveolar columnar cells and occluding the surrounding capillaries. The baby, confronted with a breast surface almost as hard as a brick wall, cannot properly apply its jaws behind the lacteal sinuses in the nipples as it should and, instead of drawing the nipple into its throat, simply champs to no purpose on the nipple itself, abrading it, making it vulnerable to infection and wholly failing to relieve the fullness of the breasts. Small wonder, then, that it loses interest and the breasts, too, take the hint and start to dry up. Waller's results (1946) in Woolwich were so remarkable that his case stands proven up to the hilt. He managed to obtain a successful lactation rate at 6 months of 83 per cent in primigravidæ and Blaikley (1953), following Waller's principles, managed to double the 6-month success rate at Guy's Hospital to 51 per cent as against only 26 per cent in a control series. Anyone who visited the British Hospital for Mothers and Babies, Woolwich, in Waller's day will have appreciated at once the reasons for his enormous success, which was due, not only to his own intensive personal supervision, but also to the wholehearted and enthusiastic support which his nursing staff supplied.

This shows what can be done when doctors, nurses and patients are all determined—an unusual combination. A review of the reasons for abandoning breast feeding within the first three months has been made by Hytten *et al.* (1958) who studied a sample of primiparæ in Aberdeen numbering 106. Seventy-four had given up by three months and all but two experienced one or more difficulties in breast feeding. The commonest complaints were of excessive crying by the baby, maternal fatigue, breast and nipple troubles and inadequate milk.

These workers agreed that the mother's attitude of mind towards the subject was of paramount importance since success in breast feeding can only be obtained in the face of a certain amount of inconvenience and occasional discomfort, more related to the modern way of life than to breast feeding *per se* (see earlier).

It is neither dignified nor profitable for the staff to engage in a battle of wills with a patient who, in her heart of hearts, has no desire or intention of breast feeding. The difficulty is to spot the losers before any conflict is about to arise and this requires a more thorough knowledge of the patient's temperament than most harassed clinicians possess in hospital practice. Bearing in mind that many cases are likely to suffer some initial discouragement in getting the baby to take an interest in what they have to provide (and some babies are insultingly sleepy when first put to the breast), one's best hope is to forestall these difficulties before they ever assume any size. It is as well to warn the mother about "fourth day puerperal blues". This is where Waller's principles, summarised later, of establishing a ready flow of milk before delivery itself and avoiding any trace of engorgement in the breast, gives lactation the chance of a flying start. Where the likelihood of failure is reinforced by an unsatisfactory psychological attitude it is better to suppress lactation from the very start.

Lactation can be suppressed by a variety of methods ranging from nothing at all to most elaborate hormone combinations. The breasts are so often literally crying out to exercise their natural function that it sometimes takes a lot of wanton effort to suppress it and the placebo technique has something punitive about it. A series of untreated cases has been compared (1965) with those receiving a homeopathic dose of 5 mg. of stilboestrol twice a day with an average stay in hospital of only 4·76 days after delivery[29]. This can hardly be called stilboestrol suppression. We ourselves have for years gone for a massive dosage scheme of stilboestrol, namely 15 mg. thrice daily followed by 10 mg. likewise, followed by 5 mg., and tapering off thereafter, and our experience accords with that of Hodge (1967) who found a 12 per cent failure rate with stilboestrol as against a 65 per cent failure rate without it. Even so the nuisance of what has been called "rebound lactation"[11] following oestrogens alone, has been found to be one of the troubles with which the general practitioner commonly has to contend after the patient comes home. For these cases an intramuscular injection of 2 ml. of Mixogen is recommended. This contains a mixture of œstradiol and testosterone, including both short and long-acting esters of each. This drug was found to work particularly well in primigravidæ if given very early in the puerperium. More recently we have had considerable success with a one-shot technique, injecting 20 mg. of œstradiol (Primogyn

1 ml.) and giving 20 mg. of frusemide (Lasix) by mouth to discourage engorgement.[30]

The use of massive dosage of œstrogens is not without its penalty often in the form of so-called secondary postpartum hæmorrhage, but, what is even more sinister, a tenfold increase in the incidence of puerperal thrombo-embolism has been reported in women whose lactation was suppressed with œstrogens as compared with those who were breast feeding.[15]

ÆTIOLOGY OF BREAST INFECTIONS

Breast abscesses are a preventable condition. Waller had only 4 such in 10,000 cases in 9 years at Woolwich, and the usual incidence which most institutions suffer does little credit to their management of lactation. The ætiology is tied up with the remarks made in the opening paragraphs, and to blame civilisation, over-sophistication or distaste for breast feeding for subsequent trouble is usually sheer nonsense. The essence of the matter lies in the state of the nipples and the prevention of overdistension of the breasts. Staphylococcal cross infection does the rest. Overdistension exposes even good nipples to traumatic suckling, but poor nipples themselves are often associated with ducts choked with colostrum. Engorgement, with its surrounding œdema, still further prevents the proper drainage of milk. The stage is now set for the access of pathogenic organisms via nipple cracks and abrasions, so that engorgement turns to mastitis and mastitis to abscess formation.

Prophylaxis in pregnancy.—Since breast infections are preventable by the satisfactory establishment and maintenance of lactation, prophylactic measures should be undertaken in pregnancy. These consist firstly in teaching the patient the art of manual expression of the breasts. This not only establishes the flow of milk and clears the ducts of colostrum blockage, but endows the patient with a skill in combating overdistension in the early days of the puerperium, which she will not then have time enough to acquire. It also means that lactation is smoothly established at the outset of the puerperium without the usual hectic course of milk coming in with a rush on the third day. This manual expression and clearance of colostrum should be kept up from the 36th week onwards. The hypothetical value of colostrum to the baby as a source of maternal antibody is insignificant in comparison with its nuisance value in causing duct blockage. Secondly, the nipples should be rendered fit for lactation. This will depend not only upon the texture of skin but more upon the property of *protraction*. In order to determine the presence of protraction or retraction it is not merely enough to tug on the nipples. They should be properly tested by pinching the areola

between finger and thumb and observing whether the nipple comes forward or tends to buckle inward. Where protraction by this simple test appears to be inadequate, the wearing of Waller glass shells during the later part of pregnancy will make a very beneficial difference. Apart from ordinary washing with soap and water, the skin of the nipples does not require any of the more traditional methods of hardening it up, for example, the use of spirit which simply encourages the later appearance of cracks and fissures.

Prophylaxis in the puerperium.—Every effort is directed to the prevention of engorgement and distension, because in this event spontaneous leakage of milk from the breast stops and the organ becomes tense and œdematous to the danger of the nipple. Breast feeding should, therefore, be stopped as soon as the breasts become tight, and manual expression should be started as soon as an outflow of milk can be obtained, shortly after which the œdema will subside and breast feeding can be resumed. Oxytocin nasal sprays have been found helpful by some by stimulating the ducts to eject milk. In breasts which tend to get rather tight, it is a good plan to perform manual expression before the feed in order that the baby has a softer breast to deal with and residual milk at the end of the feed should be expressed likewise. When suckling and expression are insufficient to relieve engorgement or the threat of it, stilbœstrol should be prescribed without hesitation, and if the breasts remain tight in spite of suckling and expression, the need for this drug is urgent. Five milligrammes of stilbœstrol should be given at once in early cases, but the dose should be adjusted at each feed time to suit individual need. One can safely give up to 20 mg. in one dose without fear of suppressing lactation, provided suckling can be quickly resumed, in which case the mechanical stimulus thereof will more than counter the inhibitory effects of the drug. The effect of stilbœstrol on the breasts lasts up to about 8 hours, so that repeated dosage may be necessary, but the effect is dramatic and the success of the treatment depends upon the promptitude with which it is instituted.

SUMMARY OF WALLER PROCEDURES

1. Teach the art of manual expression before delivery. This may make it unnecessary afterwards.

2. Encourage protraction, if necessary with the help of shells.

3. At the threat of engorgement give stilbœstrol 5 mg. four-hourly.

4. Where engorgement is rapid and severe, give up to three doses of 20 mg. of stilbœstrol four-hourly and then reduce the dose rapidly.

5. Institute manual expression of the breasts as soon as the swelling and œdema start to subside.

Waller found that stilbœstrol was needed in about 5 per cent of his cases to control milk retention.

Types of Puerperal Mastitis

Gibberd (1953) drew attention to two main types. One, the non-epidemic cellulitis, and the other, the epidemic type involving primarily the lactiferous system. In the first, infection enters via a crack or abrasion in the nipple surface, which gives rise to a spreading cellulitis with later abscess formation. It is an interlobular connective tissue cellulitis and pus cannot be expressed from the milk ducts. It is the more usual type of mastitis and may respond well to penicillin if given early and if the organisms are sensitive.

The second type is confined to hospital practice and is not found in domiciliary midwifery. It is associated with skin infections in the babies, is due to *Staph. pyogenes*, involves the lactiferous system and runs a less acute course. Since the lactiferous system is involved, pus can be expressed from the nipple, and Gibberd gave it the name of "mammary adenitis", to distinguish it from the more classical mammary cellulitis. It makes its appearance usually in the second week of the puerperium, may run a tedious course and go on to suppuration.

Non-surgical Treatment of Mammary Abscess

The antibiotics have not proved an unmixed blessing in breast infections and their indiscriminate use may mask the cardinal signs of inflammation and cause delay in surgical intervention, which is as important as ever, though the extent of operation has to some extent been modified lately. The antibiotics are admirable for aborting an infection if given early enough, but after the disease has become firmly established, they fail to secure full resolution, so that a chronic induration of the breast may be induced which may even mimic a lactation carcinoma. Ultimately in these cases one makes a belated incision, ploughing through a vascular density of inflamed tissue which bleeds furiously and only a small quantity of pus may reward one's efforts. The patient ends up with a much more persistent disability than she would have had if antibiotics had not, in the first place, delayed the decision to operate.

It is often difficult to decide whether pus is likely to be found before operating. To wait for signs of fluctuation is to wait too long, since this will only be found in neglected cases. Aspiration with a wide bore needle is not very rewarding, and it is a good rule to diagnose the presence of pus simply on the grounds of suspicion.

The baby should not be put to the breast while the infection is active and as long as pathogens can be isolated from the milk, or while the nipple is cracked. Both nipple and breast should be rested

with the help of stilboestrol and gentle manual expression, provided it is not painful. If the condition cannot be fairly smartly aborted it is better to suppress lactation outright.

SURGICAL DRAINAGE

From the above it is clear that surgical drainage is just as important as formerly and that procrastination with antibiotics interferes with its ultimate efficacy. Any breast in which inflammation does not rapidly resolve with stilbœstrol, the antibiotics and the immediate cessation of breast feeding, should be suspected of having formed pus, and the presence of a brawny œdema over the skin makes the diagnosis almost a certainty. Under a general anæsthetic a radial incision is made over the affected area and a finger is introduced into the wound to open up and drain all loculated areas. If the incision has to be placed in the upper quadrants of the breast, counter drainage through a lower incision is often necessary. The quicker pus is evacuated the less will be the disorganisation of the breast tissue and the shorter the course of the illness. Neglected cases can run a very tedious course.

Ancillary lines of treatment should not be omitted in dealing with breast abscess. All breast feeding should be stopped at once because, even though the other breast is normal, continued suckling therefrom produces cross stimulation of the inflamed breast. Stilbœstrol should be vigorously prescribed. In a great many of these cases, even though healing is very rapid, it is not possible thereafter to re-establish lactation. This takes us back to the paramount importance of the prophylactic measures outlined earlier.

THROMBOSIS

Thrombosis rears its ugly head just as much in midwifery as in general surgery, although, apart from cases delivered by Cæsarean section, the more dramatic end result, namely embolism, is relatively uncommon; nevertheless, a potent source of maternal disability lies here, and many a case of venous misery in later life owes its origin to thrombosis occurring after childbirth. The events of the puerperium rank with a family history of ulceration and the association of obesity in the ætiology of this serious disability of middle age.

There are two main varieties of thrombosis:

Ileo-femoral thrombosis.—This is segmental in nature, and may extend from the internal iliac vein as far down as the profunda femoris, and it may extend upwards into the common iliac vein. It is due to the proximity of an inflammatory process within the pelvis and it produces the acute variety of white leg. It is a true inflammatory thrombophlebitis.

Phlebothrombosis of calf.—This is the more common variety. Clotting occurs in the venous sinuses within the soleus muscle. These sinuses are without valves, and the thrombosis may spread along the veins draining into the posterior tibial vein, whereupon œdema of the ankles appears. From here the thrombosis may spread to involve the popliteal vein, resulting in considerable swelling and pain, and, finally, the femoral vein may become involved to the accompaniment of the full-blown clinical picture of white leg. Although the origin of white leg in this instance is different from the first, the condition is now hard to distinguish from that due to ileo-femoral thrombophlebitis. Thus it will be seen how the condition of white leg can arise, either as a result of inflammatory thrombophlebitis or non-inflammatory phlebothrombosis. In thrombophlebitis the infection reaches the vein along the perivenous lymphatic channels and, as a result of inflammation, the endothelium in the threatened vein is destroyed, so that thrombosis occurs. In phlebothrombosis, on the other hand, the venous endothelium is intact.

ÆTIOLOGY OF PHLEBOTHROMBOSIS

Stasis is the most important single factor, and this of course is favoured by immobility, shock and a poor venous return to the heart because of shallow post-operative respiration. Pre-operative or antepartum anæmia is also an important ætiological factor, and stasis may be caused locally by the careless use of lithotomy poles and operating table straps. There are also other contributory causes to venous stasis in the legs, namely prolonged labour, hæmorrhage, manipulations, dehydration, prolonged anæsthesia (particularly with chilling while under its influence), and the use of binders after delivery which interfere with respiration. After surgical operation, and in our case particularly after Cæsarean section, there is a marked alteration in the coagulability of the blood, the fibrinogen is increased, platelets are more numerous and they clump together more readily. The relative increase in thrombosis after Cæsarean section is therefore explained.

Ochsner and De Bakey (1940) considered that the mechanical blockage resulting from an intravascular clot or the lymphatic obstruction caused by perivenous inflammation is not enough to explain the full syndrome of white leg, and they suggested arterial vasospasm as being responsible for the full clinical picture, pointing out that ligation alone of a main vein is not followed by œdema or white leg. They consider that the arterial spasm is reflexly inducted from the thrombosed segment of vein, and were able to reproduce this spasm by causing an experimental endophlebitis with chemicals. They showed, furthermore, that this reflex arc could be blocked by

interruption of the sympathetics. As a result of the spasm, pressure within the capillaries is raised, and the endothelium, as a result of anoxia, leaks fluid into the tissues; in addition, they held that the arteriolar spasm results in a decrease in the rate of flow of lymph, causing a rise of osmotic pressure and the establishment of a vicious circle with more œdema.

THE OBJECTIVES OF TREATMENT

There are several facets to consider:

1. The prevention of further clot propagation. In the case of embolism this is vitally necessary.
2. The alleviation of symptoms which may be very severe.
3. The prevention of pulmonary embolism.
4. The prevention of residual disability and sequelæ.

In the case of ileo-femoral thrombophlebitis, the ultimate prognosis, as regards function, is often better than in severe types of phlebo-thrombosis starting in the calf. Recanalisation commonly occurs in the former, but when it occurs in the latter the patient is left with an incompetent venous system, so that, usually about two years later, she may be greatly troubled with pain in the legs on standing, œdema and later ulceration. It has to be noted that the inflammatory reaction in the leg which may be apparent in association with phlebothrombosis is a result and not a cause of clotting in a calf vein, which may have been previously normal.

Anning, in describing his 557 cases of leg ulceration, found that no less than 160 of them owed the origin of their trouble to post-partum thrombosis, and that in half of them the thrombosis occurred after the first confinement. Obstetricians tend to lose sight of the late effects of this complication of pregnancy.

METHODS OF TREATMENT

Thrombosis after delivery or operation is largely a preventable condition. Anæmia and rough handling of tissues at the time can to some extent be avoided, and hæmo-concentration can be countered by an adequate fluid intake during the early days of the puerperium. Venous stasis should be discouraged by the active use of the muscles of the extremities in bed, which is more effective than early ambula-tion, and by exercises in deep breathing which increase the rate of the venous return to the heart.

Non-specific methods.—When thrombosis threatens or appears, the affected leg, or preferably both, should be raised above the level of the heart. This can be achieved by putting the foot of the bed up on blocks. Bicycle-type exercises should be encouraged as soon as

the reduction in pain will permit their use, and massage can be instituted usually within two days. These methods alone are often all that is necessary without resorting to more elaborate lines of treatment and are effective in quickly reducing œdema and cutting short the disability. Elevating the legs by raising the foot of the bed alone will quadruple the rate of venous flow and is the most important single measure, but elevation as frequently practised by raising the leg on pillows and sandbags and, by thus immobilising it, destroys half the point of the treatment. Mobility must not be restricted.

Heparin.—This is the most important, the safest and the most certain of the anticoagulant drugs. It is prepared from mammalian lung and liver. It is one of the strongest organic acids produced within the body, bears a strongly negative electrical charge and is able to combine with various basic compounds in the blood. It acts in several ways, chiefly by preventing the action of thrombin on fibrinogen. It also acts as an antiprothrombin and reduces the conglutination of the platelets and the consequent liberation of blood-clotting enzymes. Its effect, therefore, is to prolong clotting time. Heparin should be given by intravenous injection. It should not be given intramuscularly or subcutaneously, even with the addition of hyaluronidase and 2 per cent procaine, because a hæmatoma may develop at the injection site, the extent of which may be difficult to control, and great pain will be produced. The usual dose is between 8,000 and 10,000 international units administered four-hourly, although in serious emergencies, such as massive pulmonary embolism, 25,000 international units may be injected forthwith (1 mg. equals 100 units). The effect is fully reached within about 60 seconds of administration and tails off within the next four hours, hence the need to repeat the injection. One's objective in treatment should be to increase the patient's clotting time threefold, and one should not be satisfied with a clotting time of less than twelve minutes. Subsequent doses are regulated according to the clotting time achieved. Heparin has the great advantage that the further propagation of clot is immediately suppressed and the case can be brought under control at once, so that, within 48 hours, massage can often be instituted and the patient can be got out of bed as soon as œdema and tenderness show signs of settling.

For some reason clinicians are often reluctant to use this drug, not only because of the inconvenience of giving intravenous injections, but because of the fear that a dramatic hæmorrhage may result. Fortunately a ready antidote to heparin exists in the form of a 1 per cent solution of protamine sulphate which may be given intravenously in doses of 5–10 ml. Payling Wright reckons that 1 ml. of this solution is equivalent in antidote effect to 1,000 international

units of heparin. This antidote, which should always be available when a case is being treated by heparin, acts by neutralising the negative charge on the heparin molecule. A transfusion of fresh blood should be given in addition, and any available or necessary methods adopted of arresting hæmorrhage locally. Overdosage with protamine sulphate may produce a paradoxical anticoagulant effect. It is clearly not desirable to abolish the anticoagulant effect of the heparin completely and as a rough and ready guide bleeding can be brought under adequate control by giving sufficient protamine sulphate to counteract about half the last quantity of heparin given.

Dicoumarol and allied substances.—Dicoumarol and its allies, e.g. phenindione (Dindevan), and warfarin sodium (Marevan), act upon the clotting powers of the blood by preventing the liver from synthesising prothrombin from vitamin K. They also prevent the formation of Factor VII. They are not destroyed in the stomach and can therefore be given by mouth, but their effect is somewhat indirect and delayed because at the time of first administration active prothrombin already in circulation will continue to operate for many hours.

These synthetic anticoagulants are closely related chemically to vitamin K and they probably act by competitive inhibition usurping the place of this vitamin as well as its function in the synthesis particularly of prothrombin. Dicoumarol has now given place to the more easily managed Dindevan and Marevan, the latter being more recent and having advantages of more prolonged action and more easily stabilised control in long-term treatment, but for most obstetrical cases Dindevan suffices.

It will be appreciated that these drugs do not affect the clotting time directly and the control of dosage is carried out by estimating the prothrombin time usually by the Quick one-stage method, or the prothrombin and proconvertin (P. & P.) method of Owren, and more recently the thrombotest (Owren, 1959).

Quick's method uses oxalated venous blood from which the plasma is separated. To the latter a standard thromboplastin solution is added and then calcium chloride. The time take for coagulation is recorded and either expressed as a multiple of the clotting time of a normal control plasma, e.g. $2\frac{1}{2}$ times, or as a percentage of normal prothrombin activity which is calculated by a formula:

$$\text{Prothrombin activity (percentage of normal)} = \frac{K}{PT - A} \text{ when}$$

PT is prothrombin time in seconds, and K and A are contents of 303 and 8·7 respectively.

In Owren's P. & P. method the plasma is diluted to increase sensitivity and bovine plasma, lacking in certain thromboplastin

factors but a good source of fibrinogen and Factor V (proaccelerin) is added. Calcium chloride is then added to complete the reaction and the coagulation time is noted. A graph is plotted of the prothrombin time of normal pooled plasma in a series of dilutions to express the range of times from 100 per cent to one per cent prothrombin. The result of the coagulation time of the sample under test is compared with the same time on this graph, from which can then be read off corresponding prothrombin percentage concentration. The therapeutically desired result is in the range of about 10–14 per cent of normal prothrombin concentration.

The thrombotest is designed to evaluate all four factors which these oral anticoagulants may suppress, namely Factor II (prothrombin), Factor VII (proconvertin), Factor IX (Christmas factor) and Factor X (Stuart-Prower factor). This is achieved by an all-in-one reagent (Thrombotest) containing crude cephalin, thromboplastin from ox or horse brain, adsorbed bovine plasma freed from the four factors concerned but containing the other clotting factors not affected by the anticoagulants and finally calcium chloride. This reagent is reconstituted with distilled water and can be used for testing capillary blood or venous samples.

Results are obtainable with little technical equipment or skill in 2–3 minutes and are expressed as a percentage of normal. Anticoagulant therapy should aim at about 15 per cent (range 10–25 per cent of normal).

These anticoagulants and the present methods of control are now regarded as safe, but certain factors should be borne in mind which may seriously modify the patient's response. Aspirin, and, in fact, salicylates generally exaggerate the increase in prothrombin time and should be avoided. Their even greater danger is that of an uncontrollable hæmatemesis. Broad spectrum antibiotics, by influencing the intestinal flora and thus interfering with the synthesis of vitamin K may, apparently, potentiate the anticoagulant effect. Chlorpromazine and phenylbutazone also exaggerate these effects and may have been inadvertently prescribed to control the patient's symptoms. Secondary infection, debilitating conditions and renal failure favour over-reaction, while diarrhœa and liquid paraffin may interfere with absorption and reduce the effect. Hæmaturia is usually the first sign of overdosage, and a hæmorrhagic tendency is not usually exhibited until the prothrombin falls to 20 per cent of normal.

Usually the effect of phenindione is in full swing with adequate dosage within 18 hours. Following the withdrawal of the drug, the effects persist for several days. Dosage is usually 200 mg. by mouth initially, followed by a daily dose of 100 mg., more or less, according to the results of prothrombin estimations which should be repeatedly made as long as the patient continues on this treatment. The dose

for warfarin sodium is much lower, 40–50 mg., followed by a maintenance daily dose of 3–20 mg. according to prothrombin tests. Overswings take longer to correct and stabilize.

The antidotes to overdosage are the transfusion of fresh blood and the injection of vitamin K. Vitamin K_1 (phytomenadione) is more efficient than vitamin K and, injected intravenously (5 mg.) or given orally (15 mg.), can restore a normal prothrombin level within a few hours. Severe bleeding may require up to 20 mg. intravenously (Konakion) given very slowly. Fresh blood transfusion is more rapidly effective and counteracts the drug at once, but further transfusion may be necessary later as the drug already absorbed continues to operate.

Venous ligation.—This operation is favoured by certain general surgeons and is designed to prevent pulmonary embolism, but it has little place in obstetrics and further thrombosis and embolism may arise proximal to the ligature. Recurrent embolism in spite of anticoagulant therapy may, however, necessitate it, but I would first suspect the determination with which the treatment had been pushed. I have yet to meet the case in which I was convinced of the necessity for the operation. Ligation can be performed with impunity up to the lower inferior vena cava, although later disability in the affected leg may be serious in years to come. If ligating a femoral vein, it is usually preferable, where applicable, to tie off the vein distal to the profunda femoris. The prompt treatment of embolism, however, or the threat thereof, with heparin should render this operation unnecessary.

Paravertebral block.—The rationale for this treatment has already been given in outlining the work of Ochsner and De Bakey. These workers managed to obtain relief by its use in 65 per cent of their cases with one or two treatments only, but in a few instances had to give five or six blocking injections. Pain was relieved within 20 minutes and temperature decreased within 24 hours, but the earlier the sympathetic block was performed the better. This treatment is not very frequently employed. In the first place cases must be carefully selected as suitable and the affected leg should be not only œdematous and white but also cold, thereby signifying arterial spasm. Often these criteria are not fully satisfied, and it is perhaps for this reason that although I have seen the treatment attempted on a number of occasions, I have never been very impressed with the immediate results.

OUTLINE OF TREATMENT IN SPECIFIC INSTANCES

There is no set line of treatment for thrombosis as a whole, but the following are some remarks applicable to the different varieties. **Mild cases of deep thrombosis and cases of superficial throm-**

bosis.—The treatment recommended is to raise the foot of the bed on blocks and to encourage muscle activity as soon as possible in order to defeat venous stasis and to prevent the persistence of œdema. The risk of pulmonary embolism in superficial thrombophlebitis is small in obstetrics and in our view does not justify the use of anticoagulants, except in post-operative cases, for example after Cæsarean section or if the process appears to be spreading. Phenylbutazone, dose 200 mg. thrice daily by mouth for three days and thereafter reduced to 100 mg. doses for a further two days, making a five-day course in all, produces rapid relief from pain and the signs of inflammation and œdema subside within 48 hours without confining the patient to bed. 169 such cases (10 of them antenatal) were thus treated by de Soldenhoff and Ross (1960) without incurring embolism, and in all of them resolution was sufficiently rapid not to delay dismissal from hospital. The limb was supported with crepe bandaging or elastic stocking and early ambulation was maintained.

Antenatal thrombosis.—Although this condition is not common, it is by no means rare and many cases are not reported. Wright (1951) has given an account of the treatment of the condition with anticoagulants. His scheme of treatment was to give heparin intravenously in dosages not exceeding 30,000 international units a day. The heparin molecule is too large to cross the placenta, unlike the Dicoumarol type of anticoagulants which may cause fœtal intracranial hæmorrhage. (This, however, is unlikely to occur if the prothrombin index is not reduced below 10 per cent.) Dicoumarol, therefore, should be given cautiously, and most workers feel that in antenatal thrombosis the prothrombin index should not be pushed below 30 per cent, in other words, to a level which is barely effective, anyway, and that the treatment should be stopped several days before delivery, assuming that this can be predicted. Heparin is not only more rapidly effective but very much safer. Immobility of the affected limb should be discouraged and bicycle exercises should be prescribed. Massage can be started at five days and walking should be possible within about a week. One cannot help feeling that the recovery of such patients is due to the exercises and heparin, but in no way contributed to by the dicoumarol. The most important measure of all, namely elevation of the legs above heart level, should certainly come first.

Severe cases of thrombosis and puerperal white leg.—In this condition the patient is in considerable pain at first and exercises cannot, therefore, be prescribed initially. The legs, as before, should be elevated by raising the foot of the bed and a short course of heparin is given, as outlined earlier, to prevent propagation of the clot *in situ* and the development of additional thrombosis elsewhere. Meanwhile a more prolonged course of treatment with phenindione

or warfarin is got under way. Because these drugs appear in breast milk, lactation should be suppressed. After 48 hours, with the subsidence of pain, massage and gentle movements can be started. Still keeping the legs elevated, full movements and active exercises should be in full swing after about 7 days. At no time should the legs be immobilised with sandbags and roller towels, as was so often practised in the past. The legs are kept raised until the œdema has almost disappeared, usually within about 12 days of this treatment, after which the patient may be allowed up provided a really *efficient* elastic support is applied before rising, to include the whole foot, heel and leg. This support should be used unfailingly whenever the patient is out of bed for a further six months. It is important to treat these cases very strictly, as only thereby can residual disability be prevented.

It remains now to discuss the duration of anticoagulant therapy. The general mistake is to stop too soon. Anything less than three weeks is inadequate and patients so treated and recovering would probably have done quite well without it. Treatment should be maintained for long enough to allow the clot to undergo fibrinolysis or to become thoroughly fibrosed and firmly attached to the vein wall. If pulmonary embolism has occurred the treatment should be continued for several months in order to prevent subsequent pulmonary hypertension and congestive cardiac failure.

Pulmonary embolism.—This is nowadays second only to pregnancy toxæmia as a cause of maternal death. Although it is much more common relatively after Cæsarean section than after vaginal delivery, nevertheless the Ministry of Health Confidential Enquiry Reports on Maternal Deaths (1955–57) indicated that 114 out of 157 cases of fatal embolism followed vaginal delivery and in half of them warning had been given in the form of signs of deep thrombosis or previous small emboli. The greater the physical signs in the leg the less is the risk of pulmonary embolism, and when one leg is severely affected and the patient develops an embolus, it is probable that the source is in the apparently unaffected leg. The traditional story of the patient who sits up in bed, asks for the bed pan and drops dead from pulmonary embolism is misleading in the likely sequence of events. It is more probable that the effort associated with defæcation, by distending the veins with raised intravenous pressure, is responsible for the detachment of the clot.

Seventy per cent of emboli come from the calf or the profunda system and 30 per cent from the internal iliac veins. A large embolus produces such shock and vagal inhibition that the patient dies at once. In more than half the cases, however, the immediate effects are not fatal at first, but there occurs a secondary post-embolic thrombosis within the pulmonary arteries which increases the degree

of lung infarction. Treatment must be very prompt, not only to counter the patient's immediate shock, but also to prevent this secondary thrombosis and a recurrence of fresh embolism. Clinically the patient may have a mild fever suggesting thrombosis which, sometimes after settling for a few days, is followed by a brisk rise in pulse rate and then further fever signifying minor embolism. The immediate symptoms of embolism are related mainly to hypotension, namely faintness, breathlessness and tachycardia. Pleural pain and hæmoptysis are often not present and diagnosis may be difficult, although portable chest radiography may help by demonstrating a rise in the level of the diaphragm and clouding of the costophrenic angle from partial lung collapse (Barritt and Jordan, 1961).

Emergency treatment consists in the immediate intravenous injection of morphia 15 mg. (gr. ¼) and a massive intravenous injection of heparin (25,000 international units). There is now believed to be a further beneficial effect of heparin, since it has been found that it inhibits the vasoconstrictor action of 5-hydroxytryptamine (serotonin) which is released in the early stages of clot propagation by the lysis of blood platelets.

Since the clinical signs in pulmonary embolism are out of proportion to the size of the clot or the volume of infarcted lung, and are due to the liberation of such a humoral agent, it can be seen that heparin's action transcends the prevention of further clot propagation and has the additional rôle of first-aid countering of the systemic effects of the catastrophe. Oxygen is supplied by mask. Noradrenaline may be necessary to maintain an adequate blood pressure and tachycardia is countered with digitalis. During the next 48 hours heparin is given four-hourly to maintain a clotting time of over 12 minutes. This will prevent the propagation of further clotting, and at the end of 48 hours the risk of detachment of clot already formed will have largely disappeared as a result of organisation. The feet are kept up by elevation of the foot of the bed as mentioned before and movements are encouraged as early as possible. The effect of dicoumarol is too late to make it anything more than an "also ran", and it is on heparin that we must rely for getting the case immediately under control during the first critical 48 hours. Nevertheless, warfarin treatment is instituted as soon as possible to cover the longer term treatment.

If the patient lives more than two hours after the first attack, and this is true in more than half the cases, prompt treatment along these lines will provide an excellent chance of recovery.

POSTNATAL ADVICE

There is little point in sending a patient away with instructions to return in six weeks time unless she is given advice on how to manage

meanwhile. She should be encouraged to seek official advice rather than that of her alleged friends should her breasts give trouble or should she be in doubt about baby feeding. Postnatal exercises which can be done as a matter of habit without interfering with housework should be prescribed as follows:

POSTNATAL EXERCISES

These exercises should be done each day for at least six weeks. Do exercises 1–4 six times and work up to twelve times. They can be done while working round the house. Exercises (1) and (2) are very important.

(1) Standing peeling potatoes or standing at bus stop (with legs crossed at ankles or one heel in hollow of opposite foot—ballet stance)—Press thighs together, pull up between legs, pull in abdomen and tighten seat muscles. Hold it all tight while you count four then let it all relax slowly. (This is the movement you would do if you were trying to prevent the passage of water or a bowel movement.)

(2) Standing with back against wall—pull in abdominal wall, tighten seat muscles—(imagine you are tucking your tail between your legs) and try to get lower part of back to touch the wall. This exercise can also be done in sitting position with back against chair or lying on bed with knees bent up and pressing back into bed.

(3) Standing—pull one leg up at the hip so that one leg is shorter than the other. Keep your knee straight; foot should be right off the ground. Repeat with other leg.

(4) Standing—feet together, knees together, thighs pressed together. Move along the floor for a short distance as if "twisting".

(5) Pull in abdomen before bending down to pick up anything. Always pull in abdomen before doing any housework which involves bending.

(6) Do not attempt to lift anything which is very heavy. When lifting an object of moderate weight—bend knees and keep back straight.

(7) Pram pushing. Do not crouch over pram. Keep upright and keep pram close to you. Hold the handle lightly, with elbows easy. Shoulders neither braced nor raised nor depressed but level. When pushing pram uphill lean slightly forward from the hips and bend knees slightly, but don't crouch. See that you are breathing easily.

A problem which is likely to be uppermost in the patient's mind, although one to which she may feel too reticent to confess, is the

question of resumption of marital relations and how, for the mean-time, to avoid further pregnancies. After the first month there need be no restriction with regard to the former although the patient is unlikely to be much interested and young husbands should be particularly warned that this is no unnatural phenomenon. The fear of conceiving straight away is very real. It is usual to prescribe the contraceptive pill only after the first period has re-established itself, but in the exceptionally fertile woman there is no reason why it should not be prescribed from the very first. Intra-uterine contraceptive devices have a high drop-out rate if inserted before eight weeks at least or preferably twelve.

Postpartum sterilisation, easy enough surgically during the first days of the puerperium, while the fundus of the uterus is still easily accessible through a very small incision, is an operation which I have never really liked. For one thing it is not a very suitable time for a woman to make such an irrevocable decision and for another the baby's hold on life may still be precarious. The failure rate is also higher due to recanalisation and I now much prefer to carry out the operation through a laparoscope, which makes it a very minor procedure, after three months.

Pending these measures the patient's husband should be advised to use condom contraception.

IMMUNISATION PROCEDURES

BCG vaccination against tuberculosis should be carried out within the first few days of birth. The baby should receive its first injection for diphtheria, whooping cough and tetanus at the age of three to four months followed by second and third injections at intervals of a month each. Poliomyelitis vaccine by mouth can be given at four to six months of age followed by second and third doses at intervals of four to six weeks. A booster injection for diphtheria, whooping cough and tetanus should be given at the age of eighteen months and smallpox vaccination carried out during the second year.

REFERENCES

1. ARNEIL, G. C., and KERR, MARGARET M. (1963). *Lancet*, **2**, 756.
2. ASTLEY, R. (1963). *Brit. J. Radiol.*, **36**, 2.
3. BARBER, M., HAYHOE, F. G. J., and WHITEHEAD, J. E. M. (1949). *Lancet*, **2**, 1120.
4. BARBER, M., and BURSTON, J. (1955). *Lancet*, **2**, 578.
5. BARRITT, D. W., and JORDAN, S. C. (1961). *Lancet*, **1**, 729.
6. BLAIKLEY, J. B., CLARKE, S., MacKEITH, R., and OGDEN, K. M. (1953). *J. Obstet. Gynæc. Brit. Emp.*, **60**, 657.
7. CAFFEY, J., and ROSS, S. (1956) *Pediatrics*, **17**, 642.

8. CALMAN, R. M., and GIBSON, J. (1953). *Lancet*, **2**, 649.
9. CAMPBELL, A. D., and BLAHEY, P. R. (1950). In *Modern Trends in Obstetrics and Gynæcology*. London: Butterworth & Co.
10. CAMPBELL, MARIE A., FERGUSON, ISOBEL C., HUTCHISON, J. H., and KERR, MARGARET M. (1967). *Arch. Dis. Childh.*, **42**, 353.
11. COLE, B. W., and PITTS, N. E. (1966). *Practioner*, **196**, 139.
12. COLEBROOK, L. (1936). *J. Obstet. Gynæc. Brit. Emp.*, **43**, 691.
13. COLEBROOK, L. (1955). *Lancet*, **2**, 885.
14. COLEBROOK, L., and KENNY, M. (1936). *Lancet*, **1**, 1279.
15. DANIEL, D. G., CAMPBELL, H., and TURNBULL, A. C. (1967). *Lancet*, **2**, 287.
16. DE SOLDENHOFF, R., and ROSS, A. H. M. (1960). *Practitioner*, **185**, 321.
17. DONALDSON, J. M. B. (1950). *J. Obstet. Gynæc. Brit. Emp.*, **57**, 62.
18. ELIAS-JONES, T. F., GORDON, I., and WHITTAKER, L. (1961). *Lancet*, **1**, 571.
19. GARREY, M. M., PATERSON, M. M., and EVANS, J. M. (1964). *Lancet*, **2**, 1057.
20. GIBBERD, G. F. (1953). *Amer. J. Obstet. Gynec.*, **65**, 1038.
21. GILLESPIE, W. A., SIMPSON, K., and TOZER, R. C. (1958). *Lancet*, **2**, 1075.
22. GUTHRIE, R., and WHITNEY, S. (1964). *Phenylketonuria*, Children's Bureau, Publication No. 419. Washington, D.C.: U.S. Dept. of Health, Education & Welfare.
23. HELLMAN, L. M., KOHL, S. G., and PALMER, J. (1962). *Lancet*, **1**, 227.
24. HODGE, C. (1967). *Lancet*, **2**, 286.
25. HUNTINGFORD, P. J., WELCH, G., GLASS, V., and WETHERLEY-MEIN, G. (1961). *J. Obstet. Gynæc. Brit. Cwlth.*, **68**, 179.
26. HUTCHISON, J. G. P., and BOWMAN, W. D. (1957). *Acta pædiat. (Uppsala)*, **46**, 125.
27. HYTTEN, F. E., YORSTON, J. C., and THOMSON, A. M. (1958). *Brit. med. J.*, **1**, 310.
28. KEKWICK, A. (1956). *Brit. med. J.*, **1**, 796.
29. MACDONALD, D., and O'DRISCOLL, K. (1965). *Lancet*, **2**, 623.
30. MACVICAR, J. (1968). Personal communication.
31. MANN, T. P. (1955). *Lancet*, **1**, 613.
32. MANN, T. P. (1963). *Nursing Times*, **59**, 15.
33. MANN, T. P., and ELLIOTT, R. K. (1957). *Lancet*, **1**, 229.
34. NEWSON, L. J., and NEWSON, E. (1962). *Brit. med. J.*, **2**, 1744.
35. OCHSNER, A., and DE BAKEY, M. (1940). *J. Amer. med. As.*, **114**, 117.
36. OWREN, P. A. (1959). *Lancet*, **2**, 754.
37. PLUECKHAHN, V. D. (1961). *Brit. med. J.*, **2**, 779.
38. Population Screening by Guthrie Test for Phenylketonuria in S.E. Scotland. Report by Consulting Pædiatricians & Medical Officers of Health (1968). *Brit. med. J.*, **1**, 674.
39. SHELLEY, HEATHER J., and NELIGAN, G. A. (1966). *Brit. med. Bull.*, **22**, 34.
40. STEVENSON, J. S., and SCOTT, J. (1967). *Hlth Bull (Edinb.)*, **25**, 47.
41. THEOBALD, G. W. (1959). *Brit. med. J.*, **2**, 1364.
42. WALLER, H. (1946). *Arch. Dis. Childh.*, **21**, 1.

43. WILLIAMS, R. E. O. (1958). *Publ. Hlth. Rep.* (*Wash.*), **73,** 961.
44. WILLIAMS, R. E. O. (1961). *Lancet*, **2,** 173.
45. WOLINSKY, E., LIPSITZ, P. J., MORTIMER, E. A., and RAMMELKAMP, C. H. (1960). *Lancet*, **2,** 620.
46. WRIGHT, H. P. (1951). *J. Obstet. Gynæc. Brit. Emp.*, **58,** 272.
47. WRIGHT, H. P. (1953). *Brit. med. J.*, **1,** 987.

CHAPTER XXV

POSTMATURITY AND DYSMATURITY

To the practising obstetrician the problem of post-maturity constantly recurs and it is surprising how little guidance most of the textbooks supply. How far is it a clinical entity in its own right? How much does it matter? How can one be sure that the case is postmature? What are the risks and what steps should be taken to counter them?

The difficulties arise from the absence of any fixed criteria. Size of infant alone is not enough, for the postmature baby is not always unduly large and, conversely, very large and apparently postmature babies may be born before the 40th week of pregnancy.

If postmaturity is abnormal, there should be some evidence of abnormality either in mother, child or in the process of labour, and a diagnosis by dates alone is all too often not supported by any such concrete and abnormal findings. The expected date of delivery, as reckoned by Naegele's rule, can only be calculated from the beginning of the last menstrual period and, except in rare instances, it cannot be known precisely when conception occurred.

The average duration of pregnancy so calculated is 280 days, and if this period is exceeded by 14 days or more it is reasonable to believe pregnancy to be prolonged, but this is not the same thing as saying that it is abnormal without other evidence. As Wrigley (1958) has said, there can no more be an "exact" time for gestation than an "exact" height or an "exact" weight for everyone.

Before diagnosing postmaturity with confidence, more than one criterion should be satisfied.

Finn Bøe used three standards:

1. Pregnancy had exceeded 290 days.
2. Fœtal length exceeded 54 cm.
3. Fœtal weight exceeded 4,000 g. (approx. 8¾ lb.).

All three conditions were satisfied in 2 per cent of cases which were thus classified as postmature, but only the first is ascertainable with any accuracy before the actual delivery.

The incidence of postmaturity, then, will clearly vary widely according to the arbitrary standards employed.

In Aberdeen, for example, McKiddie found that 24·6 per cent of 6,803 pregnant women went more than seven days beyond their expected date, while Rathbun in America found that 13·2 per cent

(approximately half the above percentage) had overrun their dates by more than a fortnight.

McKiddie noted no significant difference in the age groups of patients becoming "postmature". Where the provisional diagnosis of postmaturity is confirmed retrospectively by taking into account the baby's size, as regards both length and weight, the true incidence of postmaturity is certainly more in the region of 2 per cent. The babies of multiparæ tend to be heavier at birth than their elder siblings, but their length is not increased in the same ratio, so that if both factors are reckoned, postmaturity is no more likely to be confirmed.

It is probable that the incidence of true postmaturity satisfying two or more criteria would be more common were it not for the prevalence of induction of labour as a therapeutic measure to forestall it.

ÆTIOLOGY

Not much is yet known about the causes of postmaturity. The earliest beginnings of pregnancy are unlikely to provide an explanation, for it is generally agreed that the ovum can be fertilised only within the first twenty-four hours of ovulation. Coitus may, however, provoke ovulation outside the normal time limits, and although embedding of the fertilised ovum does not occur for a further five to eight days, nevertheless, it must occur at least two days before the menstrual flow would have been due or menstruation will follow; thus it will be seen that provoked ovulation later in the cycle would, at the most, account for no more than a week of apparent postmaturity.

Pregnancy can be artificially prolonged in lower animals, such as rabbits, by administering large doses of progesterone, and it is very likely that in humans endocrine influences play a large part, but progesterone in the human species has not been found capable of producing this effect.

As poor nutrition and bad social conditions can cause prematurity, so, conversely, an improved standard of living might be expected to encourage pregnancy to be prolonged, but there is nothing to suggest that it occurs to any abnormal extent. Finn Bøe noted that since 1900 there had been a tendency for the duration of pregnancy and the size of babies to be increased on average, though only to a slight degree, particularly where pregnancy mainly coincided with the summer months; but during the privations of the German occupation of Norway, pregnancy was not appreciably shortened, although birth weights tended to fall, presumably as a first result of malnutrition.

Hereditary factors are of the most certain importance and postmaturity tends to recur in successive pregnancies in the same

woman, which is a point of some prognostic significance. The condition often runs in families.

Lastly, the diabetic patient and the diabetic-prone or "prediabetic" woman tend to produce oversize and "postmature" infants.

LEGAL ASPECTS

These can be very vexing. The plaintiff is usually the supposed father who is disputing paternity on the grounds that he has had no opportunity to cohabit with his wife within the usually accepted limits of pregnancy's duration. These are not pleasant cases in which to give evidence and all the possible signs of postmaturity will have to be carefully weighed. No official upper limit has been fixed by the courts, and since the onus of proof lies with the plaintiff, the mother is likely to be given the benefit of any doubts, and doubts there will nearly always be. It is quite certain that no judicial decision will ever alter the husband's attitude and, whatever the result of the action, the child is bound to suffer in either case.

To state categorically that a pregnancy of, for example, 330 days is impossible in a given case is often beyond the competence of a medical witness to decide in the present state of our knowledge, and the courts are likely to seek subsidiary evidence of chastity, or the reverse, in the mother, in trying to reach a decision, and the case will not simply be dismissed on precedent alone.

The famous case, many years ago, of Gaskill v. Gaskill was dismissed in the mother's favour, there being no corroborative evidence whatever of lack of chastity: in this instance pregnancy was stated to have lasted for 331 days, and, if one were to be guided by precedent, it would appear that any period of gestation within that figure would, in subsequent actions, be upheld. Furthermore, advances on this figure might come to be accepted without any foreseeable limit. More recently, however, the case of Preston Jones v. Preston Jones went in the opposite direction and the stated duration of pregnancy was 360 days.

PATHOLOGY

If postmaturity is an abnormal condition it must, of course, have its own pathology.

Firstly, the fœtus is increased in size, to the possible detriment of labour. Secondly, ossification proceeds apace and results in a head which is not only larger but definitely harder and therefore less able to mould in labour. Thirdly, oxygen saturation is diminished, and though to some extent compensated for by fœtal polycythæmia, the postmature infant is liable to approach the verge of intra-uterine asphyxia.

Barcroft and Young, taking samples of blood from the anterior fontanelles of rabbit fœtuses while still *in utero* found a progressively diminished oxygen saturation level from term onwards until death occurred from asphyxia due to postmaturity. A similar mechanism has been demonstrated in humans (Walker and Turnbull, 1953; Walker, 1954).

Walker found that there was a progressive fall in the percentage level of oxygen saturation in umbilical vein blood during the second half of pregnancy from 70 per cent at about the 30th week, 60 per cent just before term and deteriorating rapidly to 30 per cent by the 43rd week—a level at which meconium-staining of the liquor, as a consequence of asphyxia, was inevitable. Furthermore, Walker and Turnbull found that this adverse trend was accelerated in cases of pre-eclamptic toxæmia or where there had been bleeding earlier in pregnancy.

From a study of the clearance rates of radio-sodium from the myometrium, Moore and Myerscough (1957) inferred that the rate of uterine blood flow was reduced in normal primigravidæ past term and that pre-eclampsia reduced the clearance rates still further. They admitted, however, a wide range of rates in normal subjects, which limits the value of the method in trying to decide which case is outliving its placental efficiency.

The influence of increasing maternal age is also reckoned by Baird (1957) to reduce placental sufficiency so that the Aberdeen school favours routine induction of labour in all primigravidæ over the age of 25 whose pregnancy runs beyond the 41st week.

An entirely opposite view stems from Belfast where Bancroft-Livingston and Neill (1957), from a careful study likewise of umbilical venous blood, showed no correlation whatever between the oxygen level thereof and either fœtal or maternal age.

Their finding would certainly indicate that the association of postmaturity and intra-uterine hypoxia has been overstressed and most authorities nowadays take an intermediate view between these rival schools of thought.

The controversy continues with unabated vigour amongst all who discuss postmaturity, which shows that the truth of the matter is neither plain nor simple.

Fœtal hæmoglobin has a greater affinity for oxygen than adult hæmoglobin, and the ratio of the fœtal to the adult variety falls progressively in later pregnancy, and presumably still more in protracted pregnancy, so that even if placental efficiency did not lessen, this of itself would contribute to anoxia.

The placenta is an ageing organ, though to what extent its functional capacity is lowered is not fully known. Although its weight is increased, much of its substance is infarcted and therefore useless.

The structural evidences of ageing, however, are not fully matched by loss of efficiency, and the rate of transfer, for example, of radio-sodium per gramme of placental weight is known to increase at least right up to term.

Microscopic examination does not help as yet in recognising placental ageing and there is scope for research here.

Calcification of the placenta is negligible in prematurity, but is more evident when the case has become postmature, whether assessed by radiography, chemistry or histological examination; nevertheless, its presence is not reliably related to adverse effects on the fœtus.

The postmature fœtus, besides being more exposed to anoxia, has also to live in a restricted environment of a progressively diminishing volume of liquor amnii, which may handicap the processes of labour. From the 37th week onwards the volume of liquor gets rapidly less (Elliott and Inman, 1961) from an average amount of about 1200 ml. until by the 43rd week it may be no more than 100 ml. in all, a clinical point which may be noticeable to the same observer supervising the case.

CLINICAL SIGNS AND DIAGNOSIS

Mistaken dates account for more errors in diagnosing post-maturity than any other factor and should be very carefully scrutin-ised. As recounted earlier, women candidates at examinations commonly assure me that less than half of all women are cast-iron sure about the date of their last period. The patient may, however, give accurate information, but conception may have occurred during a cycle which happened to be prolonged.

Normally ovulation occurs approximately fourteen days before menstruation and fertilisation of the ovum is unlikely to take place more than a day or two after it. If the menstrual cycle is one, for example, of seven weeks, this would introduce a positive error of three weeks in calculating the expected date of delivery from the onset of the last menstrual flow. It is therefore necessary to know the history of the menstrual rhythm. Where it has previously been as regular as clockwork, errors are less likely to be made, but even these cases are subject to unpredictable arrhythmia occasionally, and it is always possible that ovulation might have been delayed in any given instance. Since ovulation can be provoked, out of turn, by coitus, another source of error becomes apparent. Where a reliable history of isolated acts of intercourse can be obtained, some guidance may be forthcoming, since the ability of spermatozoa to fertilise the ovum does not usually outlive thirty-six to forty-eight hours, although living spermatozoa can sometimes be found in the cervix after as long as a week.

During antenatal supervision a record should always be made of the time of quickening, which will pin down the duration of pregnancy at that time to at least sixteen weeks. Records of the size of the uterus are far more valuable in the earlier months of pregnancy than in the later and careful notes at the time may prevent many subsequent doubts.

Normally the maternal weight stops increasing at about term and begins to fall. This is a useful sign that the case is at least mature but Browne (1962) attaches even greater importance to this sign and regards it as evidence of placental insufficiency so commonly associated with prolonged pregnancy. On examining the abdomen of the postmature case, the relative quantity of liquor to the size of the baby may appear palpably reduced. The child has increased muscle tone, giving an impression of ramrod rigidity, but this impression is largely due to the diminished amount of liquor. The value of this observation is enhanced if it is made by the same pair of hands at each visit (Wrigley, 1946).

Vaginal examination is sometimes helpful. A deeply engaged head, well applied to a thinned lower uterine segment and a ripe cervix, will suggest that the child is at least mature. The hardness of the skull cannot be very reliably assessed at this stage and the state of the fontanelles is more misleading still.

Attempts at fœtal mensuration, although of slight help in assessing prematurity, are unlikely to assist much in estimating postmaturity. The length of the fœtus in a well-flexed attitude (and herein lies the mischief) is usually double the direct distance of breech to vertex, which at term is not less than 50 cm.

Radiology may provide some help, by a study of ossification centres, though errors of up to four weeks are possible here.

The ossification centre of the cuboid usually appears at term and its appearance denotes probable maturity. The centre at the upper end of the tibia appears at about the same time but is less reliable, while the lower end of the femur usually begins to ossify somewhat earlier. Even twins, however, may show differing evidences of maturity on the basis of ossification centres (Cope and Murdoch, 1958).

Cephalometry by X-rays is often disappointing largely because it is difficult to be sufficiently certain of the distance of the fœtal head from the X-ray tube and errors are magnified on the film, and when one is dealing in significant fractions of a centimetre, it is easy to see how small errors of technique can spoil results.

The biparietal diameter, on average, increases by 0·17 cm. or more each week in the last few weeks of pregnancy. The actual attitude of the head is less important than its distance from the tube as, even though an oval shadow is cast, the smaller diameter of that oval will

correspond to the greater circular section of the head, i.e. the biparietal diameter. Our own technique of employing sonar for measuring the biparietal diameter *in utero* has been described on numerous occasions.[12, 13, 14, 34, 35] In our opinion the biparietal diameter is more closely related to maturity than it is to actual birth weight and this is a very useful point. A biparietal diameter of 9·8 cm., for example, indicates maturity at the very least and one of 10·1 cm. or over strongly suggests that the case is postmature even though the weight itself may not exceed 7 lb. In our practice, decisions as to maturity and postmaturity are more readily made by sonar than by resorting to radiography.

Diagnosis after delivery should be confirmed if only to guide one in future pregnancies, because postmaturity is often recurrent and the course of the present labour may provide very helpful information in years to come. The two most definite postpartum signs are a birth weight of over 4,500 g. (10 lb.) and a foetal length of more than 54 cm. The closure of the posterior fontanelle is too variable a sign to be trusted.

There is one important sequence of events which is worth mentioning in regard to postmaturity: occasionally a patient at or about term appears to go into labour and then, before getting properly under way, all signs of labour cease and pregnancy drags on for perhaps a week or more; hormonal influences are probably at work in discouraging true labour from establishing itself. When this happens one should be warned that maturity has been reached and overstepped and there is a strong case for not withholding induction for more than a few days because of the possibility of intra-uterine foetal death. If maternal weight is dropping at the same time, there should be even less hesitation in regarding the case as postmature.

Attempts at assessing biological maturity by cytological study of cervical and vaginal smears are being made at a number of centres, but reports are conflicting. So much depends upon the quality of the cytology. Nevertheless, this technique offers considerable hope.

More definite is a study of the cells within the liquor amnii, but this entails either deliberate amniocentesis or artificial rupture of the membranes if they have not already ruptured spontaneously. The investigation is therefore not as useful as often as its simplicity would otherwise indicate. It was noted by Brosens and Gordon that 0·1 per cent aqueous solution of Nile Blue sulphate stained mature foetal squamous cells orange. The Nile Blue test was first introduced to confirm or refute the diagnosis of premature rupture of the membranes, but it was observed that the proportion and intensity of orange-stained cells increased with the maturity. In fact between the 38th and 40th week of pregnancy there is a very sharp rise in the percentage of such cells to over 50 per cent, whereas the percentage

is less than 10 per cent at 36 weeks. Sharpe, however, found that with this test no orange-stained cells could be found in hydramnios.

Placental enzyme activity has also been studied as an index of placental ageing and therefore of significant threat from placental insufficiency. So far the enzymes studied have too wide a scatter even in normal cases to provide diagnostic evidence.

The study of pregnanediol and œstriol excretion rates (particularly the latter) may also declare diminishing placental function but unless serial records have been made over a long time and diurnal variations can be studied in sufficient detail to discount them the evidence is not likely to be of much help to the clinician faced with a given problem.

Effects and Hazards of Postmaturity

In the genuine case the risks are very real. Already short of oxygen the baby will not tolerate further hypoxia well in labour, and may die of intrapartum asphyxia. This risk is by no means uncommon and the stillbirth rate in postmaturity (5·6 per cent Rathbun) is not far short of twice that of babies born at term, largely due to this factor. In the past so much attention has been focused on the increased weight and size of the baby that this most important aspect of physiology has been sometimes overlooked.

It is true that the head is larger, and this may make labour more difficult, especially as it does not readily mould, but there is some compensation in the fact that the head is harder and therefore protects the brain better from mechanical injury. Certainly these babies stand difficult forceps deliveries rather better than most, and there should be no hesitation in applying the forceps as soon as fœtal distress (which is asphyxial) appears in the second stage of labour. Signs of fœtal distress are much commoner than usual both before and during labour.

Fortunately the neonatal death rate is not significantly altered once the postmature baby has been safely born.

Labour itself is likely to be slightly prolonged and is often associated with a deflexed fœtal attitude and a high incidence of occipitoposterior position.

Uterine inertia of one variety or another may complicate these labours. It is difficult here to distinguish cause and effect and postmaturity may even be a manifestation of uterine dysfunction as well as a cause of it.

It is not surprising, therefore, that the operative delivery rate is enormously increased, and, which is noteworthy, this particularly applies to the more serious procedures, high mid-cavity forceps applications, difficult rotations, Cæsarean section and occasionally

craniotomy. Finn Bøe quoted an operative rate of 29 per cent (44 per cent in primigravidæ), of which 19 per cent were Cæsarean sections and 6 per cent craniotomies, a figure which would hardly obtain today. The postpartum hæmorrhage rate is also greatly increased (41 per cent) and is worse in the primigravida, but the routine administration of ergometrine at the end of the second stage will help to counter this hazard. Postpartum shock and collapse are also more prevalent. These factors, together with the possibility of maternal intrapartum pyrexia, very adversely affect puerperal morbidity, and Finn Bøe in his series found maternal mortality practically trebled.

Even after safe delivery of the head, delay may occur with the shoulders in the case of a large baby and not a few are lost through this complication.

Although intracranial hæmorrhage accounts for a large proportion of fœtal deaths, the percentage of unexplained stillbirths increases with the degree of postmaturity. Malpresentations are commoner, especially breech presentation, and because the baby is larger the effects are likely to be more serious.

When labour is inert, which is often the case, especially when the head is too large to "bed down" well in the pelvis and so stimulate contractions, the risks of intrapartum asphyxia are greatly magnified, so that the need for operative delivery becomes more clamant; the relatively diminished quantity of liquor also contributes to dystocia, and the fact that the head may be well engaged and there are no signs of disproportion does not justify a complacent attitude.

In enumerating this formidable list of complications resulting from postmaturity, it may seem that the dangers have been overstressed, since the majority of cases deliver themselves satisfactorily. But a majority result is not good enough, and to foresee a risk is to go half-way towards circumventing it.

MANAGEMENT

There would be no problem if all inductions worked safely and infallibly and if prematurity never resulted by mistake. We cannot afford to lose sight of the possibility that, in postmaturity, artificial rupture of the membranes may carry with it even greater risks to the baby than those which it is hoped to prevent by such interference. Even a failed medical induction is not without its adverse effects upon the patient and the inertia in labour which may follow induction is closely bound up with demoralisation of the patient, or her obstetrician (Gibberd, 1958). Gibberd further pointed out at a discussion for general practitioners at Queen Charlotte's Hospital in 1961 that routine induction would mean that at 41 weeks 20 per

cent of patients would be induced, at 42 weeks, 10 per cent, and at 43 weeks, 3 per cent.

All are nowadays agreed, however, that the combination of postmaturity with pre-eclampsia, hypertension or any history of bleeding earlier in this pregnancy carries risks of intra-uterine fœtal anoxia, and possibly death, which far exceed those of even unsuccessful induction.

All cases therefore of hypertensive disease or of pre-eclampsia or where abortion has threatened earlier or where there has been accidental hæmorrhage, however slight, should not be allowed to overrun their dates and become postmature, but labour should be induced with determination.

The use of the Saling amnioscope[26] provides a view of the forewaters and the liquor beyond and if the liquor appears clear with flakes of clean vernix within it one is encouraged to assume that the case can safely be allowed to continue undelivered for another half week at least; in this way one's hand may be stayed from carrying out injudicious induction in the false belief that the patient was postmature. We occasionally carry out this procedure more often to reinforce a decision already taken not to induce than for any other valid reason, though, of course, amniotomy can easily be undertaken under direct vision at the same time if amnioscopy is included in the technique of induction.

If at induction the liquor is found to be stained with meconium the possibility of having to undertake Cæsarean section should be carefully considered. In such cases the foetal heart must be very vigilantly watched and if labour is not very expeditious Cæsarean section may indeed be indicated, although here again the decision may be reinforced or modified by fœtal scalp blood sampling by the Saling technique[4]. The fœtal heart may not give much warning of imminent fœtal death during labour.

For the uncomplicated case who threatens to become postmature, Wrigley has laid down a few guiding principles based upon a clinical impression of fœtal size and its relation to the amount of liquor. This is hardly exact science, but, next to sonar, it is the best that can yet be offered. He suggests that, if, at term, the baby (observed by the same person) appears to be small, the case should be watched, although he distrusts the elderly primigravida, as do all of us, and favours induction in this case.

If the fœtal size appears normal, at term he is prepared to watch the case, but for a shorter period, and is influenced by maternal age, parity, build and pelvic structure. Induction, forthwith, is advised if the fœtus appears to be large.

Wrigley's scheme is certainly to be preferred to routine induction on the evidence of dates alone, but it takes no account of placental

sufficiency. An objective measurement of this factor to indicate how near the fœtus may be to its doom is a much needed advance in obstetrics. So far all methods, mainly based upon transfer rates across the placenta of radio-active isotopes, have proved unreliable, including several months of experiments along these lines performed by the writer. (It is desirable to limit the dose of radio-sodium in pregnancy to no more than a total of 10 microcuries for all experiments in any one case. The counts so obtained, however, have far too wide a scatter to be trustworthy and the natural background count will be found to be relatively far too high.)

The use of an oxytocin drip undoubtedly raises the percentage of successful inductions of labour, but if the liquor is scanty and stained with meconium it may increase fœtal asphyxia.

Uterine irritability, as an index of the imminence of labour or of the likelihood of success following induction, can be assessed by some such test as that devised by Eddie (1963) in which minimal but increasing dosage of oxytocin, 0·01 to 0·1 units, are administered by dilute intravenous injection and the threshold of uterine response observed.

Cæsarean section should be very readily considered in all cases in which labour, following induction, persistently hangs fire or whenever signs of fœtal distress appear. One cannot escape the impression that uterine inertia and postmaturity are sometimes linked to a common disorder of uterine function and the combination should be taken seriously.

A special warning must be made about the dangers of postmaturity in the presence of a fœtal monster, including anencephaly. Many years ago Munro Kerr drew attention to the fact that about half the cases complicated by anencephaly, if left to their own devices, went postmature. In such circumstances a very dangerous situation may arise in which, when the patient ultimately goes into labour (and I had one such case who went to 46 weeks) the small "head" slips through the partially dilated cervix and comes to press on the pelvic floor and stimulate very powerful uterine contractions, so that the patient endeavours to deliver herself by bearing down before full dilation and before the shoulders can be accommodated by the undilated cervix. In the case referred to above the patient ruptured her lower uterine segment, developed an amniotic embolus and cardiac arrest, a desperate combination of circumstances, which after many hours of cardiac massage had all the unhappy ritual of death on the table and finally defeated all our efforts.

No plea is made for routine induction at 42 weeks or some such arbitrary standard, for far more mistakes are likely to be made through errors in diagnosing or assessing postmaturity than disasters are likely to be avoided thereby. It would be better stated that

when a case has overrun her dates by 14 days one ought to have concrete indications for not inducing labour.

No baby is the better for weighing more than 9 lb. at birth and the mother may ultimately be much the worse for it.

It would be as well to reiterate two rules:

1. Beware of fœtal distress.
2. Beware of delay with large shoulders.

OBSTRUCTED SHOULDERS

This problem is only likely to occur in postmaturity when delivering a very large baby, in fact it may prove the worst part of it. My sorriest experience of it concerned an elderly primigravida with a 14-lb. baby. (Her husband had weighed 15 lb. at birth—an important point to note in postmaturity and one which I overlooked in this case.) After rotating and delivering the head with Kielland's forceps I then ran into trouble with impaction of the anterior shoulder and wasted too much time trying to free it and before using the whole hand to bring down the posterior arm. In that hectic fifteen minutes of brute force, of which one could only be ashamed, the baby died. It is a nightmarish situation and one should be ready for it as soon as it is clear that the anterior shoulder is going to impact.

If not in the lithotomy position the patient must be immediately put there, or failing that, the left lateral position. The dorsal position is worse than useless as it is impossible to pull the head far enough back to free the point of the anterior shoulder. The lithotomy position allows the use of fundal pressure from above which the left lateral position does not, and is to be preferred.

The head is drawn backwards rather than pulled, remembering that the brachial plexus is vulnerable to overstretching, determined fundal pressure is applied from above and an attempt is made with the fingers to encourage rotation of the anterior shoulder under the symphysis. This usually does the trick and as soon as the point of the anterior shoulder is free the head can be lifted forwards and the posterior shoulder delivered. If this fails, general anæsthesia should be induced at once, an attempt meanwhile being made to rotate and push the shoulders round "à la Løvset", so that the posterior shoulder now becomes anterior, using a hand on the abdomen to assist rotation and trying to avoid dislodging the shoulders upwards. Too much time should not be wasted on this manœuvre which is likely to fail if the baby is really huge and tightly wedged. An alternative method is described by Holman (1963). In this method the primary attention is focused on the posterior shoulder, and the head, instead of being drawn backwards, is drawn downwards and forwards in the axis of the pelvis and, preferably with the help of a

second pair of hands, the anterior shoulder is pressed caudally in relation to the fœtus in order to reduce the transverse diameter across the shoulders. Fundal pressure is at the same time maintained.

Needless to say an episiotomy is an important adjunct to any such technique. By now, general anæsthesia should have been induced and the hand, if necessary the whole hand, is introduced to bring out the posterior shoulder or even to deliver the posterior arm. This procedure is very damaging to the maternal pelvic floor.

Sometimes, on introducing the whole hand the reason for the delay may be revealed in the form of an unsuspected gross fœtal abnormality, such as fœtal ascites, etc., and embryotomy may be required.

If the baby is already dead cleidotomy makes possible an easy delivery of impacted shoulders. Strong scissors which will not buckle are required and the most accessible clavicle, usually the anterior, is felt for and brought as far as possible within reach by traction of the head backwards. I have never performed cleidotomy in the living fœtus nor seen it done. For one thing the decision to undertake it on a living child would not be made until all other attempts at delivery had failed, by which time the baby would be dead and the immediate relation of the subclavian vessels below the clavicles is enough to discourage one.

Likewise the decision to use a hook is never made at the time as such instruments of a bygone age are never available when the emergency arises. That they would damage the brachial plexus and fracture or separate an epiphysis of the humerus is more than likely and up to the very last experience encourages one that a more normal delivery of the shoulders will yet be achieved, as is usually the case. Nevertheless, disasters from obstructed shoulders still occur and in retrospect provide some of the most mortifying recollections in obstetrics.

DYSMATURITY

This is an important subject and goes by a variety of names, including "the small for dates baby," "placental insufficiency," "intra-uterine growth retardation", and so-called "postmaturity syndrome", but "dysmaturity" is both brief and descriptive.

By international agreement all babies with birth weights below 2,500 g. (5½ lb.) are classified as premature but, as the 1958 Perinatal Mortality Survey carried out in the United Kingdom indicated, one out of three of these babies is not premature at all, but, in fact, dysmature. Dysmaturity has a totally different pathology from prematurity and a different prognosis too and taking the long view in those that survive, the premature baby, weight for weight, is likely

to fare far better, including intellectually, than its dysmature counterpart.

It is a tragic fact that dysmaturity may be a recurrent condition in some women, by no means those confined to the poorer social classes. Postmaturity and fœtal abnormality may both be associated with dysmaturity but there are certain general conditions well known to be associated with intra-uterine malnutrition and hence dysmaturity, such as pre-eclamptic toxæmia, all hypertensive conditions, recurrent antepartum hæmorrhage, chronic renal disease and many cases of heart disease. Diabetes also produces its own type of dysmaturity.

We define nowadays as dysmature any baby whose birth weight is below the tenth percentile of weight for gestation according to the Lubchenko Tables.[21, 35] These tables, based upon Caucasian types of women, were drawn up in Colorado where there are residential areas at high altitudes and the figures may be slightly less than for other parts of the Western world, but they serve to indicate dysmaturity where the gestation period is clearly known. A further distinction between dysmaturity and prematurity can be made by employing the Nile Blue sulphate stain on the cells of the liquor amnii, as it has been observed[28] that the percentage of orange-stained cells is not affected by dysmaturity and corresponds to the known gestational age.

Commonly, the dysmature infant is scraggy with poor subcutanous fat and has a poor resistance to cold. The liver reserves of glycogen are poor and these babies are particularly liable to dangerous attacks of hypoglycæmia which, if not treated promptly, may result in permanent mental damage. The brain is normally developed in accordance with the gestational age, as are the lungs, which however, are liable to the effects of meconium inhalation because fœtal distress *in utero* is common.

Ischæmia of the placental site would appear to be a factor common to most cases,[33] because experimental ischæmia of one horn of a gravid rat uterus has been shown in the second half of pregnancy to produce stunting of the fœtuses contained within it. This observation would support what is known about reduced placental blood flow in hypertensive states, for example. The placenta is not just a filter for the passage of oxygen or glucose or small molecules. In actual fact work is done by the placenta in transferring even these substances across the so-called barrier, so that placental insufficiency results not only in chronic hypoxia but also in chronic subnutrition. Normally the placenta weighs about a sixth of the weight of the infant, but in dysmaturity it may weigh appreciably less and the villous surface area is said to be much reduced.

If we could accurately assess placental function during pregnancy we would have solved one of the biggest classes of unresolved

obstetrical problems today. Attention is therefore being focused upon hormone excretion levels in the maternal urine. Of all the forms of urinary hormone assay the measure of œstrogens gives more information about the growth and development of the fœtus than any other form.[23] The ratio of the usual œstrogens, namely œstriol, œstrone and œstradiol, is usually given as 3:3:1 in the non-pregnant woman but in pregnancy the ratio goes up tenfold in the case of œstriol; in other words an enormous increase in œstriol is secreted by the placenta and gives the best biochemical index of placental function and is generally preferred to pregnanediol excretion curves. Pregnanediol levels less closely indicate blood levels of progesterone than do urinary levels of œstrogen as indices of plasma œstrogen levels. Chorionic gonadotrophin levels are even less reliable in regard to placental function. Œstriol secretion by the placenta depends upon the activity of the fœtal adrenal cortex and this, in its turn, depends upon ACTH from a functioning fœtal pituitary. The anencephalic pregnancy therefore produces very low œstriol levels.

Œstriol excretion levels as isolated tests are of very little use and proper curves should be drawn from repeated assay. Even so, low levels do not always indicate placental insufficiency and the scatter is wide. As Klopper (1965) has remarked, "It is difficult to represent the changing picture of retarded fœtal growth without producing a bewildering web of crisscross lines," and falls in œstriol output may be "reflections of an underlying disease process affecting the fœto-placental unit."

There are indeed many pitfalls in getting accurate and worth-while œstriol results even accepting the fairly wide variation in day to day excretion levels, which necessitate averaging at least two or three consecutive 24-hour collections of urine. Often bad results are due to bad specimen collection and it is usual practice to check that a urinary specimen is indeed a 24-hour collection by estimating creatinine content in the whole sample. Normally this is fairly stable within about 20 per cent per person every day; somewhere about 900 mg. a day according to the patient's weight. Any specimen which suddenly shows, for example, 500 mg. can certainly be discarded as an incomplete 24-hour collection.

Only a minority of hospitals can undertake this volume of biochemical work which is by no means easy and even we, with our extravagant facilities, have to restrict our œstriol studies to the following groups:

History of dysmaturity in previous pregnancies.
Cases where the uterus is small for known dates.
Maternal diabetes, or hypertensive conditions.
Chronic renal disease.

Recurrent antepartum hæmorrhage.
Certain cases of cardiac disease.

In addition, dysmaturity is suspected where there has been a loss of maternal weight in pregnancy or a gain of only a very few pounds. Scanty liquor is also sometimes a sign of dysmaturity.

It seems to us that growth retardation can be even more accurately and directly estimated by actually measuring fœtal growth and, as already mentioned, the use of sonar to measure the growth rate of the biparietal diameter is now increasingly employed by us.[29, 34, 35] At least with this technique the answers are immediate and any fall off in growth rate as compared with a standard chart is regarded as ominous. It is now our practice to combine biparietal diameter growth curves with œstriol excretion curves on the same chart (Fig. 1). Both techniques may reinforce unequivocally a clinical impression that intra-uterine growth is retarded and may indicate the need for elective delivery of the fœtus before it is too late. Here at least is a concentrated attack on the problem of macerated stillbirth.

What then of the survivors? As Coyle and her colleagues in Dundee have warned, a 24-hour excretion of less than 3 mg. of œstriol indicates the likelihood of intra-uterine fœtal death in the near future, although this is not invariable. In their follow up study of 14 babies whose mothers had a low œstriol excretion rate during pregnancy Wallace and Michie (1966) found that only 8 were completely normal, 2 were seriously handicapped neurologically and were mentally retarded, a third had a hemiplegia, another had retarded speech and subnormal behaviour, another was retarded and "over-active", and one had a minor neurological abnormality. These are daunting observations. Furthermore there is an increased incidence of intracranial hæmorrhage because many of these babies had thrombotest levels less than 10 per cent of normal, which even vitamin K_1 may not correct soon enough.[18] Dysmature babies therefore should be tested for clotting defects, particularly of prothrombin, and treated if there is any suspicion of intracranial hæmorrhage by fresh frozen plasma or fresh blood while waiting for vitamin K_1 to take effect. Another serious complication of dysmaturity, as already mentioned, is neonatal hypoglycæmia which has been described in the previous chapter. This must be tested for routinely and treated urgently with intravenous glucose.

It is all very well for the obstetrician to recognise dysmaturity *in utero* and to deliver the baby into a more congenial environment at the optimum moment, but if the baby is to have a real chance of being spared the hideous possible sequelæ of dysmaturity in later life he must be transferred urgently to the care of a pædiatric special department. Cases therefore of suspected dysmaturity in pregnancy

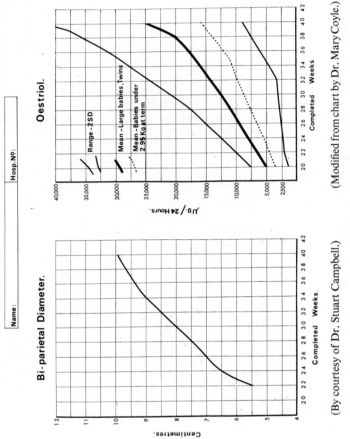

Name:　　　　　　　　Hosp.Nº:

Bi-parietal Diameter.

Centimetres.

Completed Weeks.

Oestriol.

Range - 2SD

Mean - Large babies, Twins

Mean - Babies under
2.95 Kg at term

µg·/ 24 Hours.

Completed Weeks

(By courtesy of Dr. Stuart Campbell.) (Modified from chart by Dr. Mary Coyle.)

25/Fɪɢ. 1.

should be delivered only in a highly equipped hospital with these facilities.

REFERENCES

1. BAIRD, D. (1957). *Brit. med. J.*, **1**, 1061.
2. BANCROFT-LIVINGSTON, G., and NEILL, D. W. (1957). *J. Obstet.Gynæc. Brit. Emp.*, **64**, 498.
3. BARCROFT, J., and YOUNG, I. M. (1945). *J. exp. Biol.*, **21**, 70.
4. BEARD, R. W., and MORRIS, E. D. (1965). *J. Obstet. Gynæc. Brit. Cwlth.*, **72**, 496.
5. BØE, FINN (1950). *Acta obstet. gynec. scand.*, **30**, Suppl. 1.
6. BØE, FINN (1951). *Ibid.*, **30**, 247.
7. BROSENS, I., and GORDON, H. (1965). *J. Obstet. Gynæc. Brit. Cwlth.*, **72**, 342.
8. BROSENS, I., and GORDON, H. (1966). *Ibid.*, **73**, 88.
9. BROWNE, J. C. M. (1962). *Brit. med. J.*, **2**, 1080.
10. COPE, I., and MURDOCH, J. D. (1958). *J. Obstet. Gynæc. Brit. Emp.*, **65**, 56.
11. COYLE, MARY G., GREIG, M., and WALKER, J. (1962). *Lancet*, **2**, 275.
12. DONALD, I. (1968). *Brit. med. Bull.*, **24**, 71.
13. DONALD, I., and BROWN, T. G. (1961). *Brit. J. Radiol.*, **34**, 539.
14. DONALD, I., and ABDULLA, U. (1967). *Brit. J. Radiol.*, **40**, 604.
15. EDDIE, D. A. S. (1963). *Brit. med. J.*, **1**, 723.
16. ELLIOTT, P. M., and INMAN, W. H. W. (1961). *Lancet*, **2**, 835.
17. GIBBERD, G. F. (1958). *Lancet*, **1**, 64.
18. GRAY, O. P., ACKERMAN, ANN, and FRASER, ANNE J. (1968). *Lancet*, **1**, 545.
19. HOLMAN, M. S. (1963). *S. Afr. med. J.*, **37**, 247.
20. KLOPPER, A. (1965). Research on Steroids. *Trans. 2nd Meeting International Study Group for Steroid Hormones*, pp. 63–83.
21. LUBCHENKO, LULA D., HANSMAN, CHARLOTTE, DRESSLER, MARIA, and BOYD, EDITH (1963). *Pediatrics*, **32**, 793.
22. MCKIDDIE, J. M. (1949). *J. Obstet. Gynæc. Brit. Emp.*, **56**, 386.
23. MACNAUGHTON, M. C. (1967). *Amer. J. Obstet. Gynec.*, **97**, 998.
24. MASTERS, M., and CLAYTON, S. G. (1940). *J. Obstet. Gynæc. Brit. Emp.*, **47**, 457.
25. MOORE, P. T., and MYERSCOUGH, P. R. (1957). *J. Obstet. Gynæc. Brit. Emp.*, **64**, 207.
26. MORRIS, E. D., and BEARD, R. W. (1965). *J. Obstet. Gynæc. Brit. Cwlth.*, **72**, 489.
27. RATHBUN, L. S. (1943). *Amer. J. Obstet. Gynec.*, **46**, 278.
28. SHARP, F. (1968). Experience with a test for Estimation of Foetal Maturity by Amniotic Fluid Exfoliative Cytology. (In Press.)
29. THOMPSON, H. E., HOLMES, J. H., GOTTESFELD, K. R., and TAYLOR, E. S. (1965). *Amer. J. Obstet. Gynec.*, **92**, 44.
30. WALLACE, SHEILA J., and MICHIE, EILEEN A. (1966). *Lancet*, **2**, 560.
31. WALKER, J. (1954). *J. Obstet. Gynæc. Brit. Emp.*, **61**, 162.
32. WALKER, J., and TURNBULL, E. P. N. (1953). *Lancet*, **2**, 312.

33. WIGGLESWORTH, J. S. (1966). *Brit. med. Bull.*, **22**, 13.
34. WILLOCKS, J., DONALD, I., DUGGAN, T. C., and DAY, N. S. (1964). *J. Obstet. Gynæc. Brit. Cwlth.*, **71**, 11.
35. WILLOCKS, J., DONALD, I., CAMPBELL, S., and DUNSMORE, I. R. (1967). *J. Obstet. Gynæc. Brit. Cwlth.*, **74**, 639.
36. WRIGLEY, A. J. (1946). *Proc. roy. Soc. Med.*, **39**, 569.
37. WRIGLEY, A. J. (1958). *Lancet*, **1**, 1167.

CHAPTER XXVI

PREMATURITY

"The Obstetrician delivers the baby from the Mother;
the Pædiatrician delivers the baby from the Obstetrician!"
—*Ex-Glasgow Colleague.*

ANY attempt greatly to reduce the present wastage of fœtal life calls for a successful attack upon the problems of prematurity, for no single obstetrical misfortune is more extravagant in this respect, and half of all neonatal deaths occur in premature infants. In 1956, for example, more than 11,000 babies died within the first month of life in England and Wales, and of this number nearly 7,000 weighed less than 2,500 g. There are three facets to consider, namely, the prevention of premature labour, its management when it becomes inevitable and the rearing of the infant so born. Such a child's initial handicaps are easy to appreciate when one reflects that an infant born at thirty-two weeks has lost one-fifth of the normal span of intra-uterine life, and it is surprising, therefore, that even greater degrees of prematurity than this are still compatible with full and normal subsequent development.

The responsibility for the first two sides of the problem lies with the obstetrician, but the third is now increasingly the pædiatrician's concern in any sizeable and up-to-date maternity unit, and good team work between the two services is essential.

DEFINITION

There is no satisfactory definition of prematurity, and for want of a better standard, birth weights of 2,500 g. (5½ lb.) and under have been universally accepted for the purpose of classifying births as premature. Unfortunately this definition takes no account of babies that are in fact dysmature. In other words they are small for dates and, at whatever gestational age birth occurs, their weights are considerably below average levels. This subject was dealt with in the previous chapter, but it also overlaps into the differential diagnosis of prematurity and there is much to suggest a different sort of prognosis too. Walker (1967) holds that babies below the 25th percentile up to 37 completed weeks of pregnancy should be classed as cases of poor intra-uterine growth. As mentioned previously our own standard is

that of babies below the 10th percentile, but Walker has pointed out that in a study of mixed communities there is some danger that selection will provide an excess of female babies born to small mothers and that the 10th percentile for babies of tall primigravidæ corresponds to the 25th percentile for babies of small primigravidæ. Whatever standards are used, however, there can be no doubt that dysmaturity is a syndrome in its own right and differs from prematurity, and there seems to be general unanimity with the opinion expressed by Drillien (1964) that babies born with a very low birth weight because of a shortened gestation period develop relatively better subsequently than babies born with the same low birth weight which cannot be accounted for by prematurity.

The Perinatal Mortality Survey (Butler and Bonham 1963) showed that just over one-third of low birth weight babies in fact are not prematurely born. The condition is likely to be recurrent and in Walker's Dundee series of 215 mothers with babies weighing 2,500 g. or less at 39 weeks or more, 10 per cent had had several small for date babies and a quarter of them had had at least one other child similarly dysmature. Many of these women showed a poor weight gain in pregnancy after 30 weeks.

There are certain characteristic pathological features in the dysmature baby which help to distinguish it from the premature, for example, Wigglesworth (1967) stated that histological examination of the pulmonary alveoli and renal glomeruli showed structures corresponding to the gestational age which may be of course at term or later in spite of the baby's small size. Also there is a much raised ratio of brain to liver weight from the normal figure of about 3:1 to 6:1 in these cases.[14] Their livers are not only relatively smaller but deficient in glycogen[44] and this may be the reason why they are vulnerable to hypoglycæmia[45]. This last complication may have something to do with mental retardation, and blood sugar levels below 20 mg./100 ml. are regarded as critical and worth prompt correction whether symptoms and signs are clinically present or not.

At least the accepted standard of weight is easy to apply and cannot be argued about. Admittedly there are racial differences in mean birth weight for given maturity, and in the case of males this is reputedly 100 g. greater than that of females, but these differences are not large; the greatest source of possible wrong classification is in twins who naturally tend to be underweight for their period of gestation, and this leads to the classifying of nearly half of all twins as "premature".

Incidence.—This varies between 4 and 10 per cent, and depends more upon the social and economic status of the mother than upon anything else, or rather, as Drillien (1957) has shown, the social and

economic circumstances of the mother's childhood upbringing than her state after marriage. In other words, the social grade of the baby's maternal grandfather has more influence upon its chances of being prematurely born than the grading of its own father.

Over England and Wales, as a whole, the incidence of prematurity has remained stationary at 7 per cent and the post-war rise in the general standard of living has not yet had a chance to affect it. The figure is, of course, influenced by the fact that over a third of all still-births are prematurely born; the incidence of live-born prematures is thus lower (e.g. 5 per cent in Scotland). In other words, although prematurity can be a cause of stillbirth, even more often is stillbirth a factor in producing a higher prematurity rate, although in this case premature labour is merely incidental to previous intra-uterine fœtal death. The Sub-Committee of the Central Health Services Council reporting on the prevention of prematurity and the care of premature infants (1961), regarded the problem as sufficiently large in the United Kingdom to justify the provision of at least six cots for premature infants or ill, newborn infants for every 1,000 live births. This need in any sizeable maternity unit should preferably be met by the provision of separate nurseries for premature babies born inside the Maternity Hospital and those born in domiciliary practice, because of a possible different bacteriological status.

Survival chances.—In any large series it can be seen that the chances of survival are directly proportional to the birth weight. This can only be a rough guide in assessing the prognosis in a given case, of course, and one would do better to take more note of the child's actual vigour, which is a far more reliable guide. A birth weight of under 2 lb. gives a chance of about 1 in 30 only, whereas at 3 lb. the chances are nearly 10 times as good at 1 in 3 or even better. At 4 lb. these odds are almost reversed in favour of survival, and at 5 lb. one should be able to save most of the cases.

The same Sub-Committee reported that 46 out of every 100 live premature infants weighing 1,500 g. or less (3 lb. 4 oz.) died within the first 24 hours in 1959 and that only 34 were alive at the end of the fourth week, whereas an additional 500 g. in birth weight up to 2000 g. (4 lb. 6 oz.) more than quartered the death rate within the first twenty-four hours and more than doubled the survival rate in the first month.

It is interesting to note that of those who die, nearly half do so within the first 24 hours and a further 15 per cent die within the second, so that about two-thirds of the deaths occur in under 48 hours, that is, within a period profoundly influenced by the obstetrician's management of the case in labour, since minor injuries at delivery and minor infections contracted are often sufficient to kill a premature infant.

CAUSES OF PREMATURITY

As all the factors which initiate labour are not yet known nor understood, it is often not possible to state why a particular labour should be premature, and in fact over half the cases remain un-explained. This naturally handicaps prophylaxis, and Eastman placed 75 per cent of his cases under this heading; he used two other headings, namely, cases of twins—12 per cent, and, secondly, those cases where pregnancy is complicated by some condition calling for its interruption whether by induction of labour or by Cæsarean section (13 per cent). This group therefore provides the most likely and fruitful source of improved results.

Of these complicating conditions, pre-eclamptic toxæmia is the chief offender (36 per cent), followed by hypertension 17 per cent and placenta prævia 12 per cent. With the first two a few precious extra weeks can sometimes be gained by early recognition and care-ful treatment, and in the case of placenta prævia there is already an improvement in both prematurity rate and fœtal salvage, thanks largely to Macafee's influence on the management of this condition.

It is to be noted that pre-eclamptic toxæmia is a cause of pre-maturity more through the need to terminate pregnancy than through its own direct effects on the woman, although, less often, it may kill the baby *in utero*, thus causing the premature stillbirth of a macerated fœtus.

Beyond these three chief causes listed above there are a large number of conditions each of which makes a small contribution to the prematurity rate, as follows: Hydramnios, by distending the uterus beyond what it will tolerate; accidental hæmorrhage, which may be either a manifestation of toxæmia or may be simply the ex-pression of the mechanism of abortion, though on a grander scale. Fœtal abnormalities, often a cause of miscarriage in earlier weeks, may occasionally cause a spontaneous interruption of pregnancy or, if diagnosed, may call for induction. They also are frequently associated with hydramnios. Syphilis, always quoted as a cause, particularly of premature stillbirth, is less commonly so nowadays, in fact, in far less than 1 per cent of cases, thanks mainly to routine diagnosis in early pregnancy and modern treatment. Genetic factors are also clearly responsible in certain women who seem, often re-peatedly, unable to go through to term. Cervical incompetence, or rather an undue readiness of the cervix to dilate may be a factor and justify the insertion of a Shirodkar type of stitch. (See Chapter II.)

Severe cardiac lesions predispose to premature labour and con-versely postmaturity is not common. Fibroids are often unpredict-able in their effect on pregnancy, but inasmuch as they may provoke abortion, so too they may provoke premature labour. The effect,

however, can only be regarded as mechanical when the mass of fibroids is exceptionally large, and in the average case endocrine factors are probably at work. Erythroblastosis, mainly through the changes produced in the placental villi, may terminate pregnancy early and disastrously. Trauma is responsible for a few cases, not the least common being that of external version, and for this reason, if an anæsthetic is necessary, such an operation is best postponed to within four weeks of term. Psychological shocks can bring on labour at any time in patients whose hold on pregnancy is none too secure. Chronic nephritis is now recognised as a fairly rare complication but is certainly a cause, either of itself, or through the need to terminate pregnancy.

Any serious illness, especially those producing very high temperatures, e.g. pyelitis and pneumonia, can also bring on labour, and it is important to control hyperpyrexia for this as well as for other reasons.

Of all the abdominal operations likely to be followed by premature labour, appendicectomy in a severe case associated with gross peritonitis is the most important, the peritonitis rather than the operation, of course, being the real cause. Myomectomy could be equally disastrous to continued pregnancy at this stage save that such a procedure is so seldom indicated in the later weeks.

Listeriosis (infection with *L. monocytogenes*) is now being increasingly recognised as a cause of premature stillbirth. Seeliger's monograph (1961) gave a full account of the condition. It was first noticed, about 1926, as an infection occurring in rabbits and guinea-pigs, although it can also occur in sheep, goats and rodents. If a baby is born alive having contracted such infection *in utero* it may demonstrate a confusing clinical picture of otherwise unexplained encephalitis, meningitis, septicæmia, pneumonia and conjunctivitis. The pregnant woman is believed to be very susceptible to this condition. The organism, which resembles coryza bacteria, can be cultured from meconium, conjunctival sacs, cerebrospinal fluid and throat swabs of affected babies and the infection can also be identified serologically. It is sensitive to a wide range of antibiotics although streptomycin produces resistant strains readily. An infected mother may yield listeria in blood, urine or cerebrospinal fluid. If the baby is born alive there may be pyrexia, jaundice, cyanosis, dyspnœa, signs of cerebral irritation and, at necropsy, lesions may be found in the central nervous system and foci of necrosis in lung and spleen. The placenta contains granulomatous lesions, and there may be similar lesions in the adrenals. There may be a gap of two or three months between the contraction of the infection by the mother and the delivery of an affected infant, often stillborn or frequently premature and dying in the neonatal period. Accounts of this condition from Western Ger-

many have not been matched in this country and I personally cannot recall a case in my own experience, although this may be because of previous ignorance of the condition, but our pathologists assure us that they have not missed the pathological lesion as above described. Nevertheless, in view of the experience on the European continent of this condition it would be as well to look out for its appearance in this country too.

Premature, spontaneous rupture of the membranes is usually followed by premature labour within the next ten days, but the cause of the membrane rupture is usually obscure.

There remain malnutrition and overwork, not exactly diseases in themselves, but probably more important than all the above subsidiary list put together.

It has already been said that the prematurity rate is an index of social and economic well-being. Baird, for example, showed a rate of 9·18 per cent in hospital cases, whereas the rate was only 5 per cent among those who could afford nursing-home confinements and only 3·9 per cent in those rich enough to engage the services of a specialist. There is no suggestion that the latter two groups had treatment superior to that of the hospital cases, and the differences must be due either to the food they eat or to the easefulness of their lives in pregnancy, and there is no doubt that the poorer woman is usually overworked, either through the need to keep herself in employment, or through the lack of help in household duties. Maternal diet, according to Thomson (1951), has to be very poor indeed for it to have much effect upon birth weight.

Eastman noted a higher rate among patients who did not undergo antenatal supervision, but this is probably due more to their general fecklessness as a class than to any specific virtue in antenatal care.

What is known as the Oslo Experiment is worth noting. During the years 1931–38 a home for unmarried pregnant girls, in which the inmates were cared for throughout pregnancy, showed the very low prematurity rate of 2·2 per cent, whereas the rate was 16 per cent in the case of emergency admissions of such girls not so supervised.

In spite of the war the standard of living in this country and in the U.S.A. has unquestionably risen in the poorer classes, and this factor, coupled with the development of the modern pædiatric service, has approximately halved the premature neonatal death-rate since 1926.

EFFECTS OF PREMATURITY—PATHOLOGY

These are very variable, and the apparent degree of anoxia at birth and in the first few hours of life is not necessarily paralleled by later evidences of permanent damage, so that one would be wrong to despair even in the face of repeated cyanotic attacks. Nevertheless,

no one would believe frequent or prolonged anoxia to be anything but harmful and some mental and intellectual defects can be attributed to this cause. More than five such attacks, however, signify a very bad prognosis (Donald *et al.*, 1958).

Cerebral hæmorrhage is very common and is likely to be present in over 10 per cent of premature infants however delivered, including cases born by Cæsarean section. There are many obvious reasons for this: the softness of the skull provides poor protection, allows rapid and dangerous degrees of moulding and, even without a tentorial tear being sustained, back pressure in the vein of Galen is easily induced by the stress disturbances of intracranial anatomy. Secondly, the smaller veins and capillaries are more fragile than normal and do not withstand well the engorgement of even minor degrees of asphyxia. Of the latter, massive intraventricular hæmorrhage (Figs. 1 (*a*) and (*b*) is the most characteristic lesion and is usually due to the anoxic engorgement and rupture of a vessel in the floor of one of the lateral ventricles. The blood may then track through to the subarachnoid space. This type of lesion is found in the more severe degrees of prematurity and in the ultra-premature and is entirely asphyxial in origin, having nothing whatever to do with trauma, unlike subdural bleeding (Claireaux, 1958).

The possibility that this type of bleeding may be associated with hypoprothrombinæmia should not be overlooked. This is commoner than generally recognised.[53] If this is indeed found to be present correction is achieved most rapidly by transfusion with fresh whole blood. Injections of vitamin K_1 are far more effective and safer than vitamin K analogues, but take longer than fresh blood to reverse the defect.

Throughout the body there are fewer blood vessels, a fact which favours tissue anoxia and the ready development of œdema.

Because of poor muscle development, venous return to the heart is poor. This is particularly noticeable in the relatively stagnant circulation of the extremities.

Heart failure is readily superimposed on asphyxia and pulmonary œdema develops rapidly, still further increasing anoxia and congestion. Such a baby can literally drown in its own pulmonary œdema fluids.

The fragility of the capillary vessels can be demonstrated by applying suction to an area of skin which will show hæmorrhages at about half the negative pressures necessary to provoke the same effect in the mature infant. Particularly common effects of asphyxia are subserosal hæmorrhages, especially in heart, lungs and liver, also hæmorrhages in the pia arachnoid in addition to the cerebral ventricles.

Disorders of pulmonary aeration, including atelectasis, are the commonest of all the causes of neonatal death. Asphyxial deaths thus

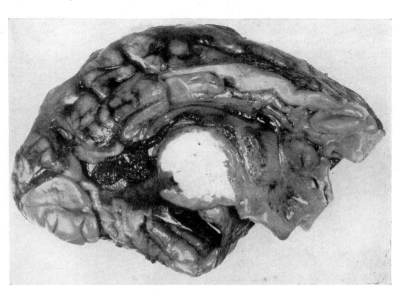

26/Fig. 1 (*a*).—Intraventricular hæmorrhage.
(By courtesy of Dr. A. E. Claireaux.)

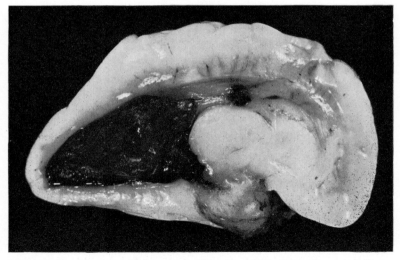

26/Fig. 1(*b*).—The area of subependymal bleeding which eventually ruptured into the ventricle is shown anterior to the clot. It is situated on the floor of the body of the lateral ventricle and the clot has been partially removed in this part of the ventricle to expose the bleeding point.

(By courtesy of Dr. Jean Scott.)

accounted for 66 per cent of the series published by us in 1958 (Donald *et al.*); any successful method of overcoming this would, of itself, make a tremendous difference to chances of survival.

It is believed that the respiratory centre is so immature that it only responds in degrees of anoxia which in themselves may be nearly lethal, and as a result of this anoxia the centres become even less sensitive, another instance of the vicious circle.

We have studied pulmonary expansion after birth in both mature and premature babies by a variety of techniques involving spirometry, electromanometry of intrathoracic pressures, and by radiography (Donald, 1954, 1957; Donald and Steiner, 1953; Donald *et al.*, 1958), and we believe that aeration of the lungs is very rapid indeed, occurring within a few minutes of the onset of vigorous crying, thus agreeing with Potter (1952) and Claireaux (1954), although it was formerly thought that expansion was not complete for many days. Vigour at birth, however, is essential and in the case of the premature baby is more important than birth weight. For the premature infant who lacks the strength to overcome the moist cohesion of the alveolar walls and the resistances of the lung tissue itself to expansion, atelectasis may persist for several days and during this critical period infection is all too liable to develop in areas of lung thus particularly predisposed, so that the case easily and often slides into one of full-blown bronchopneumonia. Poor protective coughing reflexes, furthermore, fail to deal with aspirated foreign material. Apart from pneumonia, the child is prone to all forms of sepsis, especially intestinal and skin infections, and is poorly equipped to cope with them. Much of this is preventable, but the hazards of neonatal infection are certainly greater in the premature.

Passive immunity acquired from the mother increases steadily towards term. The readiness of the tissues generally and of the infected tissues in particular to become œdematous restricts circulation in the affected part and so handicaps the fight against infection and magnifies its local effects.

Anæmia is common, largely because the main stores of iron are only laid down in the last few weeks of pregnancy. The hæmoglobin level should, therefore, be carefully watched in the neonatal period.

Fœtal shock in the course of delivery may easily occur, but is even more liable to appear as a result of handling and disturbance during the first day or two.

Jaundice comes on early and is often very deep because the liver is unable to remove bile constituents from the blood sufficiently readily; these babies are often, as a result, more than usually sleepy and reluctant to feed. The kernicterus of prematurity is independent of hæmolytic disease (see later) and may develop if the serum bilirubin is allowed to rise above 20 mg. per 100 ml. Even lower levels

than this in the vulnerable tissues of the premature baby's brain may be responsible for the lowering of the mean intelligence quotient later on in the smallest premature babies and the recognised risk of neurological sequelæ.

In the matter of metabolism generally the processes are defective in degree rather than lacking altogether, for example, the synthesis of prothrombin and of the hæmoglobin molecule is probably slow. To this factor is attributed the tendency to hæmorrhagic disease.

Because of feeding difficulties and an immature digestive metabolism, signs of malnutrition may easily develop and the premature infant is more than usually prone to rickets in later months.

Hernia, of various sorts, is more common in prematurity, for which poor muscle development is mainly responsible.

The kidneys, by reason of immaturity, are less able to excrete urine differing widely in osmotic pressure from that of blood, their concentrating power is poor and they are less able to alter water and salt excretion rates in response to the needs of the moment. It is not uncommon for no urine to be passed at all for the first day or two. The more mature the kidney the more numerous the nephron units. According to Morison, developing nephrons complete their development after birth, but no new units are formed, so that there may be a nephron deficiency.

Deficiencies in heat regulation.—The smaller the creature the greater must be the ratio of surface area, from which heat is lost, to volume and therefore the metabolic needs are correspondingly greater; for instance, a mouse will consume its own weight in food in about four days. Add to this the fact that the premature infant has very little subcutaneous fat to insulate it and the discrepancy is even more pronounced. This, however, is not all, for it is impossible, often for some weeks, for the child's digestive apparatus to cope with a quantity of food sufficient to produce the necessary number of calories. Even so, metabolism is defective to some degree, so that the fully available amount of heat is not produced, and, furthermore, the muscles whose activity is normally a very important source of heat generation are, in this case, poorly developed.

It will be seen therefore that heat is poorly generated and rapidly dissipated, rather like a budget which cannot be balanced. This simile is even more apt than at first sight, because the control mechanism is also immature and incapable of checking wild swings in temperature, which the baby's relative inability to sweat does little to stabilise.

One cannot work long with premature infants without being struck with the fantastic ranges of rectal temperature which may be demonstrated within a few hours, and more will be said of this under the section on treatment.

SIGNS AND FEATURES OF PREMATURITY

1. *Weight.* As stated before, a weight of 5½ lb. (2,500 g.) or under is the only generally accepted criterion.

2. *Length.* This is usually less than 47 cm.

3. Very little subcutaneous fat is present, a fact which gives the infant its characteristically scraggy appearance and makes the toes and fingers at first glance appear unusually long.

4. The skin, as a result of this, has a brick-reddish colour, feels very thin and wrinkles easily.

5. Lanugo, a fine downy hair, is plentiful.

6. Vernix caseosa is very scanty or absent. Vernix is composed of sebaceous material, and the glands in the skin which produce it are still immature.

7. The skull bones are very thin. This is hardly a sign of much clinical help, but is one of the most serious features of prematurity in the course of labour. It is usually said that in premature labour excessive moulding occurs to the detriment of the cranial contents, but this is not quite accurate, for when moulding occurs in mature labour the vault of the skull gradually alters its shape and maintains this alteration for some hours, and, of course, does not alter appreciably between uterine contractions. With the premature infant, however, the soft skull tends to be squeezed into a different shape with each contraction and has not the rigidity necessary fully to maintain the change in shape between each onslaught. This denies the brain and intracranial ligaments the chance to adapt themselves progressively.

On the release of pressure after delivery of the head, which may be very sudden, the damaging effects are particularly exaggerated. In the case of a breech birth, all the advantages of a small aftercoming head may be cancelled by the rapid alterations in skull shape which can occur.

8. The size of head relative to body is greater than at term; this increases the hazards of breech delivery.

9. The testicles are undescended.

10. The labia minora are exposed and apparently project because the labia majora are poorly developed, mainly through being deficient in fat.

11. Urine secreted is scanty and in fact none may be passed for up to 3 days after birth.

12. Jaundice is liable to come on early and is deep because of the slow riddance of bile pigments.

13. There is a marked tendency to hernia of various types because of poor muscle development.

14. The ears are very soft and flabby because what little cartilage they contain is particularly soft.

15. The nails are often stated not to have grown as far as the finger-tips. While long nails do not occur, this reputed shortness is, in fact, seldom seen.

16. Radiology may fail to show the ossification centres generally reputed to appear at or near term, e.g. lower end of femur and cuboid, but there is quite a wide range of variability here, often of several weeks.

The diagnosis of prematurity is therefore not difficult; what is more uncertain is to be able to assess its degree. There are, however, one or two rule-of-thumb methods which may be of some help.

According to Haas' rule, the fœtal age in lunar months can be calculated by dividing the fœtal length in centimetres by 5. This only applies after the 5th month. Before delivery, Ahlfeld's method may be tried.

The distance from breech to vertex is measured in centimetres with the help of a pelvimeter and a finger placed in the vagina. Two centimetres are subtracted, representing the thickness of the abdominal wall. Doubling this figure gives the approximate crown-heel length of the baby and makes some allowance for the usual attitude of flexion. The computed crown-heel length divided by five gives the fœtal age in lunar months (Fig. 2).

McDonald's rule for assessing the period of gestation, incidentally, consists in measuring by tape the distance from fundus uteri to symphysis pubis in centimetres. The figure obtained is multiplied by 2 and divided by 7, and this gives the maturity in lunar months. The method is not applicable before the 6th month and is likely to be upset by full engagement of the head near term.

Such rule-of-thumb methods have never been very popular, and it has to be admitted that in the absence of reliable history one can seldom do better than guesswork based on prolonged experience.

It is our view that the fœtal biparietal diameter is more closely related to maturity than to actual weight and we make increasing use of sonar for the determination of maturity on this basis during pregnancy.

LONG-TERM EFFECTS OF PREMATURITY

It is said that Sir Isaac Newton, at his birth, could have been pushed into a two-pint pot, and none would deny his intelligence; nevertheless, the chances of mental deficiency have to be carefully considered. As the treatment of prematurity continues to improve, one may well speculate upon the likelihood of burdening society with beings so handicapped mentally or physically that it might have been

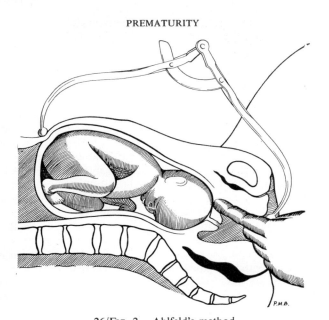

26/Fig. 2.—Ahlfeld's method.

(From Dr. C. O. McCormick's *Textbook on Pathology of Labor, the Puerperium and the Newborn*, by courtesy of C. V. Mosby Co.)

better if Nature had been allowed to take her ruthless course, but so far as modern success has gone to date this is by no means necessarily the case. If, however, the fœtus which today is regarded as previable is ever, as a matter of course, reared to full maturity and beyond, more discouraging factors may well come to light.

Surveys such as that of Knoblock *et al.* (1956) indicated an overall likelihood of neurological abnormality of approximately 8 per cent, as against 1·6 per cent in mature controls matched by social grading, birth order and race, but the mental deficiency rate was only strikingly higher (8·8 per cent) in the smaller birth weight groups of 1,500 g. (3·3 lb.) or less. These handicaps have been abundantly confirmed by Drillien (1959) who has shown that in babies weighing less than 3 lb. at birth there is not only retardation in weight and to a lesser extent in growth but, what is much worse, 14 per cent of her series in this group had an estimated I.Q. less than 70 and would be in need of special schooling, and nearly half were considered very dull. Where the birth weight was over 4½ lb. there was no difference in subsequent mental development, but below that figure the intellectual capacity of the babies would appear to be more or less inversely proportional to birth weight. Douglas (1960) likewise made a controlled study (in so far as it is possible to control such a study) of the later school

records of all children born during the first week of March, 1946, which provided 706 babies weighing less than 2,500 g. at birth, each child being matched with a control weighing more than this, but otherwise selected on the basis of sex, position in the family, the mother's age, her social grouping and home social conditions. The subsequent school records of the prematures were consistently lower than those of the controls and what is more, the handicap became more marked as the age increased; for example, from eight years to eleven, only 9·7 per cent of the premature babies gained places in Grammar Schools as compared with 22 per cent of the controls, but it was pointed out that the complex social causes of prematurity are undoubtedly a very major factor in the handicaps of these babies, rather than low birth weight *per se*.

Now, a prematurely born child may owe some of its small birth weight to one of three classes of cause. First, because of its parent's stature, it may be small for genetic reasons. Secondly, pregnancy may have been interrupted therapeutically for some obstetrical indication. Thirdly, something may have interfered with intra-uterine development. The dangers of mental retardation would appear to be mainly confined to the last group and the analysis by Douglas (1956) which was carried out on eight-year-old children by means of reading, vocabulary and intelligence testing, indicates that although premature children scored less than their controls, most markedly so in reading, the worst group were those in whom no obstetric nor genetic explanation could be found for their low birth weight. In others words, as might be expected, intra-uterine handicaps to development are more important than actual birth weight which may be the result of extraneous interference, for example, induction of labour. So far, however, it can be said that the premature infant has a very good chance of catching up in its development by the third or fourth year with four provisos:

(1) No gross or oft-repeated anoxia must be allowed to occur and so damage the central nervous system.

(2) There must be no damage to immature tissue.

(3) There must be no unfavourable genetic factors.

(4) The social grading of the parents does not fall within the lowest groups.

Obstetrical complications, *per se*, such as pre-eclamptic toxæmia, malpresentation, respiratory distress syndrome, even jaundice, convulsions and signs of cerebral irritation, are not incompatible with a subsequent reasonable intelligence quotient, provided cases of gross neurological or sensory damage are excluded.[35] In other words apparently normal children have apparently a chance of normal intellectual development.

As a matter of practical importance, therefore, it will be seen that

adequate oxygenation from the beginning is the first essential. Oxygen absorption through skin, bronchial mucous membrane and intestinal tract can only be employed as short-term expedients. The problem of atelectasis remains paramount, and as yet there is no accepted direct treatment of this condition, and all that is done at the moment is to remove as far as possible some of the factors that either favour its development or perpetuate it.

Even where anoxia has been apparently extreme, it is quite impossible to gauge how extensive will be the after effects.

RESPIRATORY DISTRESS SYNDROME
(Pulmonary Syndrome and Hyaline Membrane)

The four conditions, pulmonary syndrome of the newborn, intraventricular hæmorrhage (already described), pneumonia and birth trauma were found by Bound *et al.* (1956) to account for two-thirds of all neonatal deaths in their survey of neonatal mortality and they too noted, as I, too, had in 1954, that these conditions are not distinguishable during life by ordinary clinical methods and the baby behaves in a remarkably similar way in each. This is regrettable since, in the absence of a definitive diagnosis, specific treatment, even if it were available, cannot as yet be applied.

The term "pulmonary syndrome of the newborn" is a very useful one and was introduced by Bound and his colleagues at University College Hospital to describe cases of secondary resorption atelectasis together with one of the following: hyaline membrane, intra-alveolar hæmorrhage or pulmonary œdema. The term Respiratory Distress Syndrome (R.D.S.) is now more fashionable.

Hyaline membrane consists of an eosinophilic membrane of patchy distribution which is plastered against the walls of the air passages, especially the alveolar ducts, and which obstructs aeration (Figs. 3 and 4). Distal to these points of obstruction the alveoli collapse and become filled with fluid.

It is not yet certain what is the source or composition of the membrane, but it is believed by some to be due to particulate matter occurring in liquor amnii and possibly the inflammatory reaction so caused within the lungs. Now, although it is known that respiratory movements occur during the later part of intra-uterine life, these movements are not large, and the general belief is that deep aspiration is necessary to set the stage for the development of this membrane, for it is not to be found in the lungs of stillborn infants. The sequence of events would appear to be firstly the development of severe fœtal anoxia before or at birth resulting in the deep inspiration of liquor which is not, of itself, sufficient to obstruct subsequent breathing, but the solid matter so deposited sets up aseptic irritative changes

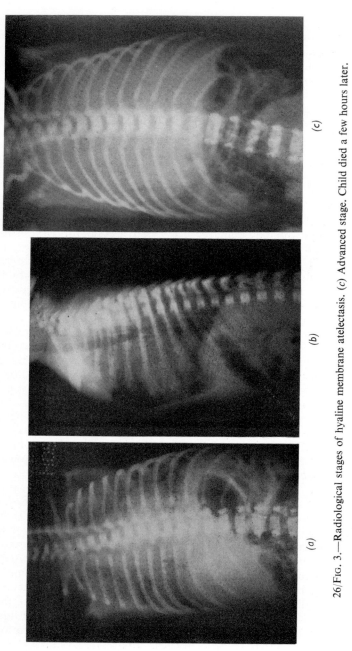

(a)

(b)

(c)

26/Fig. 3.—Radiological stages of hyaline membrane atelectasis. (c) Advanced stage. Child died a few hours later.

(By courtesy of Prof. R. E. Steiner.)

876

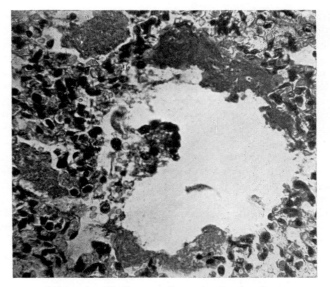

26/Fɪɢ. 4.—Hyaline membrane in alveolar duct.
(By courtesy of Dr. A. E. Claireaux.)

which differ from those of broncho-pneumonia and, as a result, this membrane, or portions of it, are to be found at autopsy. Claireaux (1953) considered that it was composed of macerated squames from the liquor. This would account for its fairly common association with conditions which produce anoxia before the membranes have ruptured, for example, antepartum hæmorrhage. If, moreover, the child is delivered by Cæsarean section without the compression of its thoracic cage by the normal processes of labour, this membrane is even more likely to develop. The other view, which is now gaining ground, is that the membrane is an exudative phenomenon from the bronchiolar and alveolar duct epithelium.

In 1959 Avery and Mead described a lipoprotein, named pulmonary surfactant, which may have something to do with preventing pulmonary collapse and which normally lines the alveoli. Others, for example, Pattle et al. (1962) have confirmed their finding that this lining substance is not present in infants dying of the respiratory distress syndrome. Prematurity is the main cause of a deficiency of surfactant. Asphyxia is also said to be a cause, either by damaging the cells in the alveoli which synthesise it or because in asphyxia there may be an exudation of fibrinogen which inactivates it.

The distribution of the membrane, plastered around the walls of the alveolar ducts, is due to the passage of air caused by the baby's

respiratory efforts. The membrane, consequently, is not found in cases of stillbirth.

While the ætiology is still in doubt, it is very likely that the persistence of the membrane within the lungs is due to a deficient pulmonary circulation, because the vascular bed within the lungs has not been adequately opened up for one reason or another, usually inadequate respiratory activity. Thus the membrane, or its precursor substance is neither absorbed nor got rid of, except in babies capable of exhibiting the necessary respiratory vigour. It is the commonest cause of secondary atelectasis.

The fact that premature infants are more than usually susceptible may be explained by their very weak powers of eliminating foreign matter from their lungs and of opening up their pulmonary circulation quickly.

As explained in the chapter on resuscitation of the newborn in the section describing the first breaths of life, the exercise of negative intrathoracic pressure by the baby in its attempts to inspire air also encourages the flow of blood into the lungs. The blood then returning from the lungs raises the left atrial pressure within the heart and closes the foramen ovale. In addition to this, it has been shown by Dawes et al. (1953–55) that there is initially a reversed flow from left to right through the ductus arteriosus which does not close functionally for the first few hours until the percentage oxygen saturation of the blood has risen from about 60 per cent at birth to over 90 per cent. In this way, blood returning from the lungs to the left atrium and ventricle is partly shunted back through the still patent ductus arteriosus into the pulmonary circulation for a second helping of oxygen—an ingenious mechanism while the lungs are still relatively inefficient from persistent atelectasis (Born et al., 1954).

It has, moreover, been shown by Lind and Wegelius (1954) that the ductus, after closure, may reopen early in the neonatal period if provoked by neonatal anoxia. In this case, if through inadequate respiratory activity the pulmonary circulation has not been sufficiently opened up, the original high resistance in the pulmonary circuit persists and blood is thereby encouraged to bypass the lungs by going from right to left through the reopened ductus. As a result, less blood returns from the lungs to the left atrium so that a pressure gradient develops between right and left atria and the foramen ovale reopens. In other words, reversion to the fœtal type of circulation has taken place and a full cyanotic attack results.

The chain of events above described explains the clinical picture in the pulmonary syndrome. The respiratory rate shortly after birth is around 70 per minute, but if this does not fall below 50 by the end of the second hour the possibility that the baby is developing the respiratory distress syndrome should be considered and a chest

X-ray obtained. Acute left heart failure may be revealed. An important alternative diagnosis may also be made by an X-ray taken at this age, namely, that of diaphragmatic hernia. In such a case transfer to a pædiatric unit with full surgical facilities is immediately necessary and oxygenation should be maintained with an endotracheal tube throughout the journey; otherwise the intestines may simply fill up, especially if oxygen is given by a mask, and the baby may become dangerously embarrassed from mediastinal displacement.

The course which is run is fairly characteristic; the baby is usually premature, practically never postmature, and appears well at birth, and may even for a time maintain a healthy colour. Crying, however, is not well sustained and within a few hours, sometimes within twenty minutes, the first signs of respiratory distress develop. These consist of whimpering and expiratory grunting and movement of the alæ nasi. Presently signs of inspiratory recession of the chest wall appear, especially in the subcostal regions and also, to a less obvious extent, in the intercostal spaces and suprasternal area. In very severe cases the whole sternum is dragged inwards by the child's inspiratory efforts.

Clearly the child is now literally fighting for its breath and Karlberg *et al.* (1954) have reckoned that in such respiratory distress the effort of breathing is between two to five times as great as normal. Our own researches encourage us in a similar view.

Radiographs taken at this time will show the developing changes which we have described as a fine miliary mottling, proceeding to coalescent areas of non-aeration and leading finally to total lung radio-opacity with only the bronchial tree outlined because of the air within it (Donald and Steiner, 1953).

After a variable number of hours the baby gives up the unequal struggle in the face of such difficulty and stops breathing. A cyanotic, or grey attack, follows. This may be the first of a series which finally ends in death, usually within two or three days, and often within twelve hours, but never in less than two hours.

We believe that milder cases of the pulmonary syndrome may survive if possessed of sufficient respiratory vigour to overcome it.

Little more is yet known, but it is believed that such membrane is cleared only with very great and prolonged difficulty, and that only those babies sufficiently vigorous to be able to manage on unaffected lung portions are likely to survive. So far, then, the treatment is not specific, and the one hope is to maintain life until respiratory compensation occurs.

PROPHYLAXIS AND PREMATURE BIRTH

Since premature birth is often deliberately brought on because of some maternal condition which either jeopardises the mother's

health or carries with it the threat of intra-uterine fœtal death, e.g. pre-eclamptic toxæmia, the only prophylactic measures that can be employed here are tied up with the early recognition of the disorder and, as far as possible, the control of its severity in order to justify prolonging pregnancy for a few more weeks. But there are many conditions which in themselves endanger neither mother nor unborn child through the continuation of pregnancy, but which carry a high prematurity rate.

Important instances in the latter group are cases of multiple pregnancy, hydramnios without demonstrable fœtal abnormality, a large mass of fibroids, severe cardiac lesions (in which induction of labour is not indicated), malnutrition and profound debility, and that group of patients who recurrently and for no apparent reason go into premature labour.

In such cases as these, notice must be taken of the liability to start labour, and an extra few weeks may be gained by keeping the patient in bed. Unless she has had a previous series of obstetrical disappointments, a healthy woman with twins is unlikely to be willing to go to bed for the last few weeks of her pregnancy on the off-chance that her children might not be prematurely born, but cases of triplets should be strongly urged to co-operate in this precaution.

Once the threat of premature labour has revealed itself by the onset of labour pains or by the rupture of membranes or a show, the patient should of course be put to bed and kept there. Even the leakage of liquor is not inevitably followed straight away by labour, although it is more than probable, and with strict care the leak may seal itself, at least temporarily, and a further ten days or more may be gained. There may be some doubt about whether the fluid draining is liquor amnii or urine from incontinence. The smell may be characteristic, but a useful method of distinguishing the two is to give methylene blue by mouth which discolours urine only. Another method to distinguish between the seepage of liquor and urine is to allow a drop of fluid to dry on an ordinary microscope slide and to look at it under low power. Aborisation crystals may be seen in the case of liquor but not in urine. Another test described by Fell (1960) is to take the soiled pad and fold it over an Albustix protein detector, and squeeze. Because of the protein in liquor amnii a positive reaction will be obtained. Unfortunately this is also true of vaginal discharges and we have found the method yields too many false positive results. We commonly employ the Nile Blue sulphate test using a 0·1 per cent aqueous solution (see previous chapter) which can be very quickly undertaken as a side-room procedure. Fœtal cells present in the liquor show up as anucleate orange-stained cells, often in clusters. Unfortunately the more premature the case the less reliable is the test and, annoyingly enough, the more premature the

case, the more serious the matter of premature membrane rupture. Undoubtedly the best of all methods is to use one's nose, a method denied to the many nicotine addicts within our profession.

During this period of trying to prolong pregnancy after early spontaneous rupture of the membranes, the bowels should be left severely alone and adequate sedatives given. Undoubtedly, morphia is the most efficient but, in the event of labour proceeding, it carries the risk that delivery may occur while the fœtus is still within the range of its effects. The barbiturates will, therefore, be found to be more generally serviceable, e.g. sodium amytal 200 mg. repeated up to three times within 24 hours or seconal in similar dosage.

The preparations for vaginal delivery include transfer of the patient, if practicable, to a hospital having an adequate pædiatric service, the preparation of a heated incubator and a suitable supply of humidified oxygen. The best incubator for the transport of the premature fœtus to hospital is its mother's uterus. Should the confinement be undertaken at home, these facilities must be improvised, and a nurse experienced in premature infant management should be in attendance. There are firms with branches in the larger cities who will supply at very short notice some admirable types of incubator on hire at very reasonable cost. Every effort within reason, however, should be made to get the baby into a properly equipped and staffed pædiatric unit at the earliest opportunity to improve its chances of healthy survival.

Conduct of Premature Labour

A somewhat limited personal experience of isoxuprine in the prevention of premature labour has not impressed me as an effective means of staving it off and this would appear to be the experience of Matthews *et al.* (1967) in a double blind trial of the drug in oral form. More reports may alter this view, possibly if given parenterally.

There is as yet no method of holding off labour with hormones, and when it is clear from the dilatation of the cervix that labour will inevitably proceed, an enema should be given, for nothing will now be gained by uterine inertia. Analgesic drugs should be used as sparingly as possible. Morphia and its derivatives, as already hinted, are poison to the premature infant, and even 10 mg. ($\frac{1}{6}$ gr.) of morphia will depress respiration in a premature infant born as much as six or seven hours later. Pethidine is preferable, although chloral and paraldehyde are safest. Premixed gas and oxygen analgesia, 50/50, for example by the Entonox apparatus is useful and perfectly safe. If labour hangs fire because of inertia we begin to fear the possibility of intra-uterine infection to which the premature fœtus is very vulnerable and we therefore give cephaloridine by intramuscular injection, 500 mg. twice daily.

Throughout labour the patient should be kept in bed, because delivery is often precipitate and unexpected.

Because of the excessively rapid and dangerous moulding which the fœtal head may undergo, its egress should be facilitated by an adequate episiotomy whenever it appears that the perineum is causing more than a moderate resistance to delivery. This can be done quite simply and quickly following local infiltration with about 8–10 ml. of 2 per cent lignocaine when the head is on the perineum. This is more than ever important with a breech delivery, and in all such cases the head should be very slowly and gently delivered, steadying the vault of the skull with the wide palm of the hand rather than with the fingers.

When the child has been born, its pharynx should be sucked out with a rubber-ended mucus-extractor at once and before dividing the cord. Swabbing out the inside of the mouth with gauze is very damaging to the lining of the cavity and should not be practised. The common types of mucus-extractor are inefficient, dirty and dangerous, because the midwife has to blow down them to clear them. A pump-driven sucker is far more satisfactory. (See chapter on Resuscitation of the Newborn.)

The cord is not divided until pulsation in it ceases, as thereby a few extra millilitres of blood are not lost to the baby. This hardly matters in a mature infant which is born with polycythæmia, but anæmia in the premature infant has to be remembered.

The child is now placed, preferably uncovered, in a warm atmosphere of oxygen in an incubator and is left alone. The skin is undoubtedly capable of absorbing appreciable quantities of oxygen, in fact it is believed that up to 10 per cent of total requirements can be met by this route, and it is surprising how quickly a combination of warmth and oxygen will revive such an infant.

The breathing is at first so shallow that it may be imperceptible, but provided the colour remains a healthy pink there is no cause for immediate concern. The cases which go grey and toneless at this stage have a bad prognosis, and many of these are the victims of intracranial bleeding. Even so, more harm results from so-called resuscitative measures than from relying solely on oxygen and warmth. Tracheal intubation is often practised, and oxygen under positive pressures of up to 30 cm. of water can be administered, but the present general view does not favour this line of treatment, except in emergency, because of the disturbance to the child which it entails, the risk of introducing infection, and damage which may be caused to the lining of the air passages. However, much depends upon the skill of the operator. It can be argued with some logic that the child well enough to stand the procedure does not need it and the child which does need it is past saving anyway. Considering how fatal

the handicaps of atelectasis may prove within the next forty-eight hours, it is possible that in expert hands intubation and some form of assisted respiration may come to be more widely used in the future. We have practised such a technique, using nylon catheters, in ultra-premature cases with some success in pulmonary aeration (Donald *et al.*, 1958), employing one of the writer's electronically controlled patient-cycled respirators. Intubation tends, after all, to be reserved for the more moribund cases and therefore the frequency of disappointment is bound to be high.

There are many indications that interest in artificial respiration in severe cases of the respiratory distress syndrome is being revived in some quarters. For example, in a small but controlled trial in Aberdeen[42] the difference in survival in cases treated by intermittent positive-pressure ventilation over many hours is striking. Our own work along these lines, using augmented respiration so as to assist a baby's own spontaneous efforts and relieve it of some of its appalling physical load in attempting to aerate atelectatic lungs, may even presently have a second innings, long after our work on the subject in the early 1950s has been forgotten.[15–19] This, of course, is no new phenomenon. It is only simple forms of treatment, after all, that manage to jump the ditch at the first attempt, and trying to maintain artificial respiration in a tiny, cyanotic and grossly atelectatic baby is hard and discouraging work. The present approach to the problem by combating respiratory and metabolic acidosis by biochemical control is described later on.

MANAGEMENT OF THE PREMATURE INFANT

There are four cardinal features in the treatment and rearing of the premature infant, and their importance runs in the following order:

(1) Maintenance of body temperature.
(2) Prevention of infection.
(3) Treatment of pulmonary atelectasis.
(4) Nutrition.

In addition, there are the more general aspects of nursing care.

MAINTENANCE OF BODY TEMPERATURE

The importance of this is often not sufficiently stressed. These babies chill off very quickly and can be seen to develop a condition of irreversible peripheral circulatory failure, the so-called grey attack, for which either pulmonary atelectasis or an inadequate supply of oxygen may be blamed, a mistake which the available but incidental evidences at autopsy tend to support. Such attacks are very liable to

follow even short periods of exposure or handling and attempts to feed. Rectal temperatures are, of course, taken as infrequently as possible in order to reduce disturbance of the child, but such information is invaluable. The surrounding cot or atmosphere temperature should be so adjusted that the baby's rectal temperature is maintained at about 96° F., which is often a difficult matter. As a general guide, if the baby is clothed the cot temperature should in the first instance be 85–90° F. near the baby's body and 75° F. in the rest of the cot. If, on the other hand, the baby is being nursed naked in an incubator, the temperature inside it should be 90–95° F. Adjustments can then be made according to the baby's temperature reactions. The dangers of overheating and burning are very great in the absence of thermostatically controlled safety cut-out switches.

Rectal temperatures are taken with special thermometers reading down to 85° F.

If the whole room can be heated to an even temperature of 80–85° F. so much the better.

The atmosphere must have a humidity of at least 75 per cent. Some incubators have special humidifiers incorporated, and in hospital units the air is automatically conditioned and humidified. In the home, however, a steam kettle should be used.

All oxygen supplied to the baby should be bubbled through warmed water, since dry, neat oxygen may act as a pulmonary irritant.

Babies, on their reception into a premature unit, are often found to have very low temperatures which must be restored carefully before irreversible changes set in. In the Glasgow series,[2] two babies with temperatures actually below 74° F. survived—surely a record!

<h3 style="text-align:center">PREVENTION OF INFECTION</h3>

There is almost no measure which can be taken to minimise this risk which could be called far-fetched, and no precaution can be safely omitted. From this point of view a premature infant is better off nursed in a good private house than in an inadequately equipped hospital. The development of premature baby units in the larger hospitals is no fanciful fad, and staffing of such units has to be on a lavish scale to make the nursing ritual possible or even tolerable for those who run it. The unit should be well separated from other departments and the nursing staff should not work elsewhere. Every member should have nose and throat swabs taken on enrolment, whenever they return to duty following any infectious illness, including the common cold for which absence from work is obligatory, and routinely every four weeks. The taking of the full holiday allowances is likewise important.

No visitors other than the baby's father, who could not reasonably

be excluded, should be allowed to enter, and of all possible visitors it must be remembered that young children are far the most dangerous.

The wearing of efficient sterilised masks is essential for everyone, and the well-disciplined habit of never touching the mask with the hands from the time it is put on until it is removed should be cultivated. If, for any reason, the mask is pulled down from the nose it should be replaced by another.

All entrants to the unit, including doctors, should put on freshly laundered coats or gowns which belong specially to the unit, because all day-to-day clothing is dirtier than one would imagine. These coats or gowns should be frequently replaced and sent to the laundry and should hang on pegs or racks not used by ordinary clothing.

Hands must be washed between handling each child.

The unit should be divided into a series of small rooms in which all the infants below 4 lb., or those not securely thriving, are strictly isolated, and each of these isolation rooms is entered through an air lock of double doors, only one of which is opened at a time. The doors should be of the swing type on springs and without handles. Each of these small rooms is centrally heated and air-conditioned to the right humidity.

The larger and older premature infants may be nursed in one room together, as it is seldom practicable to have enough isolation rooms, and the larger nursery, which is less heated, is a stepping-stone to the world outside.

Each room has its own washing and baby bathing facilities, and a separate gown is donned by the nurse for each child that she has to handle. All floors may be treated regularly with spindle oil to reduce dust-borne infection.

Milk and feeding utensils are prepared in the unit's own kitchen and feeds are prepared before and not after nappy changing.

Infants admitted from outside the hospital are particularly suspect, and should be separately nursed. For infants born following a long labour with early rupture of the membranes, ampicillin combined with cloxacillin, 50 mg. of each per Kg. of body weight, are given over 24 hours intravenously at first and later by mouth. Whatever one's views about prophylaxis with chemotherapy and its disadvantages in masking early physical signs of infection, there can be little doubt about its value in this sort of work where one cannot afford to await the signs of established disease. Nothing can so discredit a premature baby unit as the incidence of infection occurring in it. The three main types of infection encountered are bronchopneumonia, skin and conjunctival infections and gastro-enteritis. Meningeal infections should be a very rare disaster, but may follow aspiration of *E. coli* infected liquor.

No inflammatory lesion can safely be regarded as too trivial for

energetic treatment, and *Staph. pyogenes*, often penicillin-resistant, can light up an epidemic overnight.

TREATMENT OF PULMONARY ATELECTASIS

A child's first breath remains a marvel, the mechanism of which has not yet been fully explained, but very great effort (40–90 cm. H_2O) is clearly necessary to open up the alveoli, and this may prove beyond the child's power (Donald, 1957). Crying produces a sharp rise in pressure in the air passages against the resistance of the partially closed glottis, but premature infants are often too weak to cry, and under such circumstances it may take four days for full lung expansion to occur. It is remarkable at autopsy how small an amount of aerated lung can manage to support life at any rate for a few hours, but the clinical picture during life is fairly characteristic. Breathing is both shallow and rapid, in fact, respiratory rates of over 60 a minute are common, and this is mechanically inefficient and exhausting to the baby and may not be maintained. The clinical features of atelectasis and the pulmonary syndrome have already been described. Hyaline membrane accounts for very many of these cases, but is not always demonstrable.

Clearly the aspiration of meconium and mucus at birth invites atelectasis, and the first step is to remove it from the mouth and pharynx before this can occur. What is noticeable, however, is how unusual it is to find a bronchial tree blocked with mucus at autopsy in cases dying with pulmonary atelectasis; this finding weakens the case for treatment by bronchoscopic suction, which should be reserved only for the very occasional case of clinically unilateral atelectasis. This manœuvre demands the skill of one who is highly practised in it because of the disturbance and handling involved, and can only be appropriate when the blockage is high enough in the bronchus to be accessible. The natural riddance of mucus depends mainly upon an intact ciliated epithelium in the bronchial tree, and traumatic procedures, besides their general harm, can only increase reactionary œdema and produce yet more mucus. It may well be that much of the exudate blamed for non-aeration is a product rather than a cause of asphyxia.

Laryngeal spasm may at times prevent air entry, for which a small bead of mucus may be responsible.

During the first hours, the baby will often drool from its mouth large quantities of mucus, but this has probably been produced recently by the baby itself and has nothing to do with aspirated material; much of it probably comes directly from the stomach, in which organ it is very readily secreted, and for this reason and for the possible risk of subsequent aspiration, it is more logical to suck

out the stomach contents; this is a routine procedure on first receiving the baby into the unit.

The differential diagnosis of neonatal pulmonary atelectasis is often open to error. Broncho-pneumonia has already been mentioned, and often the diagnosis cannot be made before the child is beyond chemotherapeutic aid, but an equally common error is to diagnose the case as suffering from intracranial hæmorrhage. In fact, the behaviour of the baby in these conditions can be very similar, and in addition to this all three conditions may co-exist.

In recognising the reluctance of premature babies' lungs to expand, it has occurred to many workers to try to achieve adequate oxygenation by other means, though most of these methods are used chiefly for resuscitation at birth rather than during the course of the first three critical days.

One method popular for some years was to supply oxygen via the intestinal tract as described by Akerren and Furstenberg or by Yllpo's method, but is now discredited. The writer's method of augmenting respiratory effort by patient-triggered respirators encouraged us, but required unremitting supervision on a technical as well as medical level and one's principal stand-by has hitherto remained the supply of humidified oxygen in a suitable incubator aiming at concentrations of 50–60 per cent initially with very early reduction to 35 per cent as soon as possible. Higher concentrations are regarded as dangerous for prolonged periods. Oxygen is supplied in the hope that the child will oblige by breathing it, but although you can take a horse to water you cannot make it drink!

In spite of a growing amount of experimental work, theorising, talking and writing, in all of which I, too, have participated, the subject of the respiratory distress syndrome seemed to be heading for a stalemate until a fresh approach to the subject, largely under the stimulus of Usher (1961) in Montreal, altered the direction of attack, namely, an attempt to control the biochemistry of the mixed metabolic and respiratory acidosis which are lethal features of the condition. Until I heard an address by Usher to the Neonatal Society in London, I had regarded the ultimate deaths of these babies as primarily due to cardiac and peripheral circulatory failure, brought about by hypoxia and exhaustion from the mechanical difficulties of achieving and maintaining aeration of lungs whose alveolar walls, because of prematurity, were reluctant to expand and whose circulatory filling was not sufficiently encouraged by adequate respiratory effort; hence my concentration upon the technique of augmented respiration. This may be an important side of the problem but is only part of the truth. The biochemical derangement associated with the condition is profound. In both types of acidosis the pH of arterial blood may be very low, often below 7, even as low as 6·5, and in fact

most cases with a pH of less than 7 are doomed. In addition there is a low bicarbonate reserve and increased base deficit. In respiratory acidosis, moreover, the Pco_2 is very high. The normal range is between 30 and 40 mm. Hg and the case is serious if the level rises above 70 mm. Hg and hopeless if over 150 mm. Hg. Metabolic acidosis is always present and to it may be added respiratory acidosis, but there is never respiratory acidosis alone. Much of the former is probably renal in origin. Bicarbonate levels are low, for example 15 to 20 as against a normal 22 mEq/l. The additional respiratory acidosis which complicates hyaline membrane disease, for example, may show Pco_2 levels in excess of 100 mm. of mercury although the baby for a time is pink. These measurements can be made with the micro-Astrup apparatus which is capable of measuring pH, Pco_2 and plasma bicarbonate in milliequivalents per litre. Usher's recommended technique was to correct this acidosis by dripping glucose and sodium bicarbonate through an anterior scalp vein. My own pædiatric colleagues, Professor Hutchison and Dr. Margaret Kerr, have modified the technique and employed it very extensively with the most encouraging results (Hutchinson et al., 1962, 1964).

In their first series of 100 cases they included only severe cases with the following criteria common to all:

1. Expiratory grunting.
2. Tachypnœa (over 60 per minute).
3. Inspiratory recession of the chest wall.
4. Cyanosis without oxygen.
5. Characteristic radiographic changes.[17]

As well as this, all the infants showed some degree of œdema and most of them developed icterus. On clinical grounds alone therefore these babies were at very high risk.

Using heparinised samples of blood obtained by heel prick the degree of metabolic acidosis, as well as respiratory acidosis, was determined by means of the micro-Astrup apparatus. The former is correctable by intravenous sodium bicarbonate and this was given by a polythene catheter in the umbilical vein in a dose depending on the base excess and with the practical assumption that the extracellular space in the baby could be presumed to be about 35 per cent of the body weight. Using a solution, therefore, of 8·4 per cent sodium bicarbonate, as 1 mEq. is equal to 1 ml. of this mixture, the dose was calculated on the formula of:

Base excess in mEq/litre × 0·35 × the body weight in kilograms.

In other words a sort of *in vivo* titration of the baby with sodium bicarbonate. Further micro-Astrup estimations are carried out 30

minutes later and more sodium bicarbonate given as indicated, the aim being to raise the pH to between 7·35 and 7·4. Thereafter the acid base equilibrium is monitored more or less hourly and the dose of sodium bicarbonate prescribed accordingly.

Fructose, 20 per cent, is preferred to glucose because it is less damaging to the vein walls and less likely to produce thrombosis, it is metabolised independently of insulin and it is capable of replenishing the glycogen stores quickly. The total daily fluid intake is adjusted with 20 per cent fructose solution to 60 ml./Kg. An incidental beneficial effect is a likely diuresis and this is particularly helpful in the "waterlogged" baby of the diabetic mother. Very early on, hyperbaric oxygen up to 3 atmospheres absolute pressure was found to be of no benefit in cases of established respiratory distress syndrome whatever degree of oxygenation was achieved.

Unfortunately the sodium bicarbonate treatment does not relieve the high Pco_2 values which indicate severe respiratory acidosis and attempts have been made with buffer substances to raise the pH, such as THAM or TRIS which is tris-hydroxymethyl-amino-methane. The results in this respect, however, are disappointing and it still remains to be seen whether the addition of augmented respiration will improve the prognosis in these desperate cases with rising Pco_2 levels in spite of treatment. Nevertheless the biochemical correction alone of the metabolic acidosis by the above technique has resulted in a striking improvement in mortality rates from otherwise uncomplicated cases of respiratory distress syndrome, from about 45 per cent to 11·5 per cent[28, 29] and already such results have had the effect of modifying obstetrical treatment. We are now less hesitant to undertake Cæsarean section, for example, in prematurity and in conditions such as antepartum hæmorrhage and diabetes known to predispose the baby to this dreaded complication.

Formerly one would have expected at least half the cases, or more, to die. What is even more encouraging is that follow up, although necessarily short so far, has shown few complications although umbilical vein phlebitis and pyæmia were reported in 3 out of 200 cases by Scott (1965). It is now more usual to cannulate an umbilical artery, which has the additional advantage that arterial samples can easily be obtained through the same catheter.

Even a normal baby at term is born with a mild acidosis, both metabolic and respiratory, of which the respiratory element (the raised Pco_2) is eliminated presently after birth by efficient pulmonary ventilation, but the metabolic acidosis takes longer to correct and pulmonary function is the principal method by which the infant maintains its acid-base balance. When, for any reason, respiratory function fails, the derangement of metabolism becomes profound and is associated with hyperkalæmia to a lethal degree. This brings

us back to where we started and the baby that breathes and cries well gets out of its acidosis and stays out of it.

NUTRITION

A baby large and strong enough to suck should be put to the breast, six-hourly after the first day and three-hourly on the third and subsequent days until its weight has reached 6½ or 7 lb., when four-hourly feeding can be instituted. A large proportion of premature infants, however, are not sufficiently vigorous, and there remains a choice of the following methods of feeding:

(1) Tube feeding.
(2) Drop feeding with pipette.
(3) Bellcroy feeder or some similar device.
(4) Bottle feeding.
(5) Naso-gastric fine polythene tube for the seriously ill or premature.

In such an infant, each feed may be fraught with danger. In the first place the swallowing reflexes may be functionally inadequate to prevent aspiration of milk into the trachea; secondly, vomiting and regurgitation, especially common in association with cerebral irritation, may cause aspiration, and thirdly, "grey attacks" may follow the feed even without foreign matter being aspirated; this last mishap is largely provoked by the disturbance and handling entailed, but possibly reflex factors from the stomach operate as well. In addition to these immediate risks there is no doubt that more mischief is caused by feeding than through not feeding. Premature infants do not die very readily from starvation and they appear to resist dehydration well, whereas overfeeding or any attempt to force on the level of feeding easily results in gastro-enteritis, which will put the child back to worse than starting-point if not actually kill it.

Because of the aspiration risk, tube feeding is generally preferred to the other methods in the very weak and ultrapremature, and can certainly be more expeditious (Fig. 5). The utensils should of course be boiled before use and the nurse should wash her hands as in all handling manœuvres. A fine soft rubber catheter is simply passed via the mouth down to the lower end of the œsophagus, the length of tube being equal to the distance from the bridge of the nose to xiphisternum. The feed is slowly run in from a funnel. The tube should be pinched firmly on withdrawal so as to prevent any leakage of milk from its tip while passing the epiglottis. An experienced nurse can gauge well whether the baby is satisfied with the amount given.

Although there is at present some dispute about the value of delayed feeding in premature infants most feel that it is a safe rule not

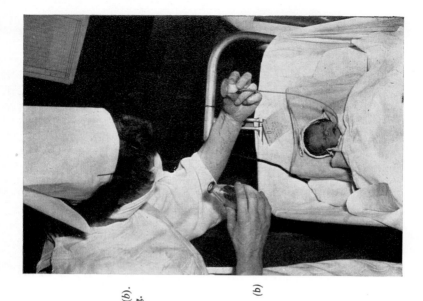

(b)

26/Fɪɢ. 5 (a) and (b).
—Tube feeding.

(a)

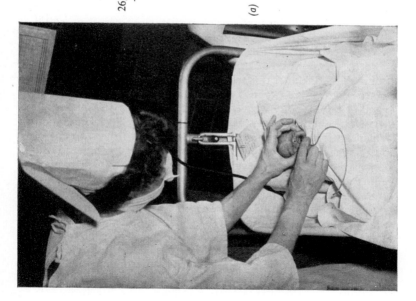

to attempt to feed until the baby demonstrates sucking movements. Another indication to start feeding is failure to pass urine for twenty-four hours after it has already been previously passed, in other words the baby is now safely dehydrated. The babies of diabetic mothers, who behave like premature babies in spite of their size, are œdematous and their peril is more or less proportional to their œdema. Nothing is more welcome in such cases than a fairly sharp loss of weight due to loss of water within the first day or two.

In recognising the dangers of feeding in the first few days, some authorities do not feed for two days or until signs of hunger are manifested. The newly recognised dangers of neonatal hypoglycæmia, especially in the dysmature, now discourage this practice. The more usual practice is to give nothing by mouth for twelve to twenty-four hours, or later if cerebral irritation is present, and then to give 1 to $1\frac{1}{2}$ drachms of 10 per cent glucose water. This will not only demonstrate the baby's ability to retain this quantity, but should vomiting and aspiration occur, its effect will be less serious. These feeds of boiled water are given three-hourly, and after the first few, full-strength breast milk is tried. The breast milk is obtained by manual expression from the mother's breast or from a bank supply and all breast milk should be boiled; pasteurisation is not sufficient in the first fortnight, because of the great danger of gastro-enteritis.

In a racily written communication by Smallpeice and Davies (1964), immediate feeding with full-strength breast milk is recommended even in those babies not interested in sucking at breast or bottle, in which case a polythene tube is passed through a nostril well down into the stomach. The tubes can be kept for as long as a week but bottle or breast feeding is encouraged as soon as the tube can be dispensed with. Under this scheme feeds are started within two hours of birth and rapidly stepped up from a total of 60 ml./Kg. of body weight (1 oz./lb. body weight) on the first day, to 150 ml./Kg. body weight ($2\frac{1}{2}$ oz./lb. body weight) on the fourth day. This quantity, divided into small frequent amounts, is put into the stomach often hourly at first in the very precarious babies, up to three hourly, as soon as possible. The advantages claimed for this early type of feeding are that it almost eradicates sympomatic hypoglycæmia and lowers the serum bilirubin. Furthermore it shortens the period taken for the baby to regain its birth weight and it is even suggested that the incidence of neurological sequalæ of prematurity may be diminished. This trial was conducted on babies weighing between 1 and 2 Kg. at birth and therefore presented quite a challenge, but the authors drove home the thrust, presumably referring to delayed feeding, that, "many well meant advances in the care of the premature baby over the last 20 years have been disastrous."

Later on when more normal feeding is established the following homely rules apply.

In assessing the amounts to give at each feeding, individual decisions must be made but a good general guide is to aim at supplying 2½ ounces daily per pound of body weight by the eighth day. This is divided into eight three-hourly feeds through day and night, and the daily increase during the first week is worked up to these figures by increments of one-eighth of this objective.

Example 1. A baby weighs 3 lb. 3 oz., i.e. 3⅕ lb.

Its average daily need by the eighth day = 3⅕ × 2½ = 8 oz.
This is divided into 8 feeds in 24 hours.
Therefore each feed = 1 oz. or 8 drachms.
The unit of increment is therefore one-eighth of this, which is 1 drachm.

Starting, therefore, with 1 drachm, each feed is increased daily by a drachm, so that by the eighth day feeds of 8 drachms are being given.

Example 2. A baby weighs 4¾ lb.

Its average daily need by the eighth day = 4¾ × 2½ = 12 oz.
At 8 feeds in 24 hours each feed = 1½ oz. or 12 drachms.
The unit of increment is one-eighth of this, which is 1½ drachms.

Starting, therefore, with feeds of 1½ drachms, a daily increase of 1½ drachms per feed brings the feeding up to desired amount by the eighth day.

This is a slow method of working up feeds, but it is also a safe method. It is a method which, with slight individual variation, will serve in nearly all cases. The ultimate aim is to build up feeds to 3½ ounces per pound body weight until the baby weighs 7 lb., because the food requirements in prematurity are proportionally greater, but it may take a few weeks to achieve this level.

When the weight has overtopped 7 lb., the usual feeding scheme can be followed and the requirements will level out to 2½ oz./lb. weight. It will be noted that no mention has been made, as yet, of artificial cows'-milk mixtures. In fact, there is no substitute to compare with human breast milk.

When, however, for some unfortunate and inescapable set of circumstances, human milk is not available, half-cream dried milk may be given at full strength, one drachm in 1 oz. and add sugar 1 drachm to each 4 oz. of mixture. Ostermilk requires no sugar, iron or other additives and is well tolerated by small premature babies.

The premature baby is born with an iron deficit which cannot be made good by natural feeding, so that after six weeks, by which

time its digestion ought to be able to cope with it, it is advisable to administer iron as follows:

Ferri et Ammon. Cit. gr. 3.
Aq Chlorof. ad ℥ 10.
Give 2 ℥ b.d. at first, increasing to 10 ℥ b.d. working up to gr. 1/lb. body weight daily.

Or the Helen Mackay mixture:

Ferrous Sulphate gr. 1½.
Hypophosphorous acid dil ℥ ¼.
Dextrose gr. 15.
Aq Chlorof. ad 1 drachm.

The above is added to some of the feeds, the aim being to give ⅛ to ½ gr. of ferrous sulphate daily per pound of body weight.

It is necessary to boil all breast milk in tube- and bottle-fed infants. All proprietary dried milks are fortified with vitamins A and D. We give Vitavel Syrup (Vitamins Ltd.) up to half a drachm daily.

Throughout all this period of assisted feeding every measure must be taken to maintain lactation in the mother, and she can, with training, become very skilful at manual expression of the breasts. Not only is her milk used in making up the feeds, but it will be needed even more when she goes home and continues breast feeding in full and the supply of surplus breast milk from the maternity unit is no longer available.

General Nursing Details

In addition to the principles already enumerated, the following points are observed:

The baby is nursed in its cot or incubator and is not bathed; in fact, cleaning is reduced to the minimum and is done with Phisohex cream. There is no need whatever, nor is it desirable, to clean off all the vernix. The routine oiling of the baby has now been abandoned.

Nappies or pieces of gauze tissue are placed under the buttocks and not round the baby, so that they can be replaced with the minimum of disturbance.

No cord dressing is applied. Such ritual, besides being useless, prevents proper inspection. No bath is given until the cord has separated and not even then unless the baby's condition warrants it. Until the first bath the baby is simply "top and tailed" with plain water when necessary.

Weighing need not be done more than twice a week and temperature taking *per rectum* is, if possible, kept down to three-hourly for the first twenty-four hours and then twice daily.

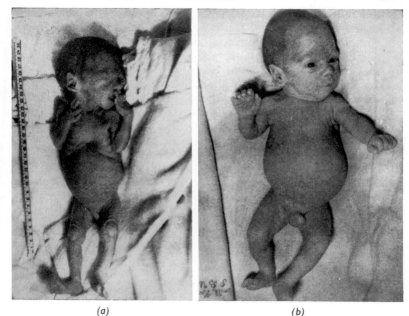

(a)   (b)

26/FIG. 6.—Gross prematurity. (a) Birth weight 1 lb. 14 oz. Note persistence of
subcostal inspiratory recession in a very premature infant at 17 days. (b) Same
infant 6 weeks later.

No routine treatment is given to eyes, ears or nostrils unless the
development of some local infection calls for it. The routine use of
eye drops as a prophylaxis against infection probably does more to
encourage the sticky eye than to prevent it, and the scouring out
of nostrils and ears with cotton-wool is both mischievous and
meddlesome.

There is probably no branch of nursing which is quite so exacting
and certainly none more important than the care of the premature
infant, but it is also one of the most rewarding.

The average stay in the unit is between six and seven weeks, but
it is doubtful if any similar period at any other time in the child's
life will have been better spent (Fig. 6).

KERNICTERUS

This is a lethal condition which is common in both hæmolytic
disease and prematurity. It refers to any type of cerebral jaundice in
which the basal nuclei of the brain become heavily stained with bile
pigments and suffer degenerative changes. The distribution and the

nature of the lesions are similar, whether associated with prematurity or hæmolytic disease. As a factor in neonatal death it is of considerable importance, and Claireaux found it responsible for 33 out of 376 deaths in infants within the neonatal period, giving an incidence of 8·8 per cent.

Kernicterus cannot occur without hyperbilirubinæmia and hyperbilirubinæmia cannot occur without jaundice. The mechanism by which this type of central nervous damage is incurred is very different in the two major conditions producing it, namely, hæmolytic disease and prematurity, but now that the metabolism of bilirubin is better understood the mechanism is clearer. The subject has been well reviewed by Claireaux (1960). Bilirubin is a natural product of red cell hæmolysis. In its unconjugated form it is highly toxic, particularly to cells within the central nervous system which for one reason or another, such as hypoxia, may be rendered vulnerable. Unfortunately bilirubin is soluble in alcohol and fat, but not in water, and until this solubility can be achieved it cannot be excreted in the bile. Conjugation, however, with glucuronic acid within the liver under the influence of the enzyme glucuronyl transferase converts it to bilirubin glucuronide which is soluble, non-toxic and readily excreted in the bile. Each gram of hæmoglobin can produce as much as 35 mg. of bilirubin on hæmolysis. Normally large quantities are therefore not produced (except in hæmolysing conditions) and are rapidly converted to the soluble and non-toxic form.

Hyperbilirubinæmia can therefore readily occur when the conversion mechanism is swamped by hæmolytic conditions or it may occur if there is some interference with this enzyme transformation. Unfortunately the latter is the case in neonates to some extent, but even more so in prematurity. The mechanism is also defective in rare conditions such as congenital non-hæmolytic jaundice (Crigler Najjar syndrome). On the other hand when jaundice is obstructive in type the bilirubin has already been converted to the harmless and soluble glucuronide before it is dammed back in the circulation and therefore kernicterus does not occur. Bilirubin is thus the responsible agent and may operate by being produced in excess as in hæmolytic disease due, for example, to the Rhesus factor, or to congenital spherocytosis (abnormal red cell fragility) or it may not be conjugated sufficiently readily, as in functional immaturity of the liver in the premature and in congenital familial non-hæmolytic jaundice.

In congenital bile duct atresia, cystic fibrosis of the pancreas and tumours, one is dealing with the more harmless obstructive variety. In galactosæmia the liver is damaged by the toxic action of one of the metabolites of galactose, because of the lack of a specific enzyme necessary for the proper breakdown of this sugar. As a result of the periportal fibrosis and cirrhosis which can thus be caused, the bile

cannuliculi contain plugs of inspissated bile and an obstructive type of jaundice results, and although mental defects may occur they do so for a different reason than from kernicterus.

When hyperbilirubinæmia is due to infection such as, for example, umbilical sepsis, or viral infections, both bilirubin and bilirubin glucuronide levels may be raised, the danger of kernicterus again coming from the former. Finally a very disturbing type of kernicterus can be due to iatrogenic hyperbilirubinæmia either because a drug increases hæmolysis directly or acts as a metabolic competitor. The analogues of vitamin K have been incriminated on both counts. Vitamin K_1, for example phytomenadione (Konakion), is both safer and more effective. This vitamin is essential for the formation within the body of prothrombin, factor VII and factor X. Vitamin K_1 is reputed to be harmless in fact and, as mentioned in the section on the Ventouse, it is our practice to carry out a thrombotest examination of the premature newborn baby's blood and because hypoprothrombinæmia is much commoner than formerly recognised. We have no hesitation in giving 5 mg. intramuscular injection repeated as necessary according to results.

It is known that bilirubin is readily bound to plasma albumin which makes it less liable to affect the cells within the central nervous system. In prematurity the level of this albumin is low. Therefore there may be an increase in the amount of dissociated bilirubin in the blood stream. Furthermore, salicylates and sulphonamides may compete with bilirubin for attachment to this albumin and may therefore enable toxic amounts of unconjugated and non-protein bound bilirubin to reach the central nervous system. Some such mechanism as this probably accounts for the fact that kernicterus may occur at different levels of serum bilirubin and that there is no critical level above which kernicterus is inevitable and below which this dreadful complication is unlikely to occur. Nevertheless, in general principle, the higher the level of bilirubin the greater the hazard. The more premature the infant the lower the bilirubin level necessary to produce kernicterus and the more damaged the brain cells by hypoxia, the more readily are they predisposed to this type of damage. In such cases Govan and Scott considered that pigmentation was a secondary factor, as they had found similar lesions in the brains of premature infants dying in the first few days of life before jaundice had made its appearance. It may well be that the cells of the nuclei have first to be damaged to make them susceptible to pigmentation, and of all the predisposing causes anoxia and prematurity operating together would appear to be the most likely.

The clinical features of the two classes of kernicterus differ mainly in the age of onset. Whereas in hæmolytic disease the jaundice usually comes on very rapidly after birth, in prematurity the jaundice ap-

pears about the third or fourth day, death occurring at about the end of the first week. In the case of hæmolytic disease, anæmia is progressive, but in the premature infant so afflicted there is often a history of asphyxia at birth or soon after; it is liable to recurrent attacks of cyanosis, is feeble and frequently œdematous. Signs of cerebral irritation are often manifest, but, serious though the condition is, premature babies often recover from severe degrees of jaundice. There remains considerable anxiety about the cerebral damage, which may have been sustained, and the chances of intellectual impairment.

Since the risk of kernicterus is to some extent proportional to the serum bilirubin level and begins to operate when this level exceeds 16 mg. per cent, becomes highly probable at 25 mg. per cent and a cast-iron certainty at 40 mg. per cent, a rising level is now accepted as an outright indication for exchange transfusion regardless of the ætiology since, at all costs, the mental damage associated with kernicterus is to be avoided. The transfusion removes the albumin/bilirubin complex and there is no other means of treating hyperbilirubinæmia. However, the exchange has to be carried further than in hæmolytic disease because this albumin/bilirubin complex is contained not only within the vascular compartment of the body, but in the extravascular fluid as well and diffusion back into the circulation may produce a sort of rebound phenomenon. The transfusion may therefore have to be repeated. In spite of the risks of exchange transfusion, particularly in the weak and premature, bilirubin levels over 20 mg. per 100 ml. are regarded by most workers as a full indication for the procedure.

A survey of the Society of Medical Officers of Health has been reported by McDonald (1962) which deals with the neurological and ophthalmic disorders in children with birth weights of 4 lb. or less (1,800 g.). Of those who had already died more than half had some neurological disorder and of those still alive nearly a quarter were found to have either a neurological or an ophthalmic disorder. How much of the former was due to kernicterus remains to be worked out by further prospective study and of the ophthalmic disorders myopia is common, and retrolental fibroplasia an even more terrible consequence of prematurity and now believed to be mainly iatrogenic in origin.

RETROLENTAL FIBROPLASIA

This condition has become a serious factor in congenital blindness. It occurs only in premature infants whose birth weight is less than 5 lb. and was first described by Terry in 1942, since when it appeared with increasing frequency on both sides of the Atlantic. The end point of the disease is blindness with searching nystagmus,

due to the presence of bilateral vascularised opaque membranes behind the lens, together with retinal detachment.

The findings of the Medical Research Council investigation have supported the popular view that the disease is caused by the too liberal use of oxygen in prematurity.

Szewczyk (1952) advanced the interesting theory that retrolental fibroplasia is a response of immature neural tissues to a rapid withdrawal from a high percentage oxygen atmosphere, without allowing sufficient time for acclimatisation to a normal atmosphere to occur. He described the development of the disease as follows: "Firstly there is a dilatation of the retinal vessels followed by tortuosity, especially in the peripheral fields. Neovascularisation is followed by the appearance of grey-white areas of œdema and exudate on the retina and, later, hæmorrhages. The retina then becomes detached and scarring and membrane formation completes the ugly process." This worker found that the early signs were reversible if he replaced the child at once in a concentration of oxygen to which it had hitherto become habituated and was able to prevent the further development of these signs by a process of slow acclimatisation to a normal atmosphere. Bembridge and his colleageus (1952) reported on the use of ACTH and cortisone. There was some evidence of benefit, but the results were variable. The Medical Research Council investigators, however, noted that the chances of spontaneous regression without treatment were 44 per cent and they doubted the real value of corticotrophin or returning the child to its former high-oxygen environment, although the number so treated was too small for firm conclusions. The likelihood of developing retrolental fibroplasia increases with the duration of oxygen therapy, but usually five days on oxygen are necessary to produce the full-blown disease. The disease is now a rarity because the dangers of injudicious oxygen therapy are today so widely recognised. Certainly concentrations of oxygen above 35 per cent for longer than a few hours are both dangerous and unnecessary.

Supervision should be maintained up to the sixth month of life at least, but if signs have not appeared by then they will not do so subsequently.

With the progressive elimination of gonococcal ophthalmia from our maternity departments, retrolental fibroplasia now constitutes the biggest single cause of blindness in children.

REFERENCES

1. AKERREN, Y., and FURSTENBERG, N. (1950·) *J. Obstet. Gynæc. Brit. Emp.*, **57**, 705.
2. ARNEIL, G. A., and KERR, MARGARET M. (1963). *Lancet*, **2**, 756.

3. AVERY, M. E., and MEAD, J. (1959). *Amer. J. Dis. Child.*, **97,** 517.
4. BAIRD, D. (1945). *J. Obstet. Gynæc. Brit. Emp.*, **52,** 217.
5. BEMBRIDGE, B. A., COXON, M., MOULTON, A. C. L., JACKSON, C. R. S., and SMALLPEICE, V. (1952). *Brit. med. J.*, **1,** 675.
6. BORN, G. V. R., DAWES, G. S., MOTT, J. C., and WIDDICOMBE, J. G. (1954). *Cold Spr. Har. Symp. quant. Biol.*, **19,** 102.
7. BOUND, J. P., BUTLER, N. R., and SPECTOR, W. G. (1956). *Brit. med. J.*, **2,** 1260.
8. BUTLER, N. R., and BONHAM, D. G. (1963). *Perinatal Mortality,* p. 142. Edinburgh: E. & S. Livingstone.
9. CLAIREAUX, A. E. (1954). *Postgrad. med. J.*, **30,** 338.
10. CLAIREAUX, A. E. (1958). In *Modern Trends in Pædiatrics,* 2nd series. London: Butterworth & Co.
11. CLAIREAUX, A. E. (1960). *Brit. med. J.*, **1,** 1528.
12. DAWES, G. S., MOTT, J. C., WIDDICOMBE, J. G., and WYATT, D. G. (1953). *J. Physiol. (Lond.)*, **121,** 141.
13. DAWES, G. S., MOTT, J. C., and WIDDICOMBE, J. G. (1954). *J. Physiol. (Lond.)*, **126,** 563; (1955). *Ibid*, **128,** 344, 361, 384.
14. DAWKINS, M. J. R. (1964). *Proc. roy. Soc. Med.*, **57,** 1063.
15. DONALD, I. (1954). *J. Obstet. Gynæc. Brit. Emp.*, **61,** 725.
16. DONALD, I. (1957). *Brit. J. Anæsth.*, **29,** 553.
17. DONALD, I., and LORD, J. (1953). *Lancet*, **1,** 9.
18. DONALD, I., and STEINER, R. E. (1953). *Lancet*, **2,** 846.
19. DONALD, I., KERR, M. M., and MACDONALD, I. R. (1958). *Scot. med. J.*, **3,** 151.
20. DOUGLAS, J. W. B. (1956). *Brit. med. J.*, **1,** 1210.
21. DOUGLAS, J. W. B. (1960). *Brit. med. J.*, **1,** 1008.
22. DRILLIEN, C. M. (1957). *J. Obstet. Gynæc. Brit. Emp.*, **64,** 161.
23. DRILLIEN, C. M. (1959). *J. Obstet. Gynæc. Brit. Emp.*, **66,** 721.
24. DRILLIEN, C. M. (1964). *The Growth and Development of the Prematurely Born Infant,* p. 77. Edinburgh: E. & S. Livingstone.
25. FELL, M. R. (1960). *Lancet*, **1,** 1295.
26. GAISFORD, W., and SCHOFIELD, S. (1950). *Brit. med. J.*, **1,** 1404.
27. GOVAN, A. D. T., and SCOTT, J. M. (1953). *Lancet*, **1,** 611.
28. HUTCHISON, J. H., KERR, M. M., MCPHAIL, M. F. M., DOUGLAS, T. A., SMITH, G., NORMAN, J. N., and BATES, E. H. (1962). *Lancet*, **2,** 465.
29. HUTCHISON, J. H., KERR, MARGARET M., DOUGLAS, T. A., INALL, J. A., and CROSBIE, J. C. (1964). *Pediatrics*, **33,** 956.
30. KARLBERG, P., COOK, C. D., O'BRIEN, D., CHERRY, R. B., and SMITH, C. A. (1954). *Acta pædiat. (Uppsala)*, **43,** Suppl. 100.
31. KNOBLOCK, H., RIDER, R., HARPER, P., and PASAMANICK, B. (1956). *J. Amer. med. Ass.*, **161,** 581.
32. LIND, J., and WEGELIUS, C. (1954). *Cold Spr. Har. Symp. quant. Biol.*, **19,** 109.
33. MCCORMICK, C. O. (1947). *Textbook on Pathology of Labor, the Puerperium and the Newborn,* 2nd edit. St. Louis: C. V. Mosby Co.
34. MCDONALD, ALISON D. (1962). *Brit. med. J.*, **1,** 895.
35. MCDONALD, ALISON D. (1964). *Brit. J. prev. soc. Med.*, **18,** 59.

36. MATTHEWS, D. D., FRIEND, J. B., and MICHAEL, C. A. (1967). *J. Obstet. Gynaec. Brit. Cwlth.*, **74**, 68.
37. MEDICAL RESEARCH COUNCIL (1955). Report of Conference on Retrolental Fibroplasia. *Brit. med. J.*, **2**, 78.
38. MINISTRY OF HEALTH, Central Health Service Council (1961). *Report of Sub-Committee on the Prevention of Prematurity and the Care of Premature Infants*. London: H.M. Staty. Office.
39. MORISON, J. E. (1952). *Foetal and Neonatal Pathology*. London: Butterworth & Co.
40. PATTLE, R. E., CLAIREAUX, A. E., DAVIES, P. A., and CAMERON, A. H. (1962). *Lancet*, **2**, 469.
41. POTTER, E. L. (1952). *Pathology of the Fetus and the Newborn*. Chicago: Year Book Publishers.
42. REID, D. M. S., TUNSTALL, M. E., and MITCHELL, R. G. (1967). *Lancet*, **1**, 532.
43. SELLIGER, H. P. R. (1961). *Listeriosis*. Basel: S. Karger.
44. SHELLEY, HEATHER J. (1964). *Brit. med. J.*, **1**, 273.
45. SHELLEY, HEATHER J., and NELIGAN, C. A. (1966). *Brit. med. Bull.*, **22**, 34.
46. SMALLPEICE, VICTORIA, and DAVIES, PAMELA A. (1964). *Lancet*, **2**, 1349.
47. SZEWCZYK, T. S. (1952). *Amer. J. Ophthal.*, **35**, 301.
48. TERRY, T. L. (1942). *Amer. J. Ophthal.*, **25**, 203, 1409.
49. THOMSON, A. M. (1951). *Brit. J. Nutr.*, **5**, 158.
50. USHER, R. (1961). *Pediat. Clin. N. Amer.*, **8**, 525.
51. WALKER, J. (1967). *Proc. roy. Soc. Med.*, **60**, 877.
52. WIGGLESWORTH, J. S. (1967). *Proc. roy. Soc. Med.*, **60**, 879.
53. WILLOUGHBY, M. L. N. (1967). Personal communication.
54. YLLPO, A. (1935). *Acta pædiat.* (*Uppsala*), **17**, Suppl. 1, 122.

CHAPTER XXVII

Rh FACTOR

THE term hæmolytic disease of the newborn has now largely supplanted the more clumsy and less euphonic name "erythroblastosis fœtalis". The essential underlying pathology is an active hæmolysis of the fœtal red cells before, at, or shortly after birth, and the three conditions, hydrops fœtalis, icterus gravis neonatorum, and hæmolytic anæmia in the newborn, are now recognised to differ only in degree and to be related to the one disease process. The discovery of the Rh factor, the recognition of its clinical importance and the practical applications of this knowledge in therapy constitute one of the great romances of modern research where theory, observation and practice have, in the space of a very few years, pieced themselves together to form a coherent picture.

In 1939 Levine and Stetson discovered an atypical immune agglutinin in a woman who had been delivered of a stillborn fœtus. In the next year Landsteiner and Wiener discovered the Rh antigen. These workers started preparing immune sera in animals by giving injections of blood from another animal, and they came thus to immunise rabbits with blood from the rhesus monkey and found that the resulting immune serum agglutinated the majority of human bloods, but by no means all. In other words, in the majority of humans there is a factor which was common to the rhesus monkey. This factor is known as the Rh factor, and those who possess it are classed as Rh-positive and those whose bloods are not agglutinated by the immune rabbit serum are called Rh-negative.

Landsteiner and Wiener in 1940 detected an Rh antibody in the serum of an Rh-negative woman who had experienced hæmolytic reactions after a transfusion with Rh-positive blood. In 1941 Levine observed the relationship between the presence of an Rh antibody in Rh-negative women whose pregnancies resulted in hæmolytic disease of the baby or in certain cases of stillbirth. From this point progress was very rapid both in the United States of America and in Great Britain, and it was soon found that there was more than one Rh factor until at last, in 1944, Fisher's CDE classification made sense out of a growing and bewildering confusion.

Iso-immunisation

Iso-immunisation has been defined as the process whereby immune antibodies are produced in one individual in response to the injection

of antigen from another individual of the same species (hence the prefix *iso*), this last individual possessing antigens which the first lacks. It follows, therefore, that there are three possible methods by which iso-immunisation can occur. The first and most obvious method is by the transfusion of unsuitable blood. In the case of the ABO groups, reactions are immediate, as immunity to the appropriate factors is inherent in the individual's make-up, although recent interest has been aroused in the possibility of anti-A reactions, but in the case of the Rh groups this immunity is actively acquired. Reaction is therefore not immediate, but immunity develops later, occasionally within a week, and repeated transfusions of unsuitable blood in respect of the Rh factor heighten the response. A second and less common method of iso-immunisation is by the intramuscular injection of unsuitable whole blood. This, in the past, has featured in the treatment of a variety of conditions, but is not numerically important. The third and most interesting method is the result of pregnancy, whereby an Rh-negative woman, pregnant with an Rh-positive child, manages by one means or another to receive into her own circulation some of her child's Rh-positive red cells which act as antigens. Any interruption, however minute, in the placental barrier between circulations of mother and child will allow the antigenic fœtal red cells to enter the maternal circulation.

The obvious time for fœtal cells to leak through into the maternal circulation, of course, is with the delivery of the placenta where damage to this organ, in the course of its separation and expulsion, may liberate cells into maternal venous sinuses sufficiently open to receive them. It is possible that the routine use of ergometrine at the beginning of the third stage may be responsible for the increase of iso-immunisation by squeezing fœtal blood cells into the maternal circulation, but this has not yet been proven. Other forms of placental accident, even minor, in the course of pregnancy, such as placental separation from any cause may likewise cause iso-immunisation even in the first pregnancy. There is now a growing weight of evidence that fœtal cells enter the circulation in small numbers even in quite normal pregnancies, since they can be recognised by their content of fœtal hæmoglobin. In many cases the ABO group of the baby is incompatible with that of the mother and the fœtal cells are immediately destroyed. Finn *et al.* (1961) found that these fœto-maternal microtransfusions were much less likely to occur in the case of women who were bearing an ABO incompatible baby. Fraser and Raper (1962) have, however, identified these ABO incompatible fœtal cells early in the puerperium, but their life in the maternal circulation is a short one. This may explain the fact that Rh iso-immunisation is less likely to occur where ABO incompatibility exists between mother and child. What is surprising is that iso-im-

munisation does not occur in every case in which an Rh-negative woman bears an Rh-positive child, but the phenomenon is doubtless dependent upon the size, quantity or repetition of the antigenic stimulus. Once the mother has become immunised, her serum will contain antibodies for most of the rest, if not all, of her life. These antibodies pass with little hindrance across the placenta in subsequent pregnancies and work havoc on the red cells of any fœtus whose blood is Rh-positive and therefore susceptible to their action. It follows, therefore, that if iso-immunisation has occurred as a result of pregnancy, the results are most likely to appear, not in that pregnancy, but in subsequent ones, although this is not always so, and any solution in placental continuity, for example from a threat to miscarry or an antepartum hæmorrhage, can provoke sensitisation in susceptible individuals. Nevertheless, it is most unlikely that a patient can become sensitised in the course of a given pregnancy before the 5th month. If, therefore, antibodies are found to be present as early as, for example, three months, previous sensitisation is indicated, and even a previous abortion occurring as early as 12 weeks may have been responsible.

The relative importance of unsuitable transfusion in iso-immunising a patient is now lessening with the more general adoption of precautions in respect of the Rh factor when transfusing women of childbearing age, so that whereas in 1950 about a third of our Rh cases with children affected with hæmolytic disease gave a history of such a transfusion in the past, the figure is now very low indeed.

The chances of iso-immunisation occurring are very much greater from unsuitable transfusion than from bearing Rh-positive children, and it has been found that a transfusion of volunteers with two spaced intravenous injections of $\frac{1}{4}$ ml. of Rh-positive blood sensitized 40 per cent of them, but that if such injections were repeated often, the figure could be raised to 90 per cent. By contrast the Rh-negative woman who has two Rh-positive babies has still only a 1 in 12 chance of being iso-immunised.

The proportion of people who are Rh-negative varies according to race. For example, in China it is most uncommon, and it might be suggested that the older civilization of the Chinese has, by a process of natural selection, bred out an undesirable gene, but in England 16·8 per cent or 17 per cent of people are in this category. Of this 17 per cent of Rh-negative women three, on average, are likely to marry Rh-negative men, so that their chances of having infants affected with hæmolytic disease are nil. Of the remaining 14, six are likely to marry homozygous Rh-positive husbands with a 1 in 12 chance of their second child being affected, and eight are likely to marry heterozygous Rh-positive husbands with a consequently reduced chance, at 1 in 15, of having an affected second child. The

more pregnancies that a woman has, who is unsuitably mated in respect of the Rh factor, the more likely is she to have, sooner or later, an affected child, and hæmolytic disease tends to be more severe with each repetition. For example, the first child to be affected has a 90 per cent chance of spontaneous survival. If the patient was not sensitised before a given pregnancy, she is practically certain not to produce a child stillborn because of hæmolytic disease, but if she has been previously sensitised, the stillbirth rate is about 30 per cent and if, having a homozygous Rh-positive husband, she has already had one stillbirth, the chances of a repetition of this disaster are as high as 80 per cent (Walker and Murray). After two Rh stillbirths the outlook indeed becomes poor.

The majority of cases of hæmolytic disease of the newborn are due to Rh incompatibilities, but there are other blood group systems which are independent of ABO or Rh grouping and which may in rare instances produce iso-immunisation. These include the MNS, P, Lutheran, Kell, Lewis, Duffy and Kidd blood group systems. When hæmolytic disease occurs, within the ABO incompatibility group it is nearly always in the case of Group O mothers with Group A babies and very occasionally Group B (Wiener *et al.*, 1960), but all these are rare phenomena compared with the Rh group of iso-immunisation. According to Walker (1959) the incidence of hæmolytic disease of the newborn due to Rh incompatibility was about six out of every thousand babies in England and Wales and until now fifteen were stillborn out of every hundred affected babies. The problem is therefore a large one.

Subgroups

The division of all humanity into the two classes, Rh-positive and Rh-negative, is an over-simplification of the facts, although in general it serves well enough. Wiener started the ball rolling by finding a serum which reacted in only 70 per cent out of the 85 per cent of known Rh-positive people, the remaining 15 per cent being unaffected. This led to the acknowledgment of at least two components of the Rh-positive group which were called Rh_1 and Rh_2, and it was not long before the study of atypical reactions led to the discovery of further subgroups such as Rh', Rh'', Rh_y, etc. Fisher's CDE classification is now more generally accepted, as it is far easier to understand, its only disadvantage being that it is inconvenient to use in speech. The CDE classification is based upon the theory that each Rh gene is made up of three components selected from three allelomorphic pairs, namely C or *c*, D or *d*, E or *e*, giving for example a gene such as C*d*E. Mathematically the possible combinations of these elements would supply us with eight Rh types of gene, but since every individual inherits genes from both parents,

the full genotype must always contain a double set of *cde* letters, for example CD*e*/*cde*. The identification of each of these six possible letters is done by means of antisera which are specific. The commonly available antisera are anti-C, anti-D, anti-E and anti-*c*. The antisera *e* and *d* are rare or not available. The accompanying table shows the relationship of the various types to each other and the more obsolete Rh₁ and Rh₂ sort of classification.

In general, the distinction between Rh-positive and Rh-negative patients is made with anti-D serum, which is the most important of the series. It will be seen that the recessive so-called Rh-negative gene has to be regarded as a definite entity possessing antigenic properties of its own, and cases have been cited in which an Rh-positive serum agglutinated all Rh-negative cells encountered by it. Such a serum might be expected to contain anti-*d*, but this is a rare phenomenon. It now appears, therefore, that when an individual lacks any one of the many Rh components, iso-immunisation may occur if this component is introduced artificially. The matter is important because, unfortunately, reactions can occur within the Rh group itself.

Other subdivisions, even of this subgrouping, continue to emerge, for example, on the C–*c* locus of the Rh gene a third alternative has been identified, namely Cᵂ. This often exists in combination with plain C. Of the four above-mentioned antisera which are fairly widely available, the anti-C is usually in the form of anti-C + Cᵂ. Pure anti-C and pure anti-Cᵂ are rarer.

In reproduction each parent hands on the first or the second half of his or her full genotype so that, for example, a case of group CD*e*/*cde* hands on either CD*e* or *cde* to the offspring. In any instance where there is a possibility of handing down a choice of either D or *d*, the case is regarded as heterozygous, and will pass on to the next generation either an Rh-positive or an Rh-negative gene, but where there is a big D in both halves of the genotype, the parent is homozygous and can only pass on an Rh-positive gene. Likewise, where there is a little *d* in both halves, the parent must breed true to type as Rh-negative. All so-called Rh-negative people must, by definition, have a little *d* in each half of the genotype and are therefore homozygous. Heterozygous persons, though in reality half Rh-positive and half Rh-negative, will always be classified as Rh-positive because D is dominant to *d*.

The practical importance in obstetrics is that the heterozygous fathers have an even chance of passing on an Rh-negative gene, so that the child of an Rh-negative mother has an even chance of being itself Rh-negative and therefore most unlikely to be the victim of hæmolytic disease. Only iso-immunisation to the less usual factors can prevent this rule from being an absolute certainty.